BIOMATERIALS ENGINEERING AND DEVICES: *HUMAN APPLICATIONS*

VOLUME 2

Orthopedic, Dental, and Bone Graft Applications

BIOMATERIALS ENGINEERING AND DEVICES: *HUMAN APPLICATIONS*

VOLUME 2
Orthopedic, Dental, and Bone Graft Applications

Edited by

Donald L. Wise, PhD
Northeastern University
Boston, MA

Joseph D. Gresser, PhD
Cambridge Scientific, Inc.
Cambridge, MA

Debra J. Trantolo, PhD
Cambridge Scientific, Inc.
Cambridge, MA

Mario V. Cattaneo, PhD
Cambridge Scientific, Inc.
Cambridge, MA

Kai-Uwe Lewandrowski, MD
Massachusetts General Hospital
Boston, MA

Michael J. Yaszemski, MD, PhD
Mayo Clinic
Rochester, MN

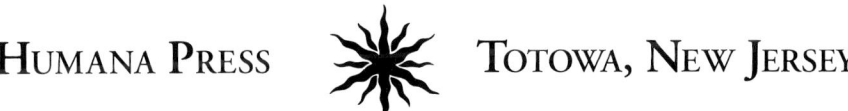

Humana Press Totowa, New Jersey

© 2000 Humana Press Inc.
999 Riverview Drive, Suite 208
Totowa, New Jersey 07512

For additional copies, pricing for bulk purchases, and/or information about other Humana titles, contact Humana at the above address or at any of the following numbers: Tel: 973-256-1699; Fax: 973-256-8341;
E-mail: humana@humanapr.com or visit our website at http://humanapress.com

All rights reserved. No part of this book may be reproduced, stored in a retrieval system, or transmitted in any form or by any means, electronic, mechanical, photocopying, microfilming, recording, or otherwise without written permission from the Publisher.

All articles, comments, opinions, conclusions, or recommendations are those of the author(s), and do not necessarily reflect the views of the publisher.

Due diligence has been taken by the publishers, editors, and author of this book to assure the accuracy of the information published and to describe generally accepted practices. The contributors herein have carefully checked to ensure that the drug selections and dosages set forth in this text are accurate and in accord with the standards accepted at the time of publication. Notwithstanding, as new research, changes in government regulations, and knowledge from clinical experience relating to drug therapy and drug reactions constantly occurs, the reader is advised to check the product information provided by the manufacturer of each drug for any change in dosages or for additional warnings and contraindications.

This is of utmost importance when the recommended drug herein is a new or infrequently used drug. It is the responsibility of the treating physician to determine dosages and treatment strategies for individual patients. Further, it is the responsibility of the health care provider to ascertain the Food and Drug Administration status of each drug or device used in their clinical practice.

The publisher, editors, and authors are not responsible for errors or omissions or for any consequences from the application of the information presented in this book and make no warranty, express or implied, with respect to the contents in this publication.

All articles, comments, opinions, conclusions, or recommendations are those of the author(s), and do not necessarily reflect the views of the publisher.

Cover design by Patricia F. Cleary.

This publication is printed on acid-free paper. ∞
ANSI Z39.48-1984 (American National Standards Institute)
Permanence of Paper for Printed Library Materials.

Photocopy Authorization Policy:

Authorization to photocopy items for internal or personal use, or the internal or personal use of specific clients, is granted by Humana Press Inc., provided that the base fee of US $10.00 per copy, plus US $00.25 per page, is paid directly to the Copyright Clearance Center at 222 Rosewood Drive, Danvers, MA 01923. For those organizations that have been granted a photocopy license from the CCC, a separate system of payment has been arranged and is acceptable to Humana Press Inc. The fee code for users of the Transactional Reporting Service is: [0-89603-859-9/00 $10.00 + $00.25].

Printed in the United States of America. 10 9 8 7 6 5 4 3 2 1

Library of Congress Cataloging-in-Publication Data

Biomaterials engineeering and devices / edited by Donald L. Wise ... [et al.].
<v. ,1->p. cm.
  Includes bibliographical references and index.
  Contents: v. 1 Fundamentals and vascular and carrier applications -- v. 2 Orthopedic, dental, and bone graft applications.
  ISBN 0-89603-858-0 (v. 1 : alk. paper) -- ISBN 0-89603-859-9 (v. 2 : alk. paper)
  1. Biomedical materials. 2. Biomedical engineering. I. Wise, Donald L. (Donald Lee), 1937-
R857.M3 B5694 2000
610'.28--dc21
                                                                99-086203

Preface

The medical device and drug industries are consistently among the strongest technological performers. Materials are a key ingredient in their dynamic growth. Development of these materials is in a constant state of activity, with the challenge of replacing old materials that cannot withstand the tests of time, and the new materials' needs coming to the forefront in modern applications. This new reference text, *Biomaterials Engineering and Devices: Human Applications*, focuses on materials used in or on the human body—materials that define the world of "biomaterials."

Biomaterials Engineering and Devices: Human Applications focuses on materials development and characterization. Chapters deal with issues in the selection of proper biomaterials from biocompatibility to biostability to structure/function relationships. Chapters also focus on the use of specific biomaterials based on their physiochemical and mechanical characterizations. Integral to these chapters are discussions of standards in analytical methodology and quality control.

The users of *Biomaterials Engineering and Devices: Human Applications* will represent a broad base of backgrounds ranging from the basic sciences (e.g., polymer chemistry and biochemistry) to more applied disciplines (e.g., mechanical/chemical engineering, orthopedics, and pharmaceutics). To meet varied needs, each chapter provides clear ancd fully detailed discussions. This in-depth, but practical, coverage should also assist recent inductees to the biomaterials circle. The editors trust that this reference textbook conveys the intensity of this fast moving field in an enthusastic presentation.

Donald L. Wise, PhD
Debra J. Trantolo, PhD
Kai-Uwe Lewandrowski, MD
Joseph D. Gresser, PhD
Mario V. Cattaneo, PhD
Michael J. Yaszemski, MD, PhD

Contents

Preface v
Contributors ix
About the Editors xiii
Contents of Volume 1 xv

PART 1 BIOMATERIALS FOR DENTAL APPLICATIONS

1 Biomaterials Used in Implant Dentistry 3
  John P. Ley, A. Norman Cranin, and Michael Katzap

2 Polymers in the Oral Environments:
  Novel Elastomers as Soft Liners 25
  Kalachandra Sid and Tetsuya Takamata

3 HA Coatings on Dental Implants 49
  Joo L. Ong, Daniel C. N. Chan, and Kazuhisa Bessho

4 Characterization of Water Inhibition
  in Light-Cured Dental Resins 61
  Kristen L. Droesch, Brian J. Love, and Virginie M. Vaubert

5 Osseointegrated Dental Implants: *Follow-up Studies* 67
  Günther Heimke and Cornelius G. Wittal

PART 2 BONY BIOMATERIALS FOR GRAFTING APPLICATIONS

6 Artificial Bone: *Hydroxyapatite Reconstruction
  of Tibial Plateau Fractures* 95
  *P. Patka, H. J. Th. M. Haarman, M. van der Elst,
  and F. C. Bakker*

7 Enhancing Cortical Allograft Incorporation Processing
  by Partial Demineralization and Laser Perforation:
  A Histological, Biomechanical, and Immunological Study 111
  *Kai-Uwe Lewandrowski, Georg Schollmeier, Axel Ekkernkamp,
  Henry J. Mankin, Hans K. Uhthoff, and William W. Tomford*

8 Synthetic Osseous Grafting:
  A Necessary Component to Oral Reconstruction 133
  Arthur Ashman and Jeffrey S. Gross

9 HA-SAL2: *Novel Bone Graft Substitute
  with Composition Mimicking Bone Mineral* 155
  *Hannah Ben-Bassat, Benjamin Y. Klein, Isaac Leichter,
  Meir Liebergall, David Segal, Frigita Kahana,
  and Sara Sarig*

10 Soluble Calcium Salts in Bioresorbable Bone Grafts 171
   *Joseph D. Gresser, Kai-Uwe Lewandrowski,
   Debra J. Trantolo, Donald L. Wise, and Yung-Yueh Hsu*

PART 3 ORTHOPEDIC FIXTURES AND CEMENTS

11 Surface Hardening of Orthopedic Implants *191*
    Ravi H. Shetty

12 Orthopedic Applications of Carbon Fiber Composites *203*
    Joseph A. Longo III and James B. Koeneman

13 Development of a Bioresorbable Interbody Fusion Device *215*
    Kai-Uwe Lewandrowski, Joseph D. Gresser, Debra J. Trantolo, Georg Schollmeier, Frank Kandziora, and Donald L. Wise

14 Follow-up-Study–Based Wear Debris Reduction with Ceramic–Metal–Modular Hip Replacements *223*
    Günther Heimke and Gerd Willmann

15 Applied Aspects of Calcium Phosphate Bone Cement Application *253*
    F. C. M. Driessens, M. G. Boltong, I. Khaïroun, E. A. P. De Maeyer, M. P. Ginebra, R. Wenz, J. A. Planell, and R. M. H. Verbeeck

16 Osteointegration and Dimensional Stability of Poly(D,L–Lactide-Co-Glycolide) Implants Reinforced with Poly(Propylene Glycol-Co-Fumaric Acid): *Histomorphometric Evaluation of Metaphyseal Bone Remodeling in Rats* *261*
    Joseph D. Gresser, Kai-Uwe Lewandrowski, Debra J. Trantolo, and Donald L. Wise

17 Particulate Metal in Late Aseptic Loosening of Cemented Total Hip Arthroplasties *281*
    Jochanan H. Boss, David G. Mendes, and Ines Misselevich

18 Injectable and Bioresorbable Poly(Propylene Glycol-Co-Fumaric Acid) Bone Cement *291*
    Debra J. Trantolo, Kai-Uwe Lewandrowski, Joseph D. Gresser, and Donald L. Wise

19 Development of a Modular Ceramic Knee Prosthesis *309*
    W. M. Payten and B. Ben-Nissan

Index *337*

Contributors

ARTHUR ASHMAN, DDS • *Department of Implant Dentistry, New York University, New York, NY*

F. C. BAKKER, MD, PhD • *Department of Surgery/Traumatology, University Hospital VU, Amsterdam, The Netherlands*

HANNAH BEN-BASSAT, PhD • *Laboratory of Experimental Surgery, Hadassah University Hospital, Jerusalem, Israel*

B. BEN-NISSAN, PhD • *Department of Chemistry, Materials, and Forensic Science, University of Technology, Sydney, Sydney, NSW, Australia*

KAZUHISA BESSHO, DDS, DMSC • *Department of Oral and Maxillofacial Surgery, Graduate School of Medicine, Kyoto University, Kyoto, Japan*

M. G. BOLTONG • *Department of Dental Materials Science, Institute of Biomedical Technologies (IBITECH), University of Gent, Gent, Belgium*

JOCHANAN H. BOSS, MD • *Department of Pathology, Bnai-Zion Medical Center; The Bruce Rapaport Faculty of Medicine, Technion—Israel Institute of Technology, Haifa, Israel*

DANIEL C. N. CHAN, DDS • *Department of Oral Rehabilitation, Medical College of Georgia, Augusta, GA*

A. NORMAN CRANIN, DDS, DEng • *Brookdale University Hospital and Medical Center, Brooklyn, NY*

E. A. P. DE MAEYER, PhD • *Department of Dental Materials Science, Institute of Biomedical Technologies (IBITECH), University of Gent, Gent, Belgium*

F. C. M. DRIESSENS, PhD • *Department of Dental Materials Science, Institute of Biomedical Technologies (IBITECH), University of Gent, Gent, Belgium*

KRISTEN L. DROESCH, BS, MS • *Department of Materials Science and Engineering, Virginia Polytechnic Institute and State University, Blacksburg, VA*

AXEL EKKERNKAMP, MD • *Department of Surgery, Berufsgenossenschaftliche Kliniken Bergmasnnsheil, Bochum, Germany*

M. P. GINEBRA, PhD • *Department of Materials Science and Metallurgy, Universitat Politecnica de Catalunya, Barcelona, Spain*

JOSEPH D. GRESSER, PhD • *Cambridge Scientific, Inc., Cambridge, MA*

JEFFREY S. GROSS, DDS • *Department of Periodontics, School of Dentistry, Case Western Reserve University, Cleveland, OH*

H. J. TH. M. HAARMAN, MD, PhD • *Department of Surgery/Traumatology, University Hospital VU, Amsterdam, The Netherlands*

GÜNTHER HEIMKE, PhD • *Nibelungenstr. 28, D-75179 Pforzheim, Germany; Department of Bioengineering, Clemson University, Clemson, SC (Retired)*

YUNG-YUEH HSU, PhD • *Cambridge Scientific, Inc., Cambridge, MA*

FRIGITA KAHANA, MSc • *Casali Institute of Applied Chemistry, The Hebrew University of Jerusalem, Jerusalem, Israel*

I. KAÏROUN, PhD • *Department of Materials Science and Metallurgy, Universitat Politecnica de Catalunya, Barcelona, Spain*

FRANK KANDZIORA, MD • *Unfall-und Wiederherstellungschirurgie, Universitatsklinikum Charite, Berlin, Germany*

MICHAEL KATZAP, DDS • *Brookdale University Hospital and Medical Center, Brooklyn, NY*

BENJAMIN Y. KLEIN, MD • *Laboratory of Experimental Surgery, Hadassah University Hospital, Jerusalem, Israel*

JAMES B. KOENEMAN, PHD • *Orthologic, Tempe, AZ*

KAI-UWE LEWANDROWSKI, MD • *Orthopedic Research Associate, Massachusetts General Hospital of Harvard Medical School, Boston, MA*

MEIR LIEBERGALL, MD • *Department of Orthopedics, Hadassah University Hospital, Jerusalem College of Technology, Jerusalem, Israel*

ISAAC LEICHTER, PHD • *Hadassah University Hospital, Jerusalem College of Technology, Jerusalem, Israel*

JOHN P. LEY, DDS • *Brookdale University Hospital and Medical Center, Brooklyn, NY*

JOSEPH A. LONGO III, MD • *World Orthopedic Research and Development Foundation, Scottsdale, AZ*

BRIAN J. LOVE, PHD • *Department of Materials Science and Engineering, Virginia Polytechnic Institute and State University, Blacksburg, VA*

HENRY J. MANKIN, MD • *Orthopedic Research Laboratories, Masschusetts General Hospital, Boston, MA*

DAVID G. MENDES • *Department of Orthopedic Surgery, Bnai-Zion Medical Center; The Bruce Rapapport Faculty of Medicine, Technion—Israel Institute of Technology, Haifa, Israel*

INES MISSELEVICH • *Department of Pathology, Bnai-Zion Medical Center; The Bruce Rapapport Faculty of Medicine, Technion—Israel Institute of Technology, Haifa, Israel*

JOO L. ONG, PHD • *Department of Restorative Dentistry, Division of Biomaterials, The University of Texas Health Science Center at San Antonio, San Antonio, TX*

P. PATKA, MD, PHD • *Department of Surgery/Traumatology, University Hospital VU, Amsterdam, The Netherlands*

W. M. PAYTEN, PHD • *Department of Chemistry, Materials, and Forensic Science, University of Technology, Sydney, Sydney, NSW, Australia*

J. A. PLANELL, PHD • *Department of Materials Science and Metallurgy, Universitat Politecnica de Catalunya, Barcelona, Spain*

SARA SARIG, PHD • *Casali Institute of Applied Chemistry, The Hebrew University of Jerusalem, Jerusalem, Israel*

GEORG SCHOLLMEIER, MD • *Arzt für Chirurgie, Berlin, Germany*

DAVID SEGAL • *Department of Orthopedics, The Hebrew University of Jerusalem, Jerusalem, Israel*

RAVI H. SHETTY, PHD • *Director, Metals Research, Zimmer, Inc., Warsaw, IN*

KALANCHANDRA SID, PHD • *NSF Science and Technology Center, High Performance Polymeric Adhesives and Composites, College of Arts and Sciences, Virginia Polytechnic Institute and State University, Blacksburg, VA; School of Dentistry—Operative Dentistry, University of North Carolina, Chapel Hill, NC; Interdisciplinary Research Center in Biomedical Materials, Queen Mary and Westfield College, University of London, London, UK*

TETSUYA TAKAMATA, DDS, PHD • *Department of Dental Diagnostic Services, Matsumoto Dental University, Hirooka, Shiojiri, Nagano, Japan; Visiting Professor, International Center for Excellence in Dentistry, Eastman Dental Institute, London, UK*

WILLIAM W. TOMFORD, MD • *Orthopedic Research Laboratories, Massachusetts General Hospital, Boston, MA*

DEBRA J. TRANTOLO, PHD • *Cambridge Scientific, Inc., Cambridge, MA*

HANS K. UHTHOFF, MD • *Bone and Joint Research Laboratory, Ottawa General Hospital, Ottawa, Ontario, Canada*

M. VAN DER ELST, MD, PHD • *Department of Surgery/Traumatology, University Hospital VU, Amsterdam, The Netherlands*

Contributors

VIRGINIE M. VAUBERT, BS, MS • *Department of Materials Science and Engineering, Virginia Polytechnic Institute and State University, Blacksburg, VA*

R. M. H. VERBEECK, PhD • *Department of Dental Materials Science, Institute of Biomedical Technologies (IBITECH), University of Gent, Gent, Belgium*

R. WENZ, PhD • *Merck Biomaterials, Darmstadt, Germany*

GERD WILLMANN, PhD • *CeramTec AG, Plochingen, Germany*

DONALD L. WISE, PhD • *Cambridge Scientific, Inc., Cambridge, MA*

CORNELIUS G. WITTAL, DDS • *Freiburg, Germany*

About the Editors

Donald L. Wise, PhD, *Senior Editor, is Cabot Professor of Chemical Engineering Emeritus at Northeastern University, Boston, MA. He is the Founder and Chairman of Cambridge Scientific, Inc., Cambridge, MA. Dr. Wise received the PhD degree from the University of Pittsburgh, Pittsburgh, PA.*

Debra J. Trantolo, PhD, *Coeditor, is President, Cambridge Scientific, Inc., Cambridge, MA. Dr. Trantolo received the PhD degree in organic chemistry from Clark University/University of Massachusetts Medical School, Worcester, MA.*

Kai-Uwe Lewandrowski, MD, *Coeditor, is an Orthopedic Research Associate at Massachusetts General Hospital of Harvard Medial School. He received the MD degree from Humboldt University in Germany.*

Joseph D. Gresser, PhD, *Coeditor, is the Senior Scientist at Cambridge Scientific, Inc., Cambridge MA. He received the PhD degree in physical chemistry from Syracuse University, Syracuse, NY.*

Mario V. Cattaneo, PhD, *Coeditor, is Director, Technology Development, Cambridge Scientific, Inc., Cambridge, MA. He received his PhD in chemical engineering from McGill University, Montreal, Canada.*

Michael J. Yaszemski, MD, PhD, *Coëditor, is Senior Associate Consultant, Department of Orthopedics, Mayo Clinic, Rochester, MN. He received the MD degree from Georgetown University School of Medicine, Washington, DC, and the PhD degree in chemical engineering from the Massachusetts Institute of Technology, Cambridge, MA.*

Contents of Volume 1

Preface
Contributors
About the Editors
Contents of Volume 2

PART 1   COMPATIBILITY AND FUNCTIONALITY ISSUES IN APPLIED BIOMATERIALS

1. The Molecular Mechanism of Biomaterial-Mediated Phagocyte Responses
   Liping Tang
2. Hypersensitivity Associated with Metallic Biomaterials
   Nadim Hallab, Joshua J. Jacobs, and Jonathan Black
3. Blood-Compatible Bioactive Polymers
   Stéphane La Barre and Catherine Boisson-Vidal
4. Novel Modification Method of Bioprosthetic Tissue for Improved Calcification Resistance
   Ki Dong Park, Young Ha Kim, and Won Kyu Lee
5. Biocompatibility of Silicone Gel Breast Implants
   Deepak V. Kilpadi and Dale S. Feldman
6. Endothelialization of Vascular Prostheses
   Gary L. Bowlin, Steven P. Schmidt, Stanley E. Rittgers, and Kristin J. Pawlowski

PART 2   DESIGN AND EVALUATION OF MATERIALS FOR VASCULAR APPLICATIONS

7. Collagen-Based Vascular Prostheses
   Jerome A. Werkmeister, Glenn A. Edwards, and John A. M. Ramshaw
8. Surface Modifications of Mechanical Heart Valves: *Effects on Thrombogenicity*
   Hoang S. Tran, Matthew M. Puc, Frank A. Chrzanowski, Jr., Charles W. Hewitt, David B. Soll, Bawa Singh, Nalin Kumar, Steven Marra, Vincent Simonetti, Jonathan Cilley, and Anthony J. DelRossi
9. The Importance of Radial Forces in Vascular Stent Design
   P. B. Snowhill, J. L. Nosher, and F. H. Silver
10. Blood Leak-proof Porous Vascular Grafts
    Jin Ho Lee, Gilson Khang, and Hai Bang Lee
11. Formation of Neointima in Vascular Prosthesis Sealed with Autologous Adipose Tissue Fragments for Femoropopliteal Bypass
    Yukio Ichikawa, Yasuharu Noishiki, Tamitaro Soma, Ichiya Yamazaki, Takayuki Kosuge, and Norihisa Karube

12 Clinical Improvement in Patients with Coronary and
    Peripheral Vascular Diseases Treated by LDL-Adsorption
    Using the Liposorber BLA-15 System
    Tetsuzo Agishi and Bruce Gordon

13 Development of a New Hybrid Coronary Stent Design
    with Optimized Biocompatible Properties
    Armin Bolz, Claus Harder, Martin Unverdorben, and Max Schaldach

PART 3   BIOMATERIALS AS CARRIERS FOR BIOACTIVE AGENTS

14 Incorporation of Active Agent into Biodegradable Cement:
    *Encapsulation of the Agent as Protection
    from Chemical Degradation
    During Cure and Effect on Release Profile*
    ***Joseph D. Gresser, Hisanori X. Nagaoka, Debra J. Trantolo,
    Pattisapu R. J. Gangadharam, Yung-Yueh Hsu,
    and Donald L. Wise***

15 New Synthetic Degradable Polymers
    as Carrier Materials for BMP
    ***Kunio Takaoka, Shimpei Miyamoto, Naoto Saito,
    and Takao Okada***

16 Use of Carrier Materials in Delivery
    of Bone Inductor Substances
    Philip J. Boyne

17 Preclinical and Clinical Evaluation
    of Osteogenic Protein-1 (BMP-7) in Bony Sites
    ***Stephen D. Cook, Samantha L. Salkeld, Laura P. Patron,
    and David C. Rueger***

18 Enzyme-Based Artificial Liver Support:
    *A Computerized Expert System for Design,
    Optimization, and Operation Control*
    Serge Guzy, Samuel Sideman, and Noah Lotan

19 Bupivacaine Release from Biopolymeric Depots
    for the Alleviation of Postoperative Pain
    ***William A. Apruzzese, Joseph D. Gresser, Daniel B. Carr,
    Louis Shuster, Donald L. Wise, and Debra J. Trantolo***

20 Biomaterial Implants for Treatment
    of Central Nervous System Diseases
    Wei Chen, Bingqing Ji, and D. Robert Lu

    Index

PART 1

BIOMATERIALS FOR DENTAL APPLICATIONS

1

Biomaterials Used in Implant Dentistry

John P. Ley, A. Norman Cranin, and Michael Katzap

1. Introduction

The implant dentist faces a plethora of biomaterials with which to become familiar, in order to properly restore the partially or completely edentulous patient. Included in these biomaterials are bone graft (BG) materials, occlusive membranes that can aid in bone augmentation, and a wide variety of implant devices that affix prosthetic teeth.

BG materials include autogenous bone, allogeneic bone, xenografts, and alloplasts. Autogenous bone is the gold standard grafting material, because of its ability to form bone by osteogenesis.

Barrier membranes are often employed in bone augmentation procedures, either alone or in conjunction with BG materials. Currently available membranes are broadly grouped into nonresorbable and resorbable varieties. Nonresorbable membranes have the longest history, but have the disadvantage of the need for removal surgery. Therefore, there has been considerable interest in the development of resorbable membranes. Most resorbable membranes are either collagen-derived or synthetically fabricated from polylactic acid (PLA) and/or polyglycolic acid (PGA).

Devices commonly referred to as dental implants can be broadly divided into subperiosteal or endosteal. The material utilized for subperiosteal designs is surgical-grade Vitallium (cobalt [Co], chromium [Cr], molybdenum [Mo]. Vitallium is utilized in this application because of its castability, a requirement of the subperiosteal implant, which is fabricated on models of the patient's bone. Endosteal implants are composed of either titanium (Ti) or Ti alloy. Hydroxyapatite (HA) coatings have been utilized in both implant designs, in an effort to increase host–implant integration.

2. BG Materials

Alveolar bone loss is a natural consequence of tooth loss. The pattern of bone loss to the edentulous ridge has been described by Lekholm and Zarb (1; Fig. 1). Dental implants placed in deficient ridges have higher failure rates, and, if successful, often result in a poor esthetic result, or they may be subjected to force vectors that are thought to be deleterious to long-term implant prognosis (2). To counter these possibly harmful results, many have advocated alveolar ridge augmentation, either prior to, or at the time of, implant placement (3–7). To accomplish this goal, the implant surgeon must be familiar with the variety of BG materials available, in order to accomplish a predictable result. Currently, there are four classes of grafting materials available: autogenous bone, allografts, xenografts, and alloplasts.

2.1. Phases of BG Healing

BG materials can influence new bone formation via three mechanisms: osteogenesis, osteoinduction, and osteoconduction.

From: *Biomaterials Engineering and Devices: Human Applications,* Volume 2
Edited by D. L. Wise, et al. © Humana Press, Inc., Totowa, NJ

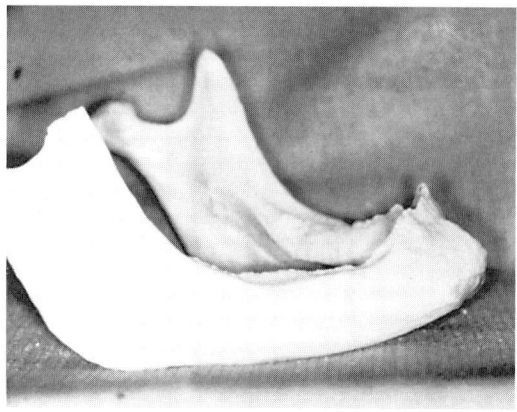

Fig. 1. Alveolar bone resorption leads to significant jaw atrophy. Its irregular pattern presents the clinician with a problematic foundation for reconstruction.

Osteogenesis represents the phase in which surviving cells of the grafted material form osteoid material *(8)*, which occurs primarily in the first 4 wk after a graft has been placed *(8)*. Because living bone cells are required for this process, autogenous BGs are the only types capable of exhibiting osteogenesis. The extent to which free autogenous grafts exhibit osteogenesis is limited *(9)*: It has been said that 80% of grafted bone cells die in the grafting process, leaving only 20% of cells remaining for osteogenesis *(10)*.

Osteoinduction is the process of inducing the conversion of undifferentiated mesenchynal cells into osteoblasts and chondroblasts *(11,12)*. By definition, this process can occur outside of the bony skeleton. Osteoinduction is thought to be the result of growth factors, such as bone morphogenic proteins (BMPs), which were first identified by Urist *(13,14)*. Osteoinduction occurs in autogenous grafts after the invasion of blood vessels and bone cells from the host into the graft. This initiates a coupled resorption–formation process that releases the BMPs from the mineral matrix of the BG *(8,15)*. The BMPs then induce the conversion of undifferentiated cells into chondroblasts and osteoblasts. Higher concentrations of BMPs have been identified in cortical bone *(14,16–18)*. Osteoinduction is also initiated in demineralized freeze-dried bone (DFDB) grafts. During the processing of DFDB, the mineral components are removed by the use of hydrochloric or nitric acids: This leaves the organic growth factors in the bone, which includes BMPs *(11,13,14,16–18)*. The osteoinduction process commences at 2 wk, peaks at 6 wk, and continues for up to 6 mo *(18)*.

Osteoconduction describes a mechanism of bone growth by apposition into and/or around a biocompatible inorganic material *(10,19)*. Osteoconduction cannot occur outside the bony skeleton, because it is completely dependent on the recipient bone bed as the source of bone cells *(8)*. Autogenous grafts, allogeneic grafts, and alloplasts all exhibit the osteoconductive phenomenon *(8)*.

2.1.1. Materials

Autogenous bone is termed the gold standard, because it exhibits all three phases of BG healing. Autogenous bone grafts can be acquired from many locations in the body. The advantage of autogenous bone is that it can be obtained in trabecular, cortical, or combined forms. Trabecular bone is advantageous, because it contains the cells for osteogenesis *(8)*. Cortical bone contains the most BMPs, and is an effective barrier to prevent tissue ingrowth *(11,14,16–18)*. Corticotrabecular grafts are useful in implant dentistry as onlay grafts *(7,20)*. Monocortical onlay grafts have been said to be the most predictable way to augment the edentulous ridge, particularly when placed prior to implant placement *(7,20)*. The disadvantage with autogenous bone is the need for a donor site and the morbidity associated with this surgery *(8,21;* Fig. 2A–F).

Allografts or allogeneic bone describes bone obtained from the same species, but different genotype, i.e., cadavers *(21)*. Allogeneic bone can be processed in a variety of manners (Table 1). The varieties of allografts include fresh-frozen, irradiated, freeze-dried (lyophilized), DFDB, and human bone ash (human-derived HA) (Fig. 3A,B).

Fresh-frozen bone is not used in implant dentistry, because of the significant concerns about possible disease transmission and possible host–graft reaction *(8,22)*. Fresh-frozen bone is osteoconductive *(8)*.

Irradiated bone is similar to frozen bone, but it has been irradiated to decrease the risk of disease transmission and antigenicity. Despite its proponents, irradiated bone is not widely used in implant

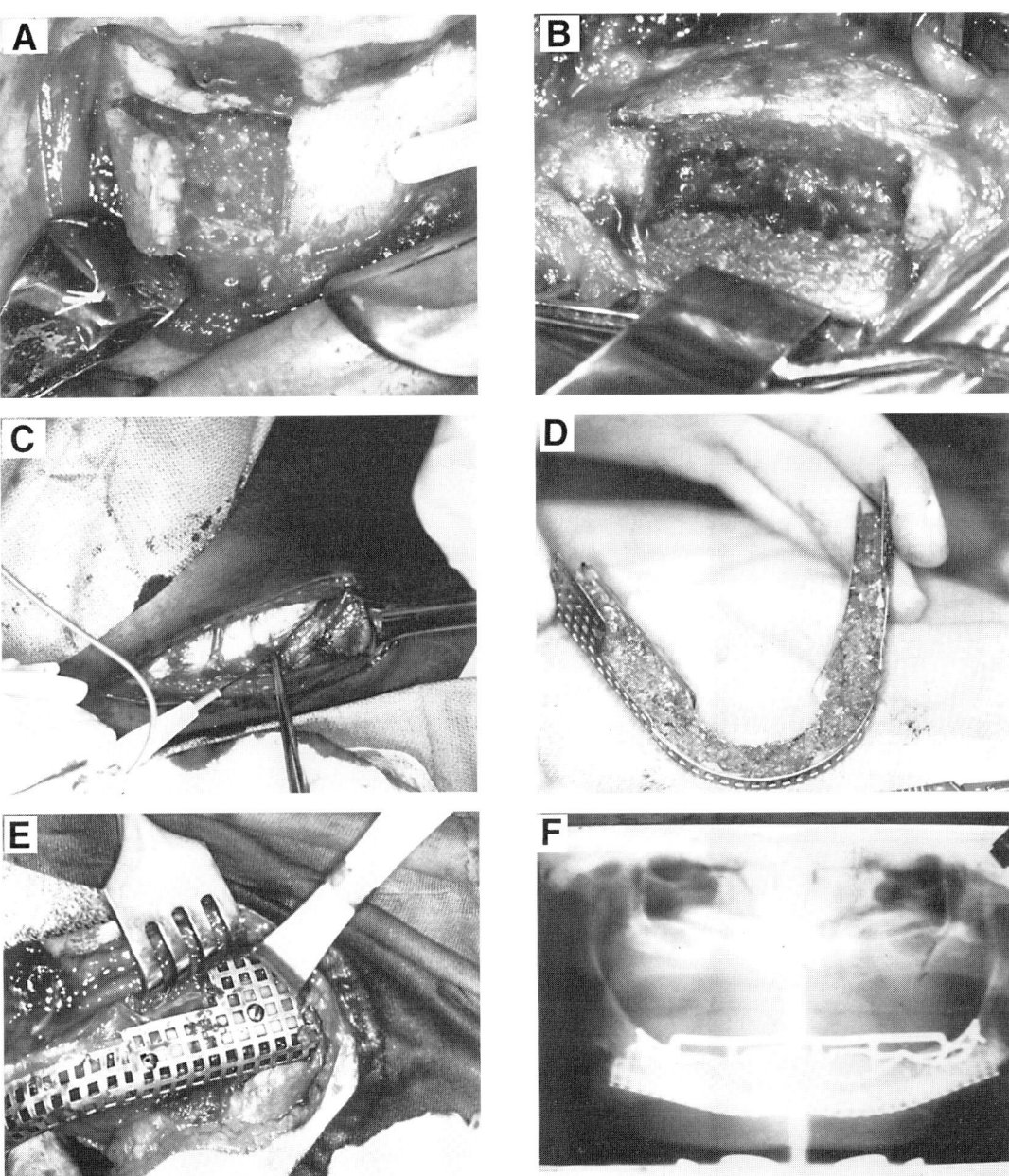

Fig. 2. Donor sites for autogenous bone grafting are retrieved from strategic sites of the skeleton: Occasionally morbid consequences accompany the retrieval. (**A**) The mandibular mental symphysis can yield as much as 15 cc of bone without sacrifice of chin morphology; however, considerable soreness and dysfunction of the lip may result on a reversible basis. (**B**) The anterior iliac crest of the pelvis can yield 3–4 × the quantity of marrow available from the chin, but patients often ambulate with discomfort for considerable periods of time. (**C**) Ribs do not offer material quantities of marrow, and as such are not particulated, but, particularly because of their curvature, serve well as mandibular substitutes. Often patients have residual chest pain and occasional pneumothorax after harvesting of the rib. (**D**) Mandibular Ti mortise form, filled with crushed autogenous bone marrow, to be used for mandibular augmentation. (**E**) Ti mortise with graft secured to mandible with screws. (**F**) This panoramic radiograph, with an autogenous BG in a Ti mortise, demonstrates the dramatic change in size that can be created using such a technique.

Table 1
Categories of Grafting Materials

	Values	Shortcomings
Autografts: This type of bone is "self-donated" by the patient. Source:		
iliac crest	Patient's own bone	Second-site morbidity
	Osteogenic	Requires general anesthesia
	Availability	Prolonged postoperative (po) recovery
Ascending ramus or symphysis of mandible	Patient's own bone	Second-site morbidity
	Osteogenic	Prolonged po recovery
	Availability	
Torus	Patient's own bone	Host site availability
	Osteoconductive	Second-site morbidity
		Cortical bone only
Rib or tibial plateau	Patient's own bone	Second-site morbidity
	Osteogenic	Requires general anesthesia
	Availability	Prolonged po recovery
Calvarium	Patient's own bone	Second-site morbidity
	Osteogenic	Requires general anesthesia
	Availability	Prolonged po recovery
Homografts/allografts: This type of bone is donated from a human source other than the patient Source: bone banks Types available:		
Demineralized freeze-dried bone[a] (DFDB)	Availability	Cost
	Osteoinductive/conductive	Patient may not accept
	Biologic acceptability	
	Replaced by patient's own bone	
Freeze-dried bone matrix	Availability	Cost
	Osteoconductive	Patient may not accept
	Biologic acceptability	
	Replaced by patient's own bone	
Irradiated bone	Availability	Cost
	Osteoconductive	Increased concerns about disease transmission because of decreased processing
	Biologic acceptability	
	Replaced by patient's own bone	
Fresh-frozen bone	Availability	Cost
	Osteoconductive	Significant risk of disease transmission and graft-host reaction
	Replaced by patients own bone	
Human bone ash (Osteomin)	Availability (Pacific Coast Tissue Bank)	Cost
	Osteoconductive (human HA)	An HA of human bone
	Resorbable	
	No risk of disease transmission	

(continued)

dentistry, because of concerns about disease transmission *(23)*. Irradiated bone acts by osteoconduction, similar to fresh-frozen bone *(23)*.

Freeze-dried bone is similar to irradiated bone, but it has been subjected to a desiccating step, and requires the action of osteoblasts to release its BMPs *(24)*. This process is unpredictable, and, as a result, freeze-dried bone acts primarily by osteoconduction *(23)*.

DFDB is subjected to a demineralization pro-

Table 1
(Continued)

	Values	Shortcomings
Xenografts: Mineralized bone matrix from a species other than man		
Source: Bovine		
Types:		
Bio-Oss, Osteograf N	Availability	Cost
	Osteoconductive	Similar to HA
	Patient acceptance	
	Biologic acceptability	
Alloplasts: These are synthetic bone materials		
Source: a variety of manufacturers		
Types:		
Nonresorbable	Availability	Cost
1. Polymer: (HTR)	Osteoconductive	Nonresorbable
	Hydrophilic	
	Patient acceptance	
	Biologic acceptability	
	Nonresorbable	
2. Ceramic: HA (i.e., Calcitite, Osteograf D, Interpore)	Availability	Cost
	Osteoconductive	Nonresorbable
	Patient acceptance	(HA component)
	Biologic acceptability	
	Nonresorbable	
3. Ceramic HA (35%) in a resorbable medium $CaSO_4$ (65%) (Hapset)	Availability	Cost
	Osteoconductive	Nonresorbable
	Patient acceptance	(HA component)
	Nonresorbable	
Resorbable	Availability	Cost
1. Ceramic (TCP) (i.e., Augmen, Synthograf)	Osteoconductive	Absorbability
	Patient acceptance	Questionable
	Biologic acceptability	Predictability
2. Ceramic (HA) (i.e., Osteogen, Osteograf LD, Osteograf N)	Availability	Cost
	Osteoconductive	Absorbability
	Patient acceptance	
	Biologic acceptability	
Bioactive Glass (i.e., Biogran, Perioglas)	Availability	Cost
	Osteoconductive	Absorbability
	Biologic acceptability	
	Patient acceptable	

Bone banks: For bone banks, *see* Appendix for members of the American Association of Tissue Banks.

^aAvailable in various forms: cortical or cancellous powder, cortical chips, monocortical or bicortical blocks, as a gel in combination with glycero: (Grafton/Osteotech), or thin cortical sheets to be used as a membrane (lambone/Pacific Coast Tissue Bank).

cess using hydrochloric or nitric acid for 6–16 h *(23)*. During this process, the calcium (Ca) and phosphate salts are removed from the bone matrix, which releases the organic growth factors (BMPs) *(12)*: Therefore, DFDB acts by osteoinduction *(11,12)*. Several authors *(25,26)* recently have questioned the amount of BMPs present in commercially available DFDB, and thus have placed its osteoinductive potential in doubt. Others *(10)* have questioned its osteoconductive

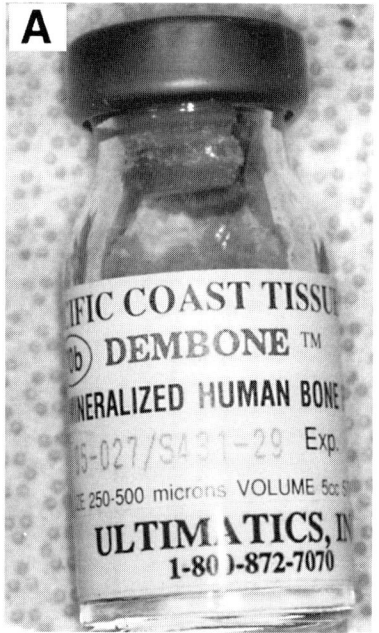

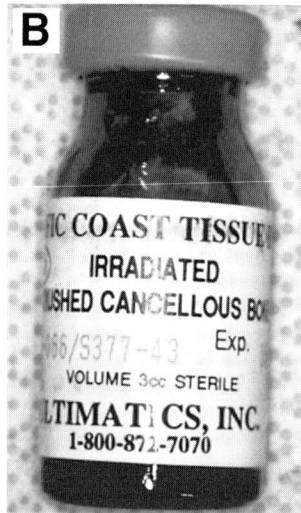

Fig. 3. **(A)** DFDB is an allograft material used for its putative osteogenic capabilities. DFDB is harvested from humans. **(B)** Irradiated cancellous bone is retrieved from human donors, and is treated by X-radiation. There may be a possibility of viral disease transmission, when using this product.

potential, because of its lack of a mineral matrix. Many *(8,10)* have suggested combining DFDB with another graft material, to increase osteoconduction and improve bone formation. DFDB is available in powder, chips, blocks, cortical, monocortical and bicortical, and thin sheets of cortical bone. The later is used as a membrane during guided bone regeneration.

Xenografts are obtained from another species. The xenografts available in dentistry today are from bovine bone, which is processed so that all the inorganic matrix is removed, leaving an inorganic component *(23)*. This is primarily HA, but may also contain other inorganic components (carbonates and tricalcium phosphate [TCP]) *(23)*. Because of their similarity to human bone, xenografts are biocompatible, and are slowly resorbed and replaced by bone *(23)*. They are particulates, and behave similarly to alloplasts, although their manufacturers state that, since these materials are natural, they are more easily recognized as bone by the human body. These materials are osteoconductive.

Alloplasts are synthetic materials that act by osteoconduction *(19,27)*. They are composed of either ceramics, glasses, polymers based on polymethylmethacrylate (PMMA) or calcium sulfate (Ca_2SO_4 [plaster of Paris]) *(19,27)*.

Bioactive ceramics are composed of calcium phosphate (Ca_2PO_4). The two primary commercially available ceramics are TCP and HA *(27;* Fig. 4A,B).

TCP has a Ca:phosphate ratio of 3:2 *(8)*. It is resorbed by osteoblasts, and replaced by new bone *(8)*. TCP has an unpredictable resorption profile *(8)*: Studies have demonstrated that TCP is not replaced by bone in a 1:1 ratio *(19)*. TCP has not been used as frequently as HA, which is the preferred CaP-based alloplast *(19,27)*.

HA is material composed of Ca and phosphorus in a 10:6 ratio *(8)*. HA is the principal inorganic component of calcified tissues of the human body. HA can be natural (allografts, xenografts), coral-based, or synthetically derived *(19,27)*. The ability of HA to act as an osteoconductive material has been well documented *(27)*. HA is synthesized from its nonceramic form by a process called sintering (heating at 700–1300°C), which fuses the crystals into a ceramic configuration *(27)*. HA has a variable resorption profile that depends on its physical and chemical properties *(8)*.

The physical properties can include surface area or shape of the product (block vs particle), porosity, and crystallinity *(8)*. The larger the particle size of the HA, the lower the resorption rate

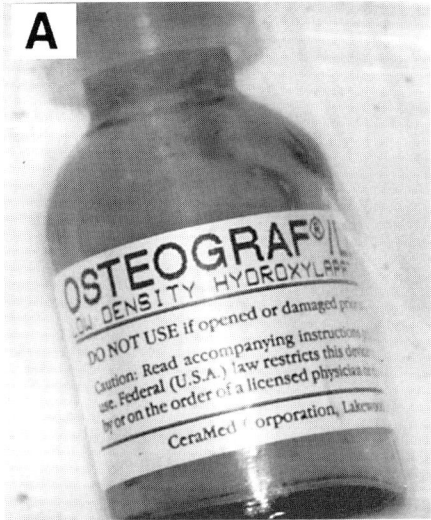
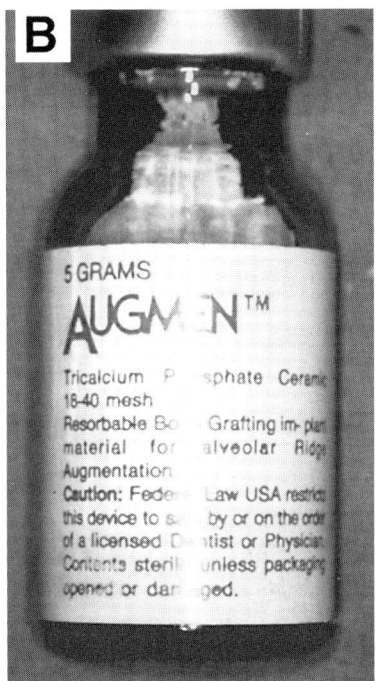
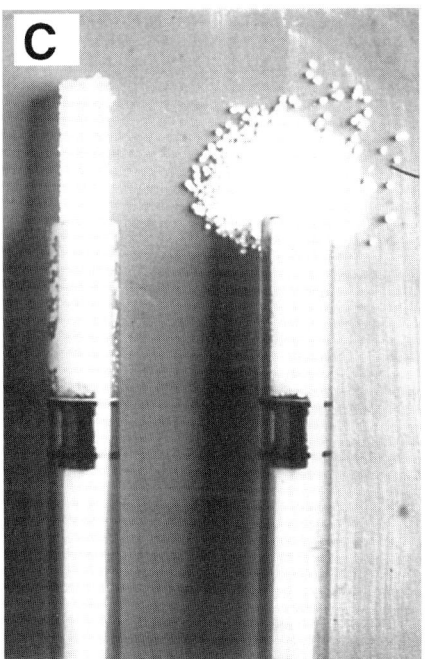
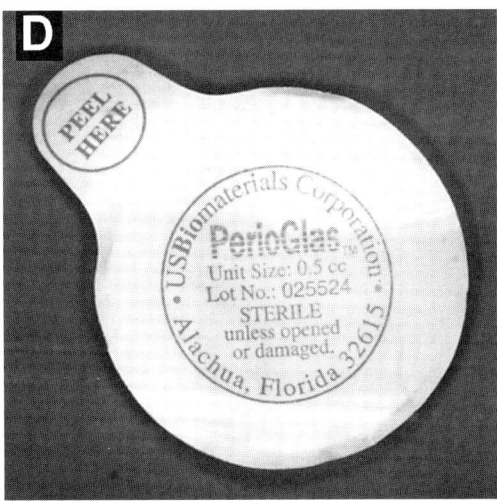

Fig. 4. **(A)** HA is used mostly for repair of small defects, in which its osteoconductive properties are beneficial. **(B)** TCP is an alloplast with no regenerative capabilities, and is used to fill defects such as extraction sockets. **(C)** Synthetic HA, available in both block and particulate form (above), is applied best when made available in a disposable syringe. When it is moistened, these 600–800-μ diameter particles have sufficient cohesion to be manageable intraoperatively (left syringe). **(D)** In addition to the passive alloplastic particulate materials listed above, surface bioactivity is attributed to this glass.

(8); the more porous the particle, the higher the resorption rate *(8,27)*. HA particles can be crystalline or amorphous *(8)*: Those of crystalline structure are less biodegradable *(8)*. The chemical properties of HA can also alter its rate of degradation. Impurities in the HA (such as Ca carbonate) act to increase solution-mediated resorption (chemical reactions); pure HA is degraded by cell-

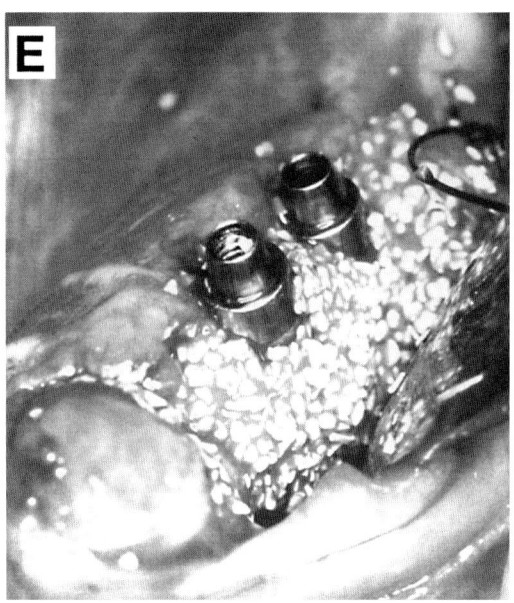

Fig. 4. (Continued) (**E**) Bone surrounding two newly placed endosteal root-form dental implants is being augmented with an osteoconductive particulate alloplast.

mediated processes (osteoclastic activity) *(8)*. HA is available in particle or block configurations *(19)*, and also in dense or porous varieties, with varying degrees of porosity *(19;* Fig. 4C).

Bioactive glasses are silicate-based alloplastic materials *(19,27)*. They are hard, solid, transparent materials composed of silicon dioxide, sodium oxide, Ca oxide, and phosphorus oxide *(28)*. Bioactive glasses undergo an interaction with bone that commences after implantation *(19,27,28)*. When exposed to a physiologic, aqueous environment, a silica-rich gel layer forms on the surface of the bioactive glass, which contains Ca and phosphate that aggregates to form HA agglomerations *(19)*. This layer is responsible for the rapid, chemical bond between bone and the glass particles *(19)*. Additionally, bioactive glass can bond to soft tissues if immobilized *(19)*. The material is available in both nonresorbable and resorbable forms *(19,27;* Fig. 4D,E).

Hard tissue replacement (HTR) is a porous polymer based on PMMA. It is biocompatible, because it is coated with polyhydroxyethylmethacryate and calcium hydroxide *(29)*. HTR is nonresorbable, serves only as a scaffold for bony ingrowth, and displays osteoconductive behavior *(19)*. It is available in both block and particulate forms.

Ca_2SO_4 is a BG material that has been used, since 1892 *(30)*, as a powder that is mixed with water, to form a dense paste that is then placed into the bone defect *(27)*. It sets by exothermic reaction to a solid mass *(27)*. The heat released during this process is not enough to damage the bone *(31)*. Ca_2SO_4 resorbs within 5–8 wk *(19)*. It has fallen out of favor as a BG alloplast, because of its unpredictable resorption profile and concerns raised regarding its release of Ca and sulfur *(27)*. A commercially available product (Hapset, Lifecore) uses Ca_2SO_4 as a carrier for nonresorbable HA. Ca_2SO_4 has also been studied as a barrier membrane for use in guided bone regeneration (GBR) procedures *(32,33)*.

2.2. Occlusive Membranes

Occlusive membranes often are employed in implant dentistry as an adjunct to augment defects in the alveolar ridge. Most often, they are accompanied by a BG material in particulate form.

The use of membranes to influence tissue growth elucidated in the 1950s *(34,35)* the use of cellulose acetate filters in nerve and tendon regeneration. Research in the 1980s *(36–45)* demonstrated the ability of membranes to allow selective repopulation of defects by the cells of the periodontal ligament and bone, in both animal and human studies.

Regeneration of the periodontal ligament and bone adjacent to defects was termed "guided tissue regeneration" (GTR) *(42)*, which was used to describe regeneration in areas without teeth, either with or without implants *(46)*. Other terms used for the use of membranes to influence bony regeneration are "selective cell repopulation" *(40)*, "controlled tissue regeneration" *(41)*, and "osteopromotion" *(47,48)*.

The phenomenon of GTR/GBR is the result of the membrane/barrier acting to exclude the apical migration of gingival epithelial and connective tissues, and to allow progenitor cells of the periodontal ligament (in GTR) or the bone (in GBR) to repopulate the defect *(46)*. The end result is the regeneration of the periodontium and/or alveolar bone. When employed in implant dentistry, membranes are often placed over particulate BG mate-

Biomaterials Used in Implant Dentistry

rials, to enhance bony regeneration in defects, either prior to or at the time of implant placement.

Studies have demonstrated the ability of occlusive membranes to enhance bone regeneration in defects adjacent to dental implants *(6,49–55)*, to augment the edentulous ridge *(4,5,56,57)* and to treat peri-implant bone destruction (peri-implantitis) *(58–60)*.

2.2.1. Materials

Membranes employed for GBR in implant dentistry can be broadly classified as nonresorbable and resorbable (Fig. 5A,B).

The nonresorbable membranes commercially available are composed of polytetrafluoroethylene (PTFE). The standard nonresorbable membrane is Gore-Tex which is composed of porous or expanded PTFE (ePTFE) *(46)*. Most other nonresorbable membranes available are of the nonexpanded or dense variety of PTFE (dPTFE).

Gore-Tex has gained preeminence in implant and grafting surgery for use in GBR *(6,49,51, 61,62)*, because of its status as the classic membrane during the development of GTR *(63,64)*. It utilizes an expanded (porous) surface, which is required to gain early connective tissue ingrowth. This feature stabilizes the overlying soft tissues *(65)*. Shortcomings of Gore-Tex have been cited, including its requirement for a second-stage surgery (and the associated morbidity) and its tendency to become exposed to the surrounding oral environment, which can result in infection and decreased bony ingrowth *(65,66)*.

dPTFE membranes have been marketed as an alternative to the expanded variety. Proponents of these membranes state that, because of their nonporous structure, they do not become integrated with the surrounding soft tissues, and become exposed during healing. This allows easy removal from its site, and acts to inhibit bacterial colonization prior to its removal *(67–69)*. Limited clinical reports indicate that these membranes function well when not primarily covered with soft tissues at the time of placement *(67,68)*. Despite promising preliminary studies *(69)*, the efficacy of dPTFE vs Gore-Tex has not been studied.

In efforts to eliminate second-stage surgery, resorbable alternatives have been studied intensively. The currently available resorbable mem-

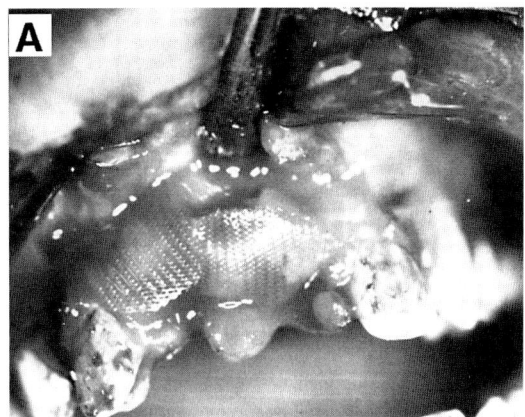

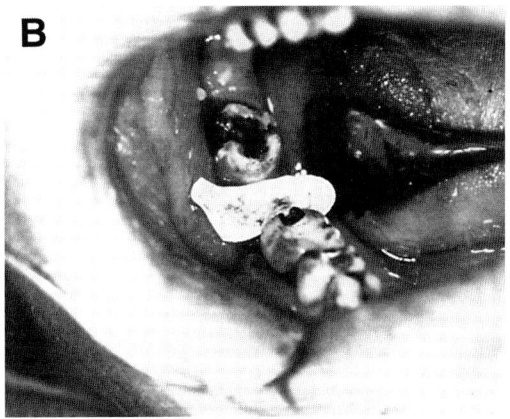

Fig. 5. GBR membranes may be resorbable or require removal in a second surgical stage. They serve to prevent epithelial downgrowth during the critical postgrafting period, when an undisturbed environment is required for mineralization. (**A**) Vicryl (PLA-PGA) mesh is predictably resorbable over a 90-d period. (**B**) Gore-Tex (PTFE) is a nonresorbable, nonporous, but reliable membrane, which requires second-stage surgery for retrieval.

branes may be divided broadly into those composed of natural or synthetic materials *(70)*.

Natural membranes presently being marketed include allogeneic tissues and collagen-based materials. The allogeneic tissue utilized as a membrane is demineralized freeze-dried cortical bone sheets (Lambone, Pacific Coast Tissue Bank). It serves both as an occlusive membrane and possibly as an osteoinductive medium for the healing bone site. Its success as a GBR membrane has been reported *(71;* Fig. 6).

Collagen has been studied as a membrane

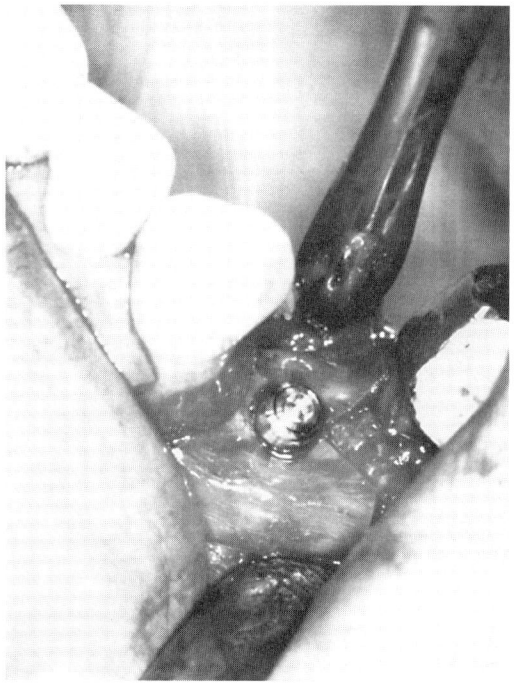

Fig. 6. Laminar bone is a natural barrier membrane made of thin layers of human cortical bone. When hydrated, it becomes soft, compliant, and versatile.

material *(72–74)*. It is currently available as derived either from bovine or porcine sources *(132)*. Collagen membranes have a fibrillar meshwork structure that acts as a conductive scaffold for colonization by host cells *(75)*. Concerns regarding potential antigenicity of collagens *(70)* resulting from contaminants and the presence of nonhelical telopeptide regions of the collagen molecule have been addressed in current-generation membranes by strict processing protocols *(76)*. Collagen is resorbed by the action of lysosomal enzymes *(77)*. When compared with ePTFE, collagen membranes show promising results *(78)*.

Synthetic membranes have been primarily composed of polymers or copolymers, PGA and/or PLA. $CaSO_4$ has also been utilized as a barrier membrane. The membranes based on PGA/PLA include Vicryl mesh, Guidor, Atrisorb, and Gore Resolute. Each of these products has PGA and/or PLA in various configurations, which result in different physical properties and resorption profiles. All of these membranes resorb by the action of hydrolysis. Studies have demonstrated the effectiveness of these materials, as compared with Gore-Tex *(48,79–87)*.

Ca_2SO_4, when used as a barrier membrane, has been shown to be successful *(88–90)*. Its effectiveness, compared with Gore-Tex, remains to be discovered.

Proper techniques for GBR have been discussed *(71)*. These include proper flap design including provision for primary passive closure of the flap, decortication of the bony walls to allow blood and bone cell infiltration, clot stabilization and maintenance of the defect (using bone grafting materials), placement of the membrane over the defect and extending to adjacent healthy bone, and stabilization of the membrane. Membrane stabilization can be aided by the use of Ti bone tacks, which affix the membrane to peripheral bone.

Criticisms of the GBR technique exist *(20)*, including questionable predictability of bone replacement, the degree of bone to implant contact when GBR is used at the time of implant placement, the quality of the newly regenerated bone, and problems associated with membrane exposure (infection and decreased bone formation). The use of barrier membranes is best when the defect is surrounded by bony walls. Larger defects are augmented more predictably by the use of autogenous bone monocortical blocks, which do not require the use of membranes.

2.3. Implant Devices

Devices termed "dental implants" commonly refer to those that support or retain one or more prosthetic teeth. Dental implants can be broadly classified as either endosseous or subperiosteal. The majority of implants placed today are of the endosseous variety. Endosseous implants are further subdivided into plate (blade) forms and root forms, the latter being the most widely used.

2.3.1. Subperiosteal Implants

Subperiosteal implants were first introduced to dentistry more than 50 yr ago *(91)*. They are fabricated by the lost-wax casting technique. The material of choice for this application has been surgical-grade Vitallium, which is composed of Co-Cr-Mo in a 66:27:7% ratio. These implants consist of a mesh-like infrastructure, which fits on the maxillary or mandibular bone in a saddle-

Biomaterials Used in Implant Dentistry

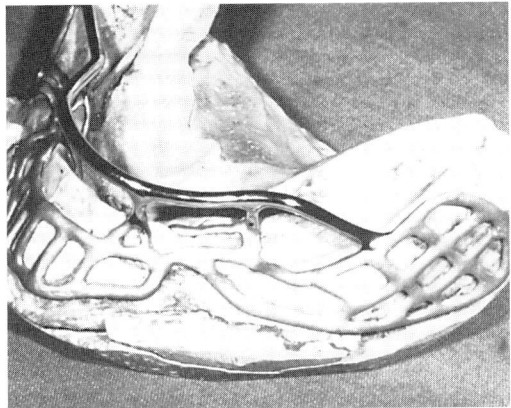

Fig. 7. Mandibular subperiosteal implant, which serves as a retaining device for prostheses for fully edentulous mandibles, is cast of Vitalium (Cr-Co-Mo alloy).

like function, and to which are attached premucosal abutments that serve as retentive devices for prostheses (Fig. 7).

The subperiosteal implant is utilized in edentulous regions of the mouth that have undergone significant bony resorption, to the extent that endosseous implants are not a viable treatment alternative. The most common application for the subperiosteal implant is in the completely edentulous mandible (Fig. 8). Subperiosteal implants also can be utilized in partially edentulous posterior regions of either the maxilla or mandible. In these applications, the prosthetic teeth, which are

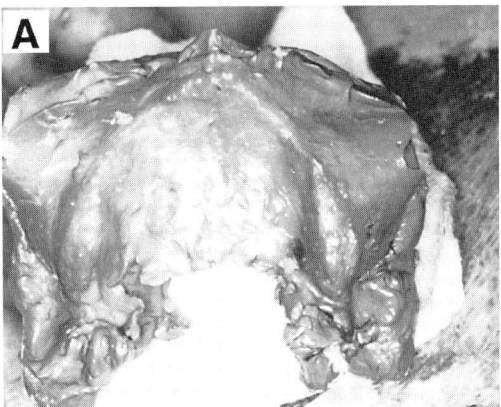

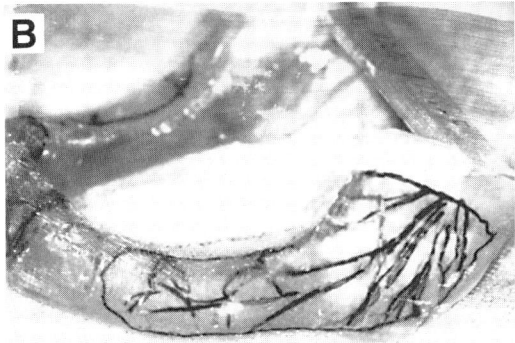

Fig. 9. (**A**) Polysulfide impression material can be used with safety and accuracy for the recording of the morphology of a jaw bone. From the model made of such an impression, a subperiosteal casting can be made using the lost wax technique. (**B**) Stereolithography is a technique used to fabricate copies of anatomic parts from CT scan images. Their high level of accurate reproducibility permits their use for casting subperiosteal implants, as well as other body replacement parts.

attached to the implant, must be rigidly connected to healthy natural teeth, in order to dissipate forces transferred to the implant. Excessive forces are detrimental to long-term implant-bone health.

Subperiosteal implants are currently fabricated from models of the bearing bone, which are obtained by one of two methods. The more traditional way, which was developed separately by Lew and Berman *(92,93)*, employs a direct bone impression, from which a stone model is made (Fig. 9A). The second method is the utilization of computer-aided design/computer-aided manufacture (CAD/CAM), by utilizing computerized tomography (CT) *(94)*. The advantage of the latter

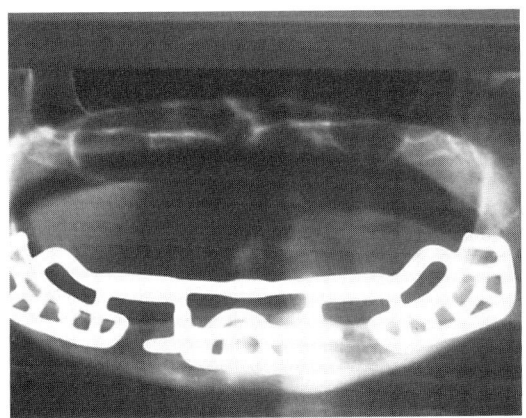

Fig. 8. Radiograph demonstrates the precision with which subperiosteal implants are adapted to the jaw.

technique is that it avoids the bone impression surgery (Fig. 9B), but critics state that it is less accurate than the direct bone impression technique. However, studies have demonstrated the long-term efficiency of subperiosteal implants fabricated on computer-generated models *(95,96).*

The original design of the subperiosteal implant has been significantly changed since its inception. Primary modification to the implant itself has been to extend the implant onto areas that do not experience the classical resorption patterns *(97).* A critical modification of the mesostructure (that which connects the implant to the prosthesis) was introduced by Cranin with the Brookdale bar *(98; see* Fig. 7). This innovation added strength to complete subperiosteal implants by joining all permucosal abutments with a rigid bar. This bar also enabled the introduction of the tripodal mandibular implant, which avoids the mental foramen region, and thus reduces the possibility of mental nerve dysesthesia.

Some clinicians have advocated coating subperiosteal implants with HA, in an effort to gain implant–bone contact and decrease the possibility of metal sensitivity *(99).* The advantage of this coating may well be outweighed by the potential soft tissue complications, if the region containing the HA becomes exposed because of infection or recession. Moreover, others *(100,101)* have reported that the primary support mechanism of subperiosteal implants is a suspensory fibrous tissue sling, a phenomenon that would be inhibited by an HA coating. There is evidence to suggest that HA-coated subperiosteal implants do not possess a fibrous sling, and do bond in spots directly with bone *(102).* Despite this finding, clinical experience suggests that the use of HA on subperiosteal implants should be approached with caution.

2.3.2. Endosteal Implants

Endosteal implants are those that are placed within the bone. After placement, the gingiva is sutured over the implant, and the implant is left undisturbed. If primary wound closure is achieved at the placement surgery, a second uncovery procedure is necessary to connect the implant to a permucosal extension, to which prosthetic teeth are attached by a variety of methods. An alternative to this technique is to affix the permucosal extension at the time of implant placement.

Endosteal implants act to provide a long-term implant–bone interface, primarily because of the bioinert (Ti or Ti alloy) or bioactive surface (HA-coated implants) present on the implant surfaces. Endosseous implants are either of the blade-form or root-form variety.

2.3.2.1. MATERIALS

2.3.2.1.1. Cobalt-Chromium-Molybdenum. Original blade designs were fabricated using Co-Cr-Mo. The long-term success of these designs was relatively poor *(103):* Several studies have demonstrated that Co-Cr-Mo does not achieve a direct bone–implant interface, but is encapsulated by a fibrous tissue envelope *(104).* The reason for this fibrous interface has been postulated to relate to the surface oxide layer present (Cr oxide), small quantities of biodegradation products, a high modulus of elasticity, or other unidentified factors *(104).* Because of this lack of a direct bone interface, Co-Cr-Mo has been abandoned in endosseous applications, particularly after the introduction of Ti, which was demonstrated to satisfy this requirement.

2.3.2.1.2. Ti and Ti alloy. Ti was introduced as a dental implant material by Brånemark, who coined the term "osseointegration" *(105),* which is defined as a direct bone–implant contact at the light microscope level. This element achieves levels of bone contact because of its bioinert surface layer of Ti oxide *(106),* which is present in both pure Ti and its alloy, commonly employed in implant designs (Ti 6-aluminum, 4-vanadium) *(106).* Both have been shown to achieve osseointegration.

Currently, Ti- and Ti-alloy-based implants are available in blade- and root-form configurations. Blade-shaped implants composed of Ti or Ti alloy are able to achieve osseointegration, if allowed to heal in an undisturbed fashion (no micromovement), as is common with root-form implant protocols *(107).*

2.3.2.1.3. HA coatings. HA has gained popularity as a coating on Ti-based endosteal implants *(121).*

Biomaterials Used in Implant Dentistry

The appeal of HA coatings is that they impart a bioactive surface to the implant *(121)*. Studies in animals have indicated that HA-coated implants achieve increased levels of bone–implant contact *(122–125)*. Studies also indicate that the HA-coated implants have increased the levels of interface attachment strength *(124)*.

Microscopic studies on HA-coated implants have demonstrated a direct bone–implant bond at the electron microscopic level *(126,127)*. This is beyond what Brånemark originally called osseointegration. In contrast, the Ti oxide–bone interface at the ultrastructural level is characterized either by an acellular and amorphic collagen-free zone, approx 500 μm in thickness, a 50-μm, of amorphous material separating the implant from an organized collagenous matrix, or by a 500–600-μm zone containing a loosely organized filamentous material separating the implant from a collagenous matrix *(128)*.

Controversies about HA coatings exist, including the possibility of resorption of the HA surface over time *(129,130)*, and there are reports of increased clinical failures (vs Ti-surfaced implants) after several years in function *(131)*. Because of these concerns, many clinicians prefer uncoated Ti or Ti alloy implants.

2.3.2.2. Designs

2.3.2.2.1. Blade Implants. Blade implants are available in a variety of configurations. They are utilized in partially edentulous regions of the maxilla or mandible that are too narrow to allow placement of root-form implants. They are tapped into the bony host site after a slot-shaped osteotomy has been prepared with a saline-cooled fissure bur. Similar to the subperiosteal implant, prosthetic teeth attached to blade implants must be rigidly connected to the natural dentition located anterior or posterior to the implant to avoid overloading, a known etiology of implant failure. Because of these limitations, root-form implants have eclipsed the blade implant as the endosteal implant of choice (Fig. 10 A,B).

2.3.2.2.2. Root-Form Implants. Root-form implants are currently the modality of choice for the vast majority of implant-borne restorations. They can be utilized in a variety of partially and fully edentulous situations, ranging from single-

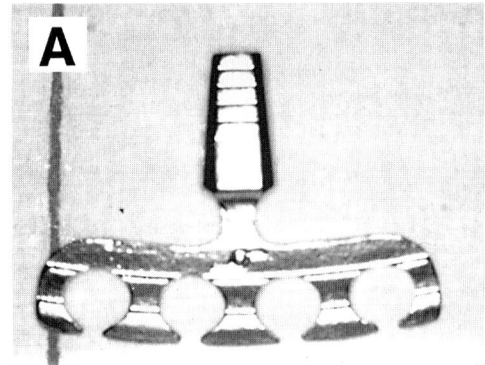

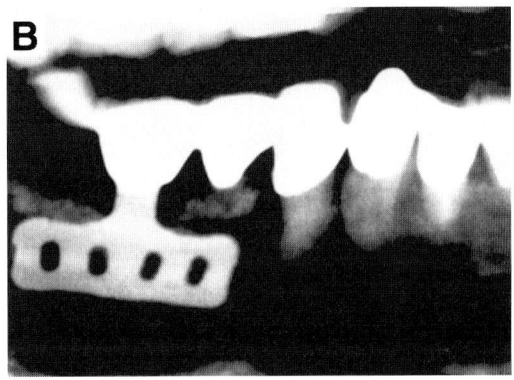

Fig. 10. **(A)** This implant was useful in areas of low ridge height or diminished buccolingual width. It is permitted to function immediately. Blades do not osseointegrate, and are not as predictable as other designs after placement. **(B)** Blades are splinted to natural teeth, which serve a symbiotic role.

tooth replacement to full-arch rehabilitation. Because of their integrated relationship to host sites, they can be prosthetically restored independent of natural teeth (single-tooth to full-arch reconstruction) (Fig. 11A–C), or, if required, they can be connected to natural teeth (Fig. 11D). Their efficacy has been well documented *(105,108–111)*, primarily because of their Ti oxide or HA surfaces, as well as by following the protocol established by Brånemark, which calls for undisturbed healing of the bone around the implant for a period of 3–6 mo *(112)*. The original operative design called for these implants to be covered by gingiva, and later to be exposed (at a second-stage procedure), to have a permucosal extension abutment placed *(112)*. The work of others *(107)* has shown that primary closure of the operative

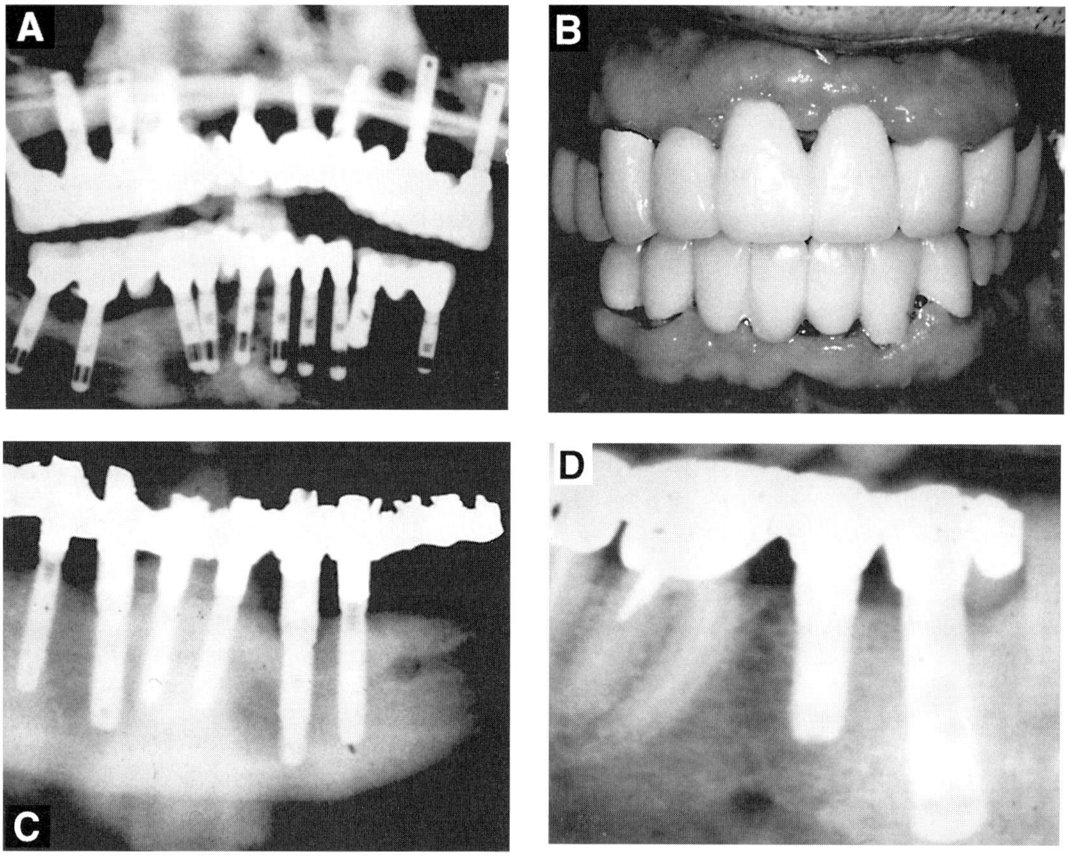

Fig. 11. **(A)** Root-form implants are designed to osseointegrate, and thus can act independently. **(B)** The same restoration viewed intraorally. The crowns can be connected to the implants, via screws or cement. **(C)** Root-form implants can be applied in fabricating nonremovable prostheses that are completely implant-supported. These may include fixed bridges (Fig. 11A), or screw-secured overdentures known as hybrids (removable by the clinician). **(D)** Root-form implants may also be used in conjunction with natural dentition to support fixed bridges.

site is not necessary, and that the lack of micromovement during healing was the critical factor. This finding has prompted some implant manufacturers to advocate single-stage surgery, at which the implant is allowed to extend through the gingiva at the time of initial placement surgery *(113–116)*. Prosthesis construction, however, must be delayed to permit osseointegration.

Root-form implants are available in a variety of lengths and widths (Fig. 12). They are available in cylindrical shapes that are tapped into position after appropriately sized osteotomies are prepared with saline-cooled drills. They may be obtained, as well, with threaded configurations that require screwing into the bone (Fig. 13A–D).

Surface finishes vary, and may be chosen on

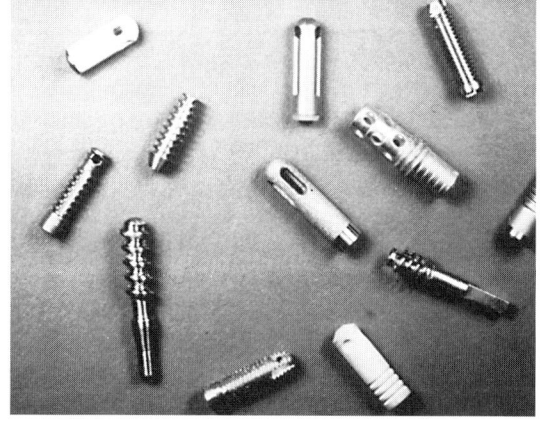

Fig. 12. A plethora of root-form implants. Two chief divisions are the screws and the cylinders.

Biomaterials Used in Implant Dentistry

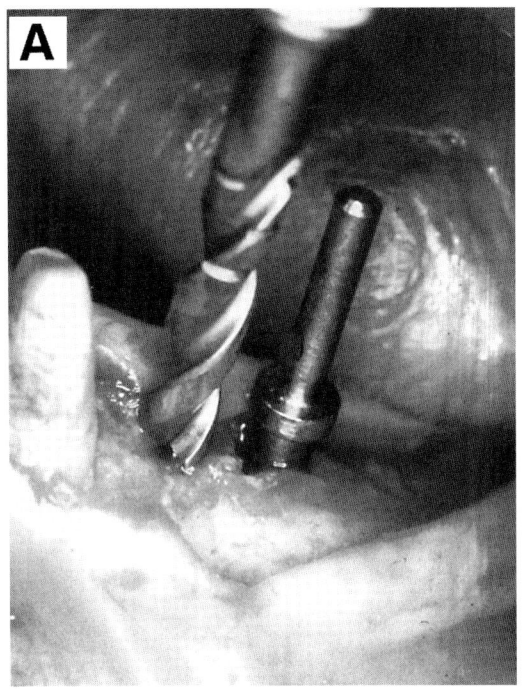
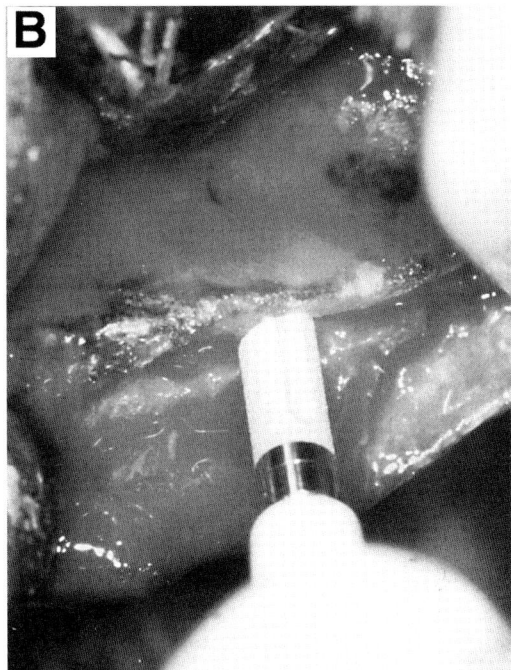
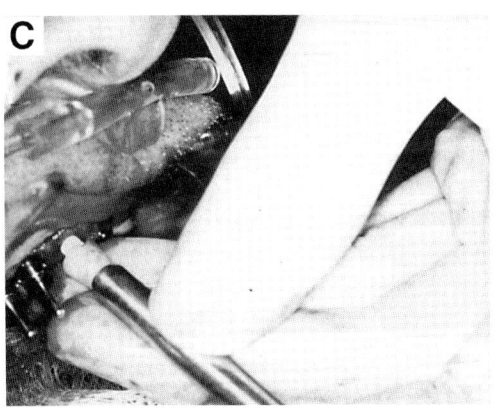
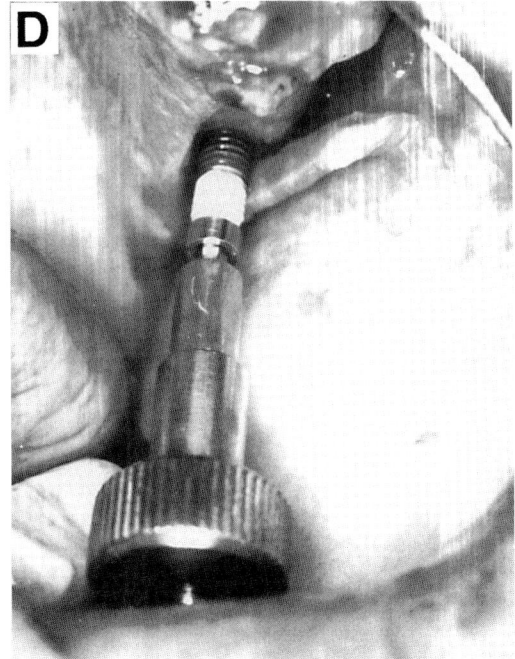

Fig. 13. **(A)** Implant sites are prepared with sequential drilling. The drills are internally irrigated, to avoid overheating of the bone. **(B)** One way to place a root-form implant is to tap it into the prepared site. This technique is limited to cylindrical implants. **(C)** The tapper engages the head of the implant. **(D)** The second method of implant placement is screwing the fixture into the bone. The operator can use hand- (shown), or motor-driven wrenches.

the basis of perceived benefit. The original Brånemark-designed implants have a machined-finished surface. Other available surfaces include grit-blasted, Ti-plasma-sprayed or porous-bead-coated. Studies indicate that surface texture affects the level of implant–bone fixation. Greater surface roughness results in increased levels of bone contact and resultant enhanced abilities to withstand

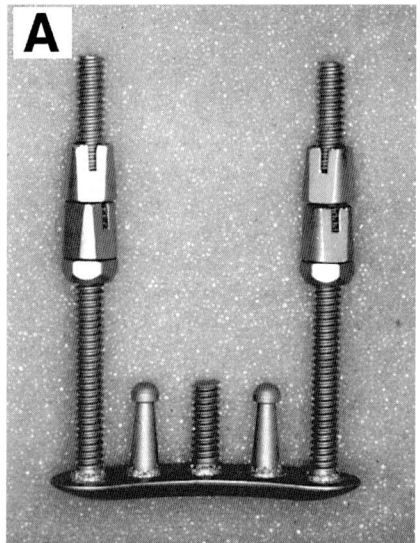

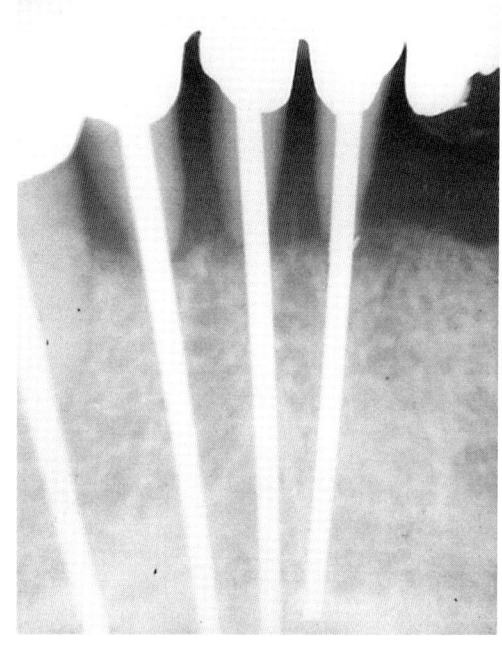

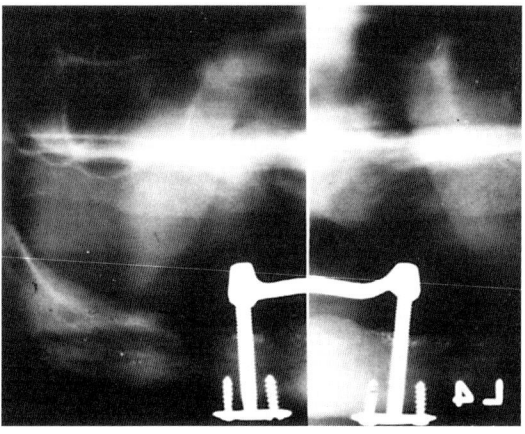

Fig. 14. **(A)** Transmandibular implant is designed to provide a stable foundation on an atrophic mandible. The surgery requires an extraoral approach. Fracture at the parasymphysis is a possibility. **(B)** Once the implant has been placed, a variety of prosthetic options are available. In the case demonstrated, a bar-supported overdenture was fabricated.

Fig. 15. Endodontic stabilizers are 1 mm in diameter. They are meant to engage the bone, yet be cemented in the tooth. Endodontic stabilizers are a viable option in cases in which the patient experiences periodontal breakdown, but cannot, for whatever reason, undergo complete periodontal and/or prosthodontic rehabilitation. Improving the crown–root ratio of the dentition will generate greater stability.

shear forces *(117–119)*. However, there appears to be an optimal range of surface roughness, beyond which bone–implant contact is diminished *(119)*. Porous, bead-coated implants are said to add an additional means of bone–implant stabilization, by facilitating bony ingrowth into the pores on the implant surface *(118,120)*. The advantage of a porous coating is that a three-dimensional bone–implant interface results. The manufacturers of these implants contend that, as a result, implants of shorter length can be used *(118)*.

2.3.2.2.3. Alternative designs. Other configurations of Ti-based endosteal implants are transmandibular implants (Fig. 14A,B), endodontic stabilizers (Fig. 15), and ramus frame implants. Their use today is limited by the dominance of the root-form design.

3. Conclusion

There is a wide variety of biomaterials available to the implant dentist. Despite advancements in allografts, xenografts, and alloplasts, autogenous bone remains the gold standard BG material, because of its ability to form bone directly within the graft by the process of osteogenesis.

Occlusive membranes are often used as a means to augment alveolar defects, either prior to or at the time of implant placement. They are often utilized in conjunction with particulate BG materials. Because of its nonresorbable nature, Gore-Tex, which is the current gold standard membrane, is being challenged by a variety of resorbable membranes of either natural or synthetic source.

Devices currently utilized as dental implants are either of the subperiosteal or endosteal variety. Subperiosteal implants are fabricated from Vitallium, and endosteal implants are composed of either Ti or Ti alloys. The current configuration of choice for implant devices is the roof-form endosteal implant. This is primarily because of its ability to maintain a tight bone–implant contact in a variety of prosthetic applications, ranging from single-tooth replacement to full-arch rehabilitation. The use of HA coatings has been employed in all implant designs, but its use is controversial, because of reports of increased long-term complications.

References

1. Lekholm U and Zarb GA. Patient selection and preparation, in *Tissue-Integrated Prostheses: Osseointegration in Clinical Dentistry*, 1985 (Branemark P-I, Zarb GA, and Albrektsson T eds), Quintessence, Chicago, pp. 199–209.
2. Jemt T and Lekholm U. Implant treatment in edentulous maxillae: a five year follow-up report on patients with different degrees of jaw resorption. *Int J Oral Maxillofac Implants* 1995; 10: 303.
3. Becker W, Schenk R, Higuchi K, et al. Variations in bone regeneration adjacent to implants augmented with barrier membranes alone or with demineralized freeze-dried bone or autologous grafts: a study in dogs. *Int J Oral Maxillofac Implants* 1995; 10: 143–154.
4. Buser D, Bragger U, Lang NP, and Nyman S. Regeneration and enlargement of jaw bone using guided tissue regeneration. *Clin Oral Implants Res* 1990; 1: 22–32.
5. Buser D, Dula K, Belser U, et al. Localized ridge augmentation using guided bone regeneration. 1. Surgical procedure in the maxilla. *Int J Periodont Restorative Dent* 1993; 13: 29–45.
6. Jovanovic SA, Spiekermann H, and Richter EJ. Bone regeneration around titanium dental implants in dehisced defect sites: a clinical study. *Int J Oral Maxillofac Implants* 1992; 7: 233–245.
7. Misch CM. Comparison of intraoral donor sites for onlay grafting prior to implant placement. *Int J Oral Maxillofac Implants* 1997; 12: 767–776.
8. Misch CE and Dietsch F. Bone-grafting materials in implant dentistry. *Implant Dent* 1993; 2: 158–166.
9. Muthukumaran N, Ma S, and Reddi AH. Dose dependence of and threshold for optimal bone induction by collagenous bone matrix and osteogenin-enriched fraction. *Collagen Rel Res* 1988; 8: 433–441.
10. Smiler DG. Bone grafting: materials and modes of action. *Pract Periodont Aesthetic Dent* 1996; 8: 413–416.
11. Urist MR and Strates BS. Bone morphogenetic protein. *J Dent Res* 1971; 50: 1392–1406.
12. Urist MR. Search for and discovery of bone morphogenetic protein, in *Bone Grafts, Derivatives and Substitutes* 1994 (Urist MR, O'Conner BT, Burwell RG, eds), Butterworth, London, pp. 315–362.
13. Urist MR. Bone: formation by autoinduction. *Science* 1965; 150: 893–899.
14. Urist MR, Silverman BF, Buring K, et al. Bone induction principle. *Clin Orthop* 1967; 53: 243–283.
15. Roberts WE, Turley PK, Brezniak N, et al. Bone physiology and metabolism. *Calif Dent Assoc J* 1987; 15: 54–61.
16. Urist MR, Hay PH, Dubue F, et al. Osteogenic competence. *Clin Orthop* 1969; 64: 194–220.
17. Urist MR, Mikulski A, and Lietze A. Solubilized and insolubilized bone morphogenetic protein. *Proc Natl Acad Sci* 1979; 76: 1823–1828.
18. Urist MR, DeLange RJ, and Finerman GA. Bone cell differentiation and growth factors. *Science* 1983; 220: 680–686.
19. Costantino PD and Friedman CD. Synthetic bone graft substitutes. Craniofac Skeletal Augmentation Replacement. 1994; 1037–1072.
20. Misch CM and Misch CE. Repair of localized severe ridge defects for implant placement using mandibular bone grafts. *Implant Dent* 1995; 4: 261–267.
21. Mellonig JT. Bone allografts in periodontal therapy. *Clin Orthop Related Res* 1996; 324: 116–125.
22. Turner DW and Mellonig JT. Antigenicity of freeze-dried bone allograft in periodontal osseous defects. *J Periodont Res* 1981; 16: 89–99.
23. Misch CE. Contemporary Implant Dentistry 1993; Mosby, St. Louis.

24. Hurt WC. Freeze-dried bone homografts in periodontal lesions in dogs. *J Periodont Dent* 1968; 39: 89.
25. Rosen V and Theis S. BMP proteins in bone formation and repair. *Trends Genet* 1992; 8: 97–102.
26. Wozney JM. Bone morphogenetic protein family and osteogenesis. *Mol Reprod Dev* 1992; 32: 160–167.
27. Hollinger JO, Brekke J, Gruskin E, and Lee D. Role of bone substitutes. *Clin Orthop Related Res* 1996; 324: 55–65.
28. Zamet JS, Darbar UR, Griffiths GS, Bulman JS, Bragger U, Burgin W, and Newman HN. Particulate bioglass as a grafting material in the treatment of periodontal intrabony defects. *J Clin Periodontol* 1997; 24: 410–418.
29. Amler MH and LeGeros RZ. Hard tissue replacement (HTR) polymer as an implant material. *J Biomed Mater Res* 1990; 24: 1079–1089.
30. Peltier LF. Use of plaster of Paris to fill defects in bone. *Clin Orthop* 1961; 21: 1–31.
31. Coetzee AS. Regeneration of bone in the presence of calcium sulfate. *Arch Otolaryngol* 1980; 106: 405–409.
32. Anson D. Calcium sulfate: a 4-year observation of its use as a resorbable barrier in guided tissue regeneration of periodontal defects. *Compendium* 1996; 17: 895–899.
33. Conner HD. Bone grafting with a calcium sulfate barrier after root amputation. *Compendium* 1996; 17: 42–46.
34. Ashley FL, Stone RS, Alonso-Artieda M, et al. Experimental and clinical studies on the application of monomolecular cellulose filter tubes to create artificial tendon sheaths in digits. *Plast Reconstr Surg* 1959; 23: 526–534.
35. Campbell JB and Bassett CAL. The surgical application of monomolecular filters (Millipore) to bridge gaps in peripheral nerves and to prevent neuroma formation. *Surg Forum* 1956; 7: 570–574.
36. Aukhil I, Petersson E, and Sugges C. Guided tissue regeneration. An experimental procedure in beagle dogs. *J Periodontol* 1986; 57: 727–734.
37. Becker W, Becker B, Berg L, et al. New attachment after treatment with root isolation procedures: report for treated class III and Class II furcations and vertical osseous defects. *Int J Periodont Restorative Dent* 1988; 3: 2–16.
38. Caffesse RG, Smith BA, Castelli WA, and Nasjleti CE. New attachment achieved by guided tissue regeneration in beagle dogs. *J Periodontol* 1988; 59: 589–594.
39. Caffesse RG, Smith AB, Duff B, et al. Class II furcations treated by guided tissue regeneration in humans: case reports. *J Periodontol* 1990; 61: 510–514.
40. Caton JG, DeFuria EL, Polson AM, and Nyman S. Periodontal regeneration via selective cell repopulation. *J Periodontol* 1987; 58: 546–552.
41. Gottlow J, Nyman S, Karring T, and Lindhe J. New attachment formation as the result of controlled tissue regeneration. *J Clin Periodontol* 1984; 11: 494–503.
42. Gottlow J, Nyman S, Lindhe J, et al. New attachment formation in the human periodontium by guided tissue regeneration. Case reports. *J Clin Periodontol* 1986; 13: 604–616.
43. Lekovic V, Kenney EB, Kovacevic K, and Carranza FA. Evaluation of guided tissue regeneration in class II furcation defects. A clinical reentry study. *J Periodontol* 1989; 60: 694–698.
44. Nyman S, Gottlow J, Karring T, and Lindhe J. Regenerative potential of the periodontal ligament. An experimental study in the monkey. *J Clin Periodontol* 1982; 9: 257–265.
45. Pontoriero R, Lindhe J, Nyman S, et al. Guided tissue regeneration in degree II furcation involved mandibular molars. A clinical study. *J Clin Periodontol* 1988; 15: 247–254.
46. Hermann JS and Buser D. Guided bone regeneration for dental implants. *Curr Opin Periodontol* 1996; 3: 168–177.
47. Linde A, Alberius P, Dahlin C, Bjurstam K, and Sundin Y. Osteopromotion: a soft-tissue exclusion principle using a membrane for bone healing and bone neogenesis. *J Periodontol* 1993; 64: 1116–1128.
48. Linde A, Thoren C, Dahlin C, and Sandberg E. Creation of new bone by an osteopromotive membrane technique: an experimental study in rats. *J Oral Maxillofac Surg* 1993; 51: 892–897.
49. Becker WB and Becker BE. Guided tissue regeneration for implants placed into extraction sockets and for implant dehiscences: surgical techniques and case reports. *Int J Oral Maxillofac Implants* 1990; 10: 377–391.
50. Becker W, Becker BE, Handlesman M, Celletti R, Ochsenbein C, Hardwick R, and Langer B. Bone formation at dehisced dental implant sites treated with implant augmentation material: a pilot study in dogs. *Int J Periodont Rest Dent* 1990; 10: 93–101.
51. Dahlin C, Sennerby L, Lekholm U, Linde A, and Nyman S. Generation of new bone around titanium implants using a membrane technique: an experimental study in rabbits. *Int J Oral Maxillofac Implants* 1989; 4: 19–26.

52. Gunay H, Skuballa C, and Neukamm FW. Experimentelle Untersuchung zur Behandlung von peri-implantaren Knochendefekten. *Z Zahnarztl Implantol* 1991; 7: 16–24.
53. Hurzeler MB and Quinones CR. Installation of endosseous oral implants with guided tissue regeneration. *Pract Periodont Aesthetic Dent* 1991; 3: 21–29.
54. Lazzara RJ. Immediate implant placement into extraction sites: surgical and restorative advantages. *Int J Periodont Rest Dent* 1989; 9: 333–343.
55. Nyman S, Lang NP, Buser D, and Bragger U. Bone regeneration adjacent to titanium dental implants using guided tissue regeneration: a report of two cases. *Int J Oral Maxillofac Implants* 1990; 5: 9–14.
56. Nevins M and Mellonig JT. Enhancement of the damaged edentulous ridge to receive dental implants: a combination of allograft and the Gore-Tex membrane. *Int J Periodont Rest Dent* 1992; 12: 97–111.
57. Siebert J and Nyman S. Localized ridge augmentation in dogs: a pilot study using membranes and hydroxyapatite. *J Periodontol* 1990; 61: 157–165.
58. Grunder U, Hurzeler MB, Schupback P, and Strub JR. Treatment of ligature-induced periimplantitis using guided tissue regeneration. A clinical and histological study in the beagle dog. *Int J Oral Maxillofac Implants* 1993; 8: 282–293.
59. Hurzeler MB, Quinones CR, Schupback P, Morrison EC, and Caffesse RG. Treatment of peri-implantitis using guided bone regeneration and bone grafts, alone or in combination, in beagle dogs. Part 2: Histologic findings. *Int J Oral Maxillofac Implants* 1997; 12: 168–175.
60. Jovanovic SA, Kenney EB, Carranza FA Jr, and Donath K. Regenerative potential of plaque-induced peri-implant bone defects treated by a submerged membrane technique: an experimental study. *Int J Oral Maxillofac Implants* 1993; 8: 13–18.
61. Dahlin C, Lekholm U, and Linde A. Membrane induced bone augmentation at titanium implants. A report on ten fixtures followed from 1 to 3 years after loading. *Int J Periodont Rest Dent* 1991; 11: 273–281.
62. Zablotsky M. Surgical management of osseous defects associated with endosteal hydroxyapatite-coated and titanium dental implants. *Dent Clin North Am* 1992; 36: 117–149.
63. Garrett S. Specific issues in clinical trials on the use of barrier membranes in periodontal regeneration. *Ann Periodontol* 1997; 2: 240–258.
64. Minabe M. Critical review of the biologic rationale for guided tissue regeneration. *J Periodontol* 1991; 62: 171–179.
65. Lundgren D, Mathisen T, and Gottlow J. Development of a bioresorbable barrier for guided tissue regeneration. *J S.D.A.* 1994; 86: 741–756.
66. Simion M, Baldoni J, Rossi P, and Zaffe D. Comparative study of the effectiveness of e-PTFE membranes with and without early exposures during the healing period. *Int J Periodont Rest Dent* 1994; 14: 166–180.
67. Bartee BK. Use of high-density polytetrafluoroethylene membrane to treat osseous defects: clinical reports. *Implant Dent* 1995; 4: 21–26.
68. Bartee BK and Carr JA. Evaluation of a high-density polytetrafluoroethylene (n-PTFE) membrane as a barrier material to facilitate guided bone regeneration in the rat mandible. *J Oral Implant* 1995; 21: 88–95.
69. Crump TB, Rivera-Hidalgo F, Harrison JW, Williams FE, and Guo IY. Influence of three membrane types on healing of bone defects. *Oral Surg Oral Med Oral Pathol Oral Radiol Endod* 1996; 82: 365–374.
70. Hutmacher D, Hurzeler MB, and Schliephake H. Review of material properties of biodegradable and bioresorbable polymers and devices for GTR and GBR applications. *Int J Oral Maxillofac Implants* 1996; 11: 667–678.
71. Fugazzotto PA. Use of demineralized laminar bone sheets in guided bone regeneration procedures: report of three cases. *Int J Oral Maxillofac Implants* 1995; 11: 239–244.
72. Chen CC, Wang HL, Smith F, Glickman GN, Shyr Y, and O'Neal RB. Evaluation of a collagen membrane with and without bone grafts in treating periodontal infrabony defects. *J Periodontol* 1995; 66: 838–47.
73. Mundell RD, Mooney MP, Siegel MI, and Losken A. Osseous guided tissue regeneration using a collagen barrier membrane. *J Oral Maxillofac Surg* 1993; 51: 1004–1012.
74. Sevor JJ, Meffert RM, and Cassingham RJ. Regeneration of dehisced alveolar bone adjacent to endosseous dental implants utilizing a resorbable collagen membrane: clinical and histologic results. *Int J Periodont Restorative Dent* 1993; 13: 71–83.
75. Pitaru S, Tal H, Soldinger M, and Noff M. Collagen membranes prevent apical migration of epithelium and support new connective tissue attachment during periodontal wound healing in dogs. *J Periodont Res* 1989; 24: 247–253.
76. Schlegel AK, Mohler H, Busch F, and Mehl A. Preclinical and clinical studies of a collagen mem-

brane (Bio-Gide). *Biomaterials* 1997; 18: 535–538.
77 Salthouse TM. Cellular enzyme activity at the polymer-tissue interface: a review. *J Biomed Mater Res* 1986; 10: 197.
78 Zitzmann NU, Naef R, and Scharer P. Resorbable versus nonresorbable membranes in combination with Bio-Oss for guided bone regeneration. *Int J Oral Maxillofac Implants* 1997; 12: 844–852.
79 Aaboe M, Pinholt EM, Hjorting-Hansen E, Solheim E, and Praetorius F. Guided tissue regeneration using degradable and nondegradable membranes in rabbit tibia. *Clin Oral Implants Res* 1993; 4: 172–176.
80 Baek SH, Broome C, Zechner W, et al. Healing of through-and-through osseous defects by membrane barrier technique in ferrets. *J Endod* 1995; 21: 228.
81 Cortellini P, Pini Prato G, and Tonetti M. Periodontal regeneration of human infrabony defects with bioresorbable membranes: a controlled clinical trial. *J Periodontol* 1995; 67: 217–223.
82 McGinnis M, Larsen P, Miloro M, and Beck FM. Comparison of resorbable and nonresorbable guided bone regeneration materials: a preliminary study. *Int J Oral Maxillofac Implants* 1998; 13: 30–35.
83 Sandberg E, Dahlin C, and Linde A. Bone regeneration by the osteopromotion technique using bioabsorbable membranes: an experimental study in rats. *J Oral Maxillofac Surg* 1993; 51: 1106–1114.
84 Simion M, Scarano A, Gionso L, and Piattelli A. Guided bone regeneration using resorbable and nonresorbable membranes: a comparative histologic study in humans. *Int J Oral Maxillofac Implants* 1996; 11: 735–742.
85 Simion M, Misitano U, Gionso L, and Salvato A. Treatment of dehiscences and fenestrations around dental implants using resorbable and nonresorbable membranes associated with bone autografts: a comparative clinical study. *Int J Oral Maxillofac Implants* 1997; 12: 159–167.
86 Stoller NH and Johnson LR. Use of the ATRISORB bioabsorbable barrier during guided tissue regeneration. *Dent Learning Syst Postgrad Dent Series* 1997; 4: 13–22.
87 Urbani G, Granziani A, Lombardo G, and Caton JG. Clinical results with exposed polyglactin 910 resorbable membranes for guided tissue regeneration. *Int J Periodont Rest Dent* 1997; 17: 41–51.
88 Pecora G, Andreana S, Margarone JE III, Covani U, and Sottosanti JS. Bone regeneration with a calcium sulfate barrier. *Oral Surg Oral Med Oral Pathol Oral Radiol Endod* 1997; 84: 424–429.
89 Sottosanti J. Calcium sulfate: a biodegradable and biocompatible barrier for guided tissue regeneration. *Compend Contin Ed Dent* 1992; 13: 226–234.
90 Sottosanti JS. Calcium sulfate-aided bone regeneration: a case report. *Periodont Clin Invest* 1995; 17: 10–15.
91 Dahl GSA. Om Mojlighoten Fur Implantation i de Kaken Av Metallskelett Som Bas Eller Retention for Fastaeller Avtagbara Proteser. *Odontol Tskr* 1943; 51: 440.
92 Berman N. Implant technique for full lower dentures. *Dent Dig* 1951; 57: 438.
93 Lew I. Full upper and lower implant dentures. *Dent Concepts* 1952; 4: 17.
94 Truitt HP, James R, and Boyne P. Non invasive technique for mandibular subperiosteal implant: a preliminary report. *J Prosthet Dent* 1986; 55: 494–497.
95 James RA, Lozada JL, and Truitt HP. Computer tomography (CT) applications in implant dentistry. *J Oral Implantol* 1991; 17: 10–15.
96 Truitt H, James RA, Altman A, and Boyne P. Use of computer tomography in subperiosteal implant therapy. *J Prosthet Dent* 1988; 59: 474–477.
97 James RA. Subperiosteal implant design based on peri-implant design based on peri-implant tissue behavior. *NY J Dent* 1983; 53: 407–414.
98 Cranin NA. Some musings on implants. *Alpha Omegan* 1975; 68: 11–15.
99 Benjamin LS. Long-term retrospective studies on the CT-scan, CAD/CAM, one-stage surgery hydroxyapatite-coated subperiosteal implants, including human functional retrievals. *Dent Clin North Am* 1992; 36: 77–93.
100 Bodine RL and Mohammed L. Macroscopic and microscopic study of a mandible with a 12-year implant in place. *Newslett Am Acad Implant Dent* 1967; 16: 8.
101 Bodine RL. Evaluation of 27 mandibular subperiosteal implant dentures after 15–22 years. *J Prosthet Dent* 1974; 32: 188.
102 Benjamin LS and Block MS. Histologic evaluation of a retrieved human HA-coated subperiosteal implant: report of a case. *Int J Oral Maxillofac Implants* 1989; 4: 63–66.
103 Cranin AN, Rabkin MF, and Garfinkel L. Statistical evaluation of 952 endosteal implants in humans. *J Am Dent Assoc* 1977; 94: 315–320.
104 Lemons JE. Dental implant interfaces as influenced by biomaterial and biomechanical proper-

ties, in *Implant Prosthodontics: Surgical and Prosthetic Techniques for Dental Implants* 1990; (Fagan MJ Jr, ed) Mosby Year Book, St. Louis, pp. 281–292.
105 Brånemark P-I, Hansson B-O, Adell R, Breine U, Lindstrom J, Hallen O, and Ohman A. Osseointegrated implants in the treatment of the edentulous jaw. Experience from a 10-year period. *Scand J Plast Reconstr Surg* 1977; 11 (Suppl 16): 1–132.
106 Masuda T, Yliheikkila PK, Felton DA, and Cooper LF. Generalizations regarding the process and phenomenon of osseointegration. Part I. In vivo studies. *Int J Oral Maxillofac Implants* 1998; 13: 17–29.
107 Brunski JB. Influence of functional use of endosteal dental implants on the tissue-implant interface: clinical aspects. *J Dent Res* 1979; 58: 1970–1980.
108 Adell R, Lekholm U, and Rockler B. 15-year study of osseointegration in the treatment of the edentulous jaw. *J Oral Surg* 1981; 10: 387–416.
109 Albrektsson T, Dahl E, Enbom I, Engevall S, Engquist B, Eriksson RA, et al. Osseointegrated implants: a Swedish multicenter study of 8139 consecutively inserted Nobelpharma implants. *J Periodontol* 1988; 59: 287–296.
110 Jemt T, Lekholm U, and Grondahl K. 3 year followup study of early single implant restorations ad modum Branemark. *Int J Periodont Rest Dent* 1990; 5: 272–281.
111 van Steenberghe D, Lekholm U, Bolender C, and Folmer T. Osseointegrated oral implants in the rehabilitation of partial edentulism: a prospective multicenter study of 558 fixtures. *Int J Oral Maxillofac Implants* 1990; 5: 272–281.
112 Brånemark PI, Breine U, Adell R, Hansson BO, Lindstrom J, and Ohlsson A. Intra-osseous anchorage of dental prostheses. I. Experimental studies. *Scand J Plast Reconstr Surg* 1969; 3: 81.
113 Babbush CA, Kent JN, and Misiek DJ. Titanium plasma-sprayed (TPS) screw implants for the reconstruction of the edentulous mandible. *J Oral Maxillofac Surg* 1986; 44: 274–281.
114 Buser D, Weber HP, and Lang NP. Tissue integration of nonsubmerged implants. 1-year results of a prospective study with 100 ITI hollow-cylinder and hollow-screw implants. *Clin Oral Implant Res* 1990; 1: 33–40.
115 Schroeder A, van der Zypen E, Stich H, and Sutter F. Reaction of bone, connective tissue and epithelium to endosteal implants with sprayed titanium surfaces. *J Maxillofac Surg* 1981; 9: 15–25.
116 Ten Bruggenkate CM, Muller K, and Oostenbeek HS. Clinical evaluation of the ITI (F-Type) hollow cylinder implant. *Oral Surg Oral Med Oral Pathol* 1990; 70: 693–697.
117 Carlsson L, Rostlund T, Albrektsson B, and Albrektsson T. Removal torques for polished and rough titanium implants. *Int J Oral Maxillofac Implants* 1988; 3: 21–24.
118 Thomas KA and Cook SD. Evaluation of variables influencing implant fixation by direct bone apposition. *J Biomed Mater Res* 1985; 19: 875.
119 Wennerberg A, Albrektsson T, and Lausmaa J. Torque and histomorphometric evaluation of c.p. titanium screws blasted with 25- and 75-mm-sized particles of AL O. *J Biomed Mater Res* 1996; 30: 251–260.
120 Deporter DA, Watson PA, Pilliar RM, Pharoah M, Smith DC, Chipman M, Locker D, and Rydall A. Prospective clinical study in humans of an endosseous dental implant partially covered with a powder-sintered porous coating: 3- to 4-year results. *Int J Oral Maxillofac Implants* 1996; 11: 87–95.
121 Kay SA, Wisner-Lynch L, Marxer M, and Lynch SE. Guided bone regeneration: integration of a resorbable membrane and a bone graft material. *Pract Periodont Aesthetic Dent* 1997; 9: 185–194.
122 Block MS, Kent JN, and Kay JF. Evaluation of hydroxyapatite-coated titanium dental implants in dogs. *J Oral Maxillofac Surg* 1987; 45: 601.
123 Cook SD, Baffes GC, and Thomas KA. Comparison of models for evaluating interface characteristics of HA-coated implants. *J Dent Res* 1991; 70: 530.
124 Cook SD, Baffes GC, and Burgess A. In vivo study of the torsional strength of HA-coated and grit-blasted implants. *J Oral Implantol* 1992; 18: 354.
125 Thomas KA, Kay JF, Cook SD, and Jarcho M. Effect of surface macrotexture and hydroxylapatite coating in the mechanical strengths and histologic profiles of titanium implant materials. *J Biomed Mater Res* 1987; 21: 1395.
126 Cook SD, Kay JF, Thomas KA, and Jarcho M. Interface mechanics and histology of titanium and hydroxyapatite-coated titanium for dental implant applications. *Int J Oral Maxillofac Implants* 1987; 2: 15–22.
127 Ogiso M, Tabata T, Ichijo T, and Borgese D. Bone calcification on the hydroxyapatite dental implant and the bone-hydroxyapatite interface. *J Long Term Effect Med Implants* 1992; 2: 137–148.
128 Linder L, Obrant K, and Boivin G. Osseointegration of metallic implants II. Transmission electron

microscopy in the rabbit. *Acta Orthop Scand* 1989; 60: 135–139.

129 Carlsson L, Regner L, Johansson C, Gottlander M, and Herberts P. Bone response to hydroxyapatite-coated and commercially pure titanium implants in the human arthritic knee. *J Orthop Res* 1994; 12: 274–285.

130 Gross KA, Berndt CC, Goldschlag DD, and Iacono VJ. In vitro changes of hydroxyapatite coatings. *Int J Oral Maxillofac Implants* 1997; 12: 589–597.

131 Wheeler SL. Eight-year clinical retrospective study of titanium plasma-sprayed and hydroxyapatite-coated cylinder implants. *Int J Oral Maxillofac Implants* 1996; 11: 340–350.

132 Yukna CN, Yukna RA. Multi-center evaluation of bioresorbable collagen membrane for guided tissue regeneration in human class II furcations. *J Periodontol* 1996; 67: 650–657.

2

Polymers in the Oral Environments

Novel Elastomers as Soft Liners

Kalachandra Sid and Tetsuya Takamata

1. Introduction

Glassy polymers are used as dental materials because their rigidity enables them to support loads and to resist forces imposed in service in the oral cavity. Glassy polymers are generally regarded as amorphous and brittle. However, classification of these materials is very much a time-dependent concept, in which a brief experimental time interval generates brittleness, but an extended time-scale can result in viscous flow. This time-dependent behavior of polymers is exemplified in the material known as "bouncing putty," which flows like a viscous fluid when left under its own weight for extended periods, but shatters like a glass when hit with a hammer. Temperature is another factor that determines whether a polymer is a glassy solid, an elastic rubber, or a viscous liquid.

2. Glass–Rubber Transition Behavior

When cyclic or repetitive motions of stress and strain are involved, it is more convenient to talk about dynamic mechanical moduli. The complex Young's modulus has the formal definition, $E^* = E' + iE''$. Where E' is the storage modulus and E'' is the loss modulus. The quantity i represents the square root of -1. The storage modulus is a measure of energy stored elastically during deformation, and the loss modulus is a measure of the energy converted to heat.

3. Distinct Regions of Viscoelastic Behavior

The states of matter of low-mol-wt compounds are well known: crystalline, liquid, and gaseous. The first-order transitions that separate these states are equally well known: melting and boiling. Another well-known first-order transition is the crystalline–crystalline transition, in which a compound changes from one crystalline form to another.

By contrast, no polymer with high molecular weight vaporizes to gaseous state: All decompose before the boiling point. In addition, no high-molecular-weight polymer attains a totally crystalline structure, except in the single-crystal form.

In fact, many important polymers do not crystallize at all, but form glasses at low temperatures. At higher temperatures, they form viscous liquids. The transition that separates the glassy state from the viscous state is known as the glass–rubber transition, which exhibits the properties of a second-order transition at very slow rates of heating or heating.

In order to provide a broader picture of the

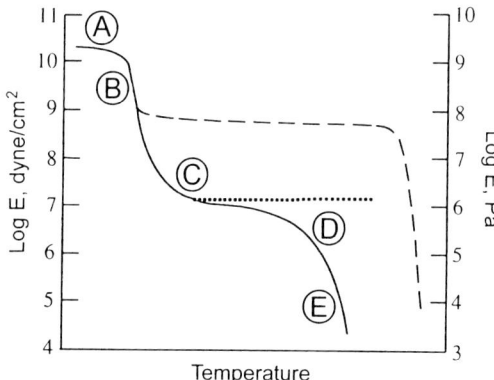

Fig. 1. Five regions of viscoelastic behavior for a linear, amorphous polymer. Also illustrated are effects of crystallinity (dashed line) and crosslinking (dotted line).

temperature dependence of polymer properties, a brief discussion of distinct regions of viscoelastic behavior is presented in the following paragraphs. The five regions of viscoelastic behavior for linear amorphous polymers (1) are shown in Fig. 1.

In region A, the polymer is glassy and frequently brittle. Typical examples at room temperature include polystyrene cups and polymethylmethacrylate (PMMA) (Plexiglas sheets). Young's modulus for glassy polymers has the value of approx 3×10^{10} dyn/cm^2 (3×10^9 Pa). In the glassy state, molecular motions are largely restricted to vibrations and short-range rotational motions.

The value of the bulk modulus was calculated in terms of the cohesive energy density (CED), which represents the energy theoretically required to move a detached segment into the vapor phase. This, in turn, is related to the square root of the solubility parameter (1). It should be noted that many hydrocarbon and not-too-polar polymers have CED values within a factor of 2 of the values for polystyrene. Region B is the glass transition region. Typically, the modulus drops a factor of approx 1000 in a 20–30°C range. The behavior of polymers in this region is best described as leathery, although a few degrees of temperature change will obviously affect the stiffness of the leather. For quasistatic measurements, the glass transition temperature, T_g, is often taken at the maximum rate of turndown of the modulus at the elbow, or d^2E/dT^2 is at a maximum. Qualitatively, the glass transition region can be interpreted as the onset of the long-range, coordinated molecular motion. In other words, at low temperatures, polymers become hard and glass-like, because the motion of the polymer chains in relation to each other is slow. The T_g itself varies widely with structure and other parameters.

Region C is the rubbery plateau region. After the sharp drop that the modulus takes in the glass transition region, it becomes almost constant again in the rubbery plateau, with typical values of 2×10^7/dyn/cm^2 (2×10^6 Pa). In the rubbery plateau region, polymers exhibit long-range rubber elasticity, which means that the elastomer can be stretched, perhaps several hundred percent, and snap back to substantially its original length, on being released.

In this region, two cases need to be discussed. First, if the polymer is linear, the modulus will drop off slowly. The width of the plateau is governed primarily by the mol wt of the polymer: the higher the mol wt, the longer the plateau. Second, if the polymer is crosslinked, the dotted line is followed and improved rubber elasticity is observed, with the creep portion suppressed. An example of a crosslinked polymer above its T_g obeying the equation, $E = 3n\mathrm{RT}$ (where n, the number of active chain segments in the network and the term RT represents the gas constant and absolute temperature). An example of a crosslinked polymer above its T_g, which obeys this relationship, is the ordinary rubber band.

The rapid, coordinated molecular motion in this region is governed by the principles of repetition and diffusion. Thus, when the elastomer is stretched, the chains deform with a series of rapid motions of the deGennes type. For crosslinked systems, the motion is thought to become a more complex affair involving the several chain segments that are bound together.

3.1. Region D: The Rubbery Flow Region

As the temperature is raised past the rubbery plateau region for linear amorphous polymers, the rubbery flow region is reached. In this region, the polymer is marked by both rubber elasticity and flow properties, depending on the time-scale of the experiment. For short time-scale experiments, the physical entanglements are not able to relax, and the material still behaves rubbery. For longer times, the increased molecular motion imparted by the increased temperature permits assemblies of chains to move in a coordinated manner (depending on the molecular weight), and hence to flow.

Region D does not occur for crosslinked polymers. That being the case, region C remains in effect up to the decomposition temperature of the polymer.

3.2. Region E: The Liquid Flow Region

At still higher temperatures, the liquid flow is reached. The polymer flows readily, often behaving like molasses. The increased energy, associated with chains, permits them to reptate out through entanglements rapidly, and to flow as individual molecules.

For semicrystalline polymers, the modulus depends on the degree of crystallinity. The amorphous portions go through the glass transition, but the crystalline portion remains hard. Thus, modulus of a composite is determined. At the melting temperature, which is always above T_g, the modulus drops rapidly to that of the corresponding amorphous material, now in the liquid flow region. Modulus and viscosity are related through the molecular relaxation time.

At a temperature range the phenomenon known as the glass transition (T_g) appears, in which the polymer possesses an intermediate modulus between glassy and rubbery behavior. The resultant viscoelastic response is usually accompanied by the dissipation of energy, which is often expressed as the loss tangent (tan δ) of the material. Loss tangent is defined as the ratio of imaginary to real moduli. At T_g, there are characteristic changes in both E' and tan δ. Below T_g, the polymer is in a glassy (rigid) state; just above T_g, it is leathery; above about T_g + 50°C, it is rubberlike. The value of E' in the rubber-like state can be used to calculate the density of elastically effective crosslinks.

Glass transition behavior is important for dental polymers, because a denture base is required to be rigid in the oral environment at temperatures approaching the boiling point of water, in the case of hot drink consumption. The major unfilled glassy polymer for such usage has, for a considerable time, been PMMA. There is also a need for polymers that exhibit rubber-like characteristics at room temperature through mouth temperature and above, such as methacrylates, into which a plasticizer is incorporated to reduce their T_g to below room temperature. These materials are used as soft liners, which can be attached to the rigid denture base, to form a soft cushion between the soft mucosa and the rigid denture. They are especially applicable to patients suffering effects of trauma or sore mouth conditions. Both the rigid and rubber-like methacrylates are available as heat or use as rigid room-temperature-curing temporary crown and bridge resins and copy dentures. Not only are these monofunctional methacrylate monomers important dental materials, but difunctional methacrylate monomers also form a large and rapidly expanding field as cosmetic composite filling materials. In this situation, the difunctional methacrylate forms the matrix phase of the filled resin. Difunctionally based methacrylate fissure sealants are also available to prevent caries forming in deep occlusal fissures, which are difficult to keep bacteria-free. Oral disease, though not dangerous to human life, affects nearly everybody, certainly in the Western world, where the field of dentistry has been identified as a priority area, in order to overcome oral diseases.

Polymeric materials for denture bases, such as vulcanite (hard rubber), and a form of agar-agar, were used occasionally as soft lining materials and elastic impression material, respectively, before the Second World War. Later, (PMMA) became the chief material of choice for full dentures, albeit with well-known defects.

Fluid room temperature vulcanizing (RTV) rubbers were developed (both silicone and polysulfide types). These were swiftly adapted for dental purposes, changing the dimensional accuracy of impressions; subsequently, other modifications of this principle followed.

4. Soft Lining Materials

There is a great demand for improved elastomeric soft lining materials that will provide longer service life, greater comfort, and improved mechanical properties and dimensional stability in the oral environment. The development of these materials has been difficult and multifactorial, and some of the factors involved in clinical failure are poorly understood. Compositions of these materials are continually being modified by manufacturers, to improve their properties and service life.

A satisfactory soft lining material is expected to have the following characteristics: It must be compatible with oral tissues; it must be compliant and resilient; it must have dimensional stability; it must adhere to PMMA dentures; it must be resistant to rupture; it must be readily wettable by saliva; it should have low and limited water uptake; and it should not support the growth of *Candida albicans (2–6)*.

It is well established that no currently available soft lining material is clinically fully satisfactory *(2,7,8)*. Much of the basic information defining the problems in the design of soft reliners for denture bases has been well documented in the literature *(4,5,9–12)*. Until recently, all soft liners fell into two classes: silicone elastomers and plasticized acrylics. Silicone polymers, in general, suffer from poor tear resistance and poor adhesion to PMMA dentures *(4)*. The earliest silicones offered for dental use suffered from several problems. Usually, these silicones were of the condensation type. Some silicone soft liners took up 60% water. Of all elastomeric polymers, silicones have the highest diffusion coefficient for water, and, since water uptake of elastomers is particularly governed by water-soluble impurities, silicones can be worse than any other polymers. There is evidence *(13,14)* that the presence of organo-tin initiators, used in some condensation silicones, causes degradation in the presence of water. Similarly, the presence of acetate ions, or residual acetic anhydride, promote the growth of *Candida (3,13)*.

So-called "soft acrylics" usually owe their compliance to the presence of a plasticizer, commonly a phthalate, although phosphates have been used. Wright *(4)* has reviewed the composition of a number of such materials. As is well known, loss of plasticizer results in hardening of the liner. At the same time, the presence of a plasticizer increases the tendency of the material to dissolve organic compounds and to discolor. However, the adhesion to PMMA is generally good.

In order to overcome the fundamental problems of hardening, peeling, and discoloration, various alternatives have been developed. Van Handell*(14)* patented a copolymer system based on an α-ω-hydroxyl-terminated silicone polymer with methacryloxypropyl trimethoxysilane as cross-linking agent, and at least one commercial product is based on this chemistry. This is not a condensation-type material, and thus avoids many of the problems associated with condensation byproducts. This material must be heat-cured. However, in the uncured state, this polymer becomes partially insoluble in solvents, with time pointing to the development of a crosslinked state. This is clearly a problem, because old batches of the material become difficult to process. Among the existing proprietary soft lining materials, Molloplast B is based on this chemistry. This is probably the best commercial product currently available, even with this shelf life problem.

Another approach is to try to exploit the good adhesion of soft acrylics, but to prevent plasticizer loss. Litchfield and Wood *(15)* patented a soft acrylic based on poly(ethylmethacrylate) polymer powder, 2-ethoxyethyl methacrylate, and a polymerizable plasticizer, di(2-ethyl hexyl) maleate. Although maleates are not very reactive, sufficient polymerization occurs to suppress leaching. A modified version of this system showed very little leaching after 7 yr *(16,17)*. Parker and Braden also described the use of powdered elastomers, doughed with a higher methacrylate (e.g., tridecyl), to give an elastomeric product with plasticizer, i.e., the problem of plasticizer leaching is largely solved *(18)*.

Gettleman, in a study of polyphosphazene materials, described the use of polyphosphazine polymers, into which methacrylate monomers had been milled to give an elastomer with good bonding, and generally satisfactory results *(19)*. The commercial product based on this approach suffered from excessive water sorption, and is not currently marketed. The use of phosphazine polymers seems very promising, and suggests that other solid industrial polymers should be examined in the same way, i.e., by milling in a suitable monomer, and then curing in the usual way. The choice of a polyphosphazine probably reflects its resistance to aging.

From the clinical point of view, the soft lining materials are shown to be successful *(20)*. Generally between 60 and 100% of patients are satisfied with their soft-lined denture *(8)*. A long-term (9-yr) study shows 12/22 Molloplast B linings still performing adequately *(12)*, the most common reason for failure being soreness (associated with the wetting characteristics of the material), followed by adhesion to the denture base. The wetting behavior of soft lining materials is a major factor in their performance, because a poorly wetted soft lining material will cause frictional damage to the oral mucosa *(8)*. The plasticized acrylic materials suffer from hardening caused by loss of plasticizer, leading to some concern over the toxicity of the phthalate plasticizer *(8)*.

Comparison of mechanical properties of soft lining materials shows wide variation, with the highest tear and tensile strengths being for the plasticized acrylic materials, and the lowest being for the silicone-based materials *(21)*.

The effect of storage in different solutions has been shown to be important in deterioration, with great reductions being observed in saliva *(22)*. Differences in laboratory and clinical results tend to reflect the inconstant nature of the mouth, with personal habits such as smoking and drinking having a profound effect on some properties, such as viscosity *(22)* and color *(12)*. The temperature cycling that the denture would be exposed to (from hot and cold drinks, and so on) has also been shown to be detrimental to the compliance of the soft lining *(23)*. The treatment of the denture during cleaning, and so on, effects the longevity of some materials, with some denture cleaning fluids leading to surface degradation *(24)* or, in the case of bleach, denture discoloration *(20)*. Despite this, the use of in vitro testing allows some degree of certainty about the material's behavior in the mouth to be determined.

The bonding of soft lining materials has recently attracted much attention, with numerous studies being conducted on commercial materials. The major factor in determining the strength of the bond is the soft lining material, rather than the type of denture base *(25)*. It is important to realize that there are three possible mechanisms of failure of material: adhesive (along the interface), cohesive (through the soft lining material), or a combination of the two. There is some concern about the testing methodology being used, with two types of tests predominating: a peel test, in which the soft lining material is peeled back on itself; and a tensile test, in which the material is sandwiched between two blocks of PMMA.

Evaluation of these two test methods has shown that both reproduce the same ordering of commercial materials *(26)*. There is, however, cause for concern about the applicability of the peel test to silicone elastomers because the orientation of the loading means the material fails cohesively, reflecting poor tear resistance *(26)*. Geometry of the tensile test makes the reference of its results to the clinical situation questionable *(8)*.

Generally, the plasticized acrylic-based materials (such as Coe Super-Soft and Vertex Soft) have the highest peel strengths, and typically fail at the adhesive joint *(25–27)*. Molloplast B is the best of the silicone-based elastomers, although it tends to fail cohesively, indicating a problem with its tear resistance *(27)*. The peel strength of Novus is between that obtained for acrylic-based materials and silicone materials, but shows a much greater sensitivity to the test method, with values almost equal to acrylic-based materials in peel, but much lower when tested by tension *(26)*. The influence of water storage has been widely investigated, because this represents the clinical situation more accurately. Here the peel strength seems to be generally high at relatively short time intervals (7 d), and lower after a more prolonged adsorption, 3 or 4 mo *(27,28)*. This is attributed to the building up of stresses at the interface and changes in the viscoelastic properties of the material *(28)*.

The water sorption of soft lining materials may explain many factors about the aging process, the plasticized acrylic-based materials (which tend to harden over time) showing a generally high uptake and high solubility, resulting from the leaching of the plasticizer *(24)*. The more durable silicones have a generally smaller uptake and lower solubility *(29)*. As previously stated, Molloplast B is perhaps the best soft lining material currently available, and this reflects its low water sorption and solubility. Thus, consideration and understanding of water uptake characteristics of these materials is of great importance.

The water sorption of PMMA and other rigid polymers is reasonably straightforward: Depending on the geometry of the specimen, a well-defined equilibrium is ultimately reached (2% for PMMA) *(21)*. The kinetics of uptake obey the laws of diffusion, and the D_{eff} can be determined *(21,30–35)*. Extensive studies have been made by Kalachandra and Turner, and Braden, et al. in predicting the water uptake of polymethacrylate systems *(32–41)*.

With most soft liners, water sorption continues for many years, even for specimens only 1 mm thick, and reaches high levels. In particular, the systems of Parker and Braden *(16,17)*, based on a polymerizable plasticizer, showed continuing uptake after 7 yr, attaining values of >10% water content. It was observed that one silicone elastomer took up more than 50 wt% water *(10)*. These high uptakes cause severe deterioration in mechanical properties. Initially, these results were surprising, because diffusion coefficients of water in elastomers are such that equilibrium should be attained in 1 d. Similar results are also seen with acrylics, even though the soft acrylics based on higher methacrylates should have lower water uptake than PMMA, because they are more hydrophobic.

Muniandy and Thomas *(42)* working on the application of natural rubber vulcanizates in marine applications, observed similar behavior. They were able to show that the high and prolonged uptake was the result of the presence of water-soluble impurities. When the penetrating water reaches an impurity site, the resultant solution droplet grows until osmotic and elastic pressures balance, i.e., the high compliance of elastomers is the essential feature. Parker and Braden *(16,17)* have shown that the same phenomenon occurs in acrylic soft lining materials. The slow continued sorption of water over an extended period is controlled by the rate of creep relaxation of the elastic pressure. Desorption, on the other hand, is diffusion-controlled and the desorption is complete in a day or so.

There are further implications in the case of soft lining materials: They are much weaker than natural rubber, and the osmotic pressures may be sufficient to cause rupture; indeed, mechanical failure was how the Parker–Braden materials failed clinically; The uptake should be less in aqueous solutions than in pure water. This was observed by Ellis *(43)* without realizing the mechanism, and has been demonstrated by Aiken *(44)*. This osmotic process is often transiently obscured by the extraction of plasticizer. In plasticized materials, the loss of plasticizer can give a false equilibrium, which occurs when water uptake is balanced by plasticizer loss.

A number of higher methacrylates have been used in soft lining materials. However, Davy and Braden *(45)* have shown that the choice is crucial. Going from polymers of n-hexyl to tridecyl methacrylate, strength drops dramatically; hence, the pentyl or hexyl ester should be used.

The following paragraphs succinctly present the findings of the authors' recent studies of soft liners (newly developed experimental and commercial) with reference to water sorption, solubility, and mechanical (dynamic mechanical) properties.

5. Study of Water Sorption of Novel Butadiene/Styrene Elastomers

The water uptake of a commercial powdered butadiene–styrene (BS) elastomer, containing a partitioning agent (i.e., antiblocking agent), was measured and compared to its purified elastomer. The water uptake was 8–12% in 6 mo for the former; the latter had only 0.5–2.5% in 6 mo *(43–49)*. The increased water uptake of BS elastomers was explained as follows: The commercial powdered BS elastomer contained a partitioning agent (talc), to prevent agglomeration on storage. The presence of water-soluble partitioning agent in the elastomers results in the formation of solution droplets at the sites of the partitioning agent. The droplets then grow, the driving force being the chemical potential gradient (osmotic pressure) between the droplet and external solution (water). In fact, the BS samples became cloudy and opaque in water, because the internal droplets scattered the light *(45)*. In order to verify that the osmotic process is indeed responsible for the high water uptake in these systems, water uptake measurements were made with n-hexyl methacrylate (HMA) and 2-ethyl hexyl methacrylate (EHMA)-based BS elastomers in saline and glucose solutions at 37°C. Lower water uptake from saline and glucose solutions was observed, compared to pure water, confirming that the process is osmotically driven. A material that has an uptake of ~6% in water, which is still increasing after 4 mo, has an uptake of only ~1% in 0.9 M saline solution at the same times. The water uptake of most of the materials from artificial saliva is less than from pure water. However, the uptake from saliva is higher than from the other solutions (0.1, 0.3, and

1.0 M NaCl and 0.1, 0.3 and 1.0 M glucose). The lowest uptake is from the saline solutions, because saline solutions of the same concentration have higher osmotic pressures than the saliva and the nonionizing glucose solutions (47,51–53).

Analysis of the data, with reference to a recent study of water uptake of soft lining materials from osmotic solutions, revealed that uptake of the two experimental materials based on 70:30 BS block copolymer, with 1 wt% of lucidol (BS1) and 1 wt% of lauryl peroxide (LP) (BS2) and Novus, was reduced in the saline solutions (0.45 and 0.9 M NaCl) relative to that observed in distilled water (53). This could explain the satisfactory clinical performance of Novus, despite its water uptake from pure water. This finding supports the theory that the high uptake of elastomeric solutions is osmotically driven (48).

In order to study the effect of the nature of the initiator on water sorption, benzoyl peroxide (BP) and lauryl peroxide initiators were used (47,51). Decomposition of BP gives benzoic acid, which is water-soluble at 37°C. However, use of LP instead of BP, in these particular formulations, did not produce any noticeable effect on water sorption, with the effect of the partitioning agent overshadowing that of the benzoic acid. A study of the effect of the extent of crosslinking on water uptake was also undertaken. It was observed that increasing the crosslinking agent (0.5 to 1.0% ethylene glycol dimethacrylate [EGDM]) in systems containing BS (47,51) resulted in a decrease in water uptake (5.4 to 5.0%), indicating that increase in crosslinking density will result in decrease in water uptake. The notable finding is that inclusion of EHMA, instead of HMA, reduced water uptake from 7.1 to 5.4%, because of the more hydrophobic character of the former (47,50), which indicates that the use of EHMA is preferred in the design of soft lining material.

Water uptake of materials prepared using an alternative BS elastomer without a partitioning agent also proved high at ~6% in 4 mo. Similarly, styrene–isoprene (SIS) elastomers produced high-water-uptake materials. These two elastomers are produced by a solution polymerization process, which results in the presence of hydroxyl groups that are hydrophilic, thus increasing the water uptake.

During the course of the water uptake investigation, it was found that some of the materials had sudden increases in water uptake after several weeks in water. This has been attributed to oxidation of the -C=C- bonds producing hydroxyl groups, which account for the increase of water uptake. It has to be noted that these materials discolored and became brittle. The rate at which this happened depended on the composition, water uptake, and immersion solution (48). The BS-based materials showed most tendency to oxidize, the SIS the least tendency. This is thought to result from some steric effect of the methyl group shielding the diene bond. Initial studies have shown that water uptake of the SIS-based materials can be reduced by increasing crosslinking, or by reinforcement with silane-treated silica. The tendency to oxidize is also reduced.

In summary, it was observed that water sorption of the samples is controlled by the nature of the samples, crosslinking density, water-soluble or hydrophilic impurities, and the osmotic pressure of the external solution.

Two types of soft lining materials were developed, based on elastomeric silicones and methacrylates.

5.1. Silicone-based Elastomers

The inherent water adsorption of both peroxy-cured and hydrosilylation-cured silicones were very small (0.5%). However, the introduction of a hydrophilic constituent as a filler increased the adsorption of water, which was attributed to the formation of droplet solutions within the material. The water uptake of the silicone materials is dependent on the filler used and its surface treatment, and on the solubility of components and additives. Use of hydrophilic filler in peroxy-cured silicone did not lead to as much increase in water sorption as anticipated, which was attributed to the siloxane in the silicone bonding or adsorbing onto the surface of the silica, and so covering with a hydrophobic siloxane (54). When calcium stearate was used to increase the wettability in these systems, the water uptake drastically increased to ~8%.

A recent study of the influence of additives in water uptake of hydrosilanized silicone rubbers found that the greater the solubility of the additive, the more prolonged the uptake and the greater the deviation from the classic diffusion theory.

**Table 1
Types of Commercial Soft Lining Materials**

Product	Material Type	Source
Molloplast B	Heat-cured silicone	Detax/Karl Huber GmbH, KG, Germany
Novus	Polyp-hosphazine	Hygienic, Akron, OH
Kurepeet	Fluoroe-lastomer	Kureha Chemical, Tokyo, Japan
Supersoft	Plasticized acrylic	Coe Laboratories, Chicago, IL

In order to obtain broadly based information on the characteristics of currently available commercial products, four commercial soft liners were selected, each representing a different type of material. These products are listed in Table 1.

6. Dynamic Mechanical Analysis (DMA)

The dynamic mechanical analyses were performed using a Perkin-Elmer (DMA)-7 Thermal Analysis System. This instrument has several design features that make it particularly useful for testing soft liners and other dental products. It is capable of operating in a compression cycling mode with a wide variety of probe tips, and permits operation with the specimen in air or immersed in water. An attempt was made to adjust the conditions of the test, to approximate, when possible, the normal conditions of use. The specimens were prepared in accordance with the manufacturer's processing instructions, and in the form of a flat sheet, 1.5-mm thick and 15-mm square. They were supported on a rigid plate and loaded with a flat-ended probe 3 mm in diameter. The probe was adjusted to maintain a static stress of 5×10^4 Pa, with a superimposed dynamic stress of 5×10^3 Pa, at a frequency of 1.0 Hz, (see Fig. 2).

Specimens were tested in both wet and dry conditions. The wet specimens had been preconditioned in 37°C water to constant weight, or for a minimum of 100 d for those specimens that failed to equilibrate. Dry specimens were tested in air; wet specimens were tested in distilled water. Each test run consisted of measurements made while heating the specimen from 5 to 95°C at 2.5°C/min. A schematic drawing showing the arrangement of the test apparatus is shown in Fig. 2; the test conditions are summarized in Table 2.

The results are obtained in the form of graphs of storage modulus (E') and tan δ vs temperature for each run. It is possible to superimpose the results from separate runs on the same graph, thus

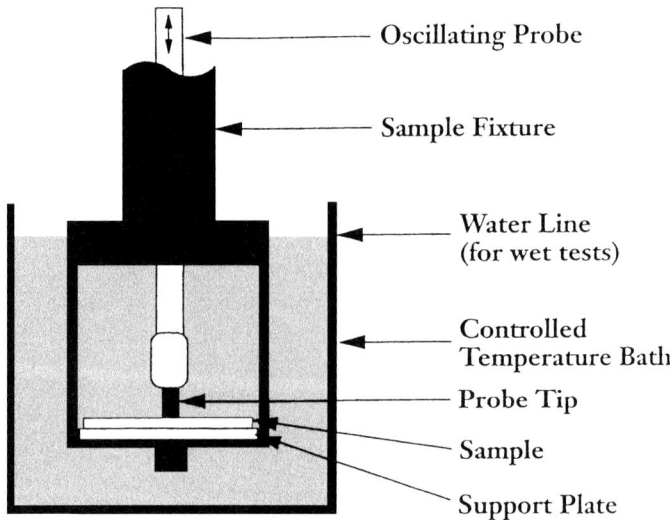

Fig. 2. A specially designed, flat-tip 3-mm diameter probe used in conjunction with Perkin-Elmer DMA-7 System.

Table 2
Dynamic Mechanical Analysis Test Conditions

Equipment	Perkin-Elmer DMA-7 Thermal Analysis System
	Probe-3 mm diameter, flat tip
Specimen	Flat sheet-15 mm/square, 1.5 mm thick
Conditions	Wet and dry
	Temperature range: 5–95°C
	Temperature rate: 2.5°C min
	Static stress: 5×10^4 Pa
	Dynamic stress: 5×10^3 Pa
	Frequency: 1.0 Hz

facilitating direct comparison of different materials or test conditions. An example of such a comparison is shown in Fig. 3, in which the results for wet and dry Supersoft are compared. These results are characteristic of the plasticized acrylic materials. A vertical line has been inserted at 37°C as an aid in evaluating the properties of the material under the condition of use. The corresponding results for Moloplast B are shown in Fig. 4. Such results are characteristic of most silicone-based soft liners.

The differences between these two sets of curves, particularly in their response to changes in temperature, can provide significant information about the structure and likely behavior of the materials. However, when comparisons are to be made among several products, it is often more convenient to tabulate the properties under the expected conditions of use. Table 3 is such a tabulation of the properties of the four materials evaluated in this study at body temperature (37°C).

Figure 5 presents the E' and tan δ measurements from an independent test of an additional dry Supersoft specimen, tested over an extended temperature range from –30°C to 150°C. Such tests can provide supplemental information to distinguish between curve deflection caused by glass transitions and melting.

The water sorption measurements (5) for commercial samples indicated that Mollosil and Evatouch had high % solubility in water (8.7 and 4.56, respectively). Novus was found to exhibit the highest water uptake (34%). The other samples with high water uptake values were Evatouch and Supersoft (6.2 and 7.35%, respectively). Molloplast B had both a low % solubility (0.37) and a low water uptake (0.4%), compared to other samples.

The DMA measurements (54) of the commercial samples indicated that changes in E' between the wet and dry samples of Molloplast B, Kurepeet, and Supersoft were insignificant. The E' of

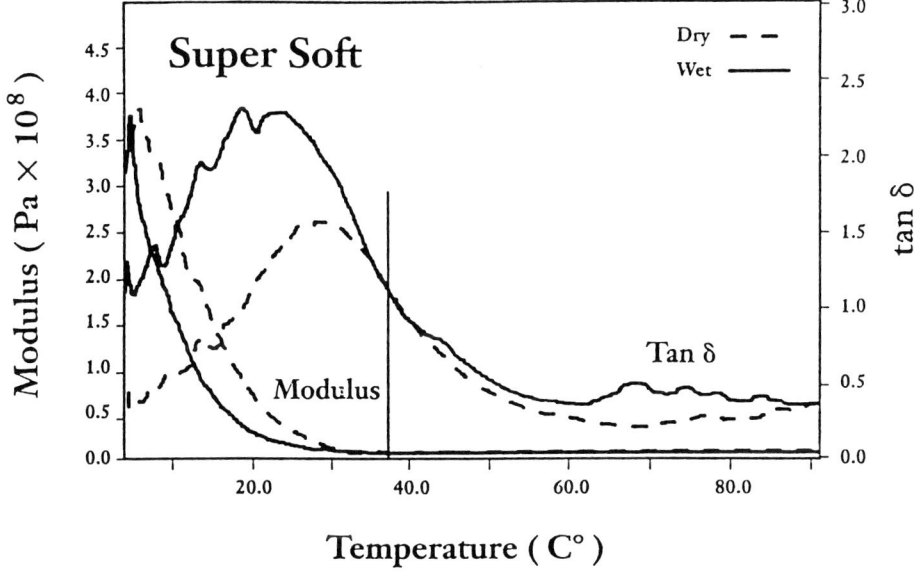

Fig. 3. DMA traces from 0 to 100°C for Supersoft in dry (– – –) and wet (——) conditions.

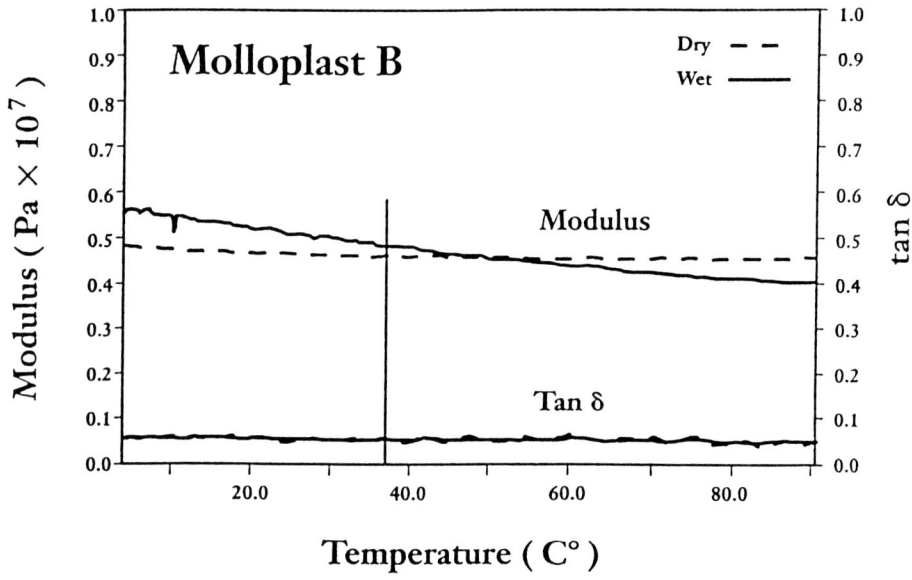

Fig. 4. DMA traces from 0 to 100°C for Molloplast B.

the wet samples of Novus, on the other hand, was about 42% lower than the dry samples, because the sorbed water (~ 34%) presumably acted as a plasticizer in the wet samples. A significant increase in tan δ of the Novus wet sample suggested that the material is capable of dissipating more energy.

No detectable correlation between tensile strengths, elongation, and the Shore durometer hardness could be found for these samples (54). Silicones and fluoroelastomer-based soft liners exhibited low tear strengths. Acrylic- and polyphosphazene-based materials had tear energies 5–10× higher. The wet samples of Molloplast B and Novus did not show any significant difference from dry samples; the acrylic Supersoft doubled in strength in the wet condition, because of stress relaxation by water.

The adhesion of these commercial soft liners were studied by measuring their peel strength (54). Molloplast B and Supersoft failed in cohesive mode; the silicones had little or no bond strength, and failed in adhesion. Novus and Kurepeet showed mixed adhesive/cohesive failure. The peel strength of Novus was found to be the greatest among all materials investigated.

6.1. Novel Silicone Materials

Although it was intended to develop silicone materials to replicate Molloplast B, this could not be achieved because of analysis and identification problems. However, alternative materials were

Table 3
DMA Properties at 37°C

Material	Chemical type	Modulus E' Dry	(Mpa), wet	Damping, dry	Tan δ, wet	Water sorption
Molloplast B	Silicone	4.8	5.1	0.005	0.005	0.5
Novus	Polyphosphazine	6.2	3.5	0.12	0.10	34.0
Kurepeet	Fluoroelastomer	5.0	5.0	0.5	0.75	2.0
Super-Soft	Plasticized acrylic	10.0	8.0	1.25	1.25	5.0

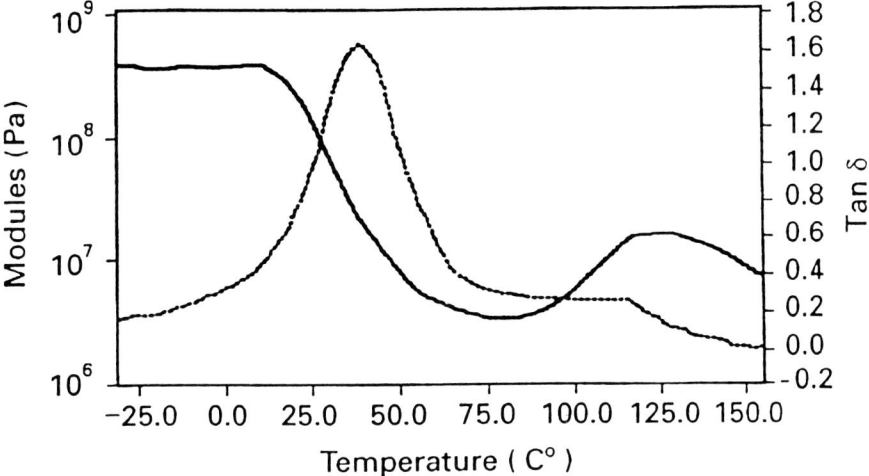

Fig. 5. DMA traces from −25 to 150°C for Supersoft.

developed that exhibited superior properties to Molloplast B. Silicone elastomers can be prepared by three different curing reactions, i.e., acetoxy, condensation, and addition. During curing, the first two processes liberate byproducts, resulting in curing shrinkage, more water sorption, and support of the colonization of the liner by *C. albicans*. Hence, it was decided to follow the addition cure method for the preparation of the silicone materials, in which both peroxy and hydrosilylation polymerization mechanisms were followed *(55)*. The properties of materials produced by both mechanisms were dependent on filler and filler surface treatment *(55)*.

6.2. Novel Elastomeric Methacrylate Systems

Systems based on the elastomers of BS copolymers, polyisoprene, and SIS copolymers have been developed. A higher alkyl methacrylate monomer (HMA or EHMA), a crosslinking agent (EGDM) and an initiator (BP or LP) were gelled with the elastomer. Then the resulting gel was reasonably stable at room temperature, so that it could be molded to the required shape, and polymerized as required. The choice of the monomers was based on their desired mechanical properties. The variations in the monomer, the elastomer:methacrylate monomer ratio, amount of crosslinking agent, and the nature of the initiator, provided adequate information about the effect of these variables on water sorption and mechanical properties *(46–50,53)*.

6.3. Viscoelastic and Mechanical Measurements

DMA measurements were made on five BS methacrylic elastomeric systems, using identical conditions (the same instrument and same technique) used for the analysis of commercial materials, in order to compare the properties *(51,52,54)*.

Increasing the amount of the crosslinking agent (from 0.5 to 1.0% EGDM) resulted in an increase in the modulus (from 15.9 to 20.9 MPa) in systems investigated with BS elastomer, EHMA monomer, and 1% LP initiator. This is apparently the effect of an increase in crosslinking density in the range studied. The incorporation of EHMA, instead of HMA, in BS elastomer-based materials resulted in reduction in dry modulus (from 19.2 to 15.9 Mpa). It also resulted in a reduction in the decrease in the modulus caused by water sorption in wet samples. This is the result of the hydrophobic nature of the EHMA monomer, which reduces the water sorption, as mentioned earlier. The developed soft liners based on BS elastomers with EHMA monomers exhibited large improvements in ultimate tensile strengths, compared to the corresponding HMA monomer systems; both systems had comparable strains *(12)*. Although

Table 4
DMA Properties and Water Sorption for SIS 5+ Experimental Materials

	E′ (MPa)	Tan δ	% water
Dry	7.4	0.39	0
Immersed in water for 4 wk DMA measurements were made	7.1	0.53	1.8

the change of initiator from BP to LP led to no apparent change in water sorption of the BS-based elastomers, a slight increase in modulus was observed with LP-initiated systems, compared to BP-initiated systems (14.0 vs 19.2 for 0.5% and 19.2 vs 20.0 Mpa for 1.0% initiator compositions). This may be attributed to the less-reactive nature of the LP, resulting in increased molecular weights. The tan δ values of these experimental materials lie within the range of accepted commercial materials. The glass transition temperatures of all the materials were observed to be below body temperature.

DMA measurements were performed for both dry and wet samples for the elastomeric materials developed *(51,52)*. Water absorption in the wet samples may act as plasticizers for these samples, reducing the I_g, E′, and compliance of the material. The use of DMA over a wide range of temperatures (0–95°C) provided ideas about the changes in viscoelastic properties of these experimental materials at various intervals of time (by preimmersing the samples from 1 wk to at least 6 mo).

Analysis of the following preliminary data (Table 4), obtained from DMA measurements on the elastomer based on SIS copolymer (SIS 5+), confirmed that the sorbed water (after 4 wk immersion) acted as a plasticizer, reducing E′ and increasing tan δ, which is consistent with expectations *(47,53)*.

Tensile strength of the elastomer-based materials was 12 MPa, with elongation to break of 800% for SIS 5+ and 400% for SBS 5+. Tear strengths were in the range 10–12 kJ/m² for both elastomers. All are well above values obtained for commercial materials *(51)*. Tear energy for peroxide-cured silicone materials were as high as 5.5 kJ/m²; the hydrosililyation-cured silicones had tensile strengths over 7 MPa and elongation to break of 400%.

6.4. Microbiology

A serious clinical concern is the propensity for some soft lining materials to become colonized by growth of indigenous oral *C. albicans* yeasts, causing allergic irritation and inflammation of the palate. In vitro microbiological tests of soft liners were performed to evaluate their interactions with *Candida* yeasts in vitro, using various growth media. When examined by scanning electron microscopy, previous exposure of soft liner materials to *Candida* species in a suitable liquid growth medium suggested that surfaces of at least one polymer were invaded by yeast cells. The following study was undertaken to repeat the tests, using two soft liner materials to explore various parameters of the study for reproducibility. The test yeasts used were American Type Culture Collection (ATCC) strains of *Candida krusei* and *C. albicans*.

A commercial brand of silicone polymer soft liner material, Molloplast B, was chosen as a representative with no acetate content, and appeared not to be attacked by yeasts. Another commercial brand of soft liner, Supersoft, was chosen as a representative of a plasticized acrylic soft liner material of liner that appeared to be attacked by yeasts, with the formation of yeast-shaped holes.

Analysis of the test results revealed the following *(55)*. The silicone polymer soft liner material, Molloplast B, and a plasticized acrylic soft liner material, Supersoft, did not appear to appreciably soften nutrients in order to support growth of the *Candida* species of yeasts; the yeasts had some ability to cling to the liner materials in a rich culture medium, but not to penetrate them; there was no indication that the yeasts could invade or digest either of the liner materials; and there was no indication that the liner materials did or could inhibit growth of the yeasts.

6.5. Relationship Between Soft Lining Materials and Yeasts

Colonization by *C. albicans* or other *Candida* strains results in poor denture hygiene, and may prevent the soft-lined denture from fulfilling the requirement of durability in the oral environment. Consequently, the evaluation of new materials should include appropriate tests of the relationship between lining materials and yeasts. This relationship may include both inhibitory effects or support of the growth of yeasts *(55)*.

This brief report outlines the method and results of the relationship between two commercial (Coe Supersoft, Novus) and three experimental (BS5+, DH5, RTV) soft lining materials and three strains of *Candida* (*C. albicans* [ATCC 24433], *Candida tropicalis* (ATCC 750), and *C. krusei* [ATCC 6258]). Tests of yeast inhibition by soft liners were performed, and the ability of soft liners to imbibe nutrients was studied *(58)*.

6.5.1. Tests of Yeast Inhibition by Soft Lining

At 24 h, inhibition was seen to occur with all *Candida* strains for RTV, and with *C. tropicalis* for BS5+. At 7 d, no further soft lining strips inhibited any *Candida* strains, and examination of the surface of the plates under the strips demonstrated some growth in every case. Even when inhibition was observed, growth of small colonies still persisted within the inhibition zones and underneath the strips. All cultures were pure. The examination of the undersurface of the strips under the dissecting microscope demonstrated heavy contamination of the lining surface via yeasts on RTV and DH5, and sparse contamination on Coe Super-Soft, Novus, and BS5+. The surface of the lining was either smooth (Novus and BS5+), smooth with some wrinkles (Coe Supersoft), smooth with small air bubbles (DH5), or rough with numerous pimples (RTV) *(55)*.

The examination of the undersurface of the strips under the scanning electron microscope is incomplete, but BS5+ with *C. albicans* demonstrated a smooth surface between the pimples and yeast cells only, and DH5 with *C. krusei* demonstrated a rough surface, but no yeast cells.

6.5.2. Ability of Soft Lining to Imbibe Nutrients

As indicated above, the results from the initial protocol showed a consistent and large increases in colony-forming units (CFU)/mL between the initial load of yeasts and the 3-d results, for both the test and control strips. Following the modification of the protocol to include washing of the yeast cells to avoid carryover of nutrient, little or no increase in CFU/mL occurred. In some cases, a reduction was found.

Analysis of the data revealed that the majority of soft lining materials neither inhibit or promote the growth of yeasts, and the materials tested here are no exception. The inhibition of growth of all *Candida* strains tested by RTV is similar to the literature data, since these are all RTV silicone rubber materials, and it is likely that the catalyst is responsible. In this case, the inhibition is not complete, and it has not been established how long this effect will last in the oral environment. No obvious relationship between the surface characteristics of the soft lining material and the contamination by yeasts can be demonstrated by these methods.

Although soft lining materials have a tendency to imbibe water, they do not appear to imbibe sufficient nutrient to encourage the growth of yeasts under the conditions of this experiment. Consequently, if good denture hygiene can be established, there is no reason for increased incidence of yeasts associated with the use of these materials *(55)*.

6.5.3. Investigation of Ability of Solid-state Nuclear Magnetic Resonance to Characterize Dental Polymers

An attempt has been made to evaluate the ability of solid-state nuclear magnetic resonance (NMR) measurements to characterize soft liners, in terms of residual monomer, water content, and the associated molecular motion as functions of chemical structure. A study of the effect of water content on the molecular motion was performed on commercial samples. Because Molloplast B absorbs little water, it was anticipated that it would not exhibit many changes in molecular motions. Hence, the study was limited to two other popular soft liners, namely, Supersoft and Novus.

The cross-polarization/magic-angle-spinning Carbon 13 (^{13}C CP/MAS) spectra did not exhibit any changes associated with water sorption for these samples. The $T_{1\rho}(^1H)$ and $T_{1\rho}(^{13}C)$ measurements also did not give any fruitful results. A limitation of this technique may be that the sample must be spun at more than 3 kHz; this restricted the experiments to be performed for samples with high water uptakes (>10%), because the sorbed water centrifuged out of the systems during the measurements. The fact that no changes were seen in the relaxation spectra is not necessarily a limitation of the technique: It may result from the nature of the systems. There are several plausible reasons why no changes were seen in relaxation times: The water did not affect the molecular motion at these water uptakes; the water affected the motion of the molecules, but it was at a frequency that does not affect the rotating frame relaxation rate, $T_{1\rho}$ (this is typically in the tens of kHz); and the water formed pools, so that it did not affect the bulk motion, but only a very small percentage of the molecules. The Novus samples are probably particularly prone to this phenomenon, because they have a highly hydrophobic portion, the polyphosphazene and more hydrophilic regions, such as the barium sulfate.

In order to detect low levels of residual monomer in a commonly used PMMA dental polymer, use of ^{13}C CP/MAS NMR technique has been made. In radiation-polymerized PMMA, amounts of methyl methacrylate (MMA) as low as 0.05%, were detected using this technique *(56,57)*.

PMMA is an extensively studied linear polymer in dental materials, particularly with reference to networks with increasing amounts of crosslinking, e.g., made by copolymerization of ethylene glycol dimethacrylate with PMMA and softliners, in which plasticized PMMA is used in order to soften the material, i.e., lower the T_g.

The following paragraphs deal with influence of mol wt and plasticizers on the sorption of water by glassy PMMA *(58–70)*.

6.6. Effect of Mol Wt on Water Sorption by PMMA

Relatively little work has been done on the influence of mol wt on the water sorption of polymers *(58–61)*. Sheppard and Newsome noted that "there is some evidence ... that the moisture regain, or water absorption, of cellulose is progressively lowered by treatments which degrade the cellulose." Degradation was monitored by measurements of solution viscosity *(65,66)*. Independently, Kargin pointed out that a decrease in mol wt may result in closer molecular packing in the glassy state, and hence in a lower sorptive capacity *(67)*. As an extreme case, he contrasted the sorption of water vapor by glasses of cellulose and by crystalline glucose. At low vapor pressures, the polysaccharide takes up water into pores, but the close-packed monosaccharide does not. Such a difference in sorptive capacity is not limited to water as penetrant, and a similar contrast was demonstrated on contacting ethyl benzene vapor with high polymers and with oligomers of styrene.

With respect to the kinetics of sorption, Rogers cited data showing that, generally, "the molecular weight of a polymer has been found to have little effect on the rates of diffusional permeation *(71–73)*.

The following paragraphs briefly describe the study of the influence of molecular weight on the sorption of water by glassy PMMA. Previously, Brauer and Sweeney *(30)* found water sorption to be little influenced by molecular weight in the range of $0.18–1.56 \times 10^6$ Daltons, at temperatures from 4 to 60°C. Bueche *(71)* found water diffusion to be independent of molecular weight in the range investigated, from $0.2–1.0 \times 10^6$ Daltons. In order to extend this work to much lower molecular weights, samples of high-molecular weight PMMA were exposed to γ-rays, which results in random fracture of the macromolecular backbone, yet with negligible concurrent crosslinking *(64)*. Previously, this technique had been used in studies of the influence of molecular weight of PMMA on fracture surface energy *(58)*, fracture morphology *(58)*, T_g, *(59)*, and tensile strength *(60)*.

A PMMA powder, described as of average mol wt 12,000 (Aldrich, Milwaukee, WI), was heated at 65°C for several weeks, in vacuum. After this treatment, the powder no longer smelled of residual monomer or transfer agent. T_gs were determined by differential scanning calorimetry (DSC), at 20°C/min, using a DuPont 990 Thermal Analyzer: before heating, $T_g = 80$°C; after heating, $T_g = 82$°C.

Another PMMA powder from Aldrich, provided as a secondary mol wt standard of M_w (weight average molecular weight) – 60,600 and M_n (number average molecular weight) = 33,200, was heated at 75°C for 6 h in vacuum.

The thinnest available sheets of PMMA were used, in order to reduce the time to water saturation to a few weeks (one-thirty-second in. Plexiglas, Rohm and Haas, Philadelphia, PA). Subsequently, this material was withdrawn from the market, and further experiments had to be curtailed. An approximate value of $M_n = 6 \times 10^5$ was calculated from solution viscosity data, assuming

Table 5
Approximate Values of M_n and T_g for Irradiated Samples of PMMA

Dose (Mrad)	0	5.7	17.7	36.6	55.5	74.7	93.9
M_n(D)	6×10^5	8.4×10^4	3.0×10^4	1.5×10^4	9.8×10^3	7.3×10^3	5.9×10^3
T_g (C)	103	–	94	87	81	75	70

a random molecular weight distribution: T_g = 103°C. Sample dimensions 7.5 × 2.5 × 0.07 cm were machined and exposed in air to γ-rays from a cesium 137 (^{137}Cs) source: The dose rate was 0.8 Mrad/h; ambient temperature = 35°C. After irradiation, samples were degassed at room temperature, in vacuum, for 1 wk. Approximate values of M_n were calculated assuming 1.7 random main-chain fractures/100 eV energy deposition (1 Mrad = 6×10^{19} eV/g) *(11)*. Approximate values of T_g were estimated from a pertinent experimental relationship between T_g and radiation dose, in the range that allows interpolation (Table 5).

6.7. Water Sorption Measurements

All samples were dried to constant weight (W_0) over anhydrous calcium sulphate (Drierite, W. R. Hammond) in air. The thickness was taken as the mean of 8-μm readings. Dried samples were immersed in distilled water at 24.2 ± 0.7°C. They were periodically removed, mopped dry, and weighed (W_t), using a Mettler Digital Balance of precision ±0.05 mg, up to a limiting value (W_∞). A few samples were studied further in a desorption cycle over the same desiccant.

A diffusion coefficient (D) was obtained by reference to Stefan's approximation of the appropriate solution of Ficks' law *(71–76)* for plane sheet geometry (Eq. 1):

$$M_t = W_t - W_0; \quad M_\infty = W_\infty - W_0,$$

$$M_t/M_\infty = -8/\pi^2 \sum_{n=0}^{n=\infty} 1/(2n+1)^2 \exp[-(2n+1)^2 \pi^2 Dt/\pi l^2] \quad (1)$$

$$M_t/M_\infty = 2(Dt/\pi l^2)^{1/2} \quad (2)$$

where M_t and M_∞ are the masses of water sorbed, or desorbed, at times t and ∞, respectively; and $2l$ is the thickness of the specimen.

Density measurements were made by Archimedes' method. Sorption data for molded samples of low molecular weight (12,000 Daltons) conform approximately to eq. 1. One sample, designated by the open circles, departed from the expected linearity of Stefan's approximation, which holds up to values of M_t/M_∞ of about 0.5. It is believed that this was caused by initiation and growth of a crack, which eventually caused separation of the sample into two fragments. The initial slope selected to represent both sets of data, is shown by the full line, and corresponds to a value of $D = 0.82 \times 10^{-8}$ cm^2/s. Values obtained for water uptake, referred to initial dry wt, of the two samples were 1.88 and 1.83 wt%. The density of the wet sample (1.1852 g/cm^3) was only slightly greater than that of the dry sample (1.1803 g/cm^{-3}). It is difficult to interpret the water sorption of samples of PMMA of low molecular weight, because volumetric changes, though small, can cause microcracking or void formation. Such changes might increase both diffusion and uptake of water. Nevertheless, there are observations from uptake data that are consistent with the occurrence of closer molecular packing. First, samples of low molecular weight (M_w = 60,600, M_n = 33,200) take up only 1.2% water, compared with samples of high molecular weight ($M_w > 10^6$) which take up to 2.0% *(61)*.

Second, although the other sample of low-molecular-weight (12,000) took up as much as 1.8–1.9% water, yet it differs from high-molecular-weight PMMA in increasing only slightly in density on saturation. In the case of high-molecular-weight PMMA, it was calculated, from changes in density, that the increase in volume accounted for only about one-half the uptake of water. The discrepancy was attributed to accommodation of about 50% of the water uptake in microvoids *(58)*. The same line of reasoning suggests that only 15% water is accommodated in microvoids in the low-molecular-weight sample. A decreased microvoid volume would be consistent with lower molecular packing. For an explicit example of the way in which a penetrant molecule might be accommodated in a microboid, the reader is referred to the work of Barrier et al. on gas sorption by glassy ethyl cellulose, which, like PMMA, has stiff and bulky macromolecules *(73)*. Their depiction of a penetrant accommodation site *(73)* can be regarded as one example of an entanglement site, mentioned in subheading 5.1. It has been concluded from the foregoing discussions that samples of PMMA of low molecular weight (110^4 Daltons) may take up less water (1.2%) than samples of normally high molecular weight (10^6 Daltons: 2.0 wt%); from density changes accompanying water sorption, it is estimated that a low-molecular-weight sample accommodated only 15% water in microvoids, compared with 50% for samples of high mol wt: Those first two conclusions are consistent with the hypothesis that, in glassy polymers, closer molecular packing may be effected in samples of low mol wt.

6.8. Effects of Plasticizers on Water Sorption of PMMA

In this subheading, some important findings made with reference to the influence of plasticizers on the water sorption of PMMA are presented. Relatively little work has been done on the influence of plasticizers on the water sorption of glassy polymers, and such work has been concentrated mostly on copolymers of vinyl chloride. Doty studied the permeation of water vapor through a copolymer of vinyl chloride and vinyl acetate containing 25% plasticizer. He was able to draw interesting conclusions from conventional analyses of temperature dependence *(75)*. This approach, at a single plasticizer content, was pursued by Kumins et al. *(76)*, who expected that placticizer would cause a physical loosening of bonds and thereby result in a decrease in activation energy, followed by a rapid increase in diffusion above T_g. A decrease in activation energy was observed, but a rapid increase in diffusion was obtained at a much higher temperature than expected. It was suggested that the copolymer had a second higher value of T_g at which the change occurred, but, in retrospect, this suggestions seems unlikely.

No systematic studies have been reported of the influence of variations in plasticizer content on the water sorption of a glass polymer. However, such studies have been reported regarding the permeability of poly(vinyl chloride) (PVC) to gases. It has been reported that plasticization of PVC results in an increase in permeability; antiplasticization results in a decrease *(63,75,77)*. In an extension of this work, Raucher and Sefcik *(78)* reported that the apparent diffusion coefficient for CO in plasticized PVC reached a minimum value, with about 10% tricresyl phosphate. The main-chain relaxation rate, determined from ^{13}C NMR spectra, reached a minimum value, with about 15% tricresyl phosphate. This correlation was interpreted as evidence for a rate-determining step, in which the jumping of CO molecules is determined by cooperative motions of the polymer main chains *(78)*, as had been described in detail by Pace and Datyner *(79)*.

Use was made of a technique in which specimens were made by high-energy irradiation of mixtures of MMA and plasticizer. Previously, this technique was found to give specimens with values of T_g that conformed to theoretical predictions of the Kelley–Bueche free-volume theory *(80)*. Also, it has been reported that inclusion of up to approx 10% dioctyl phthalate (DOP) resulted in a pronounced decrease in water uptake, which was attributed to the filling of microvoids, which, otherwise, in the absence of the plasticizer, would be available to water *(62–64)*. The chief objective of this study is to investigate whether, consistent with a physical loosening of bonds, there would be simple increases in the rate of water diffusion in the glassy state, i.e., up to T_g. An alternative possibility is that more complex behavior might be observed that would parallel antiplasticization effects, as inferred from measurements of tensile properties of PMMA plasticized with phthalates *(62,77)*.

In studies of proprietary plasticized acrylic polymers, estimation of values of diffusion coefficients was complicated by leaching out of plasticizer *(63,74)*. Plasticized PMMA was made by γ-irradiation of mixtures of monomer and various phthalates. Samples were immersed in water and uptake, and diffusion coefficients determined. More reliance was placed on determinations made in desorption, because these did not involve complications caused by loss of components of dissolution, i.e., mixtures were made of MMA (Aldrich) with both diethyl phthalate (DEP) (Aldrich) and DOP, i.e., di(2-ethylhexyl) phthalate. Mixtures of MMA and plasticizer in various proportions were polymerized by 6-h exposure to a ^{137}Cs γ-ray source (dose rate = 0.8 Mrad/h; ambient temperature = 35°C) in a nitrogen atmosphere. The plasticizer content was calculated as a volume percent, as described in previous work (62). The polymerized products, cylindrical in shape, were cut under a stream of water with a high-speed diamond band saw, to provide samples with a diameter of 1.4 cm and thickness of 0.1 cm. With up to 25% plasticizer, the products that generally were transparent appeared to be homogeneous. However, with 30% or more of DOP, products were slightly turbid. Samples were immersed in distilled water, usually at 50°C, until equilibrated with water: They were dried at room temperature over anhydrous calcium chloride, and weighed periodically. The water uptake was determined relative to the dry wt of the sample (64).

Values of T_g were estimated by DSC, as described in subheading 6.7.

The rates of desorption and sorption was analyzed by reference to conventional solutions by Fick's laws of diffusion for plane sheet geometry (Eq. 1) (68,71).

Data both in sorption and desorption conformed experimentally to Eq. 2 (Figs. 3–5). A higher rate of desorption is similar to that reported previously in studies of PMMA alone, at room temperature, and interpreted as the result of a dependence of the diffusion coefficient on water content (62,71,76). This same complexity is recognized for values of Deff obtained in the present work.

Furthermore, there is a tendency for plots to remain linear beyond the validity of the approximation in Eq. 2, i.e., at $M_t/M_\infty > 0.5$, which may indicate a time dependence of swelling on uptake of water (62). In view of these departures from ideal behavior, use of Eq. 2 provides apparent values of the diffusion coefficient, but these suffice to give a preliminary overview of trends. More reliance is placed on values of Deff calculated from desorption data up to 37°C, for which duplicate runs agreed within a few percent, but, at higher temperature, results were less reproducible (Table 6). Nevertheless, most measurements were made at 50°C, to reduce testing time.

Table 6 summarizes the data, with reference to the effect of temperature on the uptake of water and diffusion coefficient of PMMA specimens with 20% DOP.

Samples immersed in water increased in weight and reached values that are stationary, in the sense that apparently constant values were attained over a period of several days. Such stationary values are used in the present work, but it should be noted that, on prolonged immersion, a slow decrement in weight was detected, presumably caused by leaching out of plasticizer. This effect may also be a factor in accounting for the observation that estimates of water uptake by desorption are generally greater than values estimated by sorption. In the present work, uptake of water is estimated, more reliably, from desorption data.

The water uptake decreased markedly with increasing plasticizer content, up to about 10% (Fig. 6). At higher plasticizer contents, decreases were less marked, presumably because of replacement of PMMA by the more hydrophobic plasticizer. Decreases were greater for DOP than for DEP, which is consistent with a difference in water uptake: DOP, 0.18 wt%; DEP, 0.92 wt%. Water uptake increases with temperature, up to about 50°C (Fig. 6).

The influence of plasticizer on the uptake of water may be analyzed with respect to two regions, i.e., one below 10 vol% and the other above 10 vol% of the plasticizer content (Fig. 6). Above approx 10%, the influence is small and consistent with the replacement of polymer by the more hydrophobic plasticizer. Previously, the unexpected efficacy of smaller proportions of DOP was attributed to microvoid filling. This interpretation was based on evidence that PMMA, without plasticizer, takes up about 2 wt% water, but swells by only 1%. It was suggested that about one-half of the water is accommodated in microvoids. It was further suggested that DOP could also fill microvoids, and thereby exclude uptake of water. This explanation is now extended to include DEP, which is judged to be less effective as a microvoid filler. Perhaps DEP is more soluble in PMMA, and its partition into microvoids less favored. In broader perspective, similar ideas about the influence of liquid in reducing water sorption by rigid polymers can be traced back to

Table 6
Influence of Temperature on Uptake of Water and Deff of PMMA Specimens with 20% DOP

	Temperature (°C)			
	26	37	50	60
Uptake by desorption (%)	0.71	0.83	1.05	1.04
	0.60	0.84	1.08	1.07
Uptake by sorption (%)	0.71	0.53	0.91	1.04
	0.61	0.63	0.87	1.00
Diffusion coefficient, by desorption, Deff_d, (cm^2/s × 10^8)	4.90	6.5	11.1	23.8
	5.1	6.5	9.0	19.7
Diffusion coefficient, by sorption, Deff_s, (cm^2/s × 10^8)	5.6	7.7	9.6	20.6
	4.5	5.9	9.4	26.0

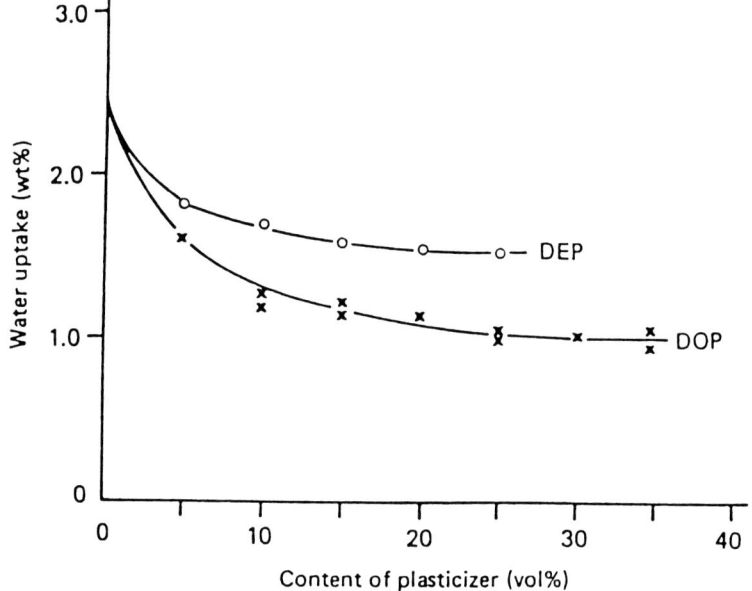

Fig. 6. Effect of plasticizers, DEP and DOP on the uptake of water by PMMA at 50°C.

Sheppard's work on cellulose and its derivatives (62,65,66).

The uptake of water in one plasticized composition (20% DOP) was found to increase with temperature (Fig. 6). It has been reported that water uptake by unplasticized PMMA (T_g = 100°C) increases above 70°C, but quantitative data are not available for comparison. In the present work, the water uptake appears to level off in the temperature range of 50–60°C (Fig. 7). For the binary composition under consideration, T_g = 66°C (Fig. 8), but this would be depressed by 1% water (T_g = −140°C) to T_g = 61°C, according to the Fox equation (65). Thus, it appears that the leveling off occurs near the T_g.

A number of factors might be expected to complicate the influence of plasticizer content on the diffusion of water through PMMA. First, differences in microvoid filling might affect results up to approx 10%. Second, antiplasticization might affect results at higher contents. In this latter respect, it has been reported that the tensile strength of PMMA at 26°C exhibits minimum and maximum values with 7 and 26% dibutyl phthalate, respectively. Notwithstanding such potential complexities, there is a relatively simple

Polymers in the Oral Environments

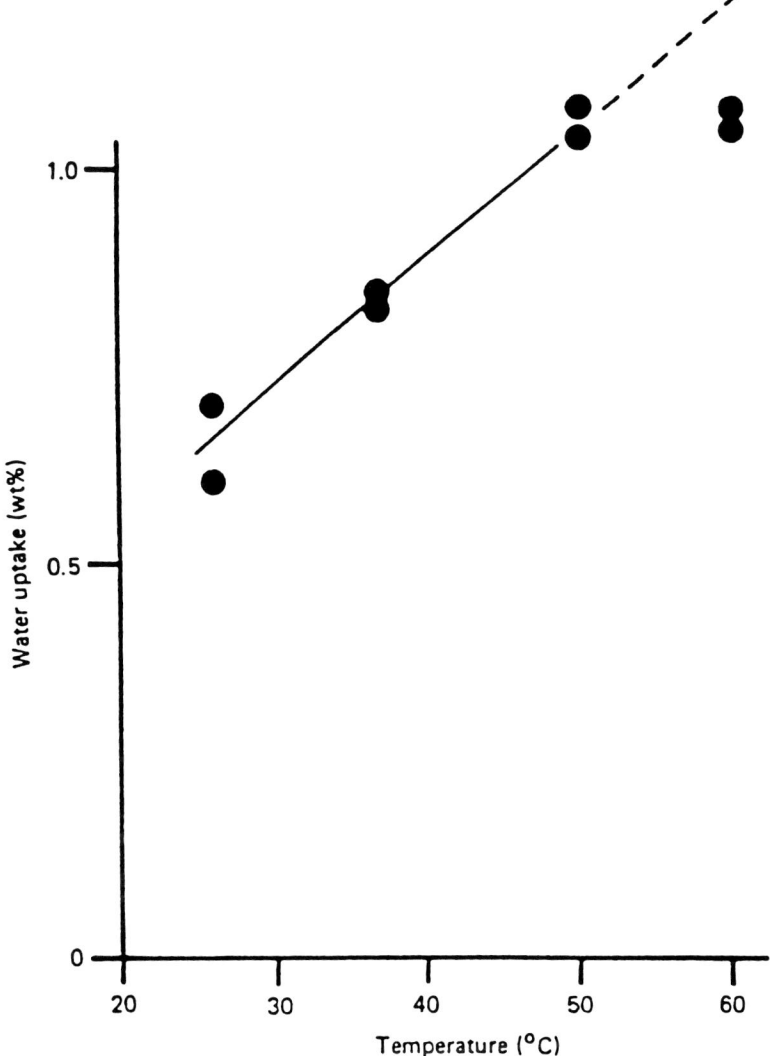

Fig. 7. Influence of temperature on water uptake: DOP 20%; PMMA, 80%.

monotonic increase in the Deff with increasing plasticizer content (Fig. 8). In the absence of any theoretical guidance, a least-squares straight line was drawn through diffusion values for all plasticized compositions judged to be in the glassy state by reference to values of T_g, i.e., with ≤20% plasticizer (Fig. 9). On this basis, it appears that the value of Deff increases more rapidly above T_g. This upturn is less marked in the case of DOP, but additional evidence of a change in mechanism was obtained in experiments on temperature dependence (Fig. 9). These indicate a higher rate of diffusion at temperatures above 50–60°C, which is near the T_g value for this composition, i.e., 61°C. The activation energy for diffusion in the glassy state is 20.5 kJ/mol. This is lower than the value reported for unplasticized PMMA (43.5kJ/mol) *(65,66)*.

There are several factors that might influence the way in which a plasticizer affects water transport in a glassy polymer. One factor is that the plasticizer molecules might increase transport by decreasing the attractive forces between segments of the macromolecules. This would have the effect of decreasing the activation energy for diffusion, as observed in the present work. Such an effort

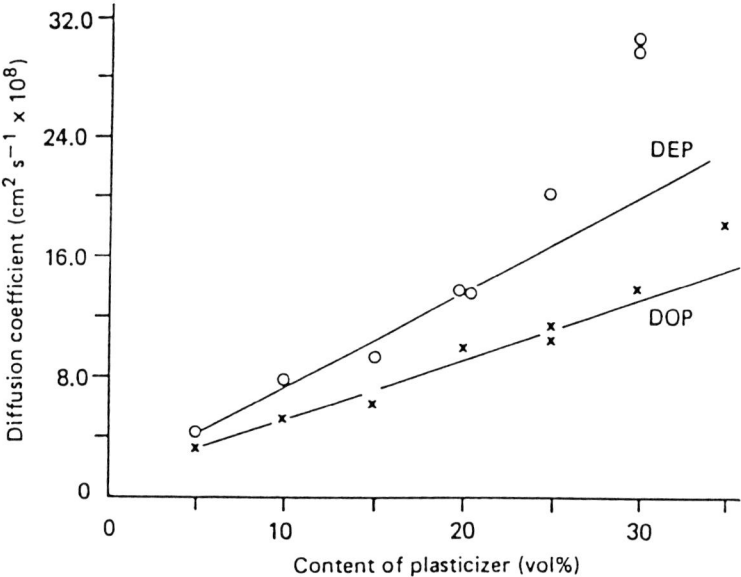

Fig. 8. Influence of plasticizer content on Deff, in desorption at 50°C.

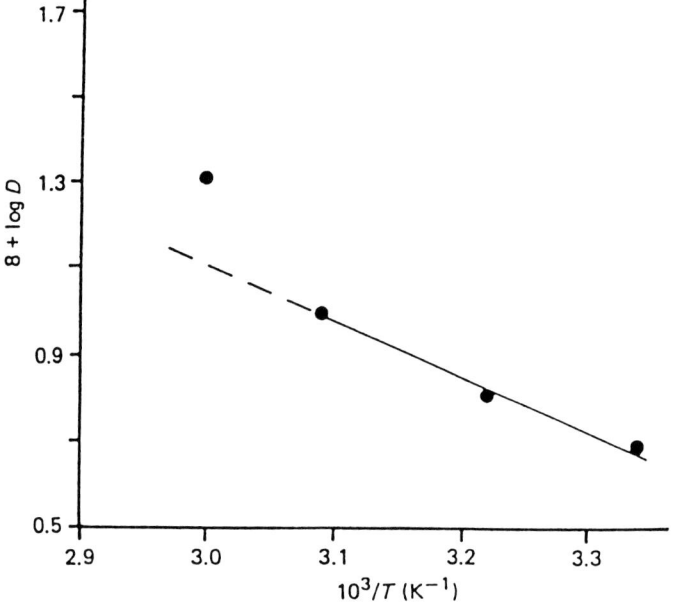

Fig. 9. Influence of temperature on Deff, in desorption: DOP, 20%; PMMA, 80%.

would also be consistent with the observed monotonic increase in the Deff up to T_g. The more marked increase in the diffusion coefficient above T_g would be consistent with transport into holes formed by main-chain motions, of the kind generally adduced to account for glass transport in glassy polymers (62). A second factor is that transport might be affected by plasticizer molecules occupying space, here termed "microvoids." Evidence for such occupancy has been presented, but

7. Conclusions

1. Two experimental materials, based on 70:30 BS block copolymer, with 1 wt% of lucidol (BS1) and 1 wt% LP (BS2), and the commercial material, Novus (based on polyphosphazine chemistry), reduced the water uptake from osmolic solutions. This could explain its good clinical performance, despite its excessive water uptake from pure water. This finding supports the theory that the high uptake of elastomeric solutions is osmotically driven.
2. It has been concluded, from the study of the relationship between soft lining materials (experimental and commercial), that these materials, studied under experimental conditions, did not support the growth of yeasts. This has been attributed to the inability of the materials to imbibe sufficient nutrients to encourage the growth of yeasts.
3. Use of CP/MAS ^{13}C NMR technique permitted detection of low levels of residual monomers (as low as 0.05%) in a commonly used PMMA dental polymer.
4. The uptake of water by PMMA is reduced by inclusion of either DOP or DEP in a way that has been interpreted to involve the filling of microvoids, which, in the absence of such additives, can accommodate water.
5. The diffusion coefficient of water in PMMA increases monotonically with increasing contents of either DOP or DEP. The diffusion coefficient increases less markedly when the plasticized polymers are in the glassy state.

Acknowledgments

The authors wish to thank Professor Howard G. Clark, Department of Biomedical Engineering, Duke University, Durham, NC, for his valuable suggestions during the preparation of this manuscript, and for constant support in research efforts.

References

1. Sperling LH. *Introduction to Physical Polymer Science* 1986; John Wiley, New York.
2. Wright PS. Soft lining materials: their status and prospects. *J Dent* 1976; 4: 247–256.
3. Wright PS. Effect of soft lining materials on the growth of *Candida Albicans*. *J Dent* 1980; 8: 144–151.
4. Wright PS. Composition and properties of soft lining materials for acrylic dentures. *J Dent* 1981; 9: 210–223.
5. Wright PS. Characterization of the adhesion of soft lining materials to poly(methyl methacrylate). *J Dent Res* 1982; 61: 1002–1005.
6. Wright PS, Young KA, Riggs P, Parker S, and Kalachandra S. Evaluating the effect of soft lining materials on growth of yeast. *J Prosthet Dent* 1998; 79: 404–409.
7. Stanford JW. Future of materials and materials research. *Adv Dent Res* 1986; 2: 187–192.
8. Braden M, Wright PS, and Parker S. Soft lining materials: a review. *Eur J Prosthodont Rest Dent* 1995; 3: 163–174.
9. Amin WM, Fletcher AM, and Ritchie GN. Nature of the interface between polymethyl methacrylate denture base materials and soft lining materials. *J Dent* 1981; 9: 336–346.
10. Braden M and Wright PS. Water adsorption and water solubility of soft lining materials for acrylic dentures. *J Dent Res* 1983; 62: 764–768.
11. Holt RA Jr, Stratton RL, and McBride C. Impression technique and laboratory procedures for a processed resilient denture liner. *Quint Dent Technol* 1986; 10: 9–12.
12. Wright PS. Observations on long-term use of soft lining material for mandibular complete dentures. *J Prosthet Dent* 1994; 72: 385–392.
13. Travaglini EA, Gibbons P, and Craig RG. Resilient liners for dentures. *J Prosthet Dent* 1960; 10: 664–672.
14. Van Handell AB. 1974; US Patent 3785054.
15. Litchfield J and Wood LG. British Patent 983817.
16. Parker S. *Development and evaluation of new elastomeric prosthetic materials*. 1982; PhD Thesis, University of London.
17. Parker S and Braden M. Water adsorption of methacrylate soft lining materials. *Biomaterials* 1989; 10: 91–95.
18. Parker S and Braden M. New soft lining materials. *J Dent* 1982; 10: 149–153.
19. Gettleman L, Guerra LR, Jameson LM, Finger IM, Agarwal A, Larson H, et al. Baseline results from two permanent soft denture reline materials. *J Dent Res* 1986; 65: 278.
20. Ryan JE. Twenty-five years of clinical application of a heat-cured silicone rubber. *J Prosthet Dent* 1991; 65: 658–661.

21 Dootz ER, Koran A, and Craig RG. Comparison of physical properties of 11 sod liners. *J Prosthet Dent* 1992; 67: 707–712.
22 Jepson NJA, McCabe JF, and Basker RM. Temporary soft lining material. *J Dent* 1995; 23: 123–126.
23 Quadah S, Huggett R, and Harrison A. Effects of thermocycling on the hardness of soft lining materials. *Quint Int* 1993; 22: 575–580.
24 Collis J. Assessment of a recently introduced fluoroelastomeric soft lining material. *Int J Prosthodont* 1993; 6(Suppl): 440–445.
25 Kutay O. Comparison of tensile end peel bond strengths of resilient liners. *J Prosthet Dent* 1994; 71: 525–531.
26 Kutay O, Bilgin T, Sakar O, and Beyli M. Tensile bond strength of a soft lining with acrylic denture base resins. *Eur J Prosthodont Rest Dent* 1994; 2: 123–126.
27 Sinobad D, Murphy WM, Huggett R, and Brooks S. Bond strength and rupture properties of some soft denture liners. *J Oral Rehab* 1992; 19: 151–160.
28 Polyzois GL. Adhesion properties of resilient lining materials bonded to light-cured denture resins. *J Prosthet Dent* 1992; 68: 854–858.
29 Kawano F, Dootz ER, Koran A, and Craig RD. Sorption and solubility of 12 soft denture liners. *J Prosthet Dent* 1994; 72: 393–398.
30 Brauer GM and Sweeney WT. Sorption of water by polymethyl methacrylate. *Modern Plas* 1955; 32: 138–143.
31 Stafford GD and Brown M. Water adsorption of some denture base polymers. *J Dent Res* 1968; 47: 341.
32 Braden M and Clark RL. Water sorption characteristics of dental microfine composite filling materials. I. Proprietary materials. *Biomaterials* 1984; 5: 369–372.
33 Braden M and Davy KWM. Water adsorption characteristics of some unfilled resins. *Biomaterials* 1986; 7: 474–476.
34 Soderholm KJM. Hydrolytic degradation of dental composites and effects of silane-treatment and filler fraction on compressive strength and thermal expansion of composites. Umea Univ Odontol Dissertations, no. 19: 1984.
35 Kalachandra S and Turner DT. Water sorption of polymethacrylate networks: BIS-GMA/TEGDM copolymers. *J Biomed Mater Res* 1987; 21: 329–338.
36 Kalachandra S and Turner DT. Water sorption of poly(methyl methacrylate): 3. Effect of plasticizers. *Polymer* 1987; 28: 1749–1752.
37 Kalachandra S and Turner DT. Influence of a plasticizer on the water sorption of polymethylmethacrylate. *J Polymer Sci Part B Polymer Phys* 1987; 25: 697–698.
38 Kalachandra S and Turner DT. Depression of the glass transition temperature of poly(methyl methacrylate) by plasticizers: conformity with free volume. *J Polymer Sci Part B Polyps Phys* 1987; 25: 1971–1979.
39 Kalachandra S. Influence of fillers on water sorption of composites. *Dent Mater* 1989; 5: 283–288.
40 Kalachandra S and Turner DT. Water sorption of plasticized denture acrylic lining material. *Dent Mater* 1989; 5: 161–164.
41 Kalachandra S, Kusy RP, Wilson TW, Shin ID, and Stejskal EO. Influence of dibutyl phthalate on the mechanical, thermal and relaxation behaviour of poly (methyl methacrylate) for denture-based soft liners. *J Mater Sci, Mater in Med* 1993; 4: 509–514.
42 Muniandy K and Thomas AG. Water adsorption in rubbers: polymers in a marine environment. *Trans I Mar E(c)* 1984; 97: 87–94.
43 Ellis B, Lamb DJ, and Saud al Nakash. Water sorption by a soft liner. *J Dent Res* 1977; 56: 1526.
44 Aiken A. Physiochemical and biological study of systems based on poly(2 ethoxy ethyl methacrylate) for use in oral and maxillofacial surgery. 1988; PhD Thesis, University of London.
45 Davy KWM and Braden M. Mechanical properties of elastomeric poly(alkylmethacrylates). *Biomaterials* 1987; 8: 393–396.
46 Parker S, Riggs P, and Martin D. Water uptake of elastomeric materials. *European Polymer Federation Symposium on Polymeric Materials,* 9–12 October, 1994; Basel, Switzerland.
47 Parker S, Riggs P, Kalachandra S, Taylor DF, and Braden MJ. Effect of composition on the mechanical properties and water sorption of a butadiene/styrene copolymer methacrylate monomer soft lining material. *Mater Sci Mater Med* 1996; 7: 245–250.
48 Riggs R, Parker S, and Kalachandra S. Influence of soluble and hydrophilic constituents on the water uptake of elastomeric materials. *Biomaterials in Medicine,* Biological Engineering Society, Dec. 6, 1995; Cambridge, UK.
49 Braden M, Parker S, Riggs PD, and Martin D. Soft lining materials in the oral environment. *Polymat '94, Biomedical Environment Session,* 19–22 September 1994; London, Imperial College, London.
50 Riggs P, Parker P, Braden M, and Kalachandra S. Mechanisms of water uptake into soft lining materials. *J Dent Res* 1996; 75: 294 (Abstract).
51 Kalachandra S, Xu D, Parker S, Riggs P, Taylor DF, and Braden MJ. Dynamic mechanical analysis

and water sorption of some experimental elastomeric soft lining materials. *J Mater Sci Mater Med* 1996; 7: 237–240.

52 Kalachandra S, Minton RF, Takamata T, and Taylor DF. Characterization of commercial soft liners by dynamic mechanical analysis. *J Mater Sci Mater Med* 1995; 6: 218–222.

53 Parker S, Riggs P, Braden M, Kalachandra S, and Taylor DF. Water uptake of soft lining materials from osmotic solutions. *J Dent* 1997; 25: 297–304.

54 Kalachandra S, Minton RJ, Taylor DF, and Takamata T. Characterization of some proprietary soft lining materials. *J Mater Sci Mater In Med* 1995; 647–652.

55 Wright PS, Young KA, Parker S, and Kalachandra S. Evaluating the effect of soft lining materials on growth of yeast. *J Prosthet Dent* 1998; 79: 404–409.

56 Kalachandra S, Turner DT, Burgess JP, and Stejskal EO. Post-irradiation reactions of monomer in poly (methyl methacrylate) by CP/MAS ^{13}C NMR: *Macromolecules,* 1994; 27: 5948.

57 Kalachandra S, Burgess JP, and Stejskal EO. Detection of monomer and dental PMMA by CP/MAS ^{13}C NMR. *J Dent Res* 1989; 68: 249.

58 Kusy RP and Turner DT. Influence of the molecular weight of poly(methylmethacrylate) on fracture surface energy is notched tension, *Polymer* 1976; 17: 161.

59 Turner DT. Glass transition elevation by polymer entanglements, *Polymer* 1978; 19: 789.

60 Turner DT. Tensile strength elevation of brittle polymers by entanglements. *Polymer* 1982; 23: 626.

61 Turner DT. Polymethyl methacrylate plus water: sorption kinetics and volumetric changes, *Polymer* 1982; 23: 197.

62 Kalachandra S and Turner DT. Water sorption of poly(methyl methacrylane) 3. Effects of plasticizers. *Polymer* 1987; 28: 1749–1752.

63 Kalachandra S and Turner DT. Influence of a plasticizer on water sorption by polymethyl methacrylate. *J Polym Sci Polym Phys Edn* 1987; 25: 697.

64 Turner DT and Abell AK. Water sorption of poly (methyl methacrylate): 2 effects of crosslinks. *Polymer* 1987; 28: 297.

65 Sheppard SE and Newsome PT. Sorption of water vapor by cellulose and its derivatives. *J Phys Chem* 1929; 33: 1817.

66 Sheppard SE. Structure of xerogels of cellulose and derivatives. *Trans Faraday Soc* 1933; 29: 77.

67 Kargin VA. Sorptive properties of glasslike polymers. *J Polym Sci* 1957; 23: 47.

68 Rogers CE. Solubility and diffusivity in *Physics and Chemistry of the Organic Solid State* 1965; Fox D, Labes MM, and Weissberger A. (eds.), Interscience, New York, pp. 509–635.

69 Rogers CE and Machin D. *CRC Critical Reviews in Macromolecular Science.* 1972; CRC, Boca Raton 245.

70 Molyneux P. Aqueous Solutions of Amphiphiles and Macromolecules, in *Water* vol. 4, 1975; Franks F (ed), Plenum, New York, pp. 703–721.

71 Bueche FJ. Diffusion of water in polymethyl methacrylate. *Polym Sci* 1954; 14: 414.

72 Barrie JA. Water in polymers, in Diffusion in Polymers. 1968; Crank J and Park GS (eds), Academic, London, pp. 259–313.

73 Crank J. The Mathematics of Diffusion. 1957; Clarendon Press, Oxford.

74 Barrer RM, Barrie JA, and Slater J. Sorption and diffusion in ethyl cellulose. Part III. Comparison between ethyl cellulose and water. *J Polym Sci* 1958; 27: 177.

75 Doty P. On the diffusion of vapor through polymers. *J Chem Phys* 1946; 14: 244.

76 Kumins CA, Rolle CJ, and Roteman J. Water vapor diffusion through vinyl chloride-vinyl acetate copolymer. *J Phys Chem* 1957; 61: 1290.

77 Olayemi JY and Oniyangi NA. Three-stage interaction of dimethyl phthalate, dibutyl phthalate and poly(vinyl acetate) with poly(methyl methacrylate). *J Appl Polym Sci* 1981; 26: 4059.

78 Raucher D and Sefcik M. Gas transport and cooperative main-chain motion in glassy polymers, in Industrial-Gas Separation. 1983; Whyte TE, Yon CM, and Wagner WH (eds), ACS Symp Ser 223, American Chemical Society, Washington, DC, pp. 89–124.

79 Pace RJ and Datyner AJ. Statistical mechanical model for diffusion of simple penetrants in polymers. I. *Theory, Polym Sci Polym Phys Edn* 1979; 17: 437.

80 Kelley FN and Bueche F. Viscosity and glass temperature relations for polymers, "Diluent Systems". *J Polymer Sci* 1961; 50: 549.

3

HA Coatings on Dental Implants

Joo L. Ong, Daniel C. N. Chan, and Kazuhisa Bessho

1. Introduction

Hydroxyapatite (HA) is one of the most biocompatible materials known and is a bioactive ceramic that has been used as a coating for metal implants, because it enhances bone healing adjacent to implants, and establishes a high interfacial bone–implant strength *(1,2)*. The rationale for the use of HA coatings on metallic implants include stimulation of bone healing, thereby expediting bone–implant stability (Fig. 1), improving the rate of osseointegration, and enhancing the bone–implant interfacial strength *(3–10)*. Thus, the use of HA coatings would speed rehabilitation of patients by decreasing the time from implant insertion to final reconstruction. However, for the past 10 yr, the use of HA-coated dental implants has initiated substantial controversy in dental implantology. The strongest argument against the routine use of HA-coated implants is the general lack of long-term documentation on HA-coated implant survival, as well as the lack of well-characterized coating prior to use. In addition, large degrees of variability between studies, involving the definition and length of implant survival/success, implant case and the site selection, surgeon experience, surgical protocols, postoperative regimens, and prosthetic restoration, makes direct interstudy comparisons problematic *(11,12)*.

2. Biological HA

One reason for investigating HA as coatings is that it is found naturally in the inorganic portions of the bone and teeth, predominantly in the impure calcium phosphate (CaP) form. Having the chemical formula $Ca_{10}(PO4)_6(OH)_2$, it is also known as calcium hydroxide phosphate *(13)*. Besides magnesium, sodium, and potassium, the mineral portion of bone consists of poorly crystallized, carbonate-containing apatite phase, plus a second CaP that is amorphous when evaluated using X-ray diffraction *(14–17)*. Table 1 shows the major compositional differences between tooth enamel and stoichiometric HA *(13,18)*.

Evidence has eluded to the fact that mineral Ca HAs are present as the chief constituent of hard tissues, with a variety of other CaP salts being present, either in early development of hard tissue or in later developmental stages *(19)*. Included in these varieties are octacalcium phosphate, monetite, and brushite.

3. HA Coating Methodology and HA Properties

HA and fluorapatite (FA) are brittle, and cannot be used as implants in load-bearing applications. Therefore, load-bearing implants have been coated with HA and FA. The objective of employing apatitic coatings is to cause earlier stabilization of the implants in surrounding bone, as well as to eliminate the use of polymethylmethacrylate bone cement around hip prostheses.

There are numerous methods for producing HA coatings on metallic implants. Foremost is a particulate deposition process known as plasma

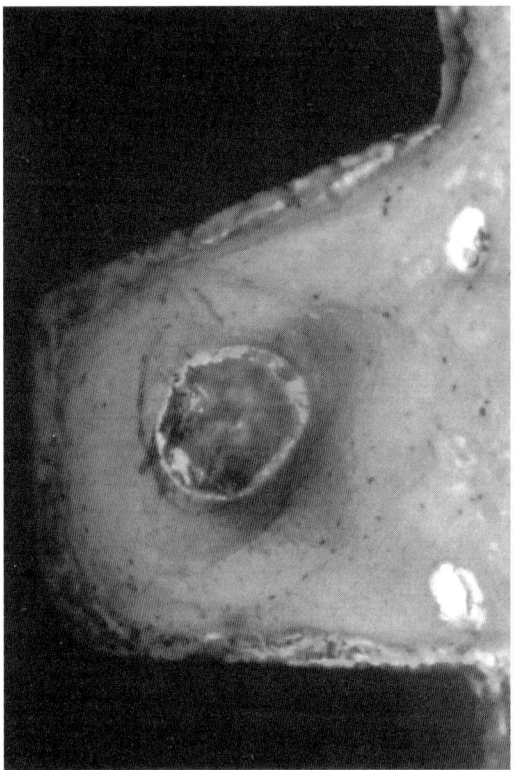

Fig. 1. Histology of marrow cavity indicating direct bone contact at the HA–bone interface (×100).

Table 1
Chemical Composition of Human Tooth Enamel and Stoichiometric HA

Constituent	Human tooth enamel (wt%)	Stoichiometric HA (wt%)
Ca	36.40	39.90
P	17.80	18.50
OH	–	3.38
CO_2	2.05	–
H_2O	≤4.00	–
Organic	0.39	–
CaP	1.58 (molar ratio)	1.67 (molar ratio)

spraying or arc plasma spraying (20). Other methods include electrophoretic co-deposition, ion implantation processes, sputter deposition, and high-velocity oxy-fuel combustion spray deposition (21–25). The plasma-spraying method is used commercially to produce coatings having a thickness >30 μm (20). The thermal spraying process utilizes a gas stream to carry HA powders, which are then passed through an electrical plasma produced by a low-voltage, high-current electrical discharge (20,26). The semimolten powders are sprayed onto the substrate, where they solidify. Advantages of plasma spraying include a rapid deposition rate and sufficiently low cost (20).

Numerous problems with the plasma-sprayed coatings have also been cited, including variation in bond strength between the coatings and the metallic substrates, nonuniformity in coating density, alterations in HA structure as a result of the process, poor adhesion between the coatings and metallic substrates, and microcracks on the HA surface (Fig. 2; 27–34). Minimal changes in the plasma-spraying technique had been reported (35) to significantly alter the structure of the HA coating. In addition, biochemical compositional analysis of HA coatings are usually performed on the precursor materials, rather than on the coated implant (36,37). Therefore, determining an optimal method for analysis of apatite surfaces remains problematic. HA coatings have been reported to be composed of varying percentages of crystalline HA, tricalcium phosphate (TCP), and amorphous CaP (5,38). Characterization of typical plasma-sprayed HA coatings revealed that the HA coating layer consisted primarily of partially dehydrated HA, with amorphous CaP along with more soluble phases, such as TCP, which are created during the high-temperature coating procedure (39–42). Investigations reported that the plasma-spray HA-coated implants were coated under normal conditions, with a crystallinity of approx 65% (43). Recent studies (43) on plasma-sprayed HA coated implants indicated that crystallinities of the coatings range between 30 and 70%, with varying percentages of crystalline HA, TCP, and amorphous caP (43a, 43b).

Thus, not all HA coatings are not the same. Currently, there are no accepted standards for manufacturing HA-coated implants (5,38,44). However, there are standards for the specification of CaP coatings for implantatable materials (American Society for Testing and Materials [ASTM] F1609) and tension-testing methods of

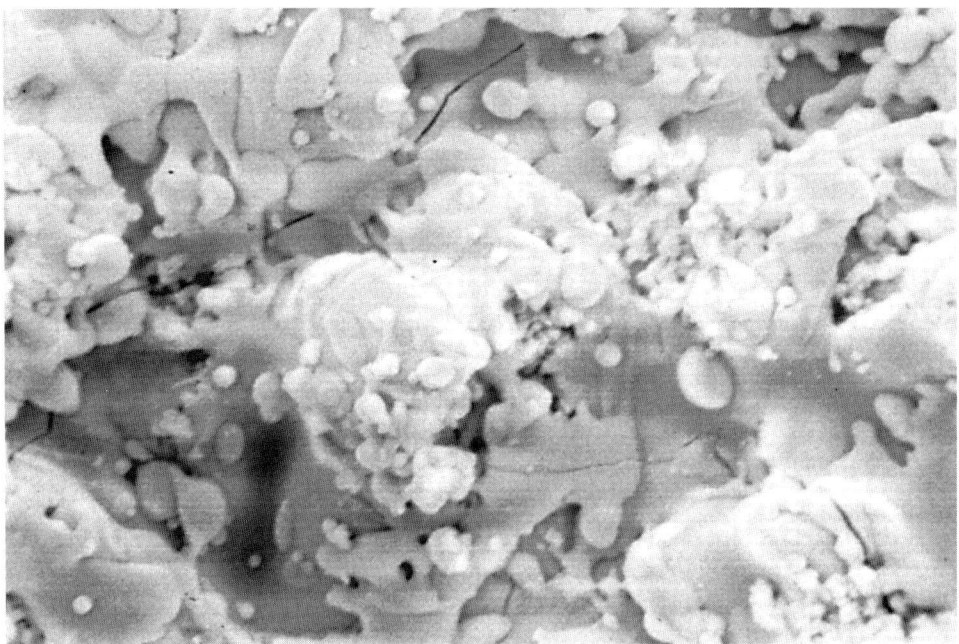

Fig. 2. Microcrack observed on the glassy-like HA surface (×3000).

CaP coatings (ASTM F1501). Other working standards in progress include the measuring crystallinity and dissolution of CaP coatings.

Physical properties of HA coatings, such as dissolution behavior or stability of the coating are critical to the implant's success *(45,46)*. It has been reported that a coating's dissolution rate is dependent on crystallinity, composition, structure, surface area, and density *(5,47,48)*. By substituting fluorine for the hydroxyl groups, FA has been reported to be more stable than HA *(47)*. It is also believed that the more crystalline HA the implant coating contains, the more resistant the coating will be to dissolution *(44)*. Conversely, increased concentrations of amorphous CaP and TCP are thought to predispose the HA coatings to dissolution *(45,49,50)*. In addition, the HA:TCP ratio has been shown to be crucial to bone regeneration in studies evaluating the regenerative potential of biphasic CaP ceramics in periodontal defects *(51)*. Other factors affecting the biological response to the HA coating have also been suggested *(52,53)*. These factors include crystallinity, content of non-HA crystalline phases, surface texture and porosity, presence of trace elements, and the bond strength of HA to the metal implant *(54)*. Of major importance in determining in vivo behavior of HA coatings may be the quantity and type of porosity in the coating. During plasma deposition, there is porosity present between, as well as within, the laminar structure of the semimolten particles, which is not squeezed out on impact with the substrate. A high porosity level, especially if the porosity is interconnected, would lead to a higher dissolution rate of the coating. One study *(55)* reported that a plasma-sprayed coating that was 100% amorphous had a much lower dissolution rate than one that was only 40% amorphous and 60% crystalline HA, because, when producing an amorphous coating for that particular study, the plasma-spray conditions were changed to give a highly melted, very fluid material with little or no porosity present in the final coating. Thus, it appears that level of porosity may be an important factor in the dissolution properties of HA coatings, to an extent not fully recognized to date.

The HA coatings were reported to have inconsistent thickness over the surfaces of the individual textured implants *(56)*. It was determined that the mean HA thicknesses were equivalent for all implant designed, ranging between 79.02 and 111.32 μm *(56)*. Most of the experimental HA-coated implants had the thickest coating in the grooves and threads. In addition, it was also reported that the addition of surface threads, grooves, and dimples did not significantly affect axial pull-out and torsional interface attachment strengths. However, the problem of low coating–metal interfacial needs to be addressed *(27)*. An average bond strength of 6.7 ± 1.5 MPa was reported for plasma-coated HA on titanium (Ti)-aluminum-vanadium (Ti-6Al-4V) substrates *(29)*. When a postheat treatment of 960°C was applied, bond strengths were increased to a range of 15.0–26 MPa.

4. In Vivo Studies on HA-coated Implants

Extensive in vivo research has cited plasma-sprayed HA coatings to be biocompatible, with reports of early skeletal attachment *(57,58)*. With plasma-sprayed FA, bone apposition has also been reported from animal studies *(59,60)*. Although fluorine plays a vital role in reducing the dissolution rate of CaP ceramics, significant amounts of fluoride may affect stromal cell proliferation *(61–63)*. Controversial observations regarding fluoride include decreased bone mineral content or improper or delayed mineralization *(64–66)*.

Early histological studies indicated direct bone contact with HA-coated implants as early as 1 mo, with 70% contact at 4 mo, and 90% contact at 10 mo. In contrast, the uncoated implants had only 50% of their surface contacting bone *(67)*. Other early studies also reported near-complete interfacial mineralization of bone directly on HA surfaces, with no fibrous tissue layer formation at 10 wk; predominantly fibrous tissue interface, with only isolated areas of direct bone contact, was observed *(68)* with commercially pure Ti implants of identical shape. Moreover, increased coronal growth of bone associated with the HA–coated implants, which was not observed with Ti implants, has been described in the animal model study *(69)*. The observation that HA-coated implants maintain osseous crest height and foster coronal apposition of bone has been supported by other studies. Maintenance of the osseous crest is of clinical significance, because it may prevent peri-implant saucerization and subsequent pocket formation *(70,71)*. Other histometric studies in animals models have also confirmed that bone adapts more rapidly to HA-coated implants than to Ti implants *(72,73)*. Three mo after implant placement, bone–implant contact at the interface in dogs was measured to be 45.7% for Ti screws, 55.0% for Ti cylinders, and 71.6% for HA-coated cylinders. A recent study confirmed the observation of higher bone contact for HA-coated screws (61.5%), compared to the commercially pure Ti screw implants (39.1%), after 3 mo implantation *(74)*. In the authors' recent implant study in dog mandibles, a significantly greater bone contact was observed with amorphous HA-type-coated cylindrical implants (50.3 ± 4.2%), compared to crystalline HA-coated (30.3 ± 6.7%) and Ti implants (33.7 ± 0.8%), after 3 wk implantation. At 12 wk, the bone contact for amorphous HA implants (70.4 ± 1.6%) remained significantly higher, compared to the crystalline HA-coated (58.2 ± 4.5%) and Ti implants (53.1 ± 7.5%). A longer implantation period in other studies indicated a 60% bone–implant contact for Ti implants, compared to 76.0% for HA-coated implants after 6 mo implantation *(75)*.

In reference to the interfacial strength, the HA-coated specimens were reported to have a push-out values of 7.28 MPa, when implanted in dog femurs; the noncoated Ti implants were reported to have a push-out value of 1.2 MPa at 10 wk *(3)*. At 32 wk, the push-out values were observed to be 5× those of the Ti implants. In a reverse-torque failure study in baboons, for a period of 3–4 mo, the HA-coated screws exhibited a greater torque removal value, compared with Ti screw implants *(76)*. HA-coated screws had values of 186.0 Ncm; Ti-6Al-4V and commercially pure Ti screws have values of 78.6 Ncm and 74.0 Ncm, respectively. In the authors' recent study, using amorphous and crystalline coatings, the HA-coated implants were observed to have greater pull-out values, compared to Ti implants. At 3 wk after implantation, the mean pull-out strength value (±1 standard error) of 250.4 ± 14.9 *N* for the amorphous-coated implants was statistically greater than the mean pull-out strength value of 139.8 ± 4.6 *N* for the crystalline HA-coated

HA Coatings on Dental Implants

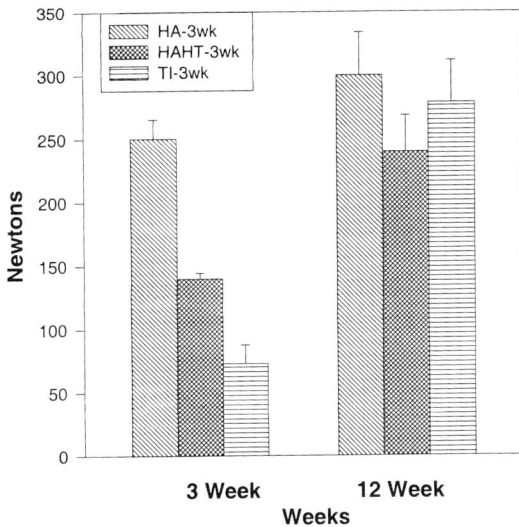

Fig. 3. Mean pull-out strength value (± 1 standard error) of amorphous coatings (HA), crystalline HA coatings (HAHT), and noncoated titanium control (TI) implants at 3 and 12 wk.

5. Considerations Associated with HA-Coated Implants

The two major concerns with using HA-coated implants are their enhanced susceptibility to bacterial colonization and their coating integrity. Other significant factors causing implant failures include microbial infection and occlusal trauma (78–80). No difference in the microbial colonization on HA-coated implant and Ti implants was reported (81,82). In addition, the sequence and composition of microbial morphotypes in the maturation of subgingival dental plaque were similar on Ti, HA, and cementum surfaces (83,84). Thus, it has been suggested that HA coatings are more susceptible to bacterial colonization than Ti implants or natural teeth, as a result of HA surface roughness and hydrophilicity, thereby enhancing plaque growth, and predisposing the implants for peri-implantitis (83,85). In the case of implant failing caused by microbial infection, successful treatment of peri-implant microflora may be complicated by HA surface roughness. When HA-coated surface is exposed to the oral environment, it becomes contaminated, and is potentially more difficult for the patient to clean than exposed Ti surfaces (86,87). A clinical case of a 50-yr-old male patient with three failing HA-coated implants is illustrated (Fig. 4–7).

Another concern with HA-coated implants is the failure of coatings as a result of dissolution (88) or coating–substrate interface fracture (77), thereby leading to implant mobility and loss (89,90). During implantation, coating resorption could also occur. However, in most studies, evaluation of HA coating resorption were performed only on stable, static, and unloaded implants. During unstable mechanical situation, an early study revealed that 65% of the 50-μm-thick HA coating was completely resorbed during the 16-wk implantation period (91). These resorptions were attributed to the dissolution of the HA surfaces and the presence of osteoclast-like cells (92–95). Although deposition of bone was most prominent on the surface of the prosthesis, there were occasional foci of bone remodeling around the implant, including osteoclast-mediated removal of the HA coating along the adjacent bone (95). Other investigations have also suggest that the increase in initial bone apposition attenuates over time, as a

implants (Fig. 3). Similarly, the pull-out strengths of amorphous and crystalline HA-coated implants were statistically greater than the mean pull-out strength of the control Ti implants (73.0 ± 14.7 N). After 12 wk implantation, the difference in mean pull-out strength values between coated implants and noncoated Ti implants decreased, with no statistical difference between the three groups tested. The mean pull-out strength value for crystalline HA-coated and control Ti implants at 12 wk was not statistically different from the amorphous-coated implants at 3 wk.

It was also reported that the success of HA-coated implants in vivo depends on the resorption of the coatings, which in turn is dependent on the surrounding condition. Marked difference in HA resorption was observed between sites in cortical bone and those in the medullary canal (8). The HA resorption rate was higher in the medullary spaces; resorption was almost absent in the areas embedded in cortical bone. Marked dissolution and resorption of HA coating and the appearance of multinucleated giant cells were observed at the areas without bone contact, suggesting a strong relationship between coating resorption and the appearance of multinucleated giant cells (77).

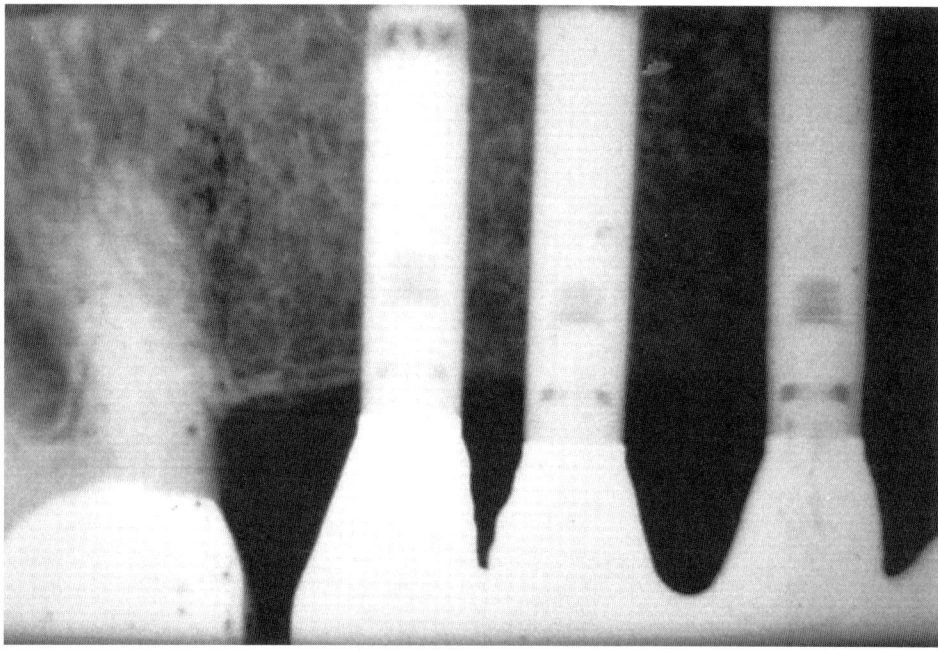

Fig. 4. Radiograph of a 55-yr-old male patient. Three HA implants were used to replace teeth 3, 4, and 5 immediate postoperation.

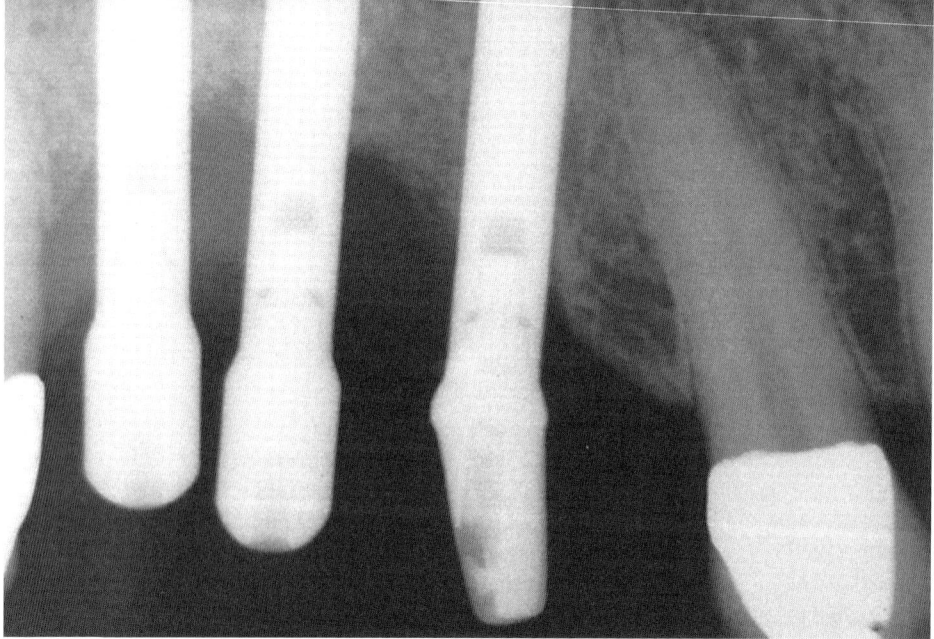

Fig. 5. Radiograph of the 55-yr-old male patient (same patient as in Fig. 4) after 4 yr implantation. Superstructure was removed showing extensive bone loss surrounding all three implants.

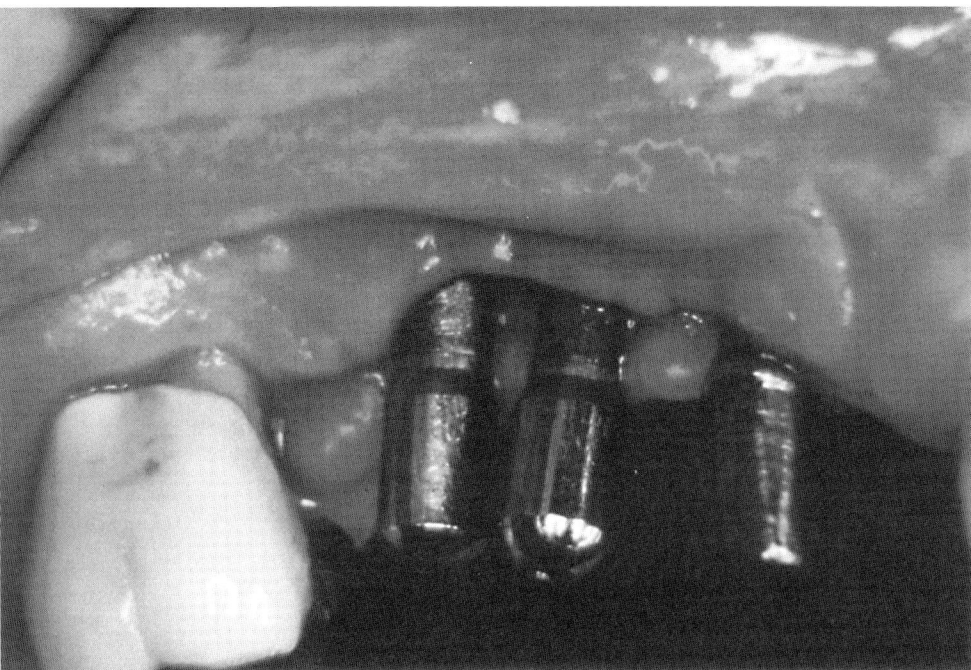

Fig. 6. When superstructure was removed, edematous tissue around the implants was clinically observed in the 55-yr-old male patient (same patient as in Fig. 4) after 4 yr implantation.

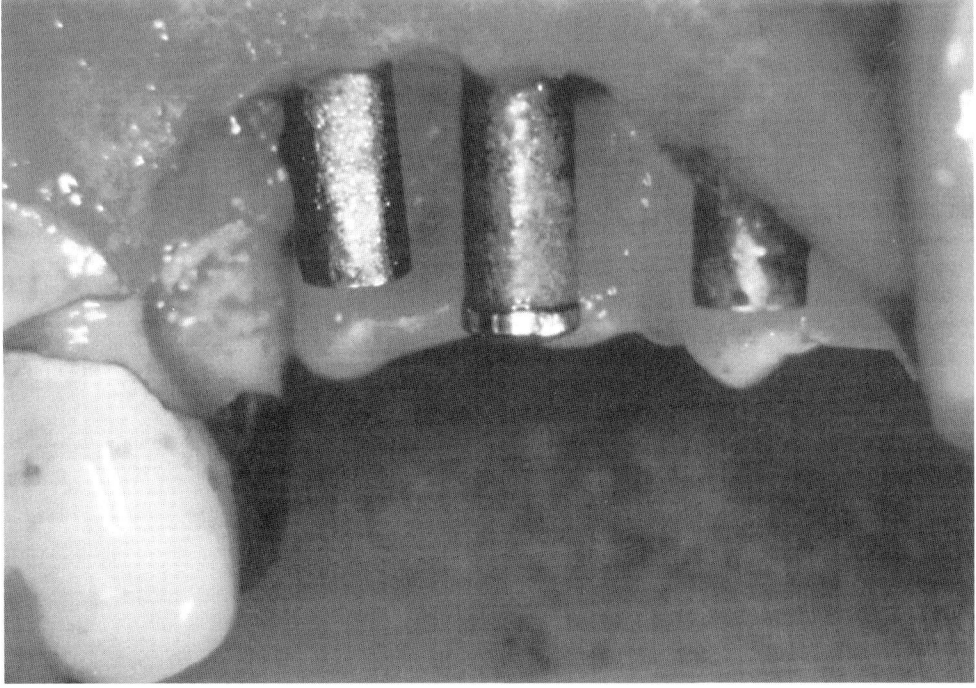

Fig. 7. After deep curettage, the patient (same patient as in Fig. 4) shows significant loss of both hard and soft tissue around the implants.

result of partial or total resorption *(96–98)*. Such a destruction of the HA coating could have damaging effects on the clinical use of these implants. Under loaded conditions, the osteoconductive effect of the HA coating is prolonged, with 7 × more bone ingrowth after 16 wk, compared to the uncoated implants *(99,100)*.

Although there is risk of coating resorption and separation from the HA-coated implants, in vivo cases of HA coating–Ti interface fractures, which are associated with implant failure, seem to be rare, especially in root-form fixtures. In multiple studies examining the 6-mo to 5-yr clinical longevity of 4133 implants, no root-form implant failures were attributed to HA coating–Ti interface fracture *(101–103)*. With HA-coated blade implants, there are occasional reports of coating separation, with several multinucleated giant cells around the exfoliated HA coatings that had no bone contact *(77,90)*. In a more recent study *(46)*, failure of the amorphous coatings in vivo has been attributed to crystallization of the coatings, thereby making the amorphous-phase brittle, and to stress accumulation within the coatings, and causing a decrease in the coating–implant interface.

6. Conclusion

Proper standardized methods for characterizing the properties of HA coatings and standard manufacturing guidelines must be established, to ensure consistent production of the coatings. In addition, the effects of crystallinity, texture, and porosity need to be evaluated experimentally, to develop HA-coated implants with optimum physical and biological properties. Although it has been generally accepted that HA coatings improve bone strength and initial osseointegration rate, optimum HA properties required to achieve maximum bone response are yet to be reported. The use of well-characterized HA implants in cell culture, animal, and clinical studies should be well documented, to avoid controversial results.

Clinically, it has been suggested that no non-coated implants should be used at the compromised site *(104)*. One clear complication in the placement of endosseous dental implants was the site with compromised quality and quantity of bone. In the compromised site, it has been reported *(102,105)* that short HA-coated implants osseointegrate more frequently than non-HA-coated implants. Thus, it has been recommended by many clinicians that the HA-coated Ti screw implants be used for the anterior maxilla and posterior mandible, where the bone depth exceeds 10 mm, and when the cortical layer is thinner and spongiosia is less dense (types 2 and 3 bone) *(102)*. In the posterior maxilla, or when the cortical layer is very thin with low density (type 4 bone), the HA-coated cylinder implants are recommended. However, long-term controlled studies are still required to validate those observations.

References

1. Kay JF. Bioactive surface coatings: cause for encouragement and concern. *J Oral Implants* 1988; 14: 43–50.
2. Bell R and Beirne O. Effect of hydroxyapatite tricalcium phosphate, and collagen on the healing of defects in the rat mandible. *J Oral Maxillofac Surg* 1988; 46: 589–594.
3. Cook SD, Kay JF, and Thomas KA. Interface mechanics and histology of titanium and HA-coated titanium for dental implant applications. *Int J Oral Maxillofac Implants* 1987; 2: 15–22.
4. de Lange GL and Donath K. Interface between bone tissue and implants of solid hydroxyapatite or hydroxyapatite-coated titanium implants. *Biomaterials* 1989; 10: 121–125.
5. LeGeros R. Calcium phosphate materials in restorative dentistry: a review. *Adv Dent Mater* 1988; 2: 164–173.
6. Jarcho M. Retrospective analysis of hydroxyapatite development for oral implant applications. *Dent Clin North Am* 1992; 36: 19–27.
7. Piattelli A, Trisi P, and Emanuelli M. Bone reactions to hydroxyapatite-coated dental implants in humans: histology study using SEM, light microscopy, and laser scanning microscopy. *Int J Oral Maxillofac Implants* 1993a; 8: 69–74.
8. Piattelli A, Cordioli GP, Trisi P, Passi P, Favero GA, and Meffert RM. Light and confocal laser scanning microscopic evaluation of hydroxyapatite resorption patterns in medullary and cortical bone. *Int J Oral Maxillofac Implants* 1993; 8: 309–315.
9. Beirne O. Reaction to the symposium, Hydroxyapatite coating on dental implants: Benefits and risks. *J Oral Implantol* 1994; 20: 240–243.
10. Ozawa S and Kasugai S. Evaluation of implant

materials (hydroxyapatite, glass-ceramics, titanium) in rat bone marrow stromal cell culture. *Biomaterials* 1996; 17: 23–29.

11. Krauser JT. Hydroxyapatite-coated dental implants: Biologic rational and surgical technique. *Dent Clin North Am* 1989; 33: 879–890.

12. Zablotsky MH. Surgical management of osseous defects associated with endosteal hydroxyapatite-coated and titanium dental implants. *Dent Clin North Am* 1992a; 36: 117–150.

13. Young RA. Biological apatite versus hydroxyapatite at the atomic level. *Clin Orthop Rel Res* 1975; 113: 249–262.

14. Bonel G, Heughebaert JC, Heughebaert M, Lacout JL, and Lebugle A. Apatitic calcium orthophosphates and related compounds for biomaterials, in *Bioceramics: Materia Characteristics Versus In Vivo Behavior* 1988; (Ducheyne P and Lemons JE, eds), NY Academy of Sciences, New York, pp. 115–139.

15. Van Mullem PJ and Maltha JC. Histology of bone: a synopsis, in *Bioceramics of Calcium Phosphate* 1983; CRC, Boca Raton, FL, pp. 53–78.

16. Posner AS. Crystal chemistry of bone mineral. *Physiol Rev* 1969; 49: 760–792.

17. Posner AS. Bone mineral on the molecular level. *Fed Proc* 1973; 32: 1933–1937.

18. Little MF and Casciani FS. Nature of water in sound human enamel. *Arch Oral Biol* 1966; 11: 565–571.

19. Termine JD. Mineral chemistry and skeletal biology. *Clin Orthop Rel Res* 1972; 85: 207–241.

20. Herman H. Plasma spray deposition processes. *MRS Bull* 1988; 12: 60–67.

21. Solieau RL. *Characterization of electrocodeposited hydroxylapatite coatings* 1991; (Master's thesis), University of Alabama, Birmingham, AL.

22. Coupe K. *Properties of Ca-P thin films produced using RF sputtering techniques* 1991; (Master's thesis), University of Alabama, Birmingham, AL.

23. Dasarathy H, Riley C, and Coble HD. Analysis of apatite deposits on subtrates. *J Biomed Mater Res* 1993; 27: 477–482.

24. Ong JL, Lucas LC, Lacefield WR, and Rigney ED. Structure, solubility and bond strength of thin calcium phosphate coatings produced by ion beam sputter deposition. *Biomaterials* 1992; 13: 249–254.

25. Haman JD, Lucas LC, and Crawmer D. Characterization of high velocity oxy-fuel combustion sprayed hydroxyapatite. *Biomaterials* 1995; 16: 229–237.

26. Bunshah RF. Deposition technologies: an overview, in (Bunshah RF, ed), *Deposition Technologies for Films and Coatings: Developments and Applications* 1982; Noyes, Park Ridge, NJ, pp. 1–18.

27. Lacefield WR. Hydroxylapatite coatings, in *Bioceramics: Material Characteristics Versus In Vivo Behavior* 1988; (Ducheyne P and Lemons JE, eds), New York Academy of Science, New York, pp. 72–80.

28. Filiaggi MJ and Pilliar RM. Interfacial characterization of a plasma-sprayed hydroxyapatite/Ti-6Al-4V implant system. *Transactions of the Tenth annual meeting of the Canadian Society for Biomaterials* June 1989; Toronto, 23–25.

29. Filiaggi MJ, Coombs NA, and Pilliar RM. Characterization of the interface in the plasma-sprayed HA coating/Ti-6Al-4V implant system. *J Biomed Mater Res* 1991; 25: 1211–1229.

30. Whitehead RY. *Structure and integrity of plasma sprayed hydroxylapatite coatings on titanium* 1991; (Master's thesis), University of Alabama, Birmingham, AL.

31. Radin S and Ducheyne P. Effect of plasma sprayed induced changes in characteristics on the *in vitro* stability of calcium phosphate ceramics. *Transactions of the 16th Annual Meeting of the Society for Biomaterials* May 20–23, 1990; Charleston. Society for Biomaterials, Birmingham, p. 128.

32. de Groot K, Geesink R, Klein C, and Serekian P. Plasma-sprayed coatings of hydroxyapatite. *J Biomed Mater Res* 1987; 21: 1375–1381.

33. de Groot K, Wolke JGC, and Jansen JA. State of the art: hydroxyapatite coatings for dental implants. *J Oral Implantol* 1994; 20: 232–234.

34. Steflik DE, Lacefield WR, Sisk AL, Parr GP, Lake FT, and Patterson JW. Hydroxyapatite-coated dental implants: descriptive histology and quantitative histomorphometry. *J Oral Implantol* 1994; 20: 201–213.

35. Zyman Z, Weng J, Liu X, Zhang X, and Ma X. Amorphous phase and morphological structure of hydroxyapatite plasma coatings. *Biomaterials* 1993; 14: 225–228.

36. Ducheyne P. Bioceramics: materials characterization versus in-vivo behavior. *J Biomed Mater Res* 1987; 21: 219–223.

37. Kay JF. Designing to counteract the effects of initial device instability: materials and engineering. *J Biomed Mater Res* 1988; 22: 1127–1132.

38. Lemons J. Hydroxyapatite coatings. *Clin Orthop* 1988; 235: 220–230.

39. Ducheyne P, van Raemdonck W, Heughebaert JC, and Heughebaert M. Structural analysis of hydroxyapatite coatings on titanium. *Biomaterials* 1986; 7: 97–103.

40. Matsui Y, Ohno K, Michi K, and Yamagata K. Experimental study of high-velocity flame-sprayed hydroxyapatite coated and noncoated titanium implants. *Int J Oral Maxillofac Implants* 1994; 9: 397–404.

41. Cheang P and Khor KA. Addressing processing problems associated with plasma spraying of hydroxyapatite coatings. *Biomaterials* 1996; 17: 537–544.

42. Tufekci E, Brantley WA, Mitchell JC, and McGlumphy EA. Microstructures of plasma-sprayed hydroxyapatite-coated Ti-6Al-4V dental implants. *Int J Oral Maxillofac Implants* 1997; 12: 25–31.

43. Geesink RG and Hoefnagels NH. Six-year results of hydroxyapatite-coated total hip replacement. *J Bone and Joint Surg (British vol)* 1995; 77: 534–547.

43a. LeGeros RZ, LeGeros JP, Kim Y, Kijkowska R, Zheng R, Bautista C, Wong JL. Calcium phosphates in plasma-sprayed HA coatings, in *Bioceramics: Materials and Applications*, vol. 48, 1994; (Fischman G, Clare A, Hench LL, eds), American Ceramic Society, Westerville, OH, pp. 173–189.

43b. Tufekci E, Brantley WA, Mitchell JC, Foreman DW, Georgette FS. Chrystallographic characteristics of plasma-sprayed calcium phosphate coatings on Ti-6Al-4V. *Int J Oral Maxillofac Implants* 1999; 14: 661–672.

44. Kay JF. Calcium phosphate coatings for dental implants. *Dent Clin North Am* 1992; 36: 1–18.

45. LeGeros R and Craig RG. Strategies to affect bone remodeling: Osseointegration. *J Bone Miner Res* 1993; 8: 583–596.

46. Ogiso M, Yamashita Y, and Matsumoto T. Process of physical weakening and dissolution of the HA-coated implant in bone and soft tissue. *J Dent Res* 1998; 77: 1426–1434.

47. Wolke JGC, Dhert WJA, Klein CPAT, de Blieck-Hogervorst JM, and de Groot K. Characterization of plasma-sprayed fluorapatite coatings for biomedical application, in (Vincenzini P, ed), *Ceramics in Substitutive and Reconstructive Surgery* 1991; Elsevier, New York, pp. 285–293.

48. Ducheyne P, Radin S, and King L. Effect of calcium phosphate ceramic composition and structure on *in vitro* behavior. I. Dissolution. *J Biomed Mater Res* 1993; 27: 25–34.

49. Nery EB, LeGeros RZ, Lynch KL, and Lee K. Tissue response to biphasic calcium phosphate ceramic with different ratios of HA/β-TCP in periodontal osseous defects. *J Periodontol* 1992; 63: 729–735.

50. Zablotsky MH. Hydroxyapatite coatings in implant dentistry. *Implant Dent* 1992; 1: 253–257.

51. LeGeros R. Calcium phosphates in oral biology and medicine, in *Monographs on Oral Science* 1991; (Meyers, HM, ed), Karger, Basel, Switzerland, pp. 154–171.

52. Lacefield WR. Characterization of hydroxyapatite coatings. *J Oral Implantol* 1994; 20: 214–220.

53. Soballe K, Hansen ES, Brockstedt-rasmussen H, and Bunger C. Hydroxyapatite coating converts fibrous tissue to bone around loaded implants. *J Bone Joint Surg Br* 1993; 75-B: 270–278.

54. Dalton JE and Cook SD. In vivo mechanical and histological characteristics of HA-coated implants vary with coating vendor. *J Biomed Mater Res* 1995; 29: 239–245.

55. Maxian SH, Zawadsky JP, and Dunn MG. In vitro evaluation of amorphous calcium phosphate and poorly crystallized hydroxyapatite coatings on titanium implants. *J Biomed Mater Res* 1993; 27: 111–118.

56. Cook SD, Salkeld SL, Gaisser DM, and Wagner WR. Effect of surface macrotexture on the mechanical and histologic characteristics of hydroxyapatite-coated dental implants. *J Oral Implantol* 1993; 19: 288–294.

57. Rivero DP, Fox J, Skipor AK, Urban RM, and Galante JO. Calcium phosphate-coated porous titanium implants for enhanced skeletal fixation. *J Biomed Mater Res* 1988; 22: 191–201.

58. Bloebaum RD, Merrell M, Gustke K, and Simmons M. Retrieval analysis of a hydroxyapatite-coated hip prosthesis. *Clin Orthop Rel Res* 1991; 267: 97–102.

59. Dhert WJA, Klein CPAT, Jansen JA, van der Velde EA, Vriesde RC, Rozing PM, and de Groot K. Histological and histomorphometrical investigation of fluorapatite, magnesium whitlockite, and hydroxyapatite plasma-sprayed coatings in goats. *J Biomed Mater Res* 1993; 27: 127–138.

60. Klein CPAT, de Blieck-Hogervorst JMA, Wolke JGC, and de Groot K. Study of solubility and surface features of different calcium phosphate coatings *in vitro* and *in vivo*: a pilot study, in *Ceramics in Substitutive and Reconstructive Surgery* 1991; (Vincenzini P, ed), Elsevier, New York, pp. 363–374.

61. Ingram GS. Some heteroanionic exchange reactions of hydroxyapatite. *Bull Soc Chim Fr* 1968; 1841–1844.

62. Kopp JB and Robey PG. Sodium fluoride does not increase human bone cell proliferation or protein

synthesis in vitro. *Calcif Tissue Int* 1990; 47: 221–229.
63. Simmons DJ, Seitz P, Kidder L, Klein GL, Waeltz M, Gundberg CM, et al. Partial characterization of rat marrow stromal cells. *Calcif Tissue Int* 1991; 48: 326–334.
64. Whyte MP, Teitelbaum SL, Bergfield M, and Avioli LV. Histomorphometric analysis of iliac crest bone from osteoporotic subjects following alternate sodium fluoride and calcium-vitamin D therapy. *Clin Res* 1978; 26: 776A.
65. Vigorita VJ and Suda MK. Microscopic morphology of fluoride-induced bone. *Clin Orthop Rel Res* 1983; 177: 274–282.
66. Likimani S, Whitford GM, and Kunkel ME. Effects of protein deficiency and fluoride on bone mineral content of rat tibia. *Calcif Tissue Int* 1992; 50: 157–164.
67. Meffert R, Block M, and Kent J. What is osseointegration? *Int J Periodont Rest Dent* 1987; 7: 9–21.
68. Thomas KA, Kay JF, Cook SD, and Jarcho M. Effects of surface macrotexture and hydroxylapatite coating on the mechanical strength and histologic profiles of titanium implant material. *J Biomed Mater Res* 1987; 21: 1395–1414.
69. Gammage DD, Bowman AE, Meffert RM, Cassingham RJ, and Davenport WA. Histologic and scanning electron micrographic comparison of the osseous interface in loaded IMZ and Integral implants. *Int J Periodont Rest Dent* 1990; 10: 125–135.
70. Kohri M, Cooper EP, Ferracane JL, and Waite DF. Comparative study of hydroxyapatite and titanium dental implants in dogs. *J Oral Maxillofac Surg* 1990; 48: 1265–1273.
71. Pilliar RM, Deporter DA, Watson PA, Paroah M, Chipman M, and Valiquette N. Effect of partial coating with hydroxyapatite on bone remodeling in relation to porous-coated titanium-alloy dental implants in the dog. *J Dent Res* 1991; 70: 1338–1345.
72. Gottlander M and Albrektsson T. Histomorphometric studies of hydroxyapatite-coated and uncoated CP titanium threaded implants in bone. *Int J Oral Maxillofac Implants* 1991; 6: 399–404.
73. Weimlaender M, Kennedy EB, Lekovic V, Beumer J, Moy PK, and Lewis S. Histomorphometry of bone apposition around three types of endosseous dental implants. *Int J Oral Maxillofac Implants* 1992; 7: 491–496.
74. Carr AB, Gerard DA, and Larsen PE. Quantitative histomorphometric description of implant anchorage for three types of dental implants following 3 months of healing in baboons. *Int J Oral Maxillofac Implants* 1997; 12: 777–784.
75. Gottlander M, Albrektsson T, and Carlsson LV. Histomorphometric study of unthreaded hydroxyapatite-coated and titanium-coated implants in rabbit bone. *Int J Oral Maxillofac Implants* 1992; 7: 485–490.
76. Carr AB, Larsen PE, Papazoglou E, and McGlumphy E. Reverse torque failure of screw-shaped implants in baboons: baseline data for abutment torque application. *Int J Oral Maxillofac Implants* 1995; 10: 167–174.
77. Takeshoita F, Ayukawa Y, Iyama A, Seutsugu T, and Kido MA. Histologic evaluation of retrieved hydroxyapatite-coated blade-form implants using scanning electron, light, and confocal laser scanning microscopies. *J Periodontol* 1996; 67: 1034–1040.
78. Rosenberg ES, Torosian JP, and Slots J. Microbial differences in 2 clinically distinct types of failures of osseointegrated implants. *Clin Oral Implants Res* 1991; 2: 135–144.
79. Verheyen CCPM, Dhert WJA, Petit PLC, Rozing PM, and deGroot K. In vitro study on the integrity of a hydroxylapatite coating when challenged with staphylococci. *J Biomed Mater Res* 1993; 27: 775–781.
80. Ichikawa T, Hirota K, Kanitani H, Wigianto R, Kawamoto N, Matsumoto N, and Miyake Y. Rapid bone resorption adjacent to hydroxyapatite-coated implants. *J Oral Implants* 1996; 22: 232–235.
81. Mombelli A, von Oosten MAC, Schurch E Jr, and Lang NP. Microbiota associated with successful or failing osseointegrated titanium implants. *Oral Microbiol Immunol* 1987; 2: 145–151.
82. Becker W, Becker BE, Newman MG, and Nyman S. Clinical and microbiological findings that may contribute to implant failure. *Int J Oral Maxillofac Implants* 1990; 5: 31–38.
83. Rams TE, Roberts TW, Feik D, Molzan AK, and Slots J. Clinical and microbiological findings on newly inserted hydroxyapatite-coated and pure titanium human dental implants. *Clin Oral Implants Res* 1991; 2: 121–127.
84. Gatewood RR, Cobb CM, and Killoy WJ. Microbial colonization on natural tooth structure compared with smooth and plasma-sprayed dental implant surfaces. *Clin Oral Implants Res* 1993; 4: 53–64.
85. Johnson BW. HA-coated dental implants: long-

term consequences. *J Calif Dent Assoc* 1992; 20: 33–41.
86. Zablotsky MH, Diedrich DL, and Meffert RM. Detoxification of endotoxin-contaminated titanium and hydroxyapatite and mechanical modalities. *Implant Dent* 1992c; 1: 154–158.
87. Zablotsky MH, Meffert R, Mills O, Burgess A, and Lancaster D. Macroscopic, microscopic and spectrometric effects of various chemotherapeutic agents on the plasma-sprayed hydroxyapatite-coated implant surface. *Clin Oral Implants Res* 1992; 3: 189–198.
88. Nancollas GH and Tucker BE. Dissolution kinetics characterization of hydroxyapatite coatings on dental implants. *J Oral Implantol* 1994; 20: 221–226.
89. Cranin AN, Mehrali M, and Baraoidan M. Hydroxyapatite-coated endosteal implants from the clinicians' perspective. *J Oral Implants* 1994; 20: 235–239.
90. Takeshoita F, Kuroki H, Yamasaki A, and Suetsugu T. Histologic observation of seven removed endosseous dental implants. *Int J Oral Maxillofac Implants* 1995; 10: 367–372.
91. van Blitterswijk CA, Grote JJ, Kuypers W, Blok-vanHoek CJ, and Daems WT. Bioreactions at the tissue/hydroxylapatite interface. *Biomaterials* 1985; 6: 243–251.
92. Muller-Mai CM, Voigt C, and Gross U. Incorporation and degradation of hydroxyapatite implants of different surface roughness and surface structure in bone. *Scan Microsc* 1990; 4: 613–624.
93. Eggli PS, Muller W, and Schenk RK. Porous hydroxyapatite and tricalcium phosphate cylinders with two different pore size ranges implanted in the cancellous bone of rabbits. *Clin Orthop Related Res* 1988; 232: 127–138.
94. Muller-Mai CM, Stupp SI, and Gross U. Nanoapatite and organoapatite implants in bone: histology and ultrastructure of the interface. *J Biomed Mater Res* 1995; 29: 9–18.
95. Bauer TW, Geesink RCT, Zimmerman R, and McMahon JT. Hydroxyapatite-coated femoral stems. *J Bone Joint Surg* 1991; 73: 1439–1452.
96. Block MS, Finger IM, Frontenot MG, and Kent JN. Loaded hydroxyapatite-coated and grit-blasted titanium implants in dogs. *Int J Oral Maxillofac Implants* 1989; 4: 219–225.
97. Maistrelli GL, Mahomed N, Fornasier V, Antonelli L, Li Y, and Binnington A. Functional osseointegration of hydroxyapatite-coated implants in a weight-bearing canine model. *J Arthroplasty* 1993; 8: 549–553.
98. Lewandowski JA and Johnson CM. Structural failure of osseointegrated implants at the time of restoration. A clinical report. *J Prosthet Dent* 1989; 62: 127–129.
99. Soballe K, Brockstedt-rasmussen H, Hansen ES, and Bunger C. Hydroxyapatite coating modifies implant membrane formation: controlled micromotion studied in dog. *Acta Orth Scand* 1992; 63: 128–140.
100. Soballe K, Hansen ES, Brockstedt-rasmussen H, and Bunger C. Tissue ingrowth into titanium and hydroxyapatite-coated implants during stable and unstable mechanical conditions. *J Orthop Res* 1992b; 10: 285–299.
101. Kent JN, Block MS, Finger KM, Guerra L, Larsen H, and Misiek DJ. Biointegrated hydroxyapatite-coated dental implants; 5 years clinical observations. *J Am Dent Assoc* 1990; 121: 138–144.
102. Saadoun AP and LeGall ML. Clinical results and guidelines on Steri-Oss endosseous implants. *Int J Periodont Rest Dent* 1992; 121: 487–499.
103. Golec TS and Krauser JT. Long-term retrospective studies on hydroxyapatite-coated endosteal and subperiosteal implants. *Dent Clin North Am* 1992; 36: 39–65.
104. Kawahara H. Biomaterials for dental implants, in *Encyclopedic Handbooks and Bioengineering* 1995; (Wise DL, et al., eds), M. Dekker, New York, pp. 1469–1524.
105. Block MS and Kent JN. Placement of endosseous implants into tooth extraction sites. *J Oral Maxillofac Surg* 1991; 49: 1269–1276.

4

Characterization of Water Inhibition in Light-Cured Dental Resins

Kristen L. Droesch, Brian J. Love, and Virginie M. Vaubert

1. Introduction

The conversion of medical resins in vivo occurs with increasing regularity, both in clinical practice and from a research perspective. In adhesive bonding for medical applications, most of these curing resin systems use a free radical polymerization mechanism to advance the chemical reaction and solidify the resin *(1)*. Chemical conversion is usually accomplished by either a light activation system, which triggers the decomposition of an activator in the resin, or by direct chemical reaction, through mixing of components in a two-part system. Inhibition of the free radical polymerization by oxygen has been reported in the literature *(1)*. Given that bony tissues, including dentin and other soft tissues, contain a substantial amount of water, the presence of water is ultimately an unavoidable circumstance in a large number of medical applications involving adhesives. Water is a key component of mineralized tissues, and cannot be readily removed without destruction of the tissue. Under ordinary circumstances, clean, dry surfaces are necessary for successful bonding. For long-term bonding in vivo, adhesives must successfully compete with water at the bond interface *(2)*. How conversion has been affected by the presence of water has not been adequately characterized, but it has generally been considered a problem. Efforts have been undertaken to reduce the overall impact of water by drying the environment in which the resin application is performed *(3)*.

In the area of dental materials, dental resins based on *bis*-glycidyl methacrylate (Bis-GMA) have been developed for a wide range of performance applications, including pit and fissure sealants, composite restoratives, and orthodontic adhesives. Pit and fissure sealants isolate tooth defects from the ingress of oral fluids and bacteria, which contribute to the initiation and propagation of caries *(4)*. Pits and fissures are an enamel fault resulting from lack of coalescence of enamel during tooth formation. Pits and fissures may extend to the dentin enamel junction, or to a lesser depth of the enamel *(3)*. There are also applications for enamel adhesives in terms of orthodontic appliance bonding *(5–7)*. Other types of acrylate-based natural tissue adhesives have been developed, and acrylic bonding cements are commonly used in a range of orthopedic bonding applications for mechanically bonding to bone *(8)*.

There already is a wealth of published work highlighting the effects of resin processing on formed properties, in terms of mechanical performance, optical quality, and, more recently, extractable resin fractions *(9)*. This work includes some of own work that indicates higher residual monomer is available as an extractable residue as the conversion process deviates from nonideality

(10–11). Whether variations in processing ultimately affect performance is an open question.

2. Experimental

2.1. Materials

Experiments were conducted to investigate the effects of polymerizing dental resin in water. Bis-GMA resin was obtained from Cook Composites and Polymers (Kansas City, MO). Three parts triethylene glycol dimethacrylate (TEGDMA) was added to one part Bis-GMA resin as a co-monomer, to reduce the viscosity of the Bis-GMA resin. Following the mixing of these resins, 2,6 dimethyl paratoluidine and camphorquinone each were added, in 2 wt% fractions, as initiator and activator for the resin, respectively. These other components were obtained from Aldrich (Milwaukee, WI). Following the mixing of these additional components, the resin was stored in a container wrapped in aluminum foil, to prevent unintended curing. This model resin formulation was chosen to minimize resin complexity and focus on conversion.

2.2. Methods

A Patterson commercial blue-light illumination system, emitting a maximum intensity near a wavelength of 440 nm, with an intensity of 250 mW, was used for resin curing. Specimens were fabricated by constructing resin molds, using silicone rubber bonded to a glass substrate, with cavities in the silicone rubber that allowed the resin to be introduced. The dimensions of each resin cavity were approx 5×14 mm. The resin volume was optimized to create specimens that were approx 1 mm thick. Once the resin cavities were filled, these samples were immediately cured, using the illumination wand. A second group was carefully lowered into a water bath, then cured using the same illumination conditions for the samples in air. Curing conditions for each resin specimen were 60 s rastered over the lateral area of the resin cavity, which led to a curing dose of 2.1 J/mm^2.

Difficulty was encountered regarding resin flow for the specimens cured under water. When the resin in the mold initially encountered the water, some resin was displaced above the cavity onto the silicone rubber, thus reducing the amount of resin in the resin cavity. This resulted in a nonuniform thickness in each mold specimen. This difficulty was attributed to surface energy of the mold–water interface, causing a layer of the mold to be wetted by the resin. Samples in the mold were sanded to provide even thickness. Resin displaced onto the mold surface was very thin, but even in thickness. Those thinner specimens allowed analysis of resin conversion directly in contact with water.

2.2.1. Dynamic Mechanical Spectroscopy

Following the curing and extraction of the specimens from the mold, the specimens were mechanically tested using dynamic mechanical spectroscopy (DMS). The authors' system, a Perkin-Elmer DMA-7 model, uses a sinusoidal strain input, and measures the dynamic force output on a beam specimen in flexure. By performing the test as a function of temperature, one can assess the variation in the phase angle between strain and load. A maximum in the phase angle is often associated with mechanical transitions in the material, such as the glass transition temperature (T_g). For this testing regimen, the maximum in the loss tangent (tan δ) curve with temperature is identified as T_g. Given that the specimens had the potential to further age after they were initially made, a maximum of 30 min was allowed between curing of the specimen and the initiation of the dynamic mechanical analysis measurements.

As a result of the thickness variations in the specimens that were fabricated, each specimen used for DMS was polished to a uniform thickness following curing. Unfortunately, the required polishing procedure also removed material that would have most closely interacted with the water on the specimen surface. As a result, these specimens represented the behavior of the subsurface material, and could not be used to assess the impact of water directly adjacent to the resin surface.

For DMS, the specimens were loaded in a three-point bend fixture with a span width of 10 mm. Once polished, the specimens were approx 0.8 mm in height and 4.1 mm in width. The specimens were held at 20°C for 2 min before the temperature was raised to 100°C, at a constant rate of 3°C/min. The static force applied was within the range of 50 to 900 mN; the dynamic force applied was in the range of 41.70 to 750 m*N*. The large variation in the applied static and dynamic forces was the result of the thickness variation caused by polishing, as well as the need to maintain an amplitude deflection of at least 5 μm.

2.2.2. Mechanical Stress Relaxation

As was indicated in subheading 2.2., wicking of resin above the resin cavity on the top of the mold surface was observed after the molds were immersed in water, but prior to curing. This material on the top of the mold surface had excellent thickness control throughout, despite its lack of thickness. Immediately following curing, this material could be removed from the surface of the silicone rubber, and, using a die, the material could be punched into dog-bone-shaped specimens. These specimens were thus adaptable for testing in a mechanical load frame.

A Polymer Laboratories (Amherst, MA) Minimat Miniature Materials Tester was employed, equipped with a 200-N load beam for tensile testing. Dog-bone specimens were punched, using a die for specimens cured in air and cured while immersed in water.

The dog-bone specimens had average dimensions of 8 mm length, 2.7 mm width, and thickness in the range of 0.29–0.70 mm. Stress relaxation experiments were performed, in which the specimens were extended to 0.6 mm strain at a strain rate of 10 mm/min, using an initial load of 6 N. The load decay was recorded and collected for each specimen, and, knowing the dimensions of each specimen, the stress relaxation data was calculated and compared between material cured in water and material cured in air.

3. Results

3.1. Dynamic Mechanical Spectroscopy

Representative curves showing the dynamic mechanical performance of light-cured resin are included for material cured in air (Fig. 1) and in water (Fig. 2). These curves show the mechanical stiffness of the elastic storage modulus and the relative phase angle (tan δ) for each material as a function of temperature. The most telling difference is a depression of an average of 6°C in the temperature, associated with the maximum in the phase angle caused by curing in water. This sug-

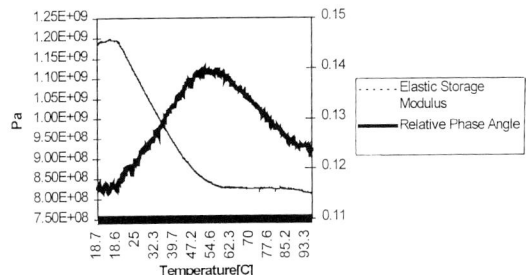

Fig. 1. DMS of Bis-GMA resin cured in air.

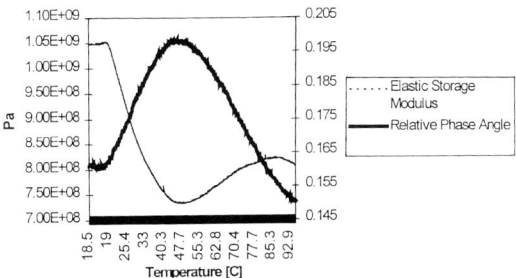

Fig. 2. DMS of Bis-GMA resin cured in water.

Table 1
Summary Comparison of T_g for Individual Resin Specimens Cured in Air, and in Water

Resin cured in air (°C)	Resin cured in water (°C)
50	44
51	50
52	40
51	

gests a measurable decrease in the overall amount of conversion as the result of curing under water. All results are shown in Table 1.

There are several factors contributing to the observed decrease in conversion: One is energy absorption, because of water in the optical pathway, between the source and the resin, decreasing the amount of energy directed at resin conversion. There is also a possibility that the water environment has increased convection that would also lead to lower overall conversion, although this likelihood is low. The other issue may be that the water somehow interferes with the resin conver-

Table 2
Summary of Constants Used to Fit Stress Relaxation Data

Sample no.	x_0	y_0	t_1	t_2	A_1	A_2	x^2
1 (Air)	9.93E-4	3.00	.137	1.74	3.47	1.75	1.04E-3
2 (Air)	−4.15E-4	2.16	.133	1.70	2.42	1.16	5.09E-4
3 (Air)	1.78E-3	3.23	.133	1.72	3.66	1.90	1.14E-3
4 (Water)	−9.93E-4	3.20	.133	1.52	3.41	1.60	1.14E-3
5 (Water)	−4.96E-3	3.39	.122	1.60	4.48	1.78	1.32E-3
6 (Water)	−1.26E-3	3.26	.137	1.68	4.50	2.08	1.61E-3

Summary of Values from Origin Used to Fit Data to $y_0 + A_1 e^{(-(x-x_0)/t_1)} + A_2 e^{(-(x-x_0)/t_2)}$.

3.2. Mechanical Stress Relaxation

Data from the stress relaxation tests were compared and analyzed using Microcal Origin 5.0. The data were empirically fit to a two-element Maxwell model, with the equation:

$$\sigma(t) = y_0 + A_1 e(-x(x-x_0)/t_1) + A_2 e(-x(x-x_0)/t_2).$$

$\sigma(t)$ is the value of stress as a function of time; x_0 corresponds to the time at which the stress relaxation test began; x corresponds to the time; additionally, t_1 and t_2 are the two corresponding time constants used for the two-element Maxwell model. The constants A_1 and A_2 relate to the vol-

sion. The direct mechanical testing would be a more telling gage.

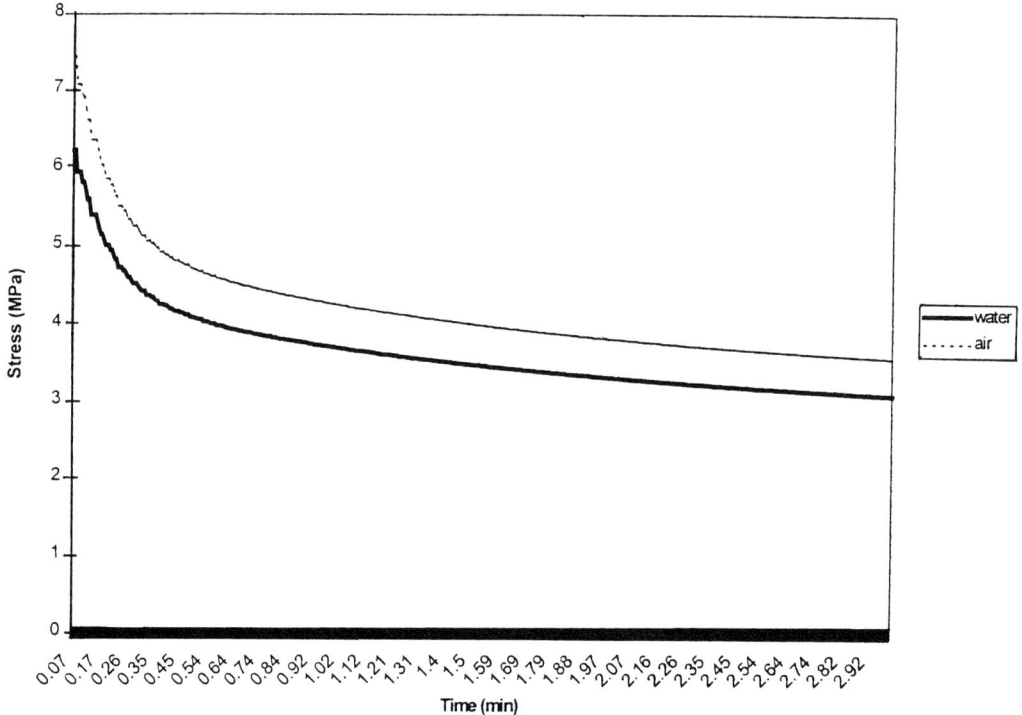

Fig. 3. Stress relaxation data for samples cured in water and in air.

ume fraction of each zone with each characteristic relaxation time. Nonviscoelastic behavior of the material is represented by the value y_0. The values calculated using this empirical fit are listed in Table 2, where χ^2 is a measure of how well the empirical model fits the raw data. Values of χ^2 close to zero denote a good fit. Figure 3 shows stress relaxation data of two specimens, each cured in air and in water. The resins cured in air had A_1 values, on average, 0.95 lower than the resins cured in water. The t_2 values of the resins cured in air were an average of 0.12 min higher than the resins cured in water. If A_1 corresponds to a fast relaxation time, the large A_1 values for specimens cured in water could be direct evidence of the decrease in conversion of material by curing in water.

Conclusions

Some effects have been observed in curing photopolymerized acrylate resins in a water environment. Nevertheless, curing is still evident, albeit with somewhat reduced conversion. The work suggests that, in other process environments, the resin is relatively robust in extending conversion. Only a slight depression in curing conversion has been observed in the authors' findings. The resin's ability to perform as an adhesive, after being exposed to water, is still being evaluated, but, with some level of substrate texturing, strength evolution is evident.

Acknowledgments

The authors would like to thank the Center for Adhesive and Sealant Science, the Adhesives and Sealants Council, the U. S. Navy, and the Department of Energy for their collective support of research in this area.

References

1 Williams D. *Concise Encyclopedia of Medical and Dental Materials*, 1990; Pergamon, New York, NY, pp. 8–14.
2 Williams D. *Biocompatibility of Dental Materials* vol. 2, 1982; CRC, Boca Raton, pp. 96–100.
3 Craig RG, O'Brien WJ, and Powers JM. *Dental Materials Properties and Manipulation* 1979; C.V. Mosby, St. Louis, MO, pp. 28–37.
4 Craig RG. *Dental Materials: a Problem Oriented Approach* 1978; C.V. Mosby, St. Louis, MO, pp. 1.
5 Meurman JH and Helminen SKJ. Effectiveness of fissure sealant 3 years after application. *Scand J Dent Res* 1976; 84: 218–233.
6 Ismail AI and Gagnon P. Longitudinal evaluation of fissure sealants applied in dental practices. *J Dent Res* 1995; 74: 1583–1590.
7 Eliades E, Eliades G, Brantley WA, and Johnston WM. Polymerization efficiency of chemically cured and visible light-cured orthodontic adhesives: degree of cure. *Am J Orthod Dentofac Orthop* 1995; 108: 294–301.
8 Eversoll DK and Moore RN. Bonding orthodontic acrylic resin to enamel. *Am J Orthod Dentofac Orthop* 1988; 93: 477–485.
9 Thompson LR, Miller EG, and Bowles WH. Leaching of unpolymerized materials from orthodontic bonding resin. *J Dent Res* 1982; 61: 989–991.
10 Vaubert VM. *Durability and Aging of Dental Fissure Sealants* 1997; MS Thesis, Virginia Polytechnic Institute and State University, Blacksburg, VA.
11 Vaubert VM, Moon PC, and Love BJ. Extractable free monomers from self cured dental sealants resulting from dispensing errors. *J Biomed Mater Res Appl Biomater* 1999; 48: 5–8.

5

Osseointegrated Dental Implants

Follow-up Studies

Günther Heimke and Cornelius G. Wittal

1. Introduction

Prospective, regular data registrations related to the essential features of surgical insertion of oral implants, their prosthodontic treatment, and follow-up examinations, as well as their eventual loss, began simultaneously with the introduction of implants that were intended for direct anchorage in their bony environment, in the late 1960s and early 1970s. Since that time, this kind of implant fixation has increasingly replaced the previous soft-tissue-encapsulated implants. This change in the intended mode of implant fixation occurred almost simultaneously in dental implantology and orthopedic reconstruction, e.g., joint replacements. It had become feasible by the observation of a particularly favorable kind of biocompatibility of titanium (Ti) and of alumina ceramics. Bony tissue directly contacting large portions of the surfaces of implants of these materials was observed. Extended studies allowed determination of the conditions for this interfacial contact and for subsequent long-term functional stability. Essentially, these conditions were found to be similar to the requirements of fracture healing, in particular, an initial press-fitting of the implant in its bony bed and the maintenance of motionlessness along the interface for a period of at least 3 mo. In animal experiments, components of total hip replacements and dental implants of these materials could be found rigidly fixed in the adjacent bone. These observations have also been seen clinically, and have been fully confirmed in thousands of cases since. The term "osseointegration" was soon coined for this kind of implant anchorage.

The results of follow-up studies of up to more than 30 yr are now available. Essentially two important studies were commenced with the introduction of two new types of implants and materials: one in Göteborg, Sweden, by Brånemark *(1)* and his team with specially designed Ti screws, in the mid 1960s, and the other in Tübingen, Germany, by Schulte et al. *(2)*, with a stepped cylindrical implant of alumina ceramic, in the mid 1970s. Publication of the early results, about 5–10 yr follow-up studies of these systems *(3–7)*, had been the first well-based documentation on the reliability of dental implants generally.

Other systems soon followed such as the International Team for Implantology (ITI) hollow cylinders, coated with Ti powders along their intraosseous portions, by Schröder et al. *(8)*, Berne, Switzerland; the Intra-Mobile Zahn (tooth) implant (IMZ) invented by Koch *(9)*, Hamburg, Germany, modified and carried on by Kirsch and

Ackermann *(10)*, Filderstadt, Germany; and the ITI titanium plasma sprayed (TPS) screws of Ledermann *(11)*, Herzogenbuchsee, Switzerland.

Although the thorough documentation of the Göteborg and Tübingen follow-up studies had been the first in this field of dentistry, and had been initiated independently, the kind and extent of data collected, as well as their methods of presentation, had been different. In addition, the two first systems initially aimed at different areas of indications: The Göteborg team aimed at the treatment of the completely edentulous jaw; the Tübingen group tried to avoid, or at least reduce, the occurrence of edentulousness, by the introduction of implants that could be inserted immediately or shortly after the loss of a tooth into an otherwise undisturbed set of teeth. Thus, e.g., the age distribution of the patients of both groups differed considerably, and so did the locations of the implants. Such basic differences limited a direct judgment of these initially different approaches into the field of dental implantology, by the comparison of simple figures of implant survival times. After their favorable initial results, however, both teams extended their ranges of indications, and, by now, have, besides their primary fields, some overlapping ranges of indication.

Obviously, the other systems had not started with such relatively confined intentions, but some inherent limitations are simply given by their geometry. The IMZ implant, e.g., can hardly be placed into a freshly exposed extraction site.

Generally, the reported success rates change when systems pass from the hands of their originators into general use. This could be observed when the application of the polymethylmethacrylate bone cement in total hip surgery left Charnley's clinic *(12)* and became routinely used, even in small country hospitals *(13)*. The osseointegrated dental implant systems were no exception.

Reports on the performance of the first-mentioned systems had established new standards in judgment of dental implant systems. The others tried to follow them. All these systems have stood the test of more than two decades of large-scale application in hospitals, clinics, and offices. Thus, they have established a high level of success rates on which evaluations of any new system, and even any intended improvement of existing systems, must be based. General agreement seemed to exist on some minimum requirements on this level of performance *(14)*, such as a survival rate of 85–90% after 5 yr and 75–80% after 10 yr, and no marked further reduction thereafter. As already mentioned, any serious and detailed discussion of the advantages or limitations of the different osseointegration-intended dental implant systems must consider many more particularities of the systems concerned.

Neither the Göteborg nor the Tübingen dental implant system had reached the aforementioned performance criteria at the beginning. Both experienced failure rates on the order of 50% during their initial periods, as can be seen from the summary in Table 1. The experiences of the two pioneering groups are available now, and must be accounted for by anyone hoping to achieve further improvements. Thus, the learning curve of any newcomer should at least be less pronounced and reach its final high level earlier.

2. Performance Criteria

The follow-up studies on the Göteborg and Tübingen implant systems were the first with reliable standards *(3–7)*, and had been designed independently. The originators of both tried to document and describe, as carefully as they could judge from their general experiences and the foregoing animal experiments, anything relevant for successful treatments and for a rational analysis of possible failures. From the beginning, the Göteborg group distinguished between *in situ* remaining implants (which they preferred to call fixtures) and bone-anchored bridges; only *in situ* remaining and functioning implants were considered successful by the Tübingen Group, and implants that had been lost or removed were considered failures. It was soon realized, however, that this straightforward description might either not allow for a sufficiently clear description of the particular features and merits of one or the other system, or might not result in a true picture. The situation became more complicated as soon as more follow-up studies were published on other implant systems, and, thus, naturally demanded performance comparisons. Of course, there may have been, and may still be, advocates of single implant systems who cannot resist defining criteria for success that favors their own system. However, such obvious

Table 1
Initial Problem Cases of Göteborg and Tübingen Implant Systems
(Percentage of Removed Fixtures or Implants)

Period	Göteborg[a]		Tübingen[b]
	Upper jaw (%)	Lower jaw (%)	(%)
First about 2 yr	50	48	54[c]
Development period (about 3 yr)	55	24	
First 5 yr accumulated			30.5[c]
First routine period (about 4 yr)	23	10	10.4
First 10 yr accumulated	37	16	23[c]

[a]Values taken from ref. 4.
[b]Values taken from refs. 6 and 7.
[c]Calculated from refs. 6 and 7 to include the failures of the clinical trial period (during the second year) with implants of different shapes and surfaces, and otherwise deviating from the original design and later routine procedure.

attempts can still contribute to evaluation if the biased aspects are carefully dismantled, so that the facts presented can be considered correctly.

The most simple method of describing the performance of an implant system is counting all implants found *in situ* after a selected period of time, and comparing this figure with the number of those originally inserted. Obviously, this would give a picture of some value only if all patients had followed the recall; otherwise, the result may be too pessimistic: Those who died or moved away, with their implants still functioning well, would not have been considered. If, on the other hand, the number of implants found *in situ* is compared with the number of patients seen in this recall, this ratio would be much too optimistic, because it would completely disregard the drop-outs, such as those who lost their implants or changed the place of treatment. Thus, any survival figure must be either corrected accordingly, or accompanied by all relevant information.

But even a correctly described survival statement can be misleading: A free-standing implant found *in situ,* but mobile, will have a considerably reduced chance of survival, and, with a high probability, will be found lost at the next examination. The same kind of implant supporting an extended bridge, together with two, three, or even more implants, can, if mobile, remain *in situ* much longer, possibly causing extended bone resorptions and severe damage to the adjacent tissue.

Many other aspects can influence the results of implant procedures besides their different indication ranges, as mentioned in the Introduction. One is the ability of an implant system to allow for treatments in particularly difficult cases, such as around fracture sites or into transplants. Another is the amount of damage remaining in the case of implant loss or removal. Thus, the pure comparison of even correctly presented survival data can give neither a complete picture nor allow for a justified judgment. In an attempt to gain a more realistic survey, some groupings of possible influences on the success rates of implants are suggested.

2.1. Material and Shape-related Criteria

The most detailed data on implant performance have become available on Ti and alumina ceramic implants. It had been the realization of the particular tissue compatibility (the bioinertness) of these materials that motivated the Göteborg *(1)* and Tübingen *(2)* teams to explore their potential for improved dental implants. In the latter system, the experiences of the first 15 yr of clinical application have allowed introduction of an additional Ti implant system preserving most of the chief design characteristics of the previous one, and avoiding its problem areas. Five yr of careful follow-up studies are available now.

For metal implants, commercially pure Ti is mostly used. Its yield strength, $Rp_{0.2} = 300$ N/mm^2, as well as its fatigue strength, $F_b = 200$ N/mm^2 *(15)* are less than half of those of the Ti-

Table 2
Grouping of Materials for Bony Reconstruction According to Their Compatibility in Bony Tissue

Degree of compatibility	Typical reactions of bony tissue	Materials
Biotolerant	Implants separated from adjacent bone by a soft tissue layer along most of the interface: distant osteogenesis.	Stainless steels; PMMA bone cements and cobalt-based alloys
Bioinert	Direct contact to bone tissue: contact osseogenesis.	Alumina ceramics; zirconia ceramics, Ti, tantalum, niobium
Bioactive	Bonding to bony tissue, in the sense of a gluing effect: bonding osteogenesis.	Ca-phosphate containing glasses and glass ceramics; HA and tri-calcium phosphate ceramics; Ti (?)

Table 3
Definitions of Terms Used for Compatibility Rating of Bone Replacement Materials

Degree of compatibility	Material influences on adjacent bony tissue	Result
Biotolerance (distance osteogenesis)	Components of the material, e.g., ions or monomers, are leaching into the surrounding tissue.	Irritation of the differentiation of precursor cells into osteoblasts, formation of a collagen-rich interlayer.
Bioinert (contact osteogenesis)	"Nothing goes into solution," leaking ions and other matter below detectability of adjacent tissue. Fast absorption of molecules from body fluent, (coating).	No biochemical influences on cell activities, no biochemical information about presence on implant. No enzyme-controlled foreign body reactions, implant camouflaged against host's immune system.
Bioactive (bonding osteogenesis)	Deposition of collagen and/or HA from the surrounding bone onto the surface of the implant.	Bond formation in the sense of a gluing effect.

6 aluminum-4-vanadium and Ti-5 aluminum-2,5 iron alloys used in orthopedic joint replacements. However, if the dimensions of the dental implants are chosen accordingly, these mechanical specifications are sufficient. Any statement on the biocompatibility of Ti and its a.m. alloys (as well as any other sufficiently bioinert material) must distinguish between two aspects: the pure material property, and possible influences of surface undulations. As far as the material properties are concerned, Ti and these alloys can be categorized as bioinert, in the sense detailed in Table 2 (suggested by Osborn [16], but modified) and Table 3. The questionable mentioning of Ti in the bioactive category indicates some caution, because this feature may rather be the result of surface modifications than an inherent material property. In the first report *(1)* on the Göteborg implants, a particular, but not precisely defined, surface roughness was mentioned as an essential feature for the achievement of a close bone contact. Similar bone contact to a Ti alloy was observed on shafts of femoral components of hip replacements by Lintner et al. *(17)*. The influences of the surface topography on the response of soft tissue, reported by Campbell and von Recum *(18)* must also be considered, because they were also seen on Ti surfaces *(19)*. Some influence by the loading on the remodeling of the bony tissue around the Göteborg implants was also observed in their early animal experiments *(1)*, but no conclusions regarding the shape of the implant were drawn.

The special kind of tissue compatibility of alumina ceramics had originally been reported by Hulbert et al. *(20)*. More detailed studies established the conditions under which implants of this bioinert material can be reliably stabilized in their bony bed (for a survey, *see* ref. 21). One surprising observation was the close similarity of the stress and strain field controlled reactions of the bony tissue in the vicinity of implants in oral and orthopedic surgery *(22)*. Thus, it is the load distribution created by the implant in its bony environment that is responsible for the results of the remodeling processes. If there are too many large interfaces along which the forces (of chewing in dentistry, or of walking in hip and knee replacements) are acting parallel, relative movements will result in interfacial motion, and a soft tissue layer will form. If, on the other hand, an interface remains either essentially load-free or is met by the forces perpendicularly (pressure), or nearly so, all processes of fracture healing can progress step by step and establish a close bone contact (within the resolution of optical microscopy), as had been shown by Griss et al. *(23)*. Figure 1 schematically demonstrates and summarizes these considerations.

This observation implies that, in a compatibility study in bony tissue, many different kinds of tissue can be found adjacent to one single test piece, depending on the stresses that had been acting during the implantation time at the site of the interface from which the tissue sample was taken. Therefore, any histologically based judgment on the biocompatibility of a material in bony tissue, not accompanied by information on the loading condition at the location concerned, is worthless *(24,25)*.

Following these design rules, the Tübingen alumina ceramic implant was supplied with steps offering interfaces that transfer the principal components of the chewing forces perpendicularly into the adjacent bony tissue. For additional stability, the implants were supplied with lacunae *(26)*, as can be seen in Fig. 2. The validity of this design concept was confirmed histologically with samples removed from human patients in three cases of accidental or bite trauma after approx 2 yr of normal functioning *(27)*. Mobility measurements of these implants point in the same direction *(28)*.

None of the osseointegration-intended implants have any design features undercutting the adjacent bone beyond the depth of the threads. This is particularly true for the Tübingen implant, with its stepped cylinders with apically decreasing diameters. If such implants are lost, the remaining

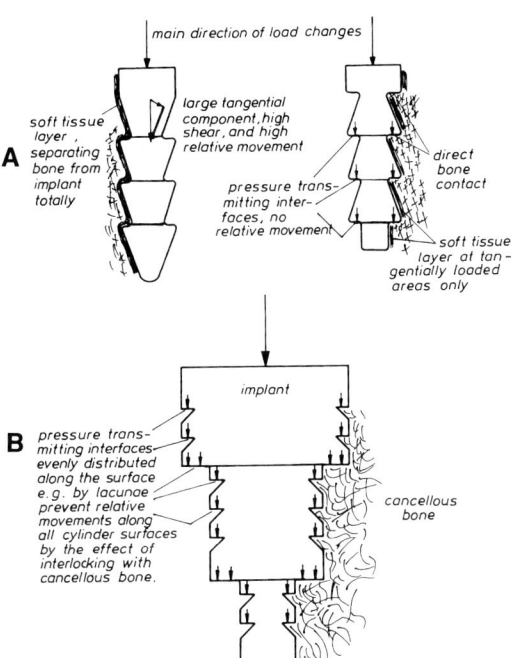

Fig. 1. Schematic presentation of the stress-and-strain-field-controlled tissue reactions around differently shaped implants. **(A)** Screw-type implant with differently oriented threads. (Left) Cross-section of threads similar to bone screws, resulting in a strong force component during screwing-in, pointing in the direction of the arrow on top. As a dental implant, however, the main components of the chewing forces meet most of the interfaces tangentially. (Right) Screw with threads offering essentially perpendicularly oriented surfaces for the transition of the chewing forces into the bony tissue. No relative movements along these pressure transmitting interfaces, and, thus, close bone contact possible. Example: Ledermann screw. **(B)** Cylindrical implant with stepwise decreasing cross-sections carrying lacunae along the surfaces of the cylinders for additional interlocking. Example: Tübingen (Frialit) implant.

cavities are not larger than any normal extraction hole. If the indications allow, these implants even can be replaced by a new implant immediately or soon afterward.

The design features discussed above for Ti and alumina ceramic implants must be regarded as a set of minimum requirements that must be met by any new implant. The survival probability of implants violating these rules is considerably reduced.

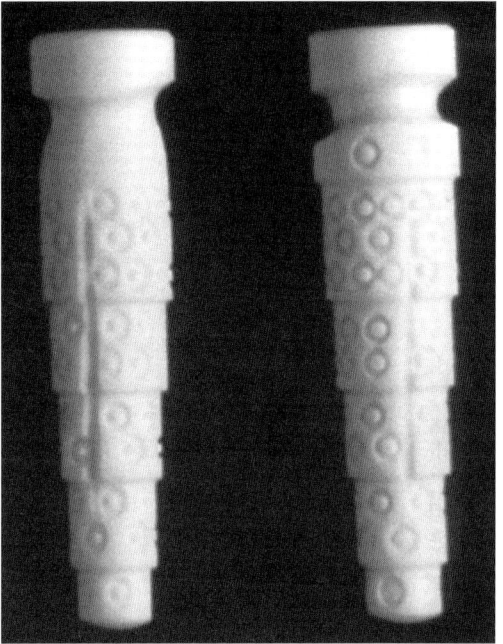

Fig. 2. Alumina ceramic implants (Frialit) with steps for essentially perpendicular load transmission and lacunae for additional stabilization by ingrown bone. (Right) Original Tübingen implant with highly polished coronal groove for the protected accommodation of the gingival margin. (Left) München (*Munic*) version with torpedo-shaped coronal portion. Its pergingival area is left in the as-fired state.

Besides the surface undulations of Ti on the threaded surfaces of the Göteborg implant and the macroscopic lacunae on the cylindrical surfaces of the Tübingen implants, essentially two other means for achieving an attachment of bony tissue along tangentially loaded interfaces have been suggested, experimentally studied, and have stood the test of at least two decades of clinical application. Both are coatings applied to the surfaces concerned, by flame- or plasma-spraying either fine Ti powders (with particle sizes on the order of a few microns) *(8,29)* or hydroxylapatite (HA) ceramics *(30,31)*. Both kinds of coatings have been applied to several dental implant systems.

Because the bioactivity of HA ceramics is the result of some chemical interaction with the surrounding body fluids and tissues, these materials cannot be regarded as completely stable *(32)*.

Therefore, a slowly progressing resorption of such coatings must be accounted for by providing these implants with design features that can maintain the osseointegration if the bioactive layers have gone.

2.2. Patient and Indication-related Criteria

Besides name, age, and sex of patients considered for implants, all major information on general health status should be considered and noted, such as poor or excessive oral hygiene, smoking habits, alcohol consumption, and medications, as well as particular observations on chewing and swelling. Any patient with more severe deviations from the average should be particularly motivated to follow the necessary precautions carefully. On recalls, the implants of such patients must be inspected with the peculiarities of these patients in mind. In case of difficulties with, or even loss of, implants, the possible influence of any of these parameters should be considered.

In addition, all relevant information concerning the oral cavity must be considered and noted, particularly the presence of inflammations of the gingiva, parodontites, paradontosis, and parafunctions. All details of the indication must also be noted carefully. The severe influences of the indications were clearly realized in the first 5-yr follow-up study of the Tübingen implant system *(6)*, as can be seen for some critical cases in Table 4.

2.3. Surgeon-related Criteria

The observation mentioned in the introduction, about a change of the success rates as soon as an implant system leaves the hands of its originator, can clearly be seen in the reports of the clinics that had been selected to join the premarket testing of the Tübingen implant system (collectively published in ref. 33). A direct demonstration of the influence of the learning effect could be found in an evaluation of 275 questionnaires returned from dentists in private offices on their experiences with Tübingen implants *(34)*. This questionnaire asked how long the system had been used in the particular office, as well as how long after insertion implant losses occurred. One of its results is reproduced in Fig. 3. Within the first 3 mo (the healing period), successes remain relatively high, but in the critical time of the supply with super-

Table 4
Critical Indications for Implantations and Their Success Rates

Indication	Success	Survival rate (%)	95% Confidential range (%)	Significance
Reimplantations	5/13	38	14–68	0.03
Adjacent cyst	13/27	48	29–68	0.02
Loss of tooth, not healed alveoli	33/39	84	69–94	0.05
Late implants	27/36	75	58–89	
Chronicle apical parodentitis	56/75	75	63–84	
Trauma	36/54	67	51–77	
Tooth fracture	36/49	73	59–85	
Root rest removed	43/61	70	57–81	
Total	178 of 256	70	63–75	

According to ref. 6.

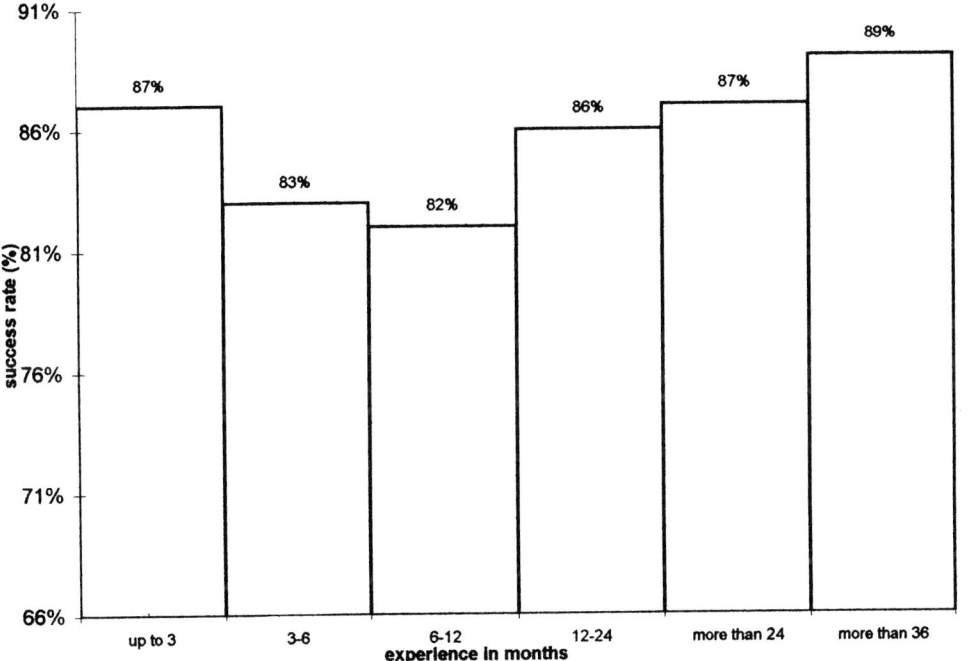

Fig. 3. The dependence of the rates of successfully accomplished implantations of Tübingen (Frialit) implants on the experience of 275 surgeons. Typical learning curve.

structures and the subsequent early loading period, implant losses are more frequent, until, for the longer periods, the typical learning effect becomes obvious.

Of course, all problems resulting from possible deviations from an optimal procedure are primarily surgeon-related (35). However, any implant system intended for application in an average dental office must account for the possibilities and limitations of this environment. Quantitative data and their correlation with an overtaxing of the average surgeon, for one or the other dental implant system, are difficult to establish and extremely rare. A comparison of the learning curves of different systems might be an approach to this problem. More of the most obviously surgeon-related problems are discussed in subheading 2.4.

2.4. Osseointegration-related Problems

Possible variations of the many single steps in the insertion of an implant are nearly unlimited for any given implant. They include the correctness of the indication, discussed above, all steps of preparation of the treatment and of the operational procedure, the guidance of the patient during the healing phase, and the choice and placement of the superstructure.

The preparation includes a careful evaluation of the situation of the gingiva and the bony tissue at the intended site of implantation. A mobile gingiva necessitates particular care. All implant systems demand particular, at least minimum, initial contact areas to the adjacent bone. If, e.g., the indication for a Tübingen implant is a traumatic tooth loss, more than half of the facial lamella must be preserved (36). An atraumatic drilling, with adequate cooling, is an absolute necessity (37) for all implants.

After the insertion of dental implants, three major kinds of treatment during the healing period must be distinguished:

1. Implant submerged underneath the gingiva. Full two-stage process (e.g., Göteborg, IMZ, Frialit-2 implants).
2. Implant perforates the gingiva, but is kept unloaded for the healing period. Protected two-stage procedure (e.g., Tübingen implant).
3. Implant perforates the gingiva, and is immediately supplied with the final superstructure, and loaded (e.g., Ledermann screw).

In the initial development study of the Göteborg system, different lengths of the protected healing period had been studied in dogs (1). In the Tübingen system, they were, additionally, clinically evaluated, with the results presented in Table 5 (6). Both data sets clearly confirm the previously mentioned comparison of the remodeling of bony tissue along the surface of a bioinert implant, with fracture healing derived from early animal studies with alumina ceramic implants.

The fact that nearly all reports about the survival rates of osseointegration-intended dental implants, as a function of time after insertion, do show a relatively high concentration of implant

Table 5
Success Rates of Tübingen Implants as Function of Length of Protected Healing in Period

Time till placement of superstructure (mo)	Success	Success rate (%)	95% Confidentiality limits (%)
0–2	9/23	39	19–61
3	16/20	80	56–94
4	39/44	89	75–96
5	31/36	86	71–95
6	29/32	91	75–98
7	16/19	84	60–97
8	12/13	92	64–99
9 or later	4–6	67	22–96

The authors note that the longer periods had been related to particularly critical cases.

losses for the healing and the early loading period, indicating that the remodeling process of the adjacent bony tissue is particularly sensitive, and must have been disturbed in these cases of early losses. As the most obvious reason, a lack of initial stability and/or a sufficient protection against loading must be assumed. This latter requirement is, obviously, much more demanding for an implant protruding through the gingiva into the oral cavity than for submerged implants.

If a sufficient bone contact had been achieved during the healing phase, it can be tested by probing the mobility of the implant, the percussive sound, and, more precisely, by the use of the Periotest method (38). The correct design and placement of the superstructure is the next critical step, as the loss rates during the initial loading period clearly indicate.

In at least one statistical evaluation of dental implant systems, however, all losses during the healing and loading phase, and, in addition, during the whole first year, had been ignored completely, and its time-scales do not commence until the placement and beginning of loading of the superstructure and after a 1-yr period (15 yr report of the Göteborg group [39]). But from the figures mentioned, at least a conclusion about the number of the early problem cases in this study is possible: From a total of 2768 insertions of implants (called fixtures in these papers), 1997 entered into their follow-up evaluation; thus 771, or 27.85%, of the initially inserted implants had not survived the first year. Obviously, the Göteborg system is no exception from the general observation of a concentration of losses during the healing and early loading period, as mention of 26% early failures in the first 10 yr report of this group *(4)* had indicated already. Rather, the early losses had increased. This was clearly confirmed in the 25-yr report, if the early losses mentioned in the previous reports for the different observation periods are accounted for. This will be discussed in some more detail in subheading 3.1.

When the superstructure is finally attached, essentially all components of the forces normally acting on the implant and deviating from the implant axis, should be kept as small as possible. A deviation of the axis of the crown of single-tooth replacements from the implant axis of more than 25 degrees results in a significant decrease in the success rate of Tübingen implants *(7)*. If large bridges or extended dentures are necessary, the deformation of the jaw under locally concentrated forces must be considered. The intramobile elements of the IMZ implants are an attempt to minimize these problems.

Most osseointegrated implants do show much-reduced loss rates after the healing and early loading periods. The vast majority of the relatively few cases of late losses can be related to events such as marginal bone loss, peri-implantites, and traumata. The Tübingen implant is more sensitive to damages by trauma, because of the inherent properties of the ceramic.

2.5. The Pergingival Portion

The parts of dental implants protruding from their endosseous portions through the subcutaneous tissue and the gingiva into the oral cavity, must provide a safe and reliable protection against any infiltration from the oral cavity. Because the majority of early tooth losses must be attributed to at least a partial reduction of this protection, the significance of this problem is obvious. From the same point of view, it is obvious that this requirement demands, for an implant and implant material, what natural teeth hardly can provide.

The much higher long-term success rates of all osseointegrated dental implants, compared to the previous, mostly soft-tissue-encapsulated implants of the same materials, can be attributed mostly to the marked reduction of mechanical irritations at this critical junction between the implants and the margins of the surrounding gingiva *(40)*. Inflammations, epithelial downgrowths, and the resulting infections caused by the unphysiologic movements of those loose implants led to an additional destruction of the surrounding bony tissue, and to still larger movements, and, thus, to a self-amplifying effect.

Although the quality of the degree of osseointegration can be tested nondestructively by indirect means, such as mobility measurements and the percussive sound only, the state of the attachment of the gingiva to the post of an implant can be assessed more directly by determining the pocket depth and the sulcus fluid flow rate (SFFR). In the first 10-yr follow-up report on the Göteborg implants *(4)*, a periabutment gingivitis was mentioned for all patients. The mean gingival index score was 1.23 ± 0.48, and a crevice of 3.72 ± 2.29 mm lingually and 2.10 ± 2.55 mm buccally, was mentioned. In the 15-yr report on the Göteborg implants, a mean clinical pocket depth of 2.6 mm ($sd = 0.9$) is reported *(39)*. The results of the first SFFR measurements, comparing the state of the gingival margin around implants and teeth of the same patient, was performed for Tübingen implants for times between 3 and 18 mo by Schareyka *(41)*, and, surprisingly, showed identical or even slightly more favorable values for osseointegrated implants than for healthy teeth of the patients. Markedly higher SFFR values were found around loose implants, indicating the influence of mechanical irritations. Measurements of both values, pocket depth and SFFR, during the first 5-yr period around Tübingen implants and natural, similarly located teeth of the same patients, showed average pocket depths of 2.2 mm and average SFFR values of 1 mm for teeth and implants alike, which remained constant during the observation period *(5)*. The SFFR measurements around osseointegrated Ti implants of similar dimensions showed higher values (average 3 mm) *(39)*. A similar difference between osseointegrated Ti and alumina ceramic implants was seen by Tetsch and Dhom *(42)* and was confirmed by Büsing and d'Hoedt *(43)*. Some results are summarized in Table 6 *(44)*.

The occurrence of plaque on the Ti Göteborg implants is described by a plaque index of 13.7

Table 6
Comparison of SFFR and Pocket Depths for Teeth and Implants of Ti and Alumina Ceramic

Details of study	Teeth	Implants		Comments
		Ceramic	Metal	
No. cases	131	66	135	Ref. 42
SFFR in relative units	7.8	5.5	12	Up to 6 yr po
No. cases	178	178[a]		Ref. 7
SFFR in mm	1	1		Up to 5 yr po
Pocket depths in mm	2.2	2.2		
No. cases	39	39[b]		Ref. 44
SFFR in mm	1	1		Up to 4 yr po
Pocket depths in mm	2.2	2.2		

[a]Round implants with diameters of 4–7 mm.
[b]Oval implants with long axis of cross-section of 6–9 mm.

($s = 21.5$) *(39)*. The occurrence of plaque on alumina ceramic implants was such a rare event that no plaque index was recorded in their follow-up studies. However, at least one case was observed and mentioned *(45)*. This behavior was, and still is, surprising, because of the high surface energy of this material and its wetting and blood clotting favoring behavior *(46)*.

The differences in the protection against loading during the healing period of the Göteborg and the Tübingen implants must also be considered in a comparison of the parameters describing the state of the gingiva adjacent to the pergingival portion of the Ti and alumina ceramic implants. Any full two-stage procedure necessitates a re-exposure of the bone and a second healing of the already irritated gingiva; in the protected two-stage procedure, this is confined to one operation only. There is another point of view still: In any full two-stage procedure, the pergingival part of the implant is a separate unit, usually fixed to the main implant body by a screw. Thus, inherently, there must exist a junction between the two parts of such an implant, which is not present in the single-piece implant of the protected two-stage and of the one-stage procedure. This junction is located in the most sensitive and critical zone of any dental implant. Any tiny crevice in this area must be regarded as critical. There is another point of view still: Usually, the main implant body and its pergingival part are of the same metal. However, because both components were subjected to different manufacturing steps, their metals had undergone at least slightly different mechanical deformations, assuming they were taken from the same ingot. Different plastic deformations of identical metals lead to slightly different electrochemical potentials. This influence will probably remain insignificant in normal cases, because of the highly protective Ti oxide surface layers on both parts. In cases of mechanical damages, or of more severe chemical disturbances by food of low pH value reaching this junction, galvanic influences amplifying ongoing tissue disturbances cannot be excluded. A similar influence was also discussed recently by Büsing et al. *(47)*.

From this point of view, osseointegrated one-piece Ti implants should show more favorable figures of merit for the gingival margin than full two-stage implants. Unfortunately, the 7-yr follow-up report of Ledermann *(48)* does not contain quantitative information on the state of the gingival margin. In a study with 872 TPS Ledermann screws in 231 patients, 49 randomly selected patients with 176 screws were carefully followed, and, besides other data, the plaque and bleeding index, the pocket depth, and the width of the fixed mucosa were recorded for up to 110 mo *(49)*. The comparative study of some implant systems of d'Hoedt and Schulte also contains gingival-margin-related values *(50)*. For the IMZ implant system, gingival-margin-related data were measured and reported by Batenburg et al. *(51)*. A comparison of their average values of pocket depth and plaque index, with the equivalent values from previously mentioned studies, is given in

Table 7
Comparison of Parameters Describing State of Gingival Margin to Different Single-piece and Full Two-stage Implants of Different Materials

Implant type	Full two-stage implants Ti		Single-piece implants	
	Göteborg	IMZ	Ti TPS screw	Alumina ceramic Tübingen
Pocket depths, mm	2.6[a]	3.6[b]	2.4[c]	2.2[d]
Plaque index	21.7[a]		1.2[c]	–

Information from: [a] ref. 39, [b] ref. 51, [c] ref. 49, [d] refs. 7 and 44.

Table 7. The intermediate values for the TPS Ledermann screw for the pocket depths and the plaque index (assuming a close-to-zero value for the Tübingen implant, as discussed above) seem to point in the direction of a possible influence of the presence of a crevice and of two electrochemically not completely identical materials in the highly sensitive immediately subgingival region. A recent experimental study of this kind of influence confirmed these clinically derived conclusions (52).

From the values presented in Tables 6 and 7, the unique position of the alumina ceramic in the pergingival portion of dental implants is correctly expressed. Thus, a composite implant, with a Ti intraosseous portion and a pergingival part made of alumina ceramic, appears to be closer to an optimal solution. Possibilities for a realization of such an implant will be discussed in subheading 4.

2.6. Esthetic and Cosmetic Aspects

The esthetics of dental implants can best be discussed from two points of view: the picture presented by the implant and the superstructure in speaking, singing, and so on, and the maintenance or restoration of the contour of the alveolar process and, thus, the facial appearance of the patient.

As far as the margin of an implant surpasses the gingiva and is not completely covered underneath or behind a crown, the white alumina ceramic has much advantage in all cosmetic aspects, compared to any metal. The importance of this point of view increases with longer survival times of implants, because of the natural, slowly progressing height reduction of the alveolar crest. For well-integrated Tübingen implants, this reduction was found to be similar to, and of the same order of magnitude as, natural teeth. In addition, the exceptional compatibility of this ceramic with gingival tissue has led to the recommendation to place all superstructures on alumina ceramic implants safely away from the gingiva, whenever cosmetics allow (36).

Following the initial concept of the Tübingen implant (also called Frialit implant, because of the trade name for the alumina ceramic of its manufacturer), many of them were inserted immediately or relatively soon after tooth losses in patients of nearly all age groups with mostly still well-preserved alveolar ridges. From the point of view of their intended osseointegration, with its completely different kind of load transition into the surrounding bony tissue compared to the situation around natural teeth, the increasingly convincing observation of a nearly identical preservation of the alveolar ridge around these implants to that around natural teeth of the same age group was by no means trivial (35). This secondary aesthetic aspect of immediate implants was subsequently also found with other implants of sufficient size, if inserted in alveolar processes that were not yet too atrophied.

Beyond the preservation of the alveolar ridge, its restoration has been attempted in cases in which it was found collapsed or resorbed to a degree no longer allowing for the insertion of an esthetically satisfying implant. Nentwig (53) employed the "bone splitting technique" for inserting his modification of the original Tübingen (Frialit) implant, shown in the left part of Fig. 2, in some cases in combination with the application of HA granules as an augmentation. This method was carried further still, using special flap techniques, by Bruschi and Scipioni (54). In following the bone remodeling processes over time, by X-ray CT scans in different levels for Tübingen implants in comparison to a neighboring ancyloted tooth, they could document the additional bone apposition around the implants and the gradual decay of this tooth.

These implants, thus, allow not only for the preservation of the alveolar processes close to their natural situation, but they even permit their reconstruction. Neither of these effects can be expressed in a usual survival rate presentation of implant systems.

3. Results of Follow-up Studies

The different influences on the performance of the two principal dental implant systems discussed throughout suggest a variety of criteria by which successes and failures can and must be judged. Thus, the pure comparison of survival figures can be as misleading as the omission of whole sets of implants placed in particular periods. However, the basics of all more detailed evaluations (their raw material), remains the summary of all inserted implants in a period concerned, in survival graphs *(55,56)* as shown for the Tübingen implants in Fig. 4. Its details, such as the distribution of implant losses over time, or comments such as those about the amount of damages to the surrounding bone caused by failed implants and their removal or their avoidance, can be used as additional criteria on the merits of one or the other system.

3.1. Figures of Merit of the First Two Systems of Osseointegrated Implants

The prospectively planned documentation of the fate of each implant inserted by the Göteborg and the Tübingen team, and the strict follow-up regime maintained for these implants, created a new standard in dental implantology. Usually, new developments undergo some trial-and-error phase until they find the most appropriate solution. The presentations of the results of the follow-up studies, and their success and failure rates, are no exception. Both teams have changed the ways of describing the survival times of their implants several times, but always allow for a tracking back to the original facts.

An example of such a modification in the presentation of the figures of merit of an implant system has been mentioned in subheading 2.4.,

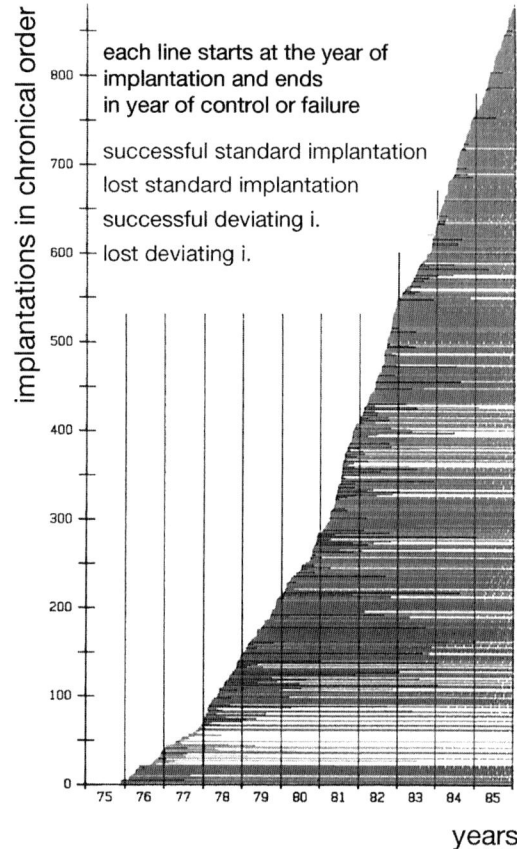

Fig. 4. Computer plot of the survival of all Tübingen (Frialit) implants inserted in the Tübingen clinic between the end of 1975 and 1986.

for a 15-yr follow-up study *(39)*. If the more than 27% first-year implant losses within the Göteborg system had not been omitted, but accounted for in the plots of their survival rate presentations, none of their numbers of implants *in situ* after 5, 10-, or 15 yr met their self-established and claimed success criteria of, e.g., at least 80% after 10 yr *(14)*. One can omit anything, and, if correctly mentioned, this may sometimes be justified and even necessary. But the numbers and trends derived from such modifications cannot at all be used for comparisons with and judgment on other systems, and definitely not for any claim of superiority *(57)*. In the 20-yr follow-up presentation of the Göteborg group *(58)*, early losses were claimed to be included. However, if compared with earlier presentations by this group, some inconsistencies remain: For example, in Table XVII on page 46 of ref. 4, 23% removed fixtures (of 503) are mentioned for the routine group period of July 1971 to June 1975, for the upper jaw. Similarly, in the 15-yr report *(39)*, 20% of mobile fixtures (implants) are mentioned in the upper jaw for the healing and 16% for the bridge-loaded period for routine group I in their Table 10 on page 404. In the 20-yr report *(58)*, the plot of the annual success rates of the fixtures in the maxillae of this same routine group claim a success rate of 80% for the same period. The graph in Fig. 4 on page 354 of ref. *58* shows, for the maxilla of routine group I, extending from July 1971 to July 1976, a success rate of 85%, for a total of 524 fixtures. If this graph is corrected for the 23% losses during the first 4 yr, the survival rates are well below 80% after 5 yr, and close to 75% after 10 yr. Note, however, that the 15-yr report considers only those implants that had survived the first year. Figure 5 is a partial reconstruction of the survival curve for the routine group I of Fig. 4 of ref. *58*. In addition, some correction appears justified also for routine group 2: In Table 4 of ref. *39*, a success rate of 88% is mentioned for the fixtures of routine group 2, in the upper jaw, after 4 yr. In the plot in Fig. 4 of ref. *58*, the 4-yr value is, for routine group 2, well above 90%. If this survival curve is extrapolated, accordingly, its 10-yr value is closer to 75% than to 80%.

The detailed discussion of the different performance criteria does not exclude the presentation of particular groups of implants. On the contrary, it even demands more sophisticated evaluations, for the sake of further improvements and an increase of the safety of implant systems. If desired, such subgroups of a total set of implants can be compared with those of sets of other implant systems, but only if these subsets are identically composed.

The originators of both of the first thoroughly documented sets of implants, those from Göteborg and from Tübingen (Frialit), soon felt the necessity of such a separate presentation of their late-placed implants from their initial ones. In this way, they accounted for what might be called their own learning phase. The Göteborg group distinguished between implants placed in their pilot period of the first 5 yr (called development group) and further 5-yr intervals (called routine groups) *(4,39,58)*. The Tübingen group separated a standard set of implants and treatments, characterized by their original material, shape, surface, and treatment protocol inserted during the first year, from implants of different shapes, surfaces, and/or treatments introduced during the second and part of the third year. The data presented in Tables 4 and 5 contain some of the results of these studies. As in the Göteborg group, parts of these variations served to define and understand the ranges and limits of indications, insertion techniques, and other details of the procedure beyond the possibilities of animal experiments. Within the third year, the Tübingen group returned to the original standard procedure. Later, the results achieved with the standard group, after the end of the development phase, were presented, in addition to those old-Frialit implants placed in Tübingen with the standard procedure.

If the modifications in the presentations of the Göteborg group are attempted to be corrected for, based on their previous statements, the approx 10-yr results of the Göteborg group, as redrawn in Fig. 5, are similar to those of the Tübingen team, as reproduced for their Frialit implants in Table 8. Both systems obviously reached a markedly reduced initial loss rate for all implants placed after the initial phases. This justifies the previously mentioned general requirements of success rates of 85–90% after 5 yr and 80–75% after 10 yr, and essentially constant success rates thereafter for all modifications of existing and new implant systems, after the completion of their development phases.

Generally, the extension of the indication range of well-proven implants must be regarded as similar to the introduction of a totally new system. If, however, the initially accumulated experiences are correctly applied, the problems encountered by the extension of the indications can be kept to a minimum, and close to the level of the original ranges. This could be achieved with Göteborg implants, in their applications to cases of partial edentulism *(59–61)*, placement in posterior maxillae *(62)*, and as single-tooth replacements *(63)*. Success rates ranged between slightly below 90% after 3 and 94% after 1 yr. The original concept of the Tübingen group with their immediate implants did not pose any restriction as to the locations of the implants in the jaws. The steps from direct,

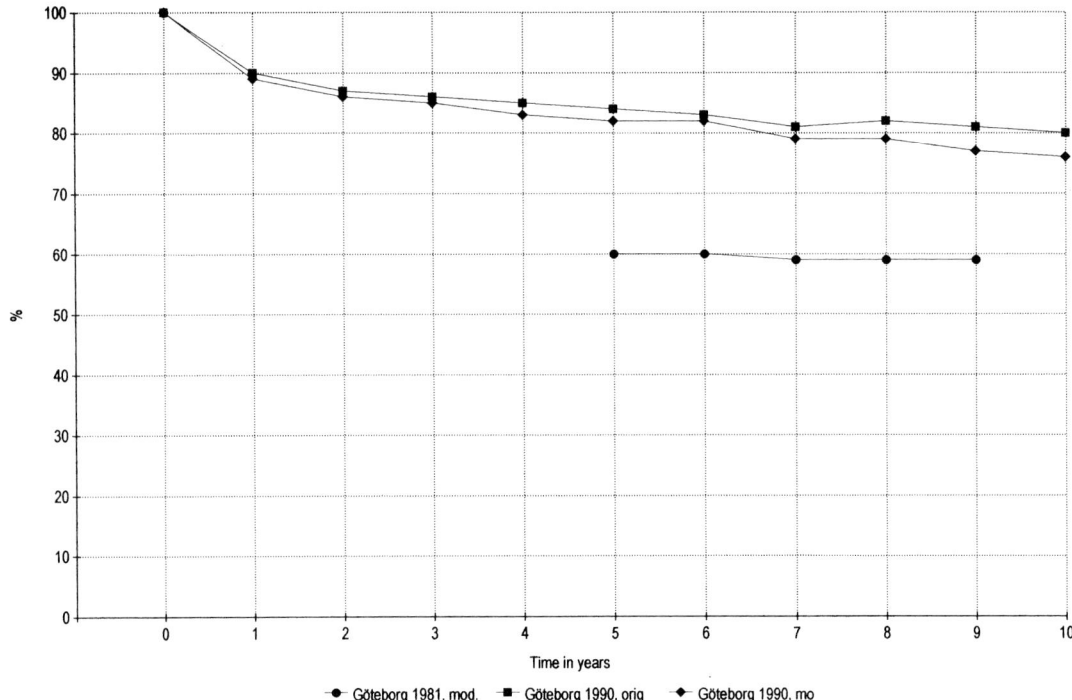

Fig. 5. Reconstruction of survival plots for the Göteborg implants (fixtures), always of their routine group 1, according to ref. *(39)*, Table 4, corrected for the 27% early losses omitted in this study, and extrapolated for intermediate values (Göteborg 1981, mod.), a direct reconstruction of the curve for fixtures in the maxillae in Fig. 5 of ref. *(57)* (Göteborg 1990, orig.), and a modification of this curve accounting for the 36 permanent losses in six patients of routine group 1 (assuming the average 6/jaw and patient) and distributing these additional approx 3.6% of the 1004 implants evenly over the observation period of the first 10 yr (Göteborg 1990, mod.).

immediate placements to delayed insertions after the healing of the extraction site, to a full late implant, were small, and were performed during the early development stages *(36)*. The Frialit implants were also supplied with many different kinds of superstructures, from single crowns to bridges and complete dentures, during the development period. Further extension of the indications, e.g., to smaller alveolar ridges, became possible with the introduction of the München variation of the original Tübingen implant and its combination with the bone-splitting technique mentioned above *(53,54)*.

Although the number of early failures of Göteborg implants gradually decreased, because of a learning effect progressing from one routine group to the next *(58)*, the number of losses during the healing phase of the Tübingen implants remained on the order of 5–10%. Two principal reasons could be detected: The protection against loading of the implants during the 3–4-mo healing periods could not be completely accomplished in all cases. Further on, histological examinations and clinical observations indicated that the growth pressure of the remodeling adjacent tissue can result in lifting the implant from its bed, because this implant does not have any undercutting portions that could oppose extroversion *(35)*. As a consequence, and in applying all experiences accumulated with the Frialit implant, the Tübingen group tested experimentally different designs, materials, and material combinations *(64)*. The Frialit-2 implant, shown in Fig. 6, was subsequently introduced for clinical trials in Tübingen. Its cylindrical sections, with the exception of the coronal one, carry self-tapping threads, with biomechanically optimized cross-sections providing purely pressure-transmitting surfaces for dis-

Table 8
Summary of Results of first 10-Yr Follow-up of All Frialit Implants Inserted in Tübingen According to Standard Procedure and Those Placed in Routine Phase

All standard implants, 1975–1985			Treatments commenced after reaching final routine, 1982–1985
	610	Total number of treatments commenced	352
	18	Disappeared from follow-up	5
(100%)	592	Treatments remaining in follow-up	347 (100%)
(15.5%)	92	Failed treatments	26 (7.5%)
	14	Attempts of reimplantation contained in these failures	5
(84.5%)	500	Successful treatments	321 (92.5%)
	28	Reimplantations contained in the successful treatments	10
(79.7%)	472	Commenced and successful treatments (regarding reimplantations as failures)	311 (89.6%)

Adapted with permission from ref. 7.

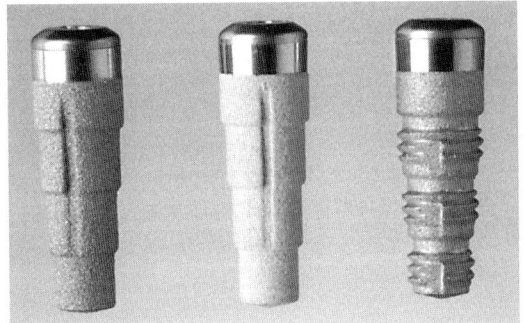

Fig. 6. Frialit-2 implants of different designs and with different surfaces. (Left) Stepped cylinder coated plasma-sprayed Ti powder. (Center) Stepped cylinder with HA coating. (Right) Stepped threaded cylinder, blasted and etched.

tally, as well as coronally, oriented forces, as schematically indicated in Fig. 7. After the preparation of the implant bed with the appropriate stepped burrs, the implants can be correctly positioned with three full turns. The implant is made of Ti, and is intended for the full two-stage procedure. Thus, it accounts for both problem fields responsible for the high early losses encountered with the original Tübingen system. Preliminary results (35) yield the expected marked reduction of early problems. The first 5-yr results confirm this (65): From a total of 696 implants placed in 376 patients, 10 implants were lost from recalls and 7 because of the death of the patient. From the

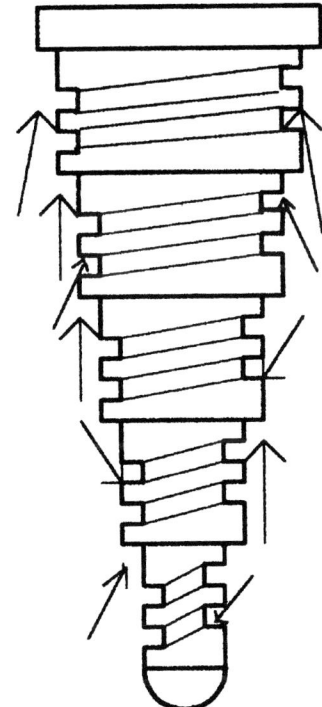

Fig. 7. Schematic presentation of the features allowing for osseointegration of Frialit-2 implants, designed to account for the stress-and-strain-field-controlled remodeling of the adjacent cancellous bony tissue. Arrows indicate the directions of possible forces. Note the down-pointing arrows, indicating some resistance to growth forces, which otherwise might lift the implant from its bed.

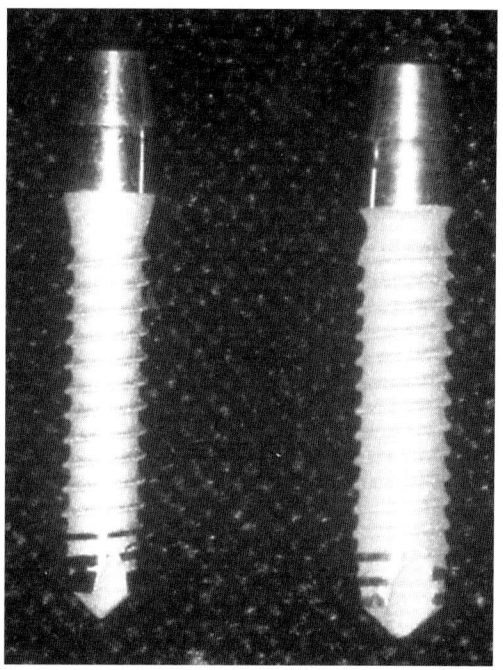

Fig. 8. Recent version of ITI Ledermann screws with HA coatings.

remaining 679 implants, 19 failed for several reasons, yielding a survival rate of more than 97%, after the observation period of 5 yr, for the oldest implant. The average pocket depth was 3 mm after 3 yr, thus was somewhat larger than for alumina ceramic implants mentioned in Tables 6 and 7. A plaque index of up to 2 was noted for 29% of the implants after 3 yr; with alumina implants, plaque was hardly observed at all. Some consequences of this observation are discussed in subheading 4.

3.2. ITI Implants

The aforementioned TPS Ledermann screw belongs to the group of ITI implants that was introduced in the late 1970s, after extended experimental studies (8,66,67). A more recent version is shown in Fig. 8. Besides this screw, the ITI system consists of implants with one or two parallel hollow cylinders connected to a pergingival post. The walls of the cylinders are perforated by relatively large holes, to allow for bony connection between the surrounding tissue and the inside core. All surfaces of the intraosseous part are coated with Ti powder by flame- or plasma-spraying. Originally, they belonged to the group 2 implants protruding through the gingiva, and remained unloaded during the healing period, with the exception of the screw type according to Ledermann, as mentioned previously.

Different results are reported in mid- and long-term follow-up studies: Ledermann (68) inserted 133 hollow cylinder implants between 1979 and 1983, of which he could follow-up 110 implants. Until 1988, 26 implants had survived, or 23.6%. One of the chief causes of failure had been infections. More favorable results are reported in a more recent multicenter study (69) on ITI hollow cylinders and screws: At three university clinics (Berne and Geneva in Switzerland and Mainz in Germany), a total of 2359 implants were consecutively inserted in 1003 patients. During the healing period, 13 implants, or 0.55%, did not successfully integrate. After a healing period of 3–6 mo, the successfully integrated implants were supplied with 393 removable and 758 fixed restorations. During follow-up, 19 implants were classified as failures for several reasons, and 17 implants (0.8%) demonstrated a suppurative peri-implant infection at the last inspection. Including 127 dropout implants (5.4% dropout rate), the 8-yr cumulative survival rates are 96.7% and 93.3%, respectively. The cumulative success rate for the screws was slightly more favorable (better than 95%) than for the hollow cylinders (91.3%), and in the mandible clearly more favorable (95%) than in the maxilla (87%). All three clinical centers had a cumulative success rate of well above 90% after these 8 yr.

In studies involving more than one kind of implant, the numbers of implants per system usually are much smaller. In one such study, including 93 ITI hollow cylinders (70) placed in partially edentulous jaws, mostly in the maxilla, 95% were still functioning after 60 mo. A few of the implants demonstrated a bone loss above 3.5 mm and a pocket depth of more than 6 mm. In another study of the Tübingen group (49,71), 19/35, or 54%, ITI implants were lost during an observation period of 5 yr. A high incidence of infections was also noted in this study. In addition, the relatively large bone losses involved with each failure of these voluminous implants demand particular care, especially in the numerous cases of infections, as had already been indicated by Tetsch *(45)*.

The results obtained with the TPS Ledermann screw do not show such a wide scatter. Ledermann himself reports about 500 implants in 146 patients, of which 476 of the implants could be followed for up to 7 years *(48)*. Forty-one of the screws, or 8.2%, had to be removed; eight patients had not been available for follow-up. The number of failures was slightly higher for women (9.44%) than for men (7.01%), in spite of the generally better oral hygiene of women. The majority of failures occurred within the first 8–12 mo. These implants were loaded immediately after their insertion, according to group 3 defined above. Krekeler et al. *(48)* found a survival probability of 77.4% for 176 TPS screws followed for 8.4 yr; however, only 65–70% had a satisfactory state of the peri-implant tissue.

In the Tübingen comparative study *(70)*, 117 TPS Ledermann screws were included, of which 12, or 10.2%, were lost in up to 9 yr. Richter et al. *(72)* report approx 36 of these screws followed for up to 7 yr, with one implant lost. The pocket depth as well as the marginal bone loss were found to be more favorable than for the IMZ implants.

A surprising feature of the TPS screws was noted by d'Hoedt and Schulte *(49)*: 5/56 implants in this study became loose temporarily, usually discerned at the 1-mo follow-up inspection, but became firmly integrated again after different periods of time. This observation can be related to the warning by Krekeler et al. *(48)* not to apply the Periotest method for determining the mobility of implants to the TPS screw within the first year po. Table 9 summarizes the data mentioned above for the ITI hollow cylinders and the TPS Ledermann screws.

3.3. IMZ Dental Implant System

The intramobile element of the cylindrical implant shown in Fig. 9 had originally been designed to at least partially substitute for the mechanical function of the desmodont, which is no longer available with a truly osseointegrated implant *(6)*, and as a kind of shock absorber. The originally plain Ti surfaces had soon been coated with Ti powder *(66)*, and later also with HA

Table 9
Summary of Survival Data of ITI Implants and TPS Ledermann Screws

Source	No. in study	Maximum follow-up period (yr)	Successes (%)
ITI cylinders			
Ledermann *(68)*	133	4	23.6
Buser et al. *(69)*	2359	8	93.3
Ellegaard et al. *(70)*	93	5	95
d'Hoedt and Schulte *(50)*			
d'Hoedt et al. *(71)*	35	5	46
TPS Ledermann screws			
Ledermann *(48)*	476	7	91.8
Krekeler et al. *(49)*	176	8.4	77.4
d'Hoedt et al. *(71)*	117	9	89.8

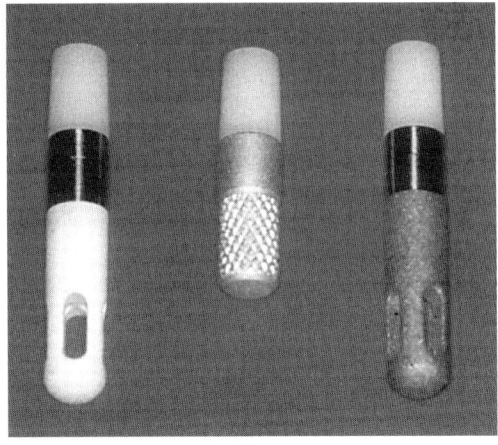

Fig. 9. IMZ implants with different coatings. (Left) HA-coated. (Right) Flame- or plasma-sprayed with Ti powder. (Center) Auxiliary parts.

ceramics *(73)* by flame- and plasma-spraying. In a report on the first 226 implants inserted within 4 yr *(29)*, the removal of six implants, and pocket depths between 1 and 4 mm, with a mean value close to 2 mm, were mentioned. An 8-yr report on all coated implants, inserted between September 1978 and June 1986, shows the loss of 36 implants, or 2.8%, of a total of 1185, placed in the maxilla, and of 10, or 1.9%, placed in the mandible *(74)*.

In a more recent study by Babbush and Shimura *(75)*, 5-yr survival rates on a total of 1059 IMZ implants are presented, of which 28 failed. The overall survival rate in totally edentulous patients, as well as in partially edentulous cases, was 96%. In the maxilla, 92%, and in the mandible, 99% of the implants surpassed the first 5 yr *in situ*. The overall success rate was 95% in this period. De Wijs et al. *(76)* found, for a total of 173 implants, a 94.4% survival rate in the maxilla after 3 yr. In all these studies, the losses were more or less equally distributed over the whole observation period. In contrast to these reports, Batenburg et al. *(50)* only saw three losses occurring during the healing period of 114 implants placed, and nothing during the follow-up to 57 mo. The data presented by Fugazzotto et al. *(77)* also show a slight concentration of their 53 failures of 2023 implants within the first 12 mo of their >60 mo follow-up time, absolute success rate, 97.4%.

But, in spite of the last two reports, a chief difference from the Göteborg, as well as from the Tübingen, system is a noticeable reduction in early losses of the implants of the IMZ system during the healing and early loading period. This was also noted by Esposito et al. *(78)*; however, their statement of an increase of the loss rate with time can be deduced neither from the survival graphs in ref. 75 nor from the figures they show. If at all, a rather constant loss rate, on the order of 0.5%/yr, appears reasonable. Thus, the total losses of IMZ implants will reach the level of the first year's failures of the other systems after about 10 yr. This was confirmed by Nagel et al. *(79)* for 7035 implants placed between 1980 and 1990 in Kirsch's private dental office, by an overall success rate slightly better than 90% after 10 yr. There are, however, reports with markedly different results: The Kaplan-Meier analysis of Dietrich et al. *(80)*, for 2017 IMZ implants inserted between 1978 and 1991, showed an overall success rate of 93.3% after 5 yr, and of 69.9% after 10 yr. None of their curves indicate a concentration of losses during the first years, but, indeed, show an increase of the loss rate with time, which is already roughly expressed by the increase of the 5- to 10-yr losses. Haas et al. *(81)* also found less-favorable total survival rates of 89.9% at 60 mo, and of 83.2% at 100 mo for 1920 implants, with particu-

**Table 10
Summary of Survival Data From
Evaluations of IMZ Implant System**

Source	No. in study	Maximum follow-up period (yr)	Successes (%)
Kirsch *(29)*	226	4	97.4
Richter et al. *(72)*	1185	8	97.2
Babbush and Shimura *(75)*	1059	5	95
de Wijs et al. *(76)*	173[a]	5.3	94.4
Batenburg et al. *(51)*	114	4.75	97.4
Friguzzotto et al. *(77)*	2023	5	97.4
Nagel et al. *(79)*	7035	10	90
Dietrich et al. *(80)*[b]	2017	10	69.9
Haas et al. *(81)*	1920	8.3	83.2

[a]All HA coated.
[b]A relatively large number of implantological beginners contributed to this study.

larly poor results in the maxillary incisor, canine, and premolar region, with survival down to less than 40% after 80 mo, and, in this single indication field, a marked increase of the failure rate over time.

All values describing the state of the gingiva around the pergingival part of the IMZ implants are similar to those of the other osseointegrated Ti implants. No marked differences between the Ti powder and the HA-coated versions have been noted. Table 10 contains a survey of the figures given above.

Generally, the IMZ system seems to have the particular advantage of avoiding most of the early problems, which, however, can be relatively easily corrected by reimplantations with the Göteborg and the Tübingen, as well as with the Frialit-2 systems. The importance of the intramobile element appears to have shifted from shock absorption back to what had been originally intended; the mobility that it provides. An unpublished estimate had shown that, with the volume available and the shock intensity acting in normal functions, the shock absorbing capacity is negligible, compared to that of all surrounding structures. A recent calculation of the shock-absorbing capacity of polyethylene liners in metal-backed sockets of total hip replacements points in the same direction *(82)*.

Additionally, the long-term successes of the Göteborg and Tübingen implants indicate that the cancellous bony structures surrounding osseointegrated implants are sufficiently deformable (have a sufficiently low modulus of elasticity), to allow for all normally necessary deformations without endangering the osseous anchorage, as had been stated by Schroeder and Ledermann (83) many years ago.

In a recent controlled clinical study by Boerrigter et al. (84) involving 62 Göteborg and 56 IMZ implants functioning for 12 mo, of which six were lost during the healing period (five Göteborg and one IMZ implant), a surprising observation was mentioned: Regarding the pocket depth, the Göteborg implants performed significantly better than the IMZ ones, but, radiographically, the IMZ did better. Regarding the pocket depth measurements, those authors point to the shape differences of the two types making it difficult to reach a deeper depth along the Göteborg implants. No explanation could be offered for the different bone losses expressed in the radiographic evaluation.

3.4. Core Vent Implants

The Core-Vent implant system was introduced with clear reference to the Göteborg system, as stated by Niznick (85,86), despite its very different design, having much more similarity with the hollow cylinders of the ITI system. More basic data on this system were not published until several years after its introduction, when Lum and Beirne (87) confirmed that bony tissue can grow through the vents to connect the core inside the cylinder to its surrounding bone, and that no soft tissue interlayer forms along the interface.

However, there are hardly any follow-up studies available on this system. Malmavist and Sennerby (88) followed 47 consecutively placed implants in 35 patients for 2–4 yr; 43 implants were available for examination; 11 of them were removed: nine because of progressive vertical bone loss; two fractured. Thus, the success rate was less than 75% within less than 5 yr. Moy, according to ref. 87, reported about 35 failures from a total of 100 implants within 3 yr. No information regarding the state of the gingival margin could be found.

3.5. Steri-Oss Implant System

The relatively new Steri-Oss system comprises several different types of Ti implants, such as screws and cylinders with various diameters and shapes, and, besides plain surfaces, with either Ti powder or HA coatings. Some of the cylinders have holes with relatively small diameters. In view of the aforementioned design rules, the plain HA-coated cylinders must be regarded critically: If the coating happens to be sucked away by the surrounding tissue after some time, there are no means for osseointegration left, thus increasing the dangers of loosenings after longer periods of time.

In a report to a conference organized by the manufacturer, Buchs et al. (89) presented a prospective clinical study of 2372 HA-coated, threaded implants, with up to 6 yr follow-up: 943 of these implants were placed into the maxilla, 1429 into the mandible. The Kaplan-Meier statistical presentation shows an overall 94.7% success rate, and 95.7% for the mandibular and 93.2% for the maxillary implants. The pocket depths ranged up to more than 7 mm, with a mean value close to 3 mm. In another study (90), 1499 implants, all of different shapes and surfaces of this system, were inserted, of which 1447 could be supplied with superstructures. Of these, 56, or 3.9%, failed during a period of up to 8 yr. However, there was a significant difference between the success rates of the Ti screws and that of the HA-coated implants, with the latter performing significantly better (97.6 and 98%) than the uncoated Ti implants (88.5%). The success rate for the cylindrical Ti plasma-sprayed implants was even higher (99.2%) than that for the HA-coated ones. There was no significant difference between the performance of HA-coated, threaded and cylindrical implants (97.6 and 98%, respectively). Because of the general dangers of a loss of the HA coating mentioned above, the results achieved with the purely cylindrical implants must be considered with care, but this does not apply to the Ti plasma-coated implants. Unfortunately, no data regarding the state of the marginal gingiva are mentioned in this report.

3.6. 3i Implant System

Like the previous system, the 3i system includes screw- and cylinder-shaped Ti implants.

Table 11
Summary of Available Figures on Success Rates of Core-Vent, Steri-Oss, and 3i Dental Implant Systems

Implant type	Success rate	Source	No. in study	Longest period of follow-up (yr)	Depths (mm)	Pocket (%)
Core-Vent	87		47	4	a	75
			100	3	a	35
Steri-Oss	89		2372	6	3	94.7
	90		1447	8	a	96.1
3i	91		1871	5	a	95

aNo values mentioned.

The intraosseous portions of the screws are very similar to those of the Göteborg system; the cylinders are close copies of the IMZ implants, and are also coated with Ti powder particles.

In a multicenter study, Lazarra et al. (91) inserted a total of 1969 of both versions of 3i implants into 653 consecutive patients during a period of 5 yr: 28 patients with 110 implants were lost during the follow-up period. The remaining 625 patients, with 1871 implants, were followed from 6 to 60 mo. During this period, 93 implants, or 5%, were considered failures. The chief causes of failure consisted of loss of osseointegration in 2.3% of the cases; crestal bone loss, requiring periodontal therapy after the first year of function in 1.7%, and mechanical problems associated with the prostheses in 0.9% of the cases. The scatter of the failure rates between the different centers was similar for both types of implants. The pocket depths are said to have been measured, but no values are given.

The statistical values on the last three implant systems are summarized in Table 11, despite the fact that their method of evaluation, as well as the types of implants involved, are rather different. Thus, the figures can only be regarded as a kind of order of magnitude information. However, even with these limitations, they give an indication of present trends and possible improvements.

4. Conclusions

The pure survival rates discussed above for the Göteborg, Tübingen, and Frialit-2 implants, and those summarized in Tables 8–11, indicate some convergence for most for the dental implant systems to values close to 95% after 5 yr, and to about 90% after 10 yr, during the last decade. If one considers some other criteria, such as, e.g., those suggested by Albrektsson (14), these data may shift to values about 5% smaller, without changing the general picture, or giving more detailed information. Because these other criteria essentially describe the state and deficiencies of the bony tissue adjacent to the implants, they give only earlier indications of implant losses that will occur in the near future, and, thus, a linear transformation of the applied scale, but without any gain regarding further improvements.

One reason is the omittance of information on the state of the gingiva, which may even be justified, because all figures available suggest some convergence of the mean values concerned for all osseointegrated, two-stage, Ti implants, on the order of magnitude of 3 mm or above. However, because some of the more recently introduced Ti implants do contain alloying elements such as vanadium and aluminum, a thorough and careful recording of these data, and their correct statistical evaluation, could possibly reveal some differences in this highly sensitive and important portion of implant performance, which no short-term study may be able to disclose.

The data on the performance of marginal gingiva, deduced from early studies (presented in Tables 6 and 7), have been confirmed by later evaluations as, e.g., given in Table 11 for the Steri-Oss system. Thus, the hierarchy of the figures of merit, describing the state of the gingival margin as a function of the material at the pergingival portion and the type of implant that can be established from the values contained in these tables, remains unchanged: Alumina ceramic in a one piece and protected two-stage implant (e.g., Tübingen); Ti in a one-piece and one-stage implant (e.g., Ledermann TPS screw); Ti in two-piece and full two-stage implants (e.g., Göteborg, IMZ, and so on).

At present, no reliable study, correlating the state of the gingival margin to the overall success rates of osseointegrated implants, could be found. Earlier, Spiekermann (40) had compared pocket depth, plaque, and gingival index to the width of soft-tissue interlayers and loosenings for osseointegrated and nonosseointegrated implants, and found a clear positive correlation. However, the better and safer the closure of the gingiva around the post of the implant, the more reduced the dangers of infections will be. Thus, generally, an near-perfect situation around the pergingival portion, approaching that around natural teeth, can be expected to prevent contamination of the highly sensitive interfaces, and to contribute to the survival expectation of implants. Such a state of the gingival margin had been found and extensively documented for osseointegrated, one-piece alumina implants, as discussed in detail in subheading 2.5.

Because the presented survival rates indicate an overall saturation for most of the screws and cylinder-shaped Ti implants with their different coatings, the only presently available general possibility for further improvements appears to rest with the combination of these Ti implants with pergingival parts, of which the side facing the gingiva is made of a medical-grade alumina ceramic. Such composite dental implants have already been suggested (92). A first approach to such a solution is shown in Fig. 10, consisting of a solid, alumina ceramic pergingival part. However, the fixation of this component requires a direct contact between the metal screw and the ceramic, involving some problems regarding metal wear and stress concentrations. Another approach aims at a pergingival part consisting of a metal core and an outside ring of alumina ceramic.

None of the procedures usually employed for joining ceramics to metals can be used directly. Gluing is to be excluded, because of the necessity for high-temperature vapor sterilization; for the same reason, mechanical means, e.g., via Morse cones as applied for the fixation of ceramic heads

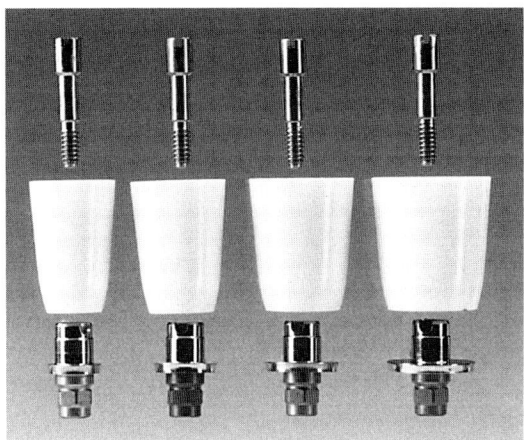

Fig. 10. Pergingival component consisting completely of alumina ceramic. (CeraBase for the Fritlit-2 implant system)

to the femoral components in hip replacements, cannot be used, and all soldering processes would require the introduction of relatively low melting and biologically critical metals, such as copper, for this delicate purpose. Therefore, a new bonding technique had to be developed.

This diffusion welding requires thin niobium and tantalum intermediate layers only. Both these metals had been shown to be as biocompatible as Ti (93). In extended studies (94–97), a mechanically strong bond and vacuum-tight seal could be achieved. The results of tests of the bend strengths of these composite implants, during which the oscillating loads were applied perpendicular to the crown, which was fixed planarly to the coronal face of the implant, are reproduced in Fig. 11, according to Petzow (98). As can be seen, even after 3×10^6 load changes, with peak values of 50 N under this unfavorable force application, none of the components of the implant were damaged. Thus, the application of this joining technique to the pergingival parts of the most successful dental implant systems can be expected to further improve their performance. In the hierarchy given above, such an implant system has the chance to be placed between level A and B, because the introduction of the alumina ceramic in the pergingival region would also remove all possible galvanic influences mentioned. The remaining handicap of any full two-stage implant,

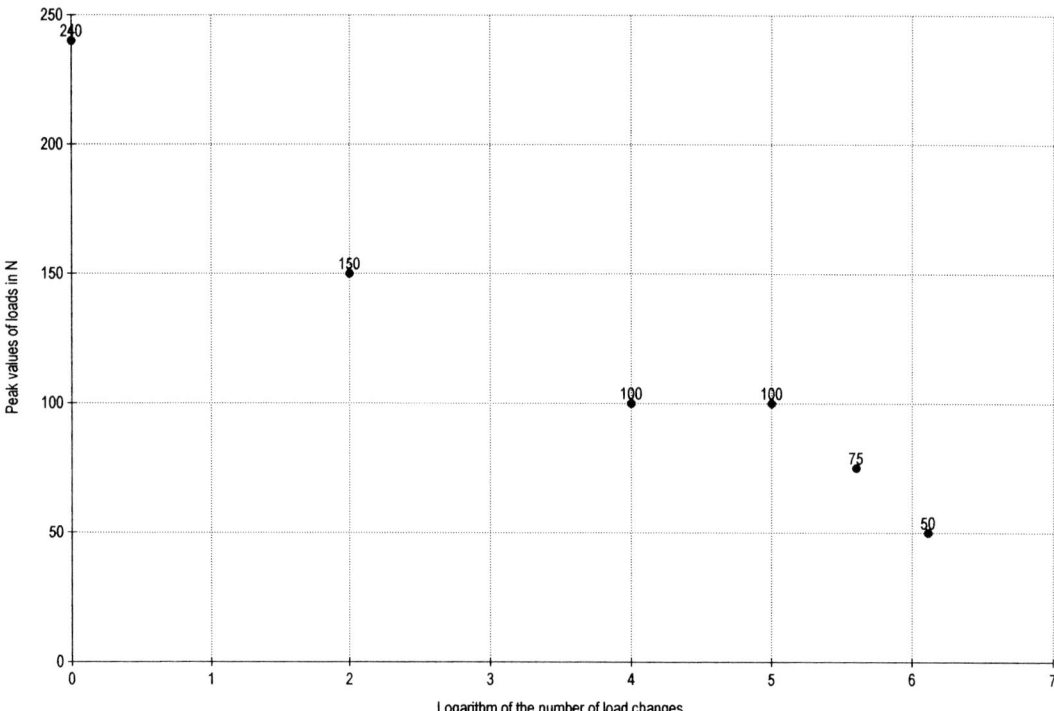

Fig. 11. Force at fracture of Ti-30 tantalum/alumina ceramic composite implants with planarly attached crowns as a function of the logarithm of load changes in Hz (number of load changes between 1 and 1,300,000 Hz) *(98)*. Force applied to top of crown, perpendicularly to the axis of the implant. The implant that had survived 1.3 million load changes had not fractured under the top load of 50 N, and did not show any sign of damage.

the gap or crevice between the pergingival portion and its intraosseous part, was studied recently in some detail by Jansen et al. *(52)*. All 13 different implant–abutment combinations tested presented microbial leakage. The proportions of tight assemblies differed between zero and 84%. The best values resulted from Frailit-2 implants that were supplied with a silicon washer between the implant body and the abutment. Whether this additional seal will stand the test of large-scale and long-term applications remains to be seen.

Of course, studies in which the conventional pure Ti and those new alumina ceramic fitted pergingival parts are compared would be particularly instructive and convincing. Unfortunately, double-blind experiments will not be possible, because no one can overlook the difference. But it is exactly this difference that will provide another advantage: The cosmetic aspect of the white color of the alumina ceramic in the pergingival portion of the front teeth region has been mentioned repeatedly.

Finally, it appears that the evaluation of some of the more important follow-up reports on osseointegrated dental implants has shown that, after more than three decades, and toward the end this century, a level of performance is achieved that is at least equivalent or even above nearly all other kinds of treatment in the different branches of dentistry, and in medicine in general. But as an additional result, guidelines could be found on which even further improvements can be based and deduced from the evaluation of existing knowledge.

Acknowledgments

Sincere thanks are due to Dipl.-Volksw. W. Hund, Friatec AG, Mannheim, for providing much of the literature and some of the figures.

References

1. Brånemark P-I, Breine U, Ardell R, Hansson BO, Lindström J, and Olsson Å. Intra-osseous anchorage of dental prostheses. I. Experimental studies. *Scand J Plast Reconstr Surg* 1969; 3: 81–100.
2. Schulte W and Heimke G. Das Tübinger Sofort-Implantat. *Quintessenz* 1976; 6: 17–23.
3. Adell R, Hansson BO, Brånemark P-I, and Breine U. Intraosseous anchorage of dental prostheses. II. Review of clinical approaches. *Scand J Plast Reconstr Surg* 1970; 4: 19–34.
4. Brånemark P-I, Hansson BO, Adell R, Breine U, Lindström J, Hallén O, and Öhman A. Osseointegrated implants in the treatment of the edentulous jaw. Experience from a 10-year period. *Scand J Plast Reconstr Surg* 1977; 11 (Suppl): 1–132.
5. Schulte W. Das Tübinger Implantat aus Frialit. Fünfjährige Erfahrungen. *Dtsch zahnärztl Z* 1981; 36: 544–550.
6. D'Hoedt B and Lukas D. Statistische Ergebnisse des Tübinger Implantates. *Dtsch zahnärztl Z* 1981; 36: 551–562.
7. d'Hoedt B. 10 Jahre Tübinger Implantat aus Frialit. Eine Zwischenauswertung der Implantatkartei. *Z Zahnärztl Implantol* 1986; 2: 6–10.
8. Schröder A, Pohler O, and Sutter F. Gewebsreaktion auf Titan-Hohlzylinderimplanatat mit Titan Spritzschichtoberfläche. *Schweiz Mschr Zahnheilk* 1976; 88: 1051–1060.
9. Koch WL. Die zweiphasige enossale Implantation von intramobilen Zylinderimplantaten: IMZ. *Quintessenz* 1976; 27: Ref. 5395 1–5.
10. Tetsch P, Ackermann KL, and Kirsch A. Experience with intramobile cylinder implants. A follow-up analysis, in *Dental Implants, Materials and Systems* 1980; (Heimke G, ed), Carl Hanser Verlag, München, pp 75–79.
11. Ledermann PH. Das titanplasmabeschichtete Schraubenimplantat als alloplastisches enossales Retentionselement im zahnlosen Problemkiefer. I. Systematischer Ablauf der Implantation bis zur Abdrucknahme am Modell. *Quintessenz Zahnärztl Lit* 1979; 30: 5.
12. Charnley J and Cupic Z. Nine and ten year results of the low friction arthroplasty of the hip. *Clin Orthop* 1973; 95: 9–25.
13. Willert HG, Semlitsch M, Kriete U, and Ziechner L. Clinical experience with Mueller total hip endoprostheses of different designs and materials, in *Mechanical Properties of Biomaterials* 1980; (Hastings GW and Williams DF, eds), Wiley, Chichester, pp. 85–101.
14. Albrektsson T, Zarb G, Worthington P, and Eriksson AR. Long-term efficacy of currently used dental implants: a review and proposed criteria of success. *J Oral Maxillofac Implants* 1986; 1: 11–25.
15. Breme J and Schmid H-J. Criteria for bioinertness of metals for osseo-integrated implants, in *Osseo-integrated Implants*, vol. 1, *Basics, Materials and Joint Replacements* 1990; (Heimke G ed), CRC, Boca Raton, pp. 31–80.
16. Osborn JF. in *Fortschritte der Kiefer- und Gesichtschirurgie XXVIII* 1983; (Pfeifer G and Schwenzer N eds), Georg Thieme Verlag, Stuttgart.
17. Lintner F, Zweymüller K, and Brand G. Die knöcherne Reaktion auf zementfrei implantierte Titaniumschäfte, in *Aktueller Stand der zementfreien Hüftendoprothetik* 1985; (Maaz B and Menge M, eds), Georg Thieme Verlag, Stuttgart, pp 44–53.
18. Campbell CE and von Recum AF. Microtopography and soft tissue response. *J Invest Surg* 1989; 2: 51–74.
19. von Recum AF. 1987; personal communication.
20. Hulbert SF, Young FA, Matthews RS, Klawitter JJ, Talbert CD, and Stelling FH. Potential of ceramic materials as permanent sceletal prostheses. *J Biomed Mater Res* 1970; 4: 433–456.
21. Heimke G. Aspects and modes of fixation of bone replacements, in Osseo-integrated Implants, Vol. I, Basics, Materials, and Joint Replacements 1990; (Heimke G, ed), CRC, Boca Raton, pp. 1–29.
22. Heimke G, Schulte W, Griss P, Jentschura G, and Schulz P. Generalization of biomechanical rules for the fixation of bone, joint, and tooth replacements. *J Biomed Mater Res* 1980; 14: 537–543.
23. Griss P, Silber R, Merkle B, Haehner K, Heimke G, and Krempien B. Biomechanically induced tissue reactions after Al_2O_3-ceramic hip joint replacement. Experimental and early clinical results. *J Biomed Mater Res Symp* 1976; 7: 519–528.
24. Heimke G, Griss P, Werner E, and Jentschura G. Effects of mechanical factors on bio-compatibility tests. *J Biomed Eng* 1981; 3: 209–213.
25. Soltesz U, Siegele D, and Baudendiestel E. Might biomechanical effects influence biocompatibility tests in bone? in *Clinical Implant Materials, Advances in Biomaterials*, vol. 9, 1990; (Heimke G, Soltesz U, and Lee AJC, eds), Elsevier, Amsterdam, pp. 657–662.
26. Heimke G, Schulte W, d'Hoedt B, Griss P, Büsing CM, and Stock D. Influence of fine surface structures on the osseo-integration of implants. *J Artif Organs* 1982; 5: 207–212.
27. Büsing CM and d'Hoedt B. Die Knochenanlagerung an das Tübinger Implantat beim Menschen. *Dtsch zahnärztl Z* 1981; 36: 563–566.
28. Scholz F. Bewegungsverhalten bei Stossanregung

des Tübinger Implantates im Vergleich zu natürlichen Zähnen. *Dtsch zahnärztl Z* 1981; 36: 567–570.
29 Kirsch A. Fünf Jahre IMZ-Implantat-System. Grundlagen, Methodik, Erfahrungen, in *Der heutige Stand der Implantologie* 1980; (Frank J, ed), Carl Hanser Verlag, München, pp. 163–181.
30 Jarchow M. Calcium phosphate as a hard tissue prosthetics. *Clin Orthop Relat Res* 1981; 157: 259–278.
31 de Groot K. *Bioceramics of Calcium Phosphate* 1983; CRC, Boca Raton.
32 Driessens FCM. Formation and stability of calcium phosphates in relation to the phase composition of the mineral in calcified tissue, in *Bioceramics of Calcium Phosphate* 1983; (de Groot K, ed), CRC, Boca Raton, FL, pp. 1–32.
33 NN. Tübingen Implant. *Dtsch Zahnärztl Z* 1981; 36: 579–608.
34 Heimke G and Hund W. Erfahrungsaustausch und kritische Wertung als Basis verbreiteter Anwendung. *Zahnarzt J* 1985; 5: 14–16.
35 Schulte W, d'Hoedt B, Axmann D, and Gomez G. First 15 years of the Tübingen implant and its further development to the Frialit®-2 system. *Z zahnärztl Implantol* 1992; 8: 3–22.
36 Schulte W. Das enossale Tübinger Implantat aus Al_2O_3 (Frialit®). Der Entwicklungsstand nach 6 Jahren. *Zahnärztl Mit* 1981; 19: 1114–1122; 20: 1181–1192.
37 Eriksson RA and Albrektsson T. Effect of heat on bone regeneration. *J Oral Maxillofacial Surg* 1984; 42: 701–711.
38 Schulte W. Messung des Dämpfungverfhaltens enossaler Implantate mit dem Periotestverfahren. Vorläufige Mitteilung. *Z Zahnärztl Implantol.* 1986; 2: 11–16.
39 Adell R, Lekholm B, Rockler B, and Brånemark P-I. 15-year study of osseointegrated implants in the treatment of the edentulous jaw. *Int J Oral Surg* 1981; 10: 387–416.
40 Spiekermann H. Clinical and animal experiences with enosseous metal implants, in *Dental Implants, Materials and Systems* 1980; (Heimke G, ed), Carl Hanser Verlag, München, pp 49–54.
41 Schareyka R. Die Sulcus-Fluid-Fließrate (SFFR) bei Tübinger Implantaten aus Aluminiumoxidkeramik. *Dtsch Zahnärztl Z* 1978; 33: 360–362.
42 Tetsch P and Dhom G. Paradontale Massnahmen bei enossalen Implantaten. *Zahnärztl Mitt* 1984; 74: 2443–2450.
43 d'Hoedt B and Büsing CM. Die Einheilung von Al_2O_3-Keramik am Beispiel des Tübinger Implantates (Frialit). *Fortschr Zahnärztl Implantol* 1985; 1: 150–162.
44 Heimke G, Schulte W, and d'Hoedt B. Influence of material and dimension on the gingival attachment to implants. *Clin Mater* 1986; 1: 147–150.
45 Tetsch P. *Enossale Implantationen in der Zahnheilkunde* 1984; Carl Hanser Verlag, München.
46 d'Hoedt B. 1986. Influence of implant materials and material surfaces on blood clotting: a scanning electron microscopic study, in Tissue Integration in Oral and Maxillofacial Surgery (D. Steenberge, ed.), *Excerpta Med,* Amsterdam, 46–50.
47 Büsing CM, D'Hoedt B, and Schulte W. Materialunabhängige Faktoren als Ursache für Mißerfolge dentaler Implantate. *Z Zahnärztl Implantol* 1987; 3: 37–40.
48 Ledermann D. Das TPS-Schraubenimplantat nach siebenjähriger Anwendung. *Quintessenz* 1984; 11: Referat 6678, 1–11.
49 Krekeler G, Schilli W, and Richter A. ITI Schraubenimplantate (TPS) zur Stegretention. Eine Langzeitstudie. *Z Zahnärztl Implantol* 1994; 10: 12–19.
50 d'Hoedt B and Schulte W. Comparative study of results with various endosseous implant systems. *Int J Oral Maxillofac Implants* 1989; 4: 95–105.
51 Batenburg RHK, van Oort RP, Reintsema H, Brouwer TJ, Raghoebar GM, and Boering G. Overdentures supported by two IMZ implants in the lower jaw. A retrospective study of peri-implant tissues. *Clin Oral Implant Res* 1994; 5: 207–212.
52 Jansen VK, Conrads G, and Richter E-J. Untersuchungen zur Dichtigkeit der Implantat-Prothetikpfosten-Verbindung. *Implantologie* 1995; 3: 229–247.
53 Nentwig G-H. Frialit implant-type München, in *Osseo-integrated Implants,* vol. II, *Implants in Oral and ENT Surgery* 1990; (Heimke G, ed), CRC, Boca Raton, pp 63–91.
54 Bruschi GB and Scipioni A. Alveolar augmentation: new applications for implants, 1990; pp. 35–61.
55 Schulte W. Frialit Tübingen implant system, in *Osseo-integrated Implants, vol. II, Implants in Oral and ENT Surgery* 1990; (Heimke G, ed), CRC, Boca Raton, pp. 1–33.
56 de Wijs FLJA, van Dongen RC, de Lange GL, and de Putter C. Front tooth replacement with Tübingen (Frialit®) implants, (de Wijs FLA, ed), *Anterior Maxillary Tooth Replacement with Implants* 1993; Thesis, Faculteit Geneskunde, Rijksuniversiteit te Utrecht, Utrecht, The Netherlands, pp. 45–63.

57. Albrektsson T. Multicenter report on osseointegrated oral implants. *J Prosthetic Dent* 1988; 60: 77–84.
58. Adell R, Eriksson B, Lekholm U, Brånemark P-I, and Jemt T. A long term follow-up study of osseointegrated implants in the treatment of totally edentulous jaws. *Int J Oral Maxillofac Surg* 1990; 5: 347–358.
59. Steenberghe D van. A retrospective multicenter evaluation of osseointegrated fixtures supporting fixed partial prostheses in the treatment of partial edentualism. *J Prosthet Dent* 1989; 61: 217–223.
60. van Steenberge D, Lekholm U, Bolender Ch, Folmer T, Henryy P, Herrmann I, et al. Applicability of osseointegrated oral implants in the rehabilitation of partial edentialism: a prospective multicenter study on 558 fixtures. *Int J Oral Maxillofac Implants* 1990; 5: 272–281.
61. Naert I, Quirnen M, van Steenberge D, and Darius P. Six-year prosthodontic study of 509 consecutively inserted implants for the treatment of partial edentulism. *J Prosthet Dent* 1992; 67: 236–245.
62. Bahat O. Treatment planing and placement of implants in the posterior Maxillae: report of 732 consecutive Nobelpharma implants. *J Oral Maxillofac Implant* 1993; 8: 151–161.
63. Engquist B, Nilson H, and Åstrand P. Single tooth replacement by osseointegrated Brånemark implants. A retrospective study of 82 implants. *Clin Oral Implant Res* 1995; 6: 238–245.
64. Gibbesch B, Elssner G, Bischoff E, and Petzow G. Ein Vergleich der $TiTa_3O/Al_2O_3$, $TiNb_4O/Al_2O_3$, und Ti/Al_2O_3 Dentalimplantatverbunde. *Z Zahnärztl Implantol* 1989; 5: 108–117.
65. Gomez-Roman G, Schulte W, d'Hoedt B, and Axmann-Krcmar D. Frialit-2 implant system: Five year clinical experience in single-tooth and immediately postextraction applications. *Int J Oral Maxillofac Implant* 1997; 12: 299–308.
66. Schroeder A. Histologische und klinische Beobachtungen bei der Erprobung von Hohlzylinder-Implantaten unter besonderer Berücksichtigung der Titanspritzschicht-Oberfäche, in *Der heutige Stand der Implantologie* 1979; (Franke J, ed), Carl Hanser Verlag, München, pp 33–48.
67. Schroeder A, Stich H, and Straumann F. Über die Anlagerung von Osteozement an einen belasteten Implantatkörper. *Schweiz Mschr Zahnheilk* 1978; 86: 713–718.
68. Ledermann PhD. ITI-Hohlzylinder nach 9 Jahren klinischer Erfahrung. *Z Zahnärztl Implantol* 1989; 5: 43–51.
69. Buser D, Mericske-Stern R, Bernard JP, Behneke A, Behneke N, Hirt HP, Belser UC, and Lang NP. Long-term evaluation of non-submerged ITI implants. *Clin Oral Impl Res* 1997; 8: 161–172.
70. Ellegaard B, Baelum V, and Karring T. Implant therapy in periodontally compromised patients. *Clin Oral Impl Res* 1997; 8: 180–188.
71. d'Hoedt B, Handtmann S, Gomez-Roman G, Axmann D, Jahn M, and Schulte W. Verweildaueranalysen nach Kaplan-Meier und Cutler-Ederer für enossale Implantate verschiedener Systeme. Langzeitergebnisse nach bis zu 18 Jahren. *Z Zahnärztl Implantol* 1996; 12: 110–120.
72. Richter E-J, Jansen V, Spiekermann H, and Jovanovic SA. Langzeitergebnisse von IMZ- und TPS-Implantaten im interforaminalen Bereich des zahnlosen Unterkiefers. *Dtsch Zahnärztl Z* 1992; 47: 449–454.
73. Osborn JF and Weiss Th. Hydroxylapatitkeramik: ein knochenähnlicher Biowerkstoff. *Acta Parodontol* 1978; 7: 1166–1171.
74. Kirsch A and Ackermann KL. Das IMZ-Implantat-System. Methoden Klinik, Ergebnisse. *ZWR Dtsch Zahnärzteblatt* 1986; 11: 1134–1144.
75. Babbush ChA and Shimura M. Five-year statistical and clinical observations with the IMZ two stage osteointegrated implant system. *Int J Oral Maxillofac Implants* 1993; 8: 245–253.
76. De Wijs FLJA, Cune MS, and De Putter C. Delayed implants in the anterior maxilla with the IMZ®-implant system. *J Oral Rehabil* 1995; 22: 319–326.
77. Fugazzotto PA, Bulbransen HJ, Wheeler SL, and Lindsay JA. Use of IMZ osseointegrated implants in partial and completely edentulous patients: success and failure rates of 2,023 implant cylinders up to 60+ months in function. *Int J Oral Maxillofac Implants* 1993; 8: 617–621.
78. Esposito M, Hirsch J-M, Lekholm U, and Thomsen P. Failure pattern of four osseointegrated oral implant systems. *J Mater Sci Mater Med* 1997; 8: 843–847.
79. Nagel R, Neugebauer J, Kirsch A, and Ackermann KL. Prognose enossaler Implantate bestimmt anhand der Daten aus einer niederlassenen Praxis am Beispiel des IMZ-Systems, in *Jahrbuch für Orale Implantologie* 1994; Quintessenz Verlag, Berlin, pp 187–190.
80. Dietrich U, Lippold R, Dirmeier Th, Behneke N, and Wagner W. Statistische Ergebnisse zur Implantatprognose am Beispiel von 2017 IMZ-Implantaten unterschiedlicher Indikation der letzen 13 Jahre. *Z Zahnärztl Implantol* 1993; 9: 9–18.
81. Haas R, Mensdorff-Pouilly N, Mailath G, and

Watzek G. Survival of 1,920 IMZ implants followed for up to 100 months. *Int J Oral Maxillofac Implants* 1996; 11: 581–588.

82 Blömer W. Design aspects of modular inlay fixation, in *Performance of the Wear Couple BIOLOX forte in Hip Arthroplasty* 1997; (Puhl W, ed), Ferdinand Enke Verlag, Stuttgart, pp. 95–104.

83 Schroeder A and Ledermann Ph. Plasmabeschichtete Titanimplantate. *Dtsch Zahnärztl Z* 1983; 38: 104–107.

84 Boerrigter EM, van Oort RP, Raghoebar GM, Stegenga B, Schoen PJ, and Boering G. Controlled clinical trial of implant-retained mandibular overdentures: clinical aspects. *J Oral Rehabil* 1996; 23: 101–109.

85 Niznick GA. Core-Vent implant system. *J Oral Implantol* 1982; 10: 379–418.

86 Niznick GA. Core-Vent implant system. The evolution of an osseoventegrated™ implant. *J Oral Implantol* 1985; 17: 1–11.

87 Lum LB and Beirne OR. Viability of the retained bone core in the Core-Vent dental implant. *J Oral Maxillifac Surg* 1986; 44: 341–345.

88 Malmqvist JP and Sennerby L. Clinical report on the success of consecutively placed Core-Vent® implants followed from 3 months to 4 years. *J Oral Maxillofac Implantol* 1990; 5: 53–60.

89 Buchs U, Hahn J, and Vassos DM. Prospective clinical study of 2,372 Steri-Oss HA-coated threaded implants. Six year post-restoration update results. *Steri-Oss International Conference;* July 1995; pp. 1–7.

90 Saadoun AP and Le Gall MG. 8-year compilation of clinical results obtained with Steri-Oss endosseous implants. *Compendium* 1996; 17: 669–688.

91 Lazzara R, Siddiqui AA, Binon P, Feldman SA, Weiner R, Phillips R, and Gonshor A. Retrospective multicenter analysis of 3i endosseous dental implants placed over a five-year period. *Clin Oral Implant Res* 1996; 7: 73–83.

92 Heimke G. Werkstoffprobleme im pergingivalen Bereich von Implantaten, in NN, *Jahrbuch für Orale Implantologie* 1993; Quintessenz, Berlin, pp 13–17.

93 Zetner K, Plenk H Jr, and Stassl H. Tissue and cell reactions in vivo and in vitro to different metals for dental implants, in *Dental Implants, Materials and Systems* 1990; (Heimke G, ed), Carl Hanser-Verlag, München, pp 15–20.

94 Korn D, Elssner G, Petzow G, and Schulte W. Neue Wege der Optimierung von Ti-Al$_2$O$_3$-Verbunden und Dentalimplantatkon-struktionen. *Z Zahnärztl Implantol* 1992; 8: 136–144.

95 Elssner G and Petzow G. Metal/ceramic joining. *ISIJ Int* 1990; 30: 1011–1032.

96 Gibbesch B, Elssner G, and Petzow G. Microstructure and mechanical properties of Ti-Ta/alumina and Ti-Nb/alumina joints for dental implants. *Int J Oral Maxillofac Implants* 1989; 4: 131–137.

97 Korn D, Müller D, Zuber K, Pudleiner M, Heiland B, Elssner G, and Petzow G. Gefüge, Grenzflächenmorphologie und mechanische Eigenschaften von Ti/Al$_2$O$_3$-Verbunden für dentale Implantate. *Praktische Metallographie, Sonderband* 1995; 26: 667–682.

98 Petzow G. Arbeits- und Ergebnisbericht. Metallkeramische Verbinungen für dentale Implantate und Untersuchungen von Material- und Material-Gewebe Grenzflächen. *Sonderforschungsbereich 175 Implantologie, Abschluβ- und Ergebnisbericht 1994–1996* 1996; Eberhard-Karls Universität Tübingen, Tübingen, Germany, pp. 241–262.

PART 2

BONY BIOMATERIALS FOR GRAFTING APPLICATIONS

6

Artificial Bone

Hydroxyapatite Reconstruction of Tibial Plateau Fractures

P. Patka, H. J. Th. M. Haarman, M. van der Elst, and F. C. Bakker

1. Introduction

Progress in the management and repair of traumatic bone defects (including those caused by malignant disease) has created a growing need for suitable material to replace bone tissue. Bone grafting is now more common than any other tissue transfer, with the exception of skin grafting and blood transfusions.

A major problem in many surgical specialties is the proper reconstruction of congenital or acquired deformities associated with severe loss of tissue. In particular, reconstruction of the joint surface requires a depot of bone tissue, to properly fill bone defects adjacent to the joint surface. Although autografts provide the best biological solution, their limitations in mechanical strength and donor site morbidity are some of the obvious disadvantages *(1–3)*.

In the elderly, there is often a lack of bone tissue that can be used for these purposes. Furthermore, the risk of complications increases with the amount of bone graft (BG) taken from the donor site *(2)*. The bone allograft's antigen (Ag) mismatch between donor and recipient affects the temporal gene expression of extracellular bone matrix, and delays new bone formation at the graft–host interface of bone allografts *(4)*. This is an important drawback of an allograft for bone healing in fractures.

The management of traumatic defects in long bones had become an increasing problem in surgery of trauma. Repair of bone defects resulted in a growing need for a suitable bone tissue replacement material. This also applies to defects caused by malignant disease, and to the necessity of bone augmentation in several surgical specialties. Many materials have been developed and used in the past *(5)*.

An ideal bone substitute must mimic the tissue it replaces in size, shape, consistency, and function. It should not be predisposed to infection, and it should not evoke a healing response that would alter its characteristics. As it disappears, it must acquire qualities of the tissue it replaced or augmented. Finally, if it does not disappear, it must be tolerated permanently.

The best material for bone defect repair seems to be an autograft. However, the available quantity is limited, and obtaining the autograft itself may cause higher morbidity *(2,5)*. Therefore, it may turn out that the best bone substitute may be allografts, and that, as the host rejection phenomenon is overcome, permanent incorporation of transplanted allografts may become possible. The present influence of genetic incompatibility, resulting in rejection of an allograft, can be reduced, but not fully eliminated, by treating these grafts by special procedures *(6)*, but such procedures influence not only the biological, but also the mechanical properties of an allograft. Within the scope of these problems, there is a continuing search for an ideal material for surgical bone repair, which combines total biological inertness with adequate mechanical properties.

Accurate reduction and stable internal fixation, followed by early mobilization, is regarded by many as the only appropriate treatment for displaced fractures of the tibial plateau *(7–11)*. For stabilization of these fractures, supporting tissue, in addition to the regular osteosynthesis materials, is necessary *(10)*.

Research on biocompatibility has brought to light ceramic materials that may be suitable for permanent bone tissue replacement. Ceramics made from the calcium phosphate (CoP) system have a unique biological profile. In particular, hydroxyapatite (HA), $Ca_{10}(PO_4)_6(OH)_2$, seems to be useful as a permanent bone substitute. This biomaterial exhibits an excellent biocompatibility with respect to bone tissue. Earlier studies on the use of HA as a hard-tissue implant showed this material to be suitable for small-volume implantation, in cases in which applied mechanical stress is either minimal or restricted to compressive physiological loads *(12)*. More recently, data have been reported on the use of apatite ceramics for repair of large defects *(13–16)*.

Previous research *(12–16)* on the use of ceramic implants for bone tissue replacement revealed that porous HA was suitable for permanent bone tissue replacement. *De novo* bone formation was observed primarily on the HA surface, without fibrous tissue interposition. The HA surface supports osteoblastic differentiation of marrow stromal stem cells, which leads to firm bone bonding *(14,15)*. Furthermore, the osteogenesis is accelerated in specific three-dimensional constitution of extracellular matrix, which makes porous HA implants favorable for osteogenetic tissue formation *(17)*. The same porous HA was used as supporting tissue in cases of the operative treatment for displaced fractures of the tibial plateau in this study. Fracture of the tibial head demands an adequate restoration of articular surface *(10)*.

2. Natural Bone Tissue

Bone is a specialized type of connective tissue, characterized by the presence of cells with long branching processes (osteocytes), which occupy cavities (lacunae) and fine canals (canaliculi) in a hard, dense matrix consisting of bundles of collagenous fibers in an amorphous ground substance (cement) impregnated with CaP complexes. The osteocytes, as well as the osteoblasts and osteoclasts, are derived by differentiation from mesenchymal cells. The osteoblasts, precursors of osteocysts, lay down the organic matrix of new bone, which subsequently is mineralized. In forming new bone, osteoblasts secrete collagen, usually apposed to a pre-existing calcified surface. The osteoclast is a multinucleated giant cell responsible for the dissolution and removal of matrix and mineral. In the steady state, this process occurs virtually simultaneously. The origin of the osteoclast is still the subject of discussion.

The bone matrix contains collagen, ground substances, and bone mineral (CaP complexes). Collagen is fibrillar in nature, having a definite arrangement of amino acid groups in a particular crystal structure. The collagen fibers demonstrate frequent crosslinkages.

Between the fibers, there is a material referred to as ground substance (cement), which is composed of protein mucopolysaccharides. The collagen supports the mineral component within the ground substance. The bone mineral contains complexes of CaP in amorphous and crystalline fractions. With aging, the crystalline fraction increases relative to the amorphous fraction. The major mineral bone component is HA. This CaP salt is nonstoichiometric, and has a Ca/phosphorus ratio of 9:6, instead of that of a stoichiometric salt, which has a ratio of 10:6. HA has a hexogonal crystal structure: The largest crystal dimension does not exceed 60 nm.

Most apatite crystals in bone are elongated along the crystallographic C-axis, and are orientated parallel to the collagen fibers. Besides plate-like crystallites, needlelike apatite crystallites have been demonstrated. The crystals first appear within the substance of the collagen fibers, then additional crystals form around the peripheries of these fibers. The final product, bone, consists mostly of collagen fibers and HA crystals. Other CaPs, present in small quantities in bone, are octacalcium phosphate, Ca pyrophosphate, and brushite.

There are two basic types of bone structure found in mammals: woven and lamellar bone. The bone cells (osteocytes) surrounded by calcified matrix are concentrically orientated to central canaliculi occupied by a capillary vessel. They form solid cylinders (osteons) around the central, longitudinally situated canals (haversian systems). The bone is built up with osteon units.

Osteogenesis or ossification is the normal manner in which bone growth occurs in the body. There are four different types of osteogenesis: enchondral osteogenesis, appositional osteogenesis, remodeling of bone, and fracture healing. Enchondral ossification is indirect bone ingrowth. Indirect bone formation means that bone is formed after, and from, the primary formation of cartilage. Direct bone formation bypasses the intermediate stage of cartilage formation. Appositional bone growth and bone remodeling are both examples of direct bone growth.

Healing of bone fractures involves direct and indirect bone formation. Following a fracture, the bone structure will be restored through several stages consisting of fibrous tissue and cartilage (callus), and finally by remodeling through simultaneous osteoblastic and osteoclastic activity. In cases of proper repositioning, fixation, and compression of a fracture with no bone tissue defect, only direct bone formation (primary osteogenesis) occurs. The bone responds to mechanical stress by placing or displacing bone elements in the direction of the applied forces, and increases or decreases in mass reflect the level of these forces. The mechanism by which mechanical forces affect the activity of the osteogenic cells is unknown. In the course of time, further thickening and reorientation of trabeculae along the lines of stress ceases, and the remodeling process gradually decreases, to the skeleton's normal rate of physiological turnover. Bone remains elastic up to about three-quarters of its breaking strain.

If one endeavours to take into account all the biological, chemical, and physical properties now known to be either mandatory or desirable in an artificial bone replacement material, then the design and production of such a material is still fraught with difficulties. At the present time, biomaterials, and especially some of the ceramics, show some of the qualities of natural bone tissue, and are the subject of experimental and clinical studies *(5,18,19)*.

3. History of Artificial Development

The oldest evidence of bone defect repair is seen in remains of trephined prehistoric skulls *(20)*. There is a report on a large defect in a bronze age skull that evidently was closed by reimplanting the removed fragment as an orthotopic bone autograft. In the specimen, the cut margin shows no sign of healing, so the operation may have been fatal.

The first successful bone defect repair was recorded by the Dutch surgeon Job van Meek'ren in 1668 *(21)*. He described the filling of a defect in a soldier's cranium with a piece of dog skull. This bone xenograft had to be removed 2 yr later on the patient's wish, since, after the transplantation, he was excommunicated and he wanted to return to the good graces of the Church.

The scientific approach to the problem of osteogenesis and bone transplantation was started by du Hamel in 1739 *(22)*. However, it took almost 200 yr before anyone was able to report large series of patients with an autogenous bone transplant. The problems of humoral and cellular immune response to bone allografts remain unsolved to this very day *(6)*.

Bone transplants are used to unite fractures, to fuse joints, and to repair skeletal defects only in those cases in which they can satisfy the criteria of mechanical stability and host incorporation without complications. The acquisition of autogenous bone transplant material is not without consequences for the patient, including additional surgical incision, weakened bone at the donor site, and increased postoperative morbidity *(2)*. Not only is the amount of autogenous bone restricted, but, furthermore, the BG may have insufficient mechanical, biological, and physiological properties.

Because of the problem of the availability of appropriate bone replacement materials, many artificial materials for bone substitution have been developed *(5,14,23,24)*. Some of them are clearly related to bone tissue. In that case, the term "transplant," as well as "implant" can be used.

According to the genetic relationship between donor and recipient, there are four classes of bone transplants:

1. Autogenous BG (autograft): donor and recipient are the same individual;
2. Isogenous BG (isograft): donor and recipient are genetically identical individuals of the same species (monozygotic twins, animals of highly inbred strain);
3. Allogenous BG (allograft): donor and recipient are genetically dissimilar individuals of the same species;
4. Xenogenous BG (xenograft): donor and recipient are individuals of different species.

Transplantation generally does not include the use of prostheses, synthetic materials, or artificial implants that may be fixed within or attached to the body, but that do not comprise human or animal cells or tissues. However, the materials could coincidentally be of similar composition to living tissue, or even be produced by living organs. An example of such a material is the porous Ca carbonate and HA skeletal structure of some marine invertebrates. In this context, the xenograft may encompass artificial implants. According to the site of implantation, transplants are termed "orthotopic" when the transplantation site and donor site are the same, and "heterotopic" when these sites are different. Grafts may be viable or nonviable when implanted.

3.1. Autogenous BG

Autogenous BG possesses maximum biocompatibility. Therefore, autogenous cancellous bone is generally considered to be the best material available for bone grafting *(5)*. Cancellous grafts are more rapidly and completely revascularized than cortical grafts.

Fundamentally, both cancellous and cortical bone are incorporated by the same process, including apposition and resorption, but there is a difference in the rate of apposition and resorption. The substitution of a cancellous BG first involves a phase of appositional bone formation and, secondarily, a resorptive phase; a cortical BG undergoes a process sometimes described as creeping substitution, and, in most cases, remains as an admixture of necrotic and viable bone *(25)*.

The mechanical strengths of cancellous and cortical autogenous BGs may be correlated with their respective repair processes. Cancellous bone autografts tend to become strong first; cortical grafts lose strength in the beginning. This weakening of cortical transplant is a function of its internal porosity, caused by the cumulative effects of increased osteoclastic and decreased osteoblastic activities, and illustrates the creeping substitution *(26)*. Experimental cortical bone transplants were shown to be approx 40–50% weaker than normal bone 6 wk–6 mo after transplantation.

Cortical bone strength was regained in approx 1–2 yr as the internal porosity approached that of normal bone. The segmental autogenous cortical bone transplant must be protected when the resorptive phase has outstripped the appositional phase. It is not precisely known when these critical phases occur in humans.

The active osteogenesis by the living cells of an autogenous bone transplant, in contrast to the inductive properties of the noncellular organic and inorganic elements of the graft, is the chief advantage of autogenous bone grafting. It is not known how much of the final incorporation of the transplant results from the tissue of the host and how much results from the remaining living cells of the graft.

Transplant failure occurs in 15–25% of autogenous segmental cortical transplants: Most of them have failed principally because they did not satisfy necessary biological, physiological, and mechanical requirements *(26)*. Adequate fixation of the graft, following its insertion, is essential, "as study of various means for these ends in such work as tree grafting will show" *(27)*.

The revascularization of bone autograft by microvascular anastomoses has been the subject of experimental studies and has become of practical importance in bone grafting. In 1923, Albee pointed out the following requirements for bone grafting from his experience of 3000 grafts: The graft should be autogenous; the marrow of the graft should be in contact with the marrow of the host bone; the graft should be the internal fixation agent, within limits (use of metal plates or other foreign material is not recommended); the graft should consist of all four bone layers, namely, periosteum, complete thickness of cortex, endosteum, and marrow; the graft should be inserted, so that corresponding cambium layers come in close contact; the graft should be strong enough that it will resist fracture during and after the period of artificial external support, until osteogenesis occurs to a sufficient degree.

Despite excellent biocompatibility, the limited availability and the higher morbidity associated with obtaining autografts remain disadvantages of autogenous BG *(2,28)*. Therefore, many bone-saving procedures, such as the use of boiled or frozen orthotopic bone autograft, have been developed in traumatology for the repair of massive loss of bone, and in oncological surgery, for after eradication of malignant or benign bone tumors. The insertion of a prosthesis to repair the continuity of bone is only a good treatment for patients with bone tumors of low-grade malignancy. Even a massive tumorous bone segment can be resected, autoclaved, and replaced to reconstruct bone continuity. However, addition of free fresh autogenous bone chips and a rigid fixation with long-term stability would be necessary. The benign, but locally destructive, bone tumor can be treated by freezing. The osteogenetic potential and the mechanical properties of bone transplants, treated this way, are not the same as those of autogenous bone.

The advantages of boiled or frozen autograft can be summarized as follows: the immediate availability of bone tissue, the graft is a good fit, sufficient stability, extensive use of bone from donor sites is not required, and reconstruction of large bone defects is possible. However, it is not always possible to save or obtain autogenous bone for bone defect repair. The defect may be too large to be filled by an autogenous BG alone. The operation required for obtaining pieces of autogenous BG may be an unnecessary additional stress for the patient *(2,28)*. In cases of facial bone defects, as well as in cases of reconstructive middle ear surgery, additional difficulties in the shaping and restoration of the normal and symmetrical facial contour may be encountered when bone chips are used. The same applies in middle ear reconstructive surgery. In such cases, some other hard-tissue substitute material is needed *(25)*. The alternative for repair of bone defects by transplantation of autogenous tissue, such as free non- or revascularized autogenous periosteum, have been reported in experimental studies *(29a)*. However, the lack of stability and the long period of time needed for bone formation from periosteum are the chief problems in the clinical use of periosteal transplant in cases of massive loss of bone.

3.2. Isogenous BG

Isogenous BG is only of theoretical importance in human bone defect repair, because of the low incidence (1:250 pregnancies) of monozygotic twins. There is no literature concerning this subject in the field of bone transplantation.

3.3. Allogenous BG

Skeletal surgery, especially bone tumor surgery, often requires additional supplies of bone, which may not be obtained in sufficient quantity and quality from the host without unacceptable risks. Therefore, allogenous and even xenogenous grafts, and, more recently, artificial materials have been considered to be alternatives to autogenous BGs.

Allogenous BGs became a relatively popular alternative to autogenous bone. However, allogenous BGs present an immunological problem. Transplants of fresh allogenous bone follow the immunological principles of other tissue allografts. The chief disadvantage of allografting is a eliciting of the immunological host response, resulting in graft rejection. Because of this allograft property, the bone autograft, even if difficult to obtain, is still preferable in bone tissue replacement.

The histocompatibility Ags of bone allografts are presumably proteins or glycoproteins on cell surfaces, although it is not certain if the bone matrix itself is able to elicit the immunological host response *(26)*. The rejections of bone allografts is considered to be a cellular, rather than a humoral, mechanism. The graft rejection is expressed by the disruption of vessels, an inflammatory reaction dominated by lymphocytes, fibrous encapsulation, peripheral graft resorption, callus bridging, nonunions, and fatigue fractures. The remodeling of allografted bone is a long-term process, including the possibility of late rejection of bone allografts.

Many techniques have been advised to minimize the antigenic differences between the donor and the recipient of a bone allograft. Destruction of the Ags within the bone allograft, blocking the host's immune response, and, recently, tissue typing, have been suggested as means of minimizing antigenic differences *(28)*. Bone allografts that are treated to destroy their antigenicity prior to implantation lack viable cells and become implants. The treatment of allografts by chemical procedures, heating or freezing, and by ionizing radiation energy causes changes in the physical and biological properties of the graft.

One of the oldest methods is boiling the BG *(29)*, which destroys the Ags of the bone, but boiled bone is less successfully incorporated in the recipient, because the cells are destroyed and the proteins are denatured. Its inductive repair capacity has been negated, but some excellent clinical results have been claimed in boiled allogenous bone implants.

Frozen BGs were frequently used as a substitute material for autografts, because they were considered to be almost nonantigenic. However, experimental and clinical findings demonstrated that bone immunogenicity was partially retained *(30a)*. Freeze-dried bone allografts were used for the clinical packing of small defects or the bridging of large defects. The final evaluation of freeze-dried bone grafting is incomplete. Long-term evaluation suggests complications similar to those found with frozen grafts *(26)*.

Treatment of an allogenous BG by chemicals may involve deproteinization, decalcification, and lipophilization. Deproteinized bone implants were obtained by ethylenediamine extraction or glycerol-ashing, but were mechanically fragile, and therefore not suitable as supportive skeletal struts. Organic decalcified bone allografts heal a skeletal defect more successfully than inorganic implants.

The temporary immunosuppression of the host, while the allograft undergoes creeping substitution and depletion of transplantation Ags, has not yet been fully investigated. This concept seems to be of limited practical value, because of the need for long-term immunosuppression and its concomitant side effects.

Histocompatibility tissue typing improves acceptance of bone allografts in experimental studies, and may be of value in clinical situations. However, the difficulties with tissue-typing procedures are still not solved *(28)*.

As an allogenous tissue, bone is antigenically active. Although many methods have been used to reduce or avoid this antigenicity, none of them has so far gained widespread acceptance. Conflicting reports regarding the boneforming efficiency of allogenous bone matrix may result from the chemical, physical, and biological treatment of bone matrix before implantation. One cannot exclude the possibility that such treatment preceding implantation may in fact render a tissue of such poor quality as to confer no particular advantage over a purely artificial substance. The conclusion may be drawn that an allogenous bone graft is not a suitable aid for restoring the continuity of a bone in adults *(30)*.

Bone allografts can also transmit human immunodeficiency virus.

3.4. Xenogenous BG

Xenogenous (hetero) grafts can be divided in two main groups: cross-species BGs and artificial material implants.

3.4.1. Cross-species BG

The cross-species (mostly bovine) BGs must be specially treated, because of genetic incompatibility, but without changing its structural characteristics *(31)*. The organic fraction (Ags, fats, mucopolysaccharides, and so on) has to be removed to allow the host's acceptance of this so-called "os purum." Ethylenediamine-treated anorganic bone has been a widely used material in bone replacement. Defatted, decalcified xenogenous bone, impregnated with fresh autologous marrow, has been used in experimental bridging of large cortical defects. However, reports on the use of this bone material have given conflicting results. Bone-inducing properties have been reported by some, but denied by others. Defatted calcified bovine graft (Kiel bone) has been used in spinal fusion. Frozen bone xenografts were used in so-called bone-banks, but were eventually discarded, because of problems arising from their genetic incompatibility.

3.4.2. Artificial Material Implants

The artificial (mostly anorganic) materials (xeno-implants) constitute a large group of metals, plastic polymers, ceramics, and composite materials. Even wooden implants have been proposed for bone tissue replacement *(32)*.

3.5. Biocompatibility

The development and application of surgical and orthopedic implants made it necessary to give increasing attention to the materials used for the manufacture of such implants. These materials, which are also referred to as biomaterials, must meet certain chemical, physical, and biological requirements, in order to ensure optimum and lasting function of the implant and success of the implantation procedure. The chemical and physical requirements include such properties as strength, wearing friction behavior, corrosion resistance, workability, and sterilizability. Acceptance by living tissues and stability within the body constitute important biological requirements.

Biocompatibility is determined by the extent of chemical and biological interaction between host and implant, and the stability (mechanical integrity) of the implant. Rapid and cheap in vitro techniques can be used to predict the quantity and cytotoxicity of moistures released by an implant. These techniques can also be used to predict changes in mechanical properties of a material during implantation, which can be important in selection of materials as candidates for definitive preclinical animal experimental and clinical studies.

A compatible implant would have no effect on the adjacent tissue, the nearby cells would show no abnormalities, no variant cell types would appear, there would be no inflammatory reactions, and there would be no cell necrosis. The histology of the tissue surrounding the implant would be altogether normal *(33)*.

The implant recognized by the recipient as a foreign body will be isolated by encapsulation. Commonly, the thickness of the encapsulating fibrous tissue membrane is often taken as a measure of the compatibility of the implant in relation to the surrounding tissue. The thinner the membrane, the better the compatibility of the implant.

Animal studies of biocompatibility are necessary, because of the complexity of chemical, biological, and physical (mechanical) implant–host interactions. Strong dependence of the tissue response on the biomechanical conditions along the interfaces has been demonstrated in experimental studies. The amount of motion between the implant and the adjacent tissues contributes greatly to the biological response. Any histological evaluation of a biomaterial for bone replacement must be accompanied by a careful description of the load and changes that have been applied to the bone–implant interface. The portion of the interface from where the histological sample was taken must be noted.

Unfortunately, methods of determination of compatibility are not standardized, which complicates any comparison of different studies of one implant material: Sometimes it makes it impossible. Therefore, it has been proposed to establish a rigid system for determining material biocompatibility by standardized test controls. Implant materials should be subjected to biological tests in a stepwise, standardized procedure. No general agreement on this has yet been reached. In general, either a material has slowly evolved to fulfill a long-established clinical need, or a new material has been tried, on an arbitrary basis, to explore clinical and commercial possibilities. Probably most biomaterials have become known in this fashion. This situation is less satisfactory than if a thoroughly scientific approach to the development of biocompatible materials had been adopted.

3.6. Biodegradable, Bioactive, and Bioinert Materials

The terms "biodegradable," "bioactive," and "bioinert" are related to the biochemical response that the implanted material provokes in the surrounding tissue, and relates to the notion of biocompatibility. Tissue reactions caused by relative movement between the implant and the adjacent tissue are not covered by these terms *(34)*.

The term "biodegradable" (bioresorbable) has been used for material that, after insertion into host tissue, is desolved without provoking any adverse tissue reaction. Some of the CaP ceramics possess such a property *(35)*.

The terms "bioactive" and "bioinert" are related to the biochemical response induced by the material at the site of implantation. Bioactive materials induce the same reaction that natural bone mineral would do at the same implant area; the bioinert materials cause no reaction at all. Bioactive ceramics can form a tight junction with the osseous tissue, analogous to the natural bone mineral. This seems to be a biochemical phenomenon, but there is still no explanation for this behavior of bioactive materials *(33,35,36)*.

3.6.1. Ceramics

Ceramics comprise heterogenous groups of related materials *(35)*. There is no universal classification for these materials. Most ceramic materials are crystalline in nature. However, there are amorphous or glassy ceramics, also. The distinction between those ceramics that are amorphous or glassy and some types of glass, which have high melting points, is difficult to draw. Different ceramics, such as CaP ceramics, crystalline variant of bioglasses, and materials such as Ca aluminates, titanates, zirconates, and alumina and silica, have been used for surgical implantation. They possess the following advantages: Many ceramic oxides are at their highest energy level and cannot be oxidized further; they are mostly insoluble in body fluids; and they are highly inert, and some of them are even bioactive *(37,38)*.

The disadvantages, however, are that ceramics are known to be brittle materials possessing no ductility, and, generally, they have an extremely high modulus of elasticity and low flexural and tensile strength. They are also difficult to manufacture, because high temperatures are required, and they are difficult to mold in applicable forms. For these reasons, in the past, very little serious consideration of ceramic materials proceeded further than the consideration of their mechanical properties, but with the development of technology and instruments for designing ceramics in applicable forms, and the development of new ceramics and composites, these disadvantages are being overcome.

In the absence of systematic guidelines, the history of the choice of ceramic materials for repair of bone defects has been one of trial and error. The first report of the use of ceramics to fill defects in bone came in 1892, from Trendelenburg's clinic in Bonn. Plaster of Paris (biodegradable Ca sulphate dihydrate) was used to fill bone cavities of different origin (tuberculosis, osteomyelitis, and enchondroma) in eight patients, with satisfactory results *(39)*. Since then, plaster of Paris has been used in a limited number of experimental and clinical studies. It has never been used widely, because of its poor mechanical properties, and because its resorption rate is too rapid to allow adequate bone ingrowth.

It has only been within the past few years that reports have appeared on the use of ceramic materials for internal prosthetic application, and also on the repair of skeletal defects. In 1963, almost 70 yr after the first use of plaster of Paris to fill a bone defect, a porous ceramic material with good tissue compatibility was proposed for bone replacement.

The first applications of these materials were in dentistry, and in oral and maxillofacial surgery. Later, various methods were used to replace bone with different ceramic materials in surgery and orthopedics. Ceramics have been injected as a solution, or implanted as granules, to stimulate osteogenesis; they have been used as a filler that is resorbed at approximately the same rate that new bone regenerates. They have also been used as a compact material in places of atrition, or as a porous implant that would invite osseous proliferation into open pores. A most important observation has been the high degree of compatibility between the host bone and some of the ceramic materials *(14)*.

The use of porous ceramics in soft tissue replacement, such as tracheal prostheses, or in the cardiovascular system as valve replacement, had not been generally recommended because of the high infection rate, and because of their severe thrombogenic activity when in direct contact with blood *(40)*. Still, dense ceramics, such as vitreous carbon, have found wide application in replacement of heart valves.

Currently, the ceramics used as bone tissue replacement material show encouraging experimental and clinical results. The cell and tissue compatibility of many ceramic materials has been improved in these studies. Particularly, HA displays an attractive profile that features its excellent biocompatibility *(14)*. Porous ceramics, with a pore size greater than 100 µm, show significant ingrowth of natural bone when these implants are in contact with host bone tissue. These ceramics have already been developed as commercially available implants, and are used in clinical praxis. Reduced mechanical resilience appears to be the only disadvantage that might restrict its clinical application. The search continues for an ideal ceramic material for surgical implants that would combine complete biological inertness with adequate mechanical strength.

3.6.2. Composite Materials

A composite material is simply a combination of two or more different materials. In order to design a composite material having a certain set of properties, the following characteristics of the compounds must be considered: biodegradability, biocompatibility, elastic moduli, mechanical strength, and binding tendencies between the components. These variables interact in a complex manner, and a detailed consideration of each is necessary to anticipate the behavior of various components when combined to form a composite material. Modern composites try to imitate nature. Bone is a composite of the strong but soft protein, collagen, and the hard but brittle mineral, HA. Modern composites try to achieve similar results by the combination of strong fibers, of a material such as carbon, in a soft matrix. The new materials provide strength, stiffness, and lightness, and are also inert.

Most composite materials include a ceramic component, because of the biocompatibility and the biodegradability of ceramics. The other component can be metal or plastic. A familiar example is Cerosium (alumina and epoxy resin) and Fiberglass (fiber-glass-reinforced plastic). An unscratched ceramic can be very strong, but flaws enable it to be easily cracked. If the ceramic is divided into minute pieces, as in powder, a crack present cannot find a continuous path through the material. For the particles, or, more usually, fibers, to form a useful structural material, they must be bound together in a matrix. The properties of the matrix are of great importance. The matrix must not scratch the fibers and introduce cracks. It must transmit stress to the fibers, be plastic and adhesive to immobilize the fibers securely, and, finally, it must deflect and control cracks within the composite. Under tensile load, virtually all the stress is carried by the fibers, so that the matrix makes a negligible contribution to the breaking strength of the composite.

Under stress, the fibers with cracks may break, but the soft matrix hinders propagation of the crack. The fibers do not fail at one plane, so that the progression of the crack completely across the material occurs only if the fibers are withdrawn from the matrix. If the adhesion between matrix and fibers is low, the crack that initially runs at right angles to the fibers will be deflected along the weak interface and rendered harmless, as far as the tensile strength of the composite is concerned. For resistance to tension, shear stress, and compression, multiple orientation of fibers provides moderate strength in many directions, although the absolute strength in any axis will be compromised. For internal reconstruction of the skeleton, the absolute strength of the implant would be no advantage, because it would be so different from that which is present in bone. To use rigid implant materials, some method of providing a gradual transmission in stiffness across the bone–implant interface would be necessary. At present, composites are under consideration that may provide both superior metals and polymers for implantation *(38)*.

Early composite materials for bone replacement were developed from plaster of Paris. In 1960, plaster of Paris was mixed with epoxy resin to achieve better strength for the filling of large osseous defects. The epoxy resin, however, made this material incompatible with living tissue.

Compositions of apatite powder and a collagen matrix, with the same ratio of these components as exists in bone, have been developed recently *(38)*. However, lack of mechanical stability still prevents the use of this material (Collapat) in bone replacement surgery. This material, with its bone-like composition, may become an important bone substitute in the future. Currently, there is no synthetic composite material available that possesses both biocompatibility and mechanical properties necessary for segmental bone replacement.

4. Clinical Bone Substitution

4.1. Materials and Methods

The authors' prospective clinical study consisted of filling bone defects with HA implants, to support the tibial plateau, after operative treat-

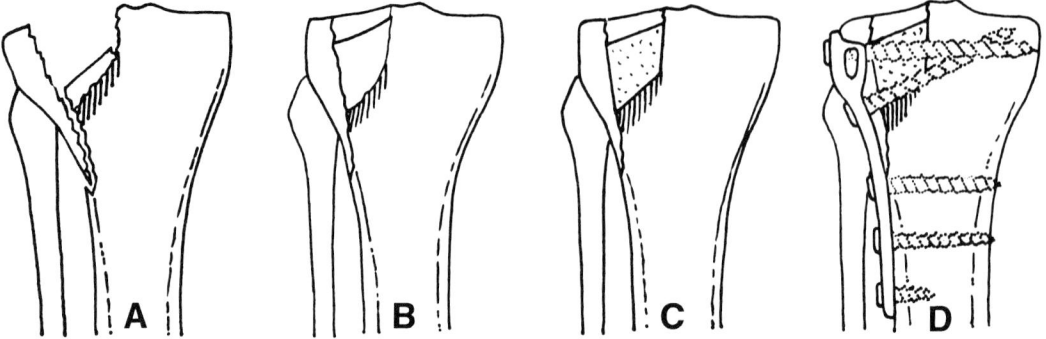

Fig. 1. Restoration of articular congruity of the tibial plateau.

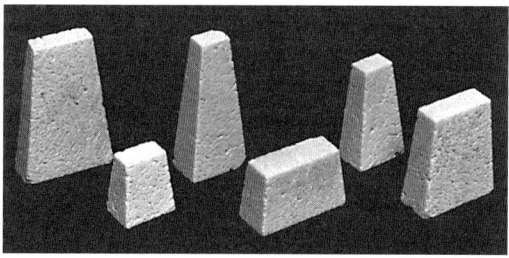

Fig. 2. HA implants of different shape and volume.

ment in cases of displaced fractures (Fig. 1). Open reduction was performed only in local-depression fractures displaced more than 1 cm. Depressed tibia plateau fragments were elevated (Fig. 1B), the resulting bone defect was filled with HA implants of appropriate volume and shape (Fig. 1C), and the fracture was stabilized with plate and screws (Fig. 1D).

Sixty-one patients, mean age 46 yr (18–76 yr), were treated and followed-up for at least 3 yr (3–12 yr). Rigid internal fixation was achieved in part by support of the fracture with HA implants, and allowed immediate postoperative mobilization of the knee joint. The operative procedure was open in 47 patients; in 14 patients, an arthroscopic guided technique was used.

HA material for clinical use was prepared by the same procedure as for experimental study, but the ^{45}Ca level was not used, and the implant shape was pyramidal in 11 patients. However, HA granula were used in 50 patients *(14–37)* (Fig. 2).

4.2. Results

The clinical study provided radiographical long-term results, up to 12 yr, in 61 patients. All of them had only minor loss of knee motion; normal extension and flexion not less than 130°. One patient died because of a myocardial infarction 2 wk postoperatively. Knee flexion had already exceeded 1201 with a normal extension range. This patient provided the only tissue for macroscopic and microscopic observation (Fig. 3). Sixty remaining patients recovered within 2 wk of hospitalization. Weight bearing was allowed gradually, starting 6 wk after surgery. Full weight bearing was achieved 12 wk postoperatively in all patients. No changes in the HA implants were observed up to 11 yr after implantation, as seen on the radiographs (Fig. 4), nor were there physical changes in the function of the operated limb.

4.3. Discussion

There is a growing need for a suitable material that is directly available and can be supplied in unlimited quantities in the reconstruction of bone defects, especially for bone defects remaining after the restoration of local depression of articular surface. In these cases, the proper support of repaired articular surface makes it possible to mobilize the damaged joint immediately after surgery, which is desirable for the ultimate result. Tibial plateau fracture may contribute to irregularity of the articular surface, angular deformity, ligament laxity, and tearing of the meniscus. The radiographic appearance usually does not reflect

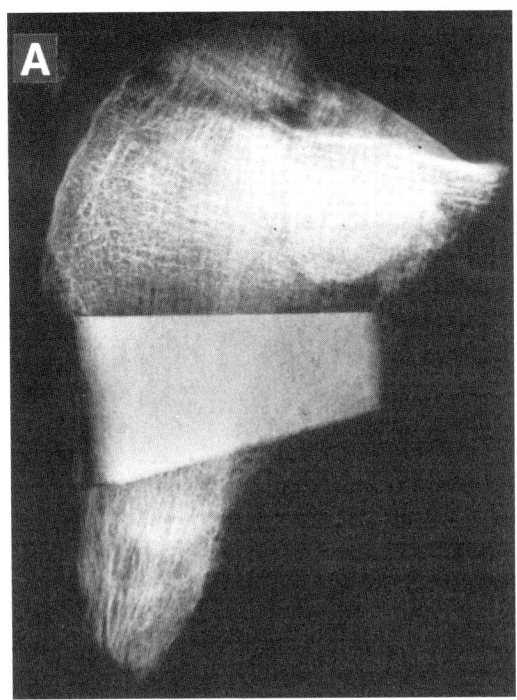
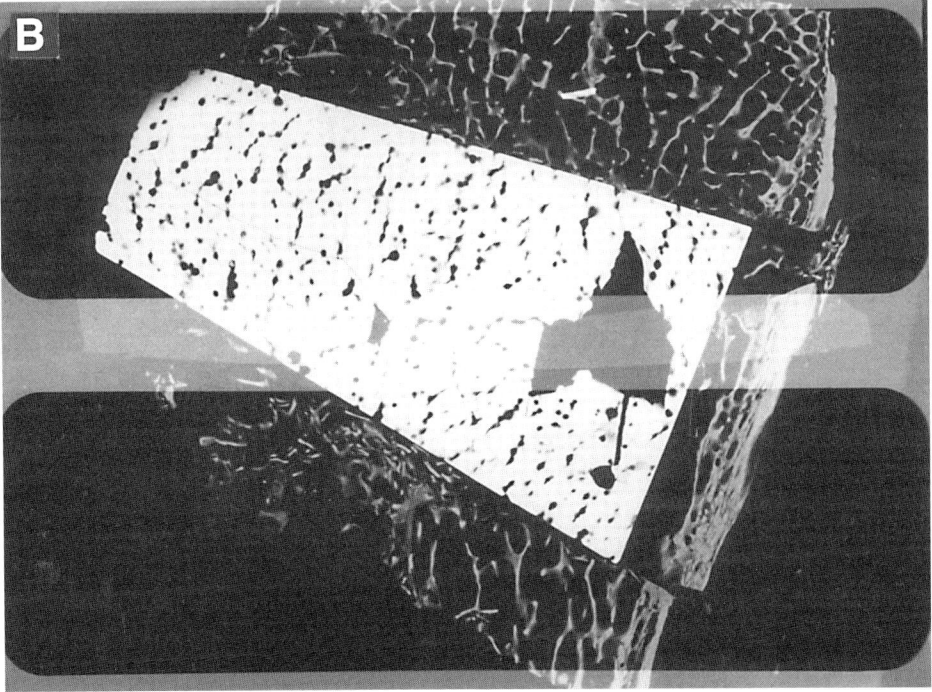

Fig. 3. Radiograph (**A**) and micrograph (**B**) of HA implants 2 wk after implantation.

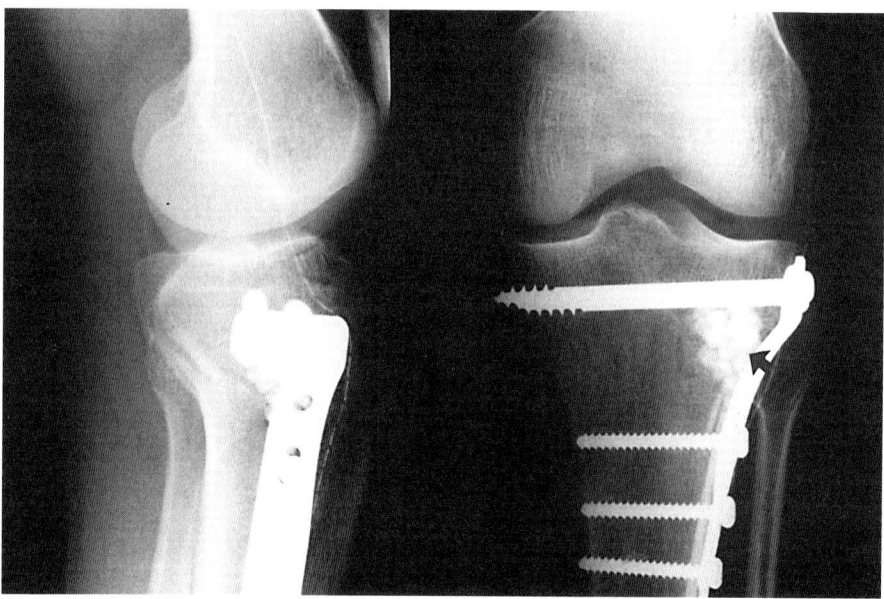

Fig. 4. Radiograph of a HA implant in tibial head 5 yr after implantation.

the final clinical result. The prognosis has been shown to be most closely related to the residual displacement of the articular surface and the angular deformity. To avoid the poor outcome leading to late resurfacing procedures *(41,42)*, or making the elevating osteotomies for posttraumatic deformaties necessary *(43)*, primary operative treatment of tibial plateau fractures should be performed in displacements exceeding 1 cm *(44)*. However, this treatment results in knee stiffness, when the joint is not mobilized immediately after surgery *(7)*.

Early active motion of the knee joint is the most important step in obtaining optimum results in the treatment of fractures of the tibial condyle *(44)*. This necessitates the use of stable internal fixation, which implicates the use, among others, of materials to fill bone gaps. The HA has been proven to be useful for this purpose. It withstands the compression forces, fills bone cavity, supports the joint surface, and makes no second surgery necessary to obtain an autogenous BG *(45–49)*.

Carbonated HA, which can be molded during the operative procedure, and is suitable in a paste consistency for easy filling of bone gaps, has recently been developed. This poorly crystalline apatitic CaP is prepared as an injectable paste, at room temperature, and hardens by the endothermical setting reaction at 37°C after implantation *(50;* Fig. 5). Experience with this promising variant of solid HA is limited, especially concerning its resorbability.

5. Conclusion

A suitable material of proper quality, which is readily available, is still needed for surgical repair of bone defects. Some ceramics and some ceramic composite materials are being investigated, because of their biocompatibility and similarity to normal bone.

Ceramics, as oxides, are not subject to the oxidative corrosion to which all metals are susceptible; neither do they evoke the tissue reaction characteristic of many polymers. The open porosity of these structures allows ingrowth of living tissues within the interstices of the material, thereby encouraging its active fixation. Furthermore, even osteoconductivity has been reported, in the case of some ceramics.

Although abrasion resistance may be comparable to that of metals, and strength in compression far superior, the tensile strength of conventional ceramics is far below the requirements for an

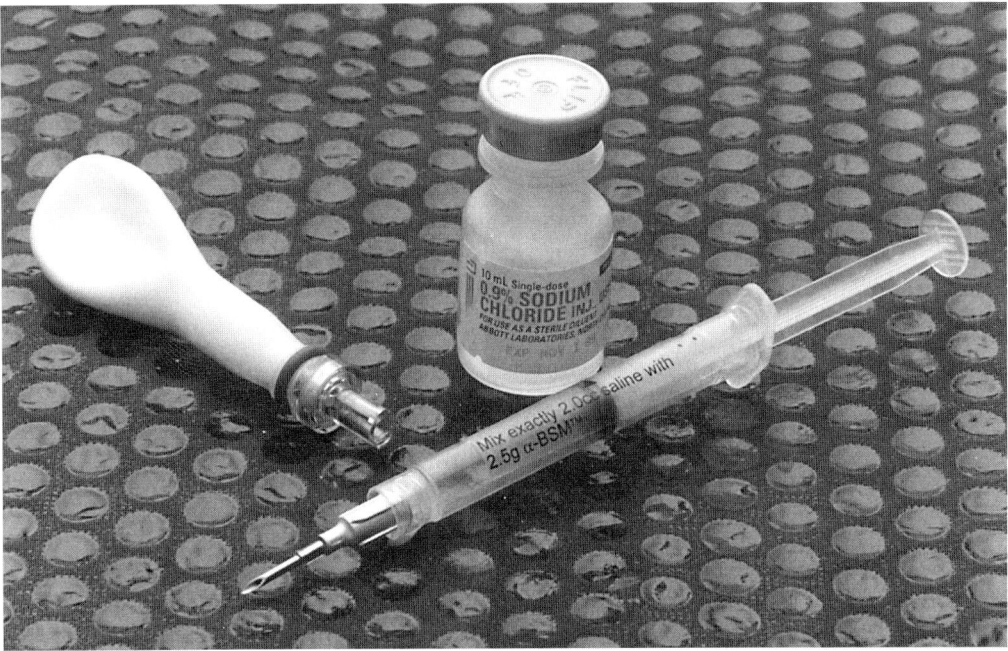

Fig. 5. Apatitic CaP paste for bone substitution.

implant material in bone tissue. Therefore, the clinical use of ceramics is still limited to parts of the skeleton that are exposed only to compression forces. The possibility of impregnating a brittle ceramic material with a ductile and resilient material, to improve its mechanical properties, is the subject of many investigations. At this moment, the ideal combination has not yet been discovered.

Acknowledgments

The authors gratefully acknowledge the contribution to this study of Dr. J. G. C. Wolke from the Department of Biomaterial Sciences, Nÿmegen University, The Hague, The Netherlands, CAM-implants, for providing help with manufacturing implants.

References

1. Enneking WF, Eady JL, and Burchhardt H. Autogenous cortical bone grafts in the reconstruction of segmental skeletal defects. *J Bone Joint Surg* 1980; 62: 1039.
2. Grob D. Autologous bone transplantation: problems at the donor site. *Unfallchirurg* 1986; 89: 339–345.
3. Weiland AJ, Moore JR, and Daniel RK. Vascularised bone autografts: experience with 41 cases. *Clin Orthop* 1983; 174: 87.
4. Virolainen P, Vuono E, and Aro HT. Different healing rates of bone autografts, syngeneic grafts, and allografts in experimental rat model. *Arch Orthop Trauma Surg* 1997; 116: 486–491.
5. Damien ChJ and Parsons JR. Bone graft and bone graft substitutes: a review of current technology and applications. *J Appl Biomater* 1991; 2: 187–208.
6. Dijk BA van, Stassen J, Kunst VAJM, Slooff TJJH, and Hoorn JR van. Rhesus immunisation after bone allografting. *Acta Orthop Scand* 1988; 59: 482.
7. Gausewitz S and Hohl M. Significance of early motion in the treatment of tibia plateau fractures. *Clin Orthop Relat Res* 1986; 202: 135–138.
8. Rasmussen PS. Tibial condylar fractures; impairment of the knee joint stability as an indication for surgical treatment. *J Bone Joint Surg* 1973; 55A: 1331–1350.
9. Wagner HE and Jacob PP. Problems involved in plate osteosynthesis in bicondylar tibial fractures. *Unfallchirurg* 1986; 89: 304–311.
10. Kotter A and Ruter A. Tibiakopffracturen. *Unfallchirurg* 1997; 90: 742–749.

11 Blattert TR, Weckbach A, Kuntz E, and Wagner R. Consequences of injury and succeeding joint-impairment after fracture dislocation of the tibial head. *Zentralbld Chir* 1997; 122: 986–993.

12 Holmes R, Mooney V, Bucholz R, and Tencer A. Coralline hydroxyapatite bone graft substitute: preliminary report. *Clin Orthop Rel* 1984; 188: 252–262.

13 Holmes RE, Bucholz RW, and Mooney V. Porous hydroxyapatite as a bone-graft substitute in metaphyseal defects. *J Bone Joint Surg* 1986; 68A: 904–911.

14 Patka P, Otter G den, Groot K de, and Driessen AA. Reconstruction of large bone defects with calcium phosphate ceramics: an experimental study. *Neth J Surg* 1985; 37: 38–44.

15 Wipperman BW. *Hydroxylapatite Keramik als Knochenersatzstoff* 1996; Springer Verlag, Heidelberg.

16 Bucholz RW, Carlton A, and Holmes R. Interporous hydroxyapatite as a bone graft substitute in tibial plateau fractures. *Clin Orthop Rel Res* 1989; 24: 53–62.

17 Kawai N, Niwa S, Sato M, Sato Y, Sawa Y, and Ichihara I. Bone formation by cells from femurs cultured among three-dimensionally arranged hydroxyapatite granules. *J Biomed Mater Res* 1997; 37: 1–8.

18 Hulbert SF and Young FA. *Use of Ceramics in Surgical Implants* 1978; Gordon and Breach, London.

19 Recum AF von. Academic environment of biomaterials science and engineering. *J Appl Biomater* 1992; 3: 63–71.

20 Parry TV. Trephination of the living human skull in prehistoric times. *Br Med J* 1923; 1: 457–460.

21 Meek'ren J. *Heel-en Geneeskonstige Aanmerkingen* 1668; Casparus Commelijn, Amsterdam, Collection of The Museum of Leiden, The Netherlands.

22 Hamel M du. *Sur le Developpement et la Crue des Os des Animaux* 1742; Mem d l'Acad Roy Sciences, Paris, 55: 354–370.

23 Rubin RL. *Biomaterials in Reconstructive Surgery* 1983; CV Mosby, London.

24 Hollinger JO, Mark DE, Goco P, et al. A comparison of four particulate bone derivates. *Clin Orthop Rel Res* 1991; 267: 255–263.

25 Enneking WF, Burchardt H, Puhl JJ, and Piotrowski G. Physical and biological aspects of repair in dog cortical B bone transplants. *J Bone Joint Surg* 1975; 57A: 237–252.

26 Burchardt H and Enneking WF. Transplantation of bone. *Surg Clin N Am* 1978; 58: 403–427.

27 Albee Th. Fundamentals in bone transplantation. Experience in three thousand bone graft operations. *JAMA* 1923; 81: 1429–1432.

28 Blakmore ME. Fractures at cancellous bone graft donor sites. *Injury* 1983; 14: 519–522.

29 Kirkup JR. Traumatic femoral bone loss. *J Bone Joint Surg* 1965; 47B: 106–110.

29a van den Wildenberg, FA, Goris RJ, Boetes L. Revascularized periosteum in transplantations. *Eur Surg Res* 1983; 15: 110–113.

30 Habal MB and Reddi AH. *Bone Grafts and Bone Substitutes* 1992; W.B. Saunders, London.

31 Karges DE, Anderson KJ, Dingwall, and Jowsey J. Experimental evaluation of processed heterogenous bone transplants. *Clin Orthop* 1963; 29: 230–247.

31a Bos GD, Goldbergh VM, Powel AE, Heiple KG, and Zika JM. The effect of histocompatibility matching on canine frozen bone allografts. *J Bone Joint Surg* 1983; 65A: 89–96.

32 Colville J. Carbonised wood: an experimental bone implant. *J Bone Joint Surg* 1980; 62B: 259.

33 Clark AE, Hench LL, and Paschall HA. Influence of surface chemistry on implant interface histology: a theoretical basis for implant materials selection. *J Biomed Mater Res* 1976; 10: 161–174.

34 Williams DF. *Definition in Biomaterials*. 1987; Elsevier, Amsterdam.

35 Ducheyne P and Lemons JE. Bioceramics: material characteristics versus in vivo behavior. *Ann NY Sci Acad* 1988; 523.

36 Osborn JF and Newesely H. Material science of calcium phosphate ceramics. *Biomaterials* 1980; 1: 108–111.

37 Patka P, den Hollander W, den Otter G, Heidendal GAK, and de Groot K. Scintigraphic studies to evaluate stability of ceramics (hydroxyapatite) in bone replacement. *J Nucl Med* 1985; 6: 263–271.

38 Clarke KI, Graves SE, Wong ATC, Triffitt JT, Francis MJO, and Czernuszka JF. Investigation into the formation and mechanical properties of a bioactive material based on collagen and calcium phosphate. *J Mater Sci Mater Med* 1993; 4: 107–110.

39 Dreesmann H. Veber knochenplombierung. *Beitr Klin Chir* 1892; 9: 804–810.

40 Vos GA, Patka P, Klein CAPT, Hoitsma HFW, and de Groot K. Trachael reconstruction with hydroxyapatite tracheal prosthesis. *Life Support Syst* 1986; 4: 283–287.

41 Bömler J and Arnold CC. Resurfacing of depression fractures of the lateral tibial condyle. *Acta Orthop Scand* 1981; 52: 231–232.

42 Locht RC, Gross AE, and Langer F. Late osteo-

chondral allograft resurfacing for tibial plateau fractures. *J Bone Joint Surg* 1984; 6-A: 325–328.

43 Kleming R and Hax PM. Intraligamentous elevating osteotomies for posttraumatic deformities about the knee. In Corrective Osteotomies of the Lower Extremity After Trauma 1985; (Hierholzer G and Muller KH, eds), Springer Verlag, Berlin, pp. 323–328.

44 Hohl M and Luch JV. Fractures of the tibial condyle. *J Bone Joint Surg* 1956; 38-A: 1001–1018.

45 den Hollander W, Patka P, Klein CPAT, and Heidendal GAK. Macroporous calcium phosphate ceramics for bone substitution: a tracer study on biodegradation with ^{45}Ca tracer. *Biomaterials* 1991; 12: 569–573.

46 Hollinger JO, Brekke J, Gruskin E, and Lee D. Role of bone substitutes. *Clin Orthop Rel Res* 1996; 324: 55–65.

47 Klein CPAT, Patka P, and den Hollander W. Macroporous calcium phosphate bioceramics in dog femora: a histological study of interface and biodegradation. *Biomaterials* 1989; 10: 59–62.

48 Lobenhoffer P. Mininvasive Kniegelenkschirurgie. *Zentralbl Chir* 1997; 122: 974–985.

49 Nunes CR, Simski SJ, Sachdeva R, and Wolford LM. Long-term ingrowth and apposition of porous hydroxylapatite implants. *J Biomed Mater Res* 1997; 37: 560–563.

50 Knaack D, Goad EB, Aiolova M, Tofighi, Jacobs K, Rey Ch, and Lee D. Novel fully resorbable calcium phosphate bone substitute. *J Bone Miner Res* 1997; 12: S1,202.

7

Enhancing Cortical Allograft Incorporation Processing by Partial Demineralization and Laser Perforation

A Histologic, Biomechanical, and Immunological Study

Kai-Uwe Lewandrowski, Georg Schollmeier, Axel Ekkernkamp, Henry J. Mankin, Hans K. Uhthoff, and William W. Tomford

1. Introduction

The management of large skeletal defects continues to present a major challenge to orthopedic surgeons, particularly when the problem arises in young patients, in whom artificial devices and joint implants are likely to fail early. Both cemented *(1,2)* and uncemented *(3–5)* devices have significant complications in children and young adults. Therefore, development of a system that provides a biologic alternative seems eminently worthwhile.

Allogeneic musculoskeletal tissues are increasingly used in reconstructive orthopedic surgery. Their clinical use shows promise, but problems such as fracture, nonunions, and infection persist and their incorporation into host bone remains slow and unpredictable. Evidence for this statement is the marked increase in the use of large frozen cortical bone allografts in limb-sparing procedures for the treatment of bone tumors *(6–16)*, of massive traumatic injuries *(17,18)*, or avascular necrosis *(6)*. Moreover, these types of grafts are increasingly used in revisions of failed joint arthroplasties, in which extensive bone loss, caused by osteolysis, is commonly encountered *(19–24)*.

Continued study of the procedure and analysis of causes of failure have led us to conclude that most of these complications result from slow and unpredictable incorporation, which itself may be secondary to antidonor immune responses. Even though the overall success rate for massive cortical bone allografts (defined as return to work and engagement in relatively normal activities, without crutches or braces) is approx 75–85%, only 50% of these patients have an entirely uncomplicated postoperative (po) course. About one quarter of the total group requires further surgery, such as autologous grafting or replating for stress fractures *(25–28)* or delayed union *(11,12,26,28, 29,30–32)*. Some patients require graft excision, because of infection *(33–35)*; others require reimplantation, long-term bracing, or amputation. Clearly, problems still exist with this procedure.

The authors report on experimental results of the use of cortical bone allografts that were modified by a new processing method of controlled partial hydrochloric acid (HCl) demineralization and laser perforation. The objective of these studies was to develop a new type of cortical bone allograft with improved osteoinductive properties. On the basis of cumulative histologic, biomechanical, and immunological data of in vitro and in vivo studies, the authors are currently developing partially demineralized and laser-perforated cortical bone allografts for clinical use.

2. Processing of Cortical Bone Allografts: Historical Considerations

In 1881, a report of the first human homograft transplant was published *(36)* and soon thereafter methods for processing of musculoskeletal tissues began to be investigated, to assure adequate storage. Research on bone and cartilage storage was performed, with the earliest publications originating from Europe. In 1910, Bauer *(37)* published studies on storage of bone at refrigerator temperatures (4–10°C). He claimed, after a series of animal experiments, that bone refrigerated for as long as 3 wk would serve as a successful transplant. In 1911, Tuffier *(38),* working in Paris, reported successful incorporation of bones placed into an animal model after being preserved at similar temperatures for up to 2 mo. Tuffier also evaluated clinical transplants of cartilage, but he found that these fared well in storage for only up to 5 d, beyond which time they deteriorated quickly after transplantation *(39).*

Alexis Carrel *(40)* is generally credited with the earliest studies performed in North America on the storage of musculoskeletal tissues. He discussed the use of cadavers for tissue donation, and noted that fresh cadavers might serve as an almost limitless source of transplants. Carrel showed that, after death, tissue degradation occurred rapidly at body temperatures, but could be delayed or decreased if the body was stored at temperatures of −1 or −2°C. He therefore recommended that, if cadavers were used as donors, they should be put into cold storage.

Albee *(41)* was using stored bone in his clinical surgery as early as 1910. In 1915, Albee published his ideas on the preservation of bone. He recommended that cadaver bone should be rinsed in a normal salt solution immediately after recovery, wrapped in gauze, placed in a jar of Vaseline, and put into cold storage at 4–5°C.

In 1914, Gallie *(43)* reported that, because all cells in bone grafts (BGs) die, except perhaps surface osteoblasts in autogenous grafts, there was little reason not to use stored allografts. Gallie believed that bone could be transplanted in almost any form, and, in 1918, he reported on the use of boiled bone in patients with Pott's disease *(44).* He obtained grafts at autopsy, shaped them, and boiled them before clinical use. He even made bone plates and bone screws from boiled allograft.

Other investigators, however, were more concerned about the survival of cells in grafts and the best method of storage to promote cell survival. In 1916, Dobrowolskaja *(45)* reported that storage of bone in plasma was helpful in promoting cell survival. In 1922, Lewis and McCoy *(46)* evaluated survival of cells after tissue retrieval and found that muscle cells died upon retrieval, and brain cells died about an hour after retrieval, but cartilage cells survived up to 240 h when kept at temperatures of 4–6°C.

In 1923, Haas reported that osteoblastic cells survived up to 19 h in air at room temperature *(47)*; in 1925, he reported experiments on freezing bone *(48)* in which he found that bone stored at temperatures near freezing (0–6°C), for up to 5 d showed signs of proliferation of osteogenic cells when used as bone transplants in animal experiments. Haas recommended the use of frozen bone, and suggested that boiling was not a satisfactory means of treatment of a BG *(49).*

Controversy over the ideal type of preparation of a BG continued into the 1930s. Some investigators supported the idea that any allograft was essentially dead, and that treatment before or during storage did not adversely affect its clinical value as a transplant. After Gallie's reports on the use of boiled bone, Groves removed diseased bones from patients, boiled them, and then used them as autografts. He found evidence of incorporation of these types of bones within a few months after transplantation.

After World War II, in the middle and late 1940s, several reports appeared on the use of banked bone allografts and the methods of storage of human bones. Much of this work was performed in New York hospitals. While working at

New York Orthopaedic Hospital in the middle 1940s, Bush *(50)* reported that he had transplanted fresh BGs from living donors into recipients in simultaneous operations. The donor provided bone that was termed "homologous" (allogenic), if the donor and recipient were unrelated, and "syngeneous," if the donor and recipient were related (e.g., father and son). Bush was probably also the first investigator to use deep freezing for storage of large numbers of BGs for clinical use. Together with Garber, who was a pathologist at New York Hospital, Bush *(50)* found, in experiments with chinchilla rabbits, that homogenous bone, frozen at −25°C, healed in a fashion similar to fresh homogenous bone. Based on the results of these studies, Bush decided to bank bones by freezing, which he believed would provide a better long-term storage method than refrigeration.

In 1949, Weaver *(51)* reported on his experiences in procurement of bone from cadavers. To develop a source of bone other than surgical patients, Weaver began to recover tissues from fresh cadavers or young adults who died in traumatic circumstances, and from whom bone could be removed within 2 h of death. Weaver recommended that all cadaver donors be reviewed for infection, cancer, and "blood dyscrasias," and be tested serologically for syphilis. He recommended that all recoveries be performed under aseptic conditions in a morgue. He processed bone by removing soft tissues, but leaving the periosteum. Cortical bone was fashioned into strips, cancellous bone was crushed or used as blocks, and carpal and tarsal bones were used for replacement of similar bones. Weaver wrapped bone in cotton cloth and sterile silk wraps, and stored the grafts in a deep freezer, using dry ice. Later, he began to place grafts into sealed glass bottles and store them in an ice cream storage cabinet at approx −20 − −25°C. Weaver used massive cortical BGs as onlays or inlays, bone pegs, and dual grafts. Smaller grafts were used for packing and arthrodeses.

The next major development in bone processing and banking was a change in the general type of bank from small hospital-based banks to large region-based banks. This change began in the late 1940s, when George Hyatt, an orthopedist serving in the US Navy, perceived a potential need for a large supply of stored bone and tissues, such as skin and dura mater, during wartime. Assigned to the National Naval Medical Center in Bethesda, MD, Hyatt began a bone bank there by storing bone by freezing *(52)*. In 1950 and 1951, partly in response to a stimulus provided by injuries that occurred during the Korean conflict, such as mandibular and facial injuries, for which no satisfactory source of autogenous bone was available, Hyatt established a formal center for the recovery, processing, storage, and shipment of bone, to provide grafts to naval medical facilities throughout the world.

First, Hyatt realized that shipment of bone stored by freezing was difficult, because of the need to maintain allografts in a frozen state during shipping. To solve this problem, he developed procedures for storing bone by lyophilization, or freeze-drying *(53)*. This method was chosen, because it had been successfully applied to the storage of human blood plasma during World War II, and was shown to be applicable to human skin *(47,54)*. In developing methods of freeze-drying bone, Hyatt collaborated with Earl W. Flosdorf, who was the Director of Research and Development at the F. J. Stokes Machine Company in Philadelphia, PA *(55)*, which specialized in the manufacture of freeze-drying equipment. Flosdorf was the author of a text, and an expert on freeze-drying *(56)*. Under Hyatt's direction, the Navy Tissue Bank began to freeze-dry almost all of its tissues. It subsequently perfected this process, which is now used by tissue banks throughout the world, and is the storage method of over 95% of stored bone allografts.

Perhaps the most important stimulus to tissue and bone banking in the United States was the development of the American Association of Tissue Banks (AATB) in the mid-1970s. The AATB held its first meeting in the spring of 1975 in Washington, DC. Although processing of cadaver bone allografts is essentially still done with techniques similar to those originally described by Hyatt, the major contribution to bone banking made by the AATB has been its influence on quality assurance in tissue preparation.

3. Background and Significance

In an attempt to enhance incorporation of cortical bone allografts into host bone, previous research focused on the development of a new processing method consisting of controlled partial demineralization and laser perforation. The approach of using HCl demineralization was chosen because it is known to result in the exposure of osteoinductive noncollagenous bone matrix factors to the surrounding soft tissues *(57)*. Such factors include the transforming growth factor (TGF-β), bone morphogenetic proteins (BMPs) *(57–63)*, and sialoproteins, including osteopontin *(64)*, bone Gla protein *(65)*, osteocalcin *(66–69)*, and others. They contribute to the tranformation of mesenchymal cells into the osteogenic and chondrogenic cells *(20)* required for induction of bone resorption and formation of new bone *(70)*.

Immune responses to bone allografts have been implicated in causing adverse biological outcomes. *In vivo* and *in vitro* experiments have provided evidence of both humoral and cellular-mediated rejection *(71–79)*. Other studies *(74,76, 80–82)* have suggested that the predominant response of the host to the bone allograft is a cellular-mediated response to the major histocompatibility complex (MHC) class I and II cell surface antigens (Ags) recognized by responding T-lymphocytes in the host.

Most knowledge of immune responses to cortical bone allografts is based on rodent studies, which have demonstrated that bone allografts are a potent stimulus of donor-specific immune responses *(81,83–92)*. Immunological studies in dogs have suggested that modulation of immune responses may favorably influence incorporation of vascularized cortical bone allografts *(91–96)*. In numerous other animal models, high immunogenicity (i.e., highly mismatched, fresh grafts) has correlated with poor biologic outcome. In contrast, low immunogenicity (i.e., MHC Ag-matched and/or frozen/freeze-dried grafts) was associated with improved outcome *(82,97–100)*. These observations support the hypothesis that immune responses against BG-related Ags have biologic significance in animals.

The influence of immune responses on these large grafts in humans is less clear. Small, fresh-frozen *(76,101)* and freeze-dried *(102,103)* grafts have been shown to elicit humoral and cellular immune responses, but their effect on incorporation was questionable. In studies of large grafts, 85% of bone allograft recipients were found to have an antibody (Ab) response against a cell standard panel *(104)*. However, an almost identical percentage was found in a control population (possibly secondary to transfusions or pregnancy *(104)*. Other studies have failed to correlate the degree of donor–recipient histoincompatibility with clinical complications *(105–112)*. Their incidence is therefore probably related more to a delayed incorporation *(99)*.

Clinical complications are multifactorial in origin. The effect of factors such as graft fit, internal fixation device application, mechanics of the extremity, vascularity of the tissue bed, and use of adjuvant radiation or chemotherapy must be included in any assessment of the causes of graft failure. Studies to date have failed to adequately define the effect of immune responses on bone allograft outcomes in humans, in part because of their lack of consideration of these variables. Therefore, further immunological assessment of partially demineralized and laser-perforated transplants was indicated, to determine how and if the immune system affects their incorporation into host bone.

Studies *(113–118)* have attempted to improve host incorporation by altering the geometric surface configuration of cortical bone. The mechanisms by which the presence of laser holes promoted osteogenesis and incorporation in partially demineralized grafts include the greater surface area of partially demineralized bone and/or increased access to vascular tissue. Previous studies have indicated that the geometry of an implant may influence the extent of bone formation. The osteoconductive potential of cortical bone allografts so treated has been attributed, at least in part, to its morphometric similarity to cancellous bone.

Gendler *(114)* used fully demineralized diaphyseal allogeneic struts perforated by use of a mechanical drill. In comparison, O'Donnell et al. *(116)* used demineralized calvarial cortical bone. Bernick et al. *(113)* characterized the inductive cellular events in a similar system. Scanlon *(117)* implanted demineralized canine femoral strut allografts in an orthotopic model. The latter two studies used an erbium:yttrium-scandium-gallium-garnet (Er:YSGG) laser for drilling of cortical bone allografts, thereby increasing the bone porosity and allowing demineralization to proceed in areas normally inaccessible to the demineralization process. When reimplanted, these grafts may therefore be more osteogenic than cortical grafts without holes. An advantage of the erbium-yttrium-aluminum-garnet (Er:YAG) laser over mechanical drilling is that thermal bone damage does not occur. Tissue is removed by explosive vaporization *(119,120)*. Furthermore, laser ablation is a noncontact process permitting sterile handling of the grafts. Finally, it allows the drilling of a large number of very small holes in a uniform pattern.

Although demineralization has been successful in improving osteoinductive properties of bone in experimental *(121–125)* and clinical studies *(70,75,126–128)*, fully demineralized cortical bone has found limited clinical application in long bone reconstruction. The primary reason for this is that cortical bone, once subjected to extensive demineralization, loses its essential biomechanical properties. However, sufficient mechanical strength of these grafts is necessary, in order to withstand skeletal forces when used in long bone reconstruction. Demineralization of cortical bone yields a geometric surface configuration that is less advantageous for bony ingrowth when compared with cancellous bone, because cortical bone is less porous and has a comparatively low surface area:volume ratio.

4. Hypotheses

On the basis of the rationales presented above, the authors have tested the following hypotheses:

1. Partial demineralization improves osteoinductive properties of cortical bone allografts, which should result in acceleration of incorporation into host bone.
2. Partial demineralization is controllable, allowing production of grafts that retain sufficient mechanical strength for use in long bone reconstruction.
3. Drill holes modify cortical bone allografts into more porous scaffolds, facilitating development of focal centers of bone resorption and new bone formation. If the net result of these concurrent processes is in favor of new bone formation, the graft should be fully replaced by the recipient's own bone.
4. Acid demineralization leads to depletion from the graft of cellular components that express transplantation Ags.
5. Therefore, the effect of demineralization on graft incorporation potentially may be twofold: It should improve osteoinduction and reduce graft rejection.

These hypotheses have stimulated the investigation of the process of cortical bone demineralization. Mathematical models predicting demineralization kinetics were developed, which in turn allowed control of mechanical properties of such treated grafts by deriving mechanical models. Good fit to mechanical models was determined by measuring flexural rigidity and compression strength of partially demineralized and laser-perforated diaphyseal bone allografts. As described in the following subheadings, these methods were employed in orthotopic transplantation studies in rats and later in sheep. These studies showed improved incorporation of partially demineralized and laser-perforated cortical bone allografts, and suggested that both processes may be applicable to clinical bone allografts.

5. In Vitro Studies

Because fully demineralized cortical bone grafts have lost their ability to withstand normal skeletal forces, initial research in this laboratory focused on how to control the demineralization process: a method hitherto unknown.

Several investigators had characterized the demineralization process with the "classic shrinking-core reaction model *(129–131)*; a model that is generally applied to fluid–solid diffusion systems *(132)*. This theory implies the existence of a sharp reaction front that, in the case of demineralization of cortical bone, separates the demineralized from the mineralized portion. Because no study visually demonstrating this reaction front has been published, the authors began to investigate the morphology of the demineralization process with electron microscopy. Verification of the existence of this sharp reaction front was impor-

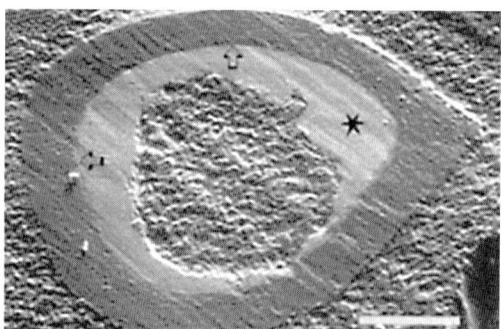

Fig. 1. SEM of a cross-section of a partially demineralized rat tibia diaphysis embedded in epon (E), showing a circumferential band of demineralized bone surrounding the inner undecalcified core. The * indicates undemineralized cortical bone (bar = 500 µm).

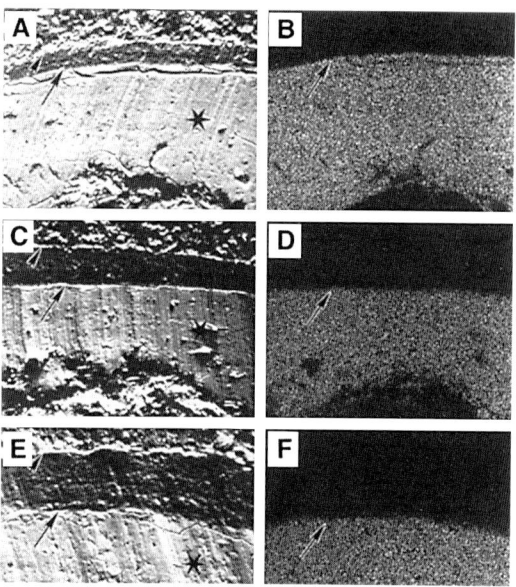

Fig. 2. SEMs of a cross-section of rat tibia diaphyses (2A,C,E), with corresponding calcium X-ray dot maps (2B,D,F) demonstrating the reduction of the bone-mineral-containing cortical bone core (*). Short arrowhead at the periosteal surface of the cortex, long arrowhead at the interface. Demineralization was performed in 0.5 N HCl for increasing immersion time: (2A,B) 10 min, demineralization depth ≈ 70 mm; (2C,D) 20 min, demineralization depth ≈ 95 mm; (2E,F) 60 min, demineralization depth ≈ 150 mm. The length of the bar on the bottom of the figure equals 100 mm.

tant for modeling purposes, to predict the demineralization process and the biomechanical properties of a bone allograft after the demineralization process.

5.1. Electron Microscopy Studies

5.1.1. Methods and Results

Scanning electron microscopy (SEM) demonstrated the process of cortical bone demineralization (Fig. 1) *(133)*. The authors confirmed that HCl demineralization of cortical bone results in a sharp advancing interface separating the outer demineralized bone from the inner cortical bone core (Fig. 2A–F). The thickness of the interface at the reaction front was approx 20 µ in the specimens studied.

5.1.2. Conclusion

These observations were critical for controlled modification of cortical bone grafts in current clinical use, because they suggested that the structural strength of long bone allografts after demineralization is predictable. In fact, it is provided by the strengths of the inner residual mineralized core, whose properties can be described as those of a bone with reduced outer dimensions *(134)*.

5.2. Demineralization Kinetics Studies

Once the existence of a sharp reaction front during the process of acid demineralization of cortical bone was established, the authors investigated ways to determine the position of this reaction front as a function of the immersion time in HCl, a method that would ultimately allow control of the demineralization process.

5.2.1. Methods

The authors considered the sharp interface between the outer demineralized and the inner mineralized portion to be a reaction front of bone mineral breakdown that is typical of diffusion-rate-limited processes *(132)*, in which the acid reacts instantaneously with the bone mineral upon arrival at the reaction front *(131,135)*. Consequently, the acid concentration at the reaction front would equal zero at any given time, and the advance of the reaction front would be solely dependent on the diffusivity of the bone. These assumptions were used to analyze the time dependencies of demineralization of human, rat, bovine, and sheep cortical bone.

5.2.2. Results

Mathematical models were derived for predicting the demineralization kinetics of cortical bone *(131,135)*. For planar geometry, the depth of demineralization process as a function of the immersion time t in acid, $\delta(t)$ *(cm)*, is given by:

$$\delta = \sqrt{2DC_0 t/10^3 \lambda} \quad (1)$$

where D is the effective mass diffusivity of HCl into the bone [cm²/s], C_0 is the acid concentration [mol/L], t the immersion time in the HCl acid bath (s), and λ the mols of acid necessary to demineralize 1 cm³ of cortical bone completely (mol/cm³).

In cylindrical geometry, the time dependence of the depth of demineralization can also be expressed analytically, but no longer has the simple square root of immersion time dependence found in planar geometry. Using dimensionless variables, r_d^* and t^*, the time dependence of the radial penetration depth of the demineralization process $\delta(t)$ with $d = r_0 - r_d$ is given by:

$$t = \sqrt{10^3 \delta r_0^2 / 4 C_0 D} \left(2\sqrt{r_0 - \delta^2/r_0^2} \ln \frac{\sqrt{r_0 - \delta/r_0}}{\sqrt{r_0 - \delta^2/r_0^2} + 1} \right) \quad (2)$$

where r_0 is the initial radius of a cylindrical bone and r_d the radial position of the demineralization front. The immersion time in HCl, required to obtain a certain demineralization depth, depends on the initial radius of a cylindrical bone. The solution presented in Eq. 2 is therefore normalized for this dependence. In order to fit the experimental data to the analytical models, the values of the effective mass diffusivities, D, at different acid concentrations, and the value of δ as the minimum mols of HCl required for complete demineralization of a specific volume of cortical bone, were determined.

5.2.3. Conclusion

The authors demonstrated that the planar model can be considered the most practical approximation for BGs with irregular planar shapes, such as cortical struts; the cylindrical model approximates grafts with primarily curved surfaces, such as occur in long diaphyseal BGs *(131)*. The use of these two simple mathematical models *(131)* for planar and cylindrical geometry allows accurate prediction of the demineralization of cortical bone allografts of most sizes and shapes. They provided us with the theoretical basis for modifying currently used cortical bone allografts to cortical bone transplants with a surface layer of highly osteoinductive demineralized bone, while retaining biomechanical strength required for stable reconstruction.

5.3. Biomechanical Studies

5.3.1. Methods

Because control of the biomechanical properties of demineralized diaphyseal bone allografts is required for their clinical application, the authors then investigated the changes in whole-bone flexural rigidity in human fibulae, as a function of the demineralization depth, using a nondestructive four-point bending test *(134)*. Starting at the facies medialis, the flexural rigidity was determined in 24 planes at 15-degree sequential angular increments. This allowed data collection around the circumference of the bone. Test bones included four pairs of left and right human fibulae and 15 single fibulae. The elliptical distribution of the flexural rigidity of left and right fibulae and single fibulae before and after demineralization was compared. The stiffness index (*SI*) was defined as a parameter to describe the mechanical status of the test bones.

5.3.2. Results

The rigidity of diaphyseal bones was strongly dependent on the reduction of their cortical thickness by demineralization. A mathematical model allowing prediction of the reduction of the rigidity of diaphyseal bone grafts, as a function of the demineralization depth, was derived:

$$SI^* = r_{df}^4 - n^4/r_o^4 - r_i^4 \quad (3)$$

where r_o is the outer radius of the graft, r_i the inner radius of the graft, and r_{df} the radial position of the demineralization front.

The experimental *SI* values fitted well ($R = 0.98$) to the analytical model presented in Eq. 3 based on the sharpness of the reaction front seen in the electron microscopic studies, which suggested that the structural strength of long BGs after demineralization is predictable. This was confirmed by the authors' biomechanical studies *(134)*, which showed that the strength of a partially demineralized diaphyseal BG is in fact provided by the residual mineralized core, whose properties can be described as those of a bone with reduced outer dimensions. Based on observation of a wide range of left–right variability of flexural rigidity found in human fibula pairs *(134),* and on biological data in animals *(121,136,137),* the authors proposed that a reduction of rigidity by 20–30% may be the maximum feasible range for partial demineralization of diaphyseal bone grafts.

Using the same nondestructive four-point bending and compression tests, additional biomechanical studies on sheep bones showed that laser-drilling alone, with a hole diameter of 300 µm and a distance of 2 mm between holes, results in a 3–5% reduction of whole-bone flexural rigidity *(138).* The combination of partial demineralization (20% reduction of flexural rigidity) and laser-drilling resulted in an overall reduction of flexural rigidity by 35–40%. In compression testing, laser-perforated and partially demineralized bone specimens showed a marked decrease in the ultimate failure stress. The observed increase in failure strain appeared to be related to compression of the laser holes.

5.3.3. Conclusion

The findings of these biomechanical studies suggest that partial demineralization and laser perforation can be applied to diaphyseal BGs, and that their decreased mechanical properties are a function of changes in bone geometry produced by both processes.

6. In Vivo Studies

The focus of subsequent animal studies in rats and sheep, using orthotopic tibial transplantation models, was to apply these methods of controlled partial demineralization and laser perforation to cortical bone allografts, and to evaluate their effect on the incorporation process.

6.1. Transplantation Studies in Rats
6.1.1. Methods

Initial animal studies in Sprague-Dawley rats used diaphyseal tibial cortical bone allografts from rats of the same outbred strain *(136,137, 139).* Grafts were prepared by partial demineral-

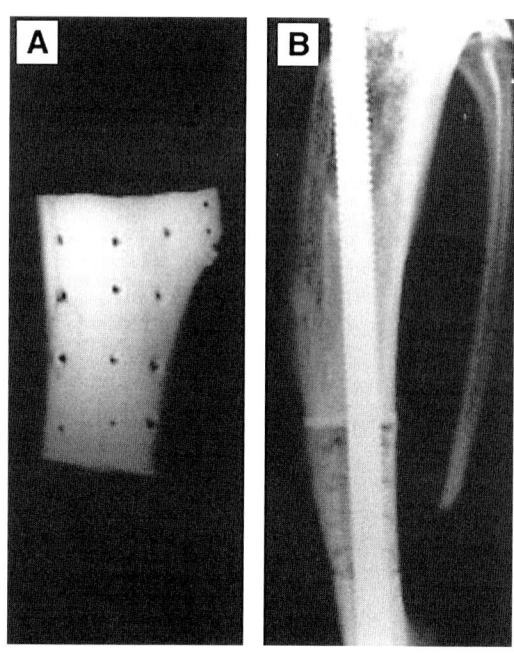

Fig. 3. **(A)** Photograph of a laser-ablated (type IV) diaphyseal rat tibia graft. **(B)** Orthotopic implantation after resection of mid-diaphyseal segment of the same length. Fixation was achieved with 0-062 in. threaded K-wire. The fibula was osteotomized.

ization and drilling of 0.3-mm diameter holes, with a pulsed, 2.94-µm wavelength Er:YAG laser. Six types of grafts were analyzed, including eight rats per type and time-point: untreated (type I); demineralized 25 µm deep (type II); demineralized 150 µm deep (type III); laser-perforated (type IV, fig. 3A); laser-perforated, and then demineralized 25 µm deep (type V); and laser-ablated, and then demineralized 150 µm deep (type VI).

Grafts were stripped of soft tissues, and, after removal of the bone marrow by multiple washings in saline, were stored at –80°C. At time of surgery, grafts were thawed in a solution containing polymyxin B sulfate (500,000 U/L) and bacitracin (50,000 U/L), and then were orthotopically transplanted into the tibia of adult Sprague-Dawley rats. Animals were followed for up to 4 mo. A total of 96 rats, in two sets of 48 animals each, was operated. Each set included six groups of eight rats per graft type. Animals were sacrificed at four (set 1) and 16 (set 2) wk postoperatively. Grafts were evaluated throughout the study by high-resolution radiography, to exclude patholog-

Processing Cortical Allografts

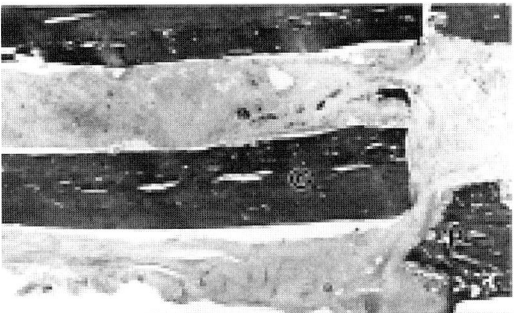

Fig. 4. Longitudinal section through a type I rat graft (untreated control) retrieved at po wk 16 (H&E, ×1.25) showing the graft (G) in the center and portions of the adjacent proximal (P) and distal (D) host bone. The graft is not incorporated. There is minimal osteoclastic activity at the proximal end of the graft, but no endochondral callus or bone formation at either junction site. There is moderate periostal bone formation (PF) at proximal junction site.

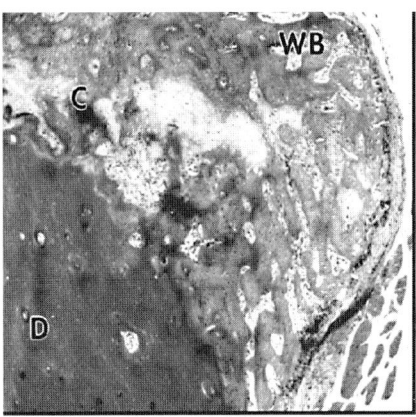

Fig. 5. Photomicrograph of a longitudinal section taken from distal junction site (D) of a type II (minimally demineralized) rat graft (G) retrieved at po wk 16 (H&E, ×5) showing endochondral callus formation (C) with periosteal woven bone (WB).

ical fractures. X-rays were taken immediately postoperatively, and at 4-wk intervals, using a specimen X-ray unit (Microfocus 50E6310F/G; Xerox, Rochester, NY). Histological evaluation of grafts was performed at one and 4 mo postoperatively with use of hematoxylin and eosin (H&E) staining.

6.1.2. Results

The control grafts (type I) of group 1 showed no incorporation (Fig. 4).

New bone growth was confirmed in type II (Figs. 5 and 7), type III (Fig. 6), type V (Fig. 9), and type VI (Fig. 10) grafts; laser drilling alone resulted only in bone resorption (Fig. 8). The amount of new bone growth was estimated by comparing graft bone mineral density prior to implantation to values obtained after graft retrieval. These measurements were correlated to histomorphometric analysis of graft incorporation.

6.1.3. Conclusion

Results in rats showed that the process of partial demineralization ($p < 0.000001$) and laser ablation with partial demineralization ($p < 0.000001$) were both significant in enhancing bone growth in this model (data not shown) *(136,137,139)*. New bone growth was already significantly increased when grafts were prepared with minimal demineralization ($p < 0.015$; data not shown).

This study in rats demonstrated that osteogenesis in orthotropically transplanted cortical BGs could be fostered by laser perforation and additional minimal partial demineralization. The efficacy of these techniques in maintaining structural integrity, while improving osteoinductive properties, represented an advance in understanding how osteogenesis in cortical BGs could be improved.

6.2. Transplantation Studies in Sheep

The rodent study described above showed improved incorporation following partial demineralization, and suggested that minimal surface demineralization was sufficient to achieve this effect. A large animal study, using sheep, was then conducted *(106,140–142)*.

6.2.1. Methods

Outbred 1-yr-old black-faced mismatched dew sheep were used both as donors and recipients. The grafts were 30 mm long, and were used to replace a defect of similar size created in the midshaft tibia of the left hind leg. Fixation was achieved with an intramedullary nail and with two proximal and two distal locking screws. This provided excellent rotational stability and

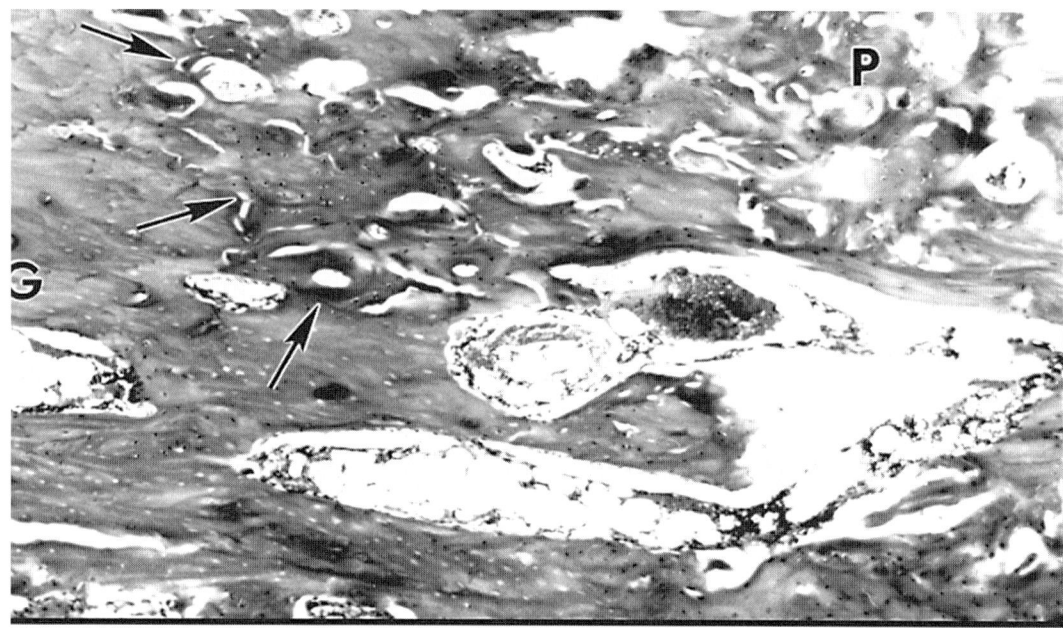

Fig. 6. Photomicrograph of a longitudinal section made at the proximal junction site of a type III (extensively demineralized) rat graft retrieved at po wk 16 (H&E, ×5). Note complete healing between proximal host bone (P) and graft bone (G) by new bone formation. There is a sharp interface (arrowheads) between newly formed woven bone and graft bone. Note osteoclastic and osteoblastic activity at the interface.

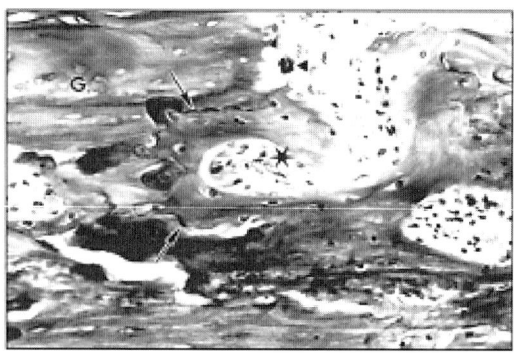

Fig. 7. Photomicrograph of a longitudinal section made at the periphery of the cortex of the shaft of a type II (minimally demineralized) rat graft (G) retrieved at po wk 16 (H&E, ×20). Note incorporation involving formation of osteoclastic resorption lacunae (——→) from the periphery into the cortex. There are resorption lacunae filled with woven bone (arrowheads at cement lines). Note ingrowth of endothelial cells forming capillaries filled with erythrocytes(✶).

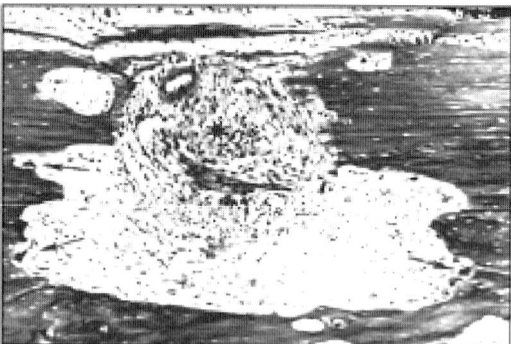

Fig. 8. Photomicrograph of a longitudinal section made at the cortex of a type IV (laser-ablated only) rat graft retrieved at po wk 16 (H&E, ×10). The laser hole is cut axially. The original size of the laser hole (✶) was 330 µm. Osteoclastic activity (arrowheads) is present, indicating that enlargement of the hole has occurred. There was no evidence of new bone formation.

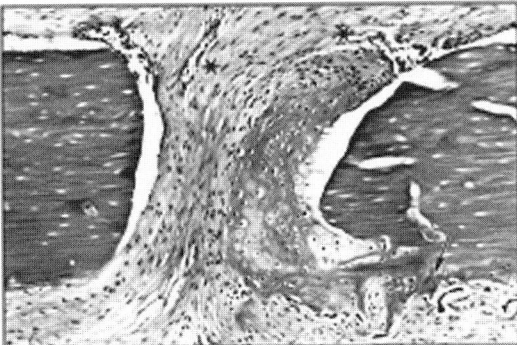

Fig. 9. Photomicrograph of a longitudinal section made at the cortex of a type V rat graft (laser-ablated, then minimally demineralized) retrieved at po wk 4 (H&E, ×10). Note ingrowth of vascular tissue (✱), cartilage and woven bone (arrowhead) evident within the laser holes.

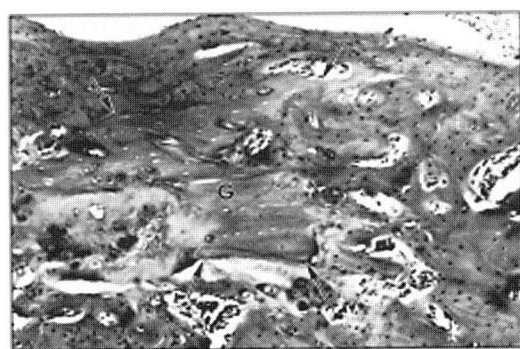

Fig. 10. Photomicrograph of a longitudinal section made at the cortex of a type VI (laser-ablated, then extensively demineralized) rat graft retrieved at po wk 16 (H&E ×5). Laser holes to left and right from the graft (G) filled with new woven bone and some cartilage. Remnant of the original graft outlined by arrowheads. Incorporation from the laser holes seemed to have occurred.

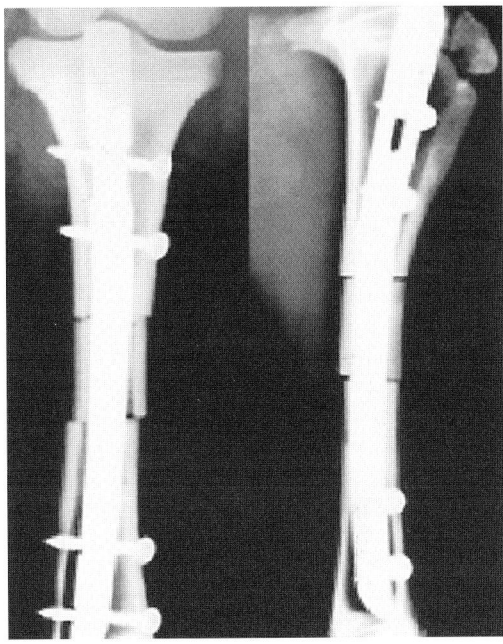

Fig. 11. Immediate po X-ray of a sheep tibia transplanted with an intercalary bone allograft: (Left) AP view; (Right) lateral view.

Table 1
Group Design and Graft Types of Sheep Study

Group	Graft type and treatment
1	Fresh-frozen control graft, no other treatment
2	Fresh-frozen graft, additionally treated by partial demineralization
3	Fresh-frozen graft, additionally treated by partial demineralization and laser perforation

reduction at the host–bone allograft junction sites (Fig. 11).

As indicated in Table 1, different types of bone transplants were used in three groups of eight animals each: group 1. fresh-frozen control allografts; group 2. partially demineralized bone allografts (reduction of flexural rigidity by 20%); group 3. laser-perforated and partially demineralized bone allografts (same extent of demineralization as in group 2). In group 3 transplants, laser holes were drilled at a distance of 2.5 mm from each other. Thus, an average of 80 holes was drilled around the circumference of the graft, through the entire thickness of the cortex. Thereafter, demineralization was performed as noted previously (131).

Prior to transplantation, allografts were thawed in a solution containing polymyxin B sulfate (500,000 U/L) and bacitracin (50,000 U/L). Peridural anesthesia (4 mL 0.5% xylocaine) was used during surgery. Animals were followed by monthly radiographs, and were sacrificed at 9 mo postoperatively. Sequential fluorochrom labeling was done at 2 and 7 mo postoperatively, allowing

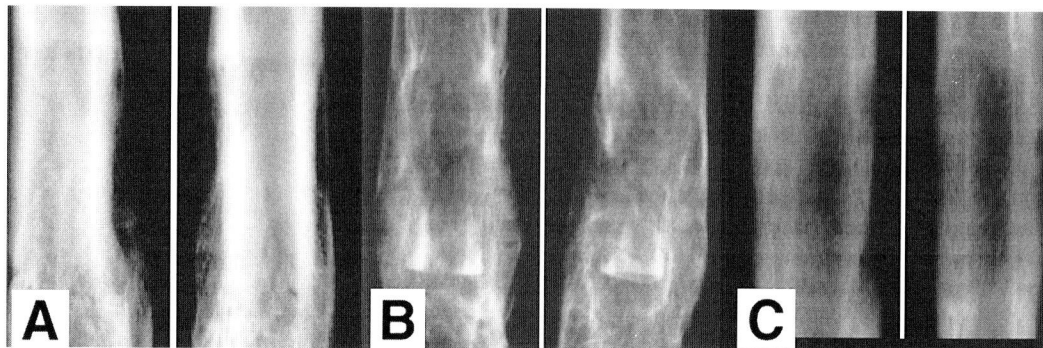

Fig. 12. Radiographs taken 9 mo postoperatively, after sacrifice and removal of the intramedullary fixation device. Anteroposterior view on the left, lateral view on the right. (**A**) fresh-frozen control allograft: scant radiographic evidence of incorporation, graft identifiable, arrow at periosteal bone cuff surrounding the graft; (**B**) partially demineralized allograft; graft underwent excessive resorption, arrow at allograft remnant; (**C**) laser-perforated and partially demineralized bone allograft; graft completely incorporated, with very smooth transition at both the proximal and the distal junction site.

evaluation of serial undecalcified and decalcified histological sections. T-cells were obtained from donor peripheral blood. Recipient serum was collected at 4-wk intervals, to determine the development of an antidonor immune response. Immediately after sacrifice, transplanted bones were analyzed with use of a high-resolution computed tomography (CT) (slice thickness, 2 mm), allowing morphometric measurement of the remaining allograft bone. Prior to histological analysis, biomechanical testing was done using the same nondestructive four-point bending test as described in subheading 5.3.

6.2.2. Results
6.2.2.1. Radiographic Follow-up

Monthly radiographic follow-up and radiographs taken after sacrifice demonstrated integrity of the host–bone allograft construct throughout the entire PO period. No pathological fractures were observed in any of the 24 operated animals.

Fresh-frozen control bone allografts showed little radiographic evidence of incorporation (Fig. 12A). Even though healing at the junction sites generally occurred 3–4 mo postoperatively, grafts of this group were clearly identifiable on X-rays taken at 9 mo postoperatively, and after sacrifice *(141)*. Control grafts, used in group 1 animals, showed little radiographic evidence of bone resorption. In addition, periosteal bone was noted to have grown from the adjacent host bone over the bone transplant, forming a periosteal bone cuff (arrow in Fig. 12A).

Compared to control grafts, partially demineralized bone allografts, used in group 2 animals, showed progressive resorption of the bone transplant, generally starting at 2 mo postoperatively, and with most of the graft resorbed at time of sacrifice (Fig. 12B). Bone resorption was followed by extensive periosteal bone formation, which ultimately led to closure of the defect and formation of a bridging bone between the proximal and distal host bone. However, the formation of persistent resorption lacunae was frequently noted.

Laser-perforated and partially demineralized bone transplants, used in group 3 animals, were noted to stimulate early bone resorption and new bone formation, which started between 4 and 8 wk postoperatively. At 2 mo postoperatively, enlargement of the laser holes was radiographically evident in most animals of this group. This was closely followed by new bone formation within the laser holes, leading to an increasing incorporation of these grafts during the remaining po period (Fig. 12C).

Quantitative analysis of high resolution CT scans (after sacrifice and removal of the intramedullary nail) was used to determine percentage rates of remaining bone allograft volume. This study revealed that allografts were replaced by newly formed bone in all group 3 animals, which were

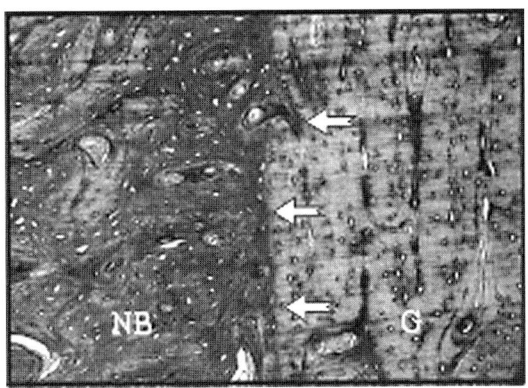

Fig. 13. Photomicrograph made at a cross-section of the cortex of a sheep tibia control allograft retrieved at 9 mo postoperatively (Heidenheins Azan, ×4), showing a periosteal bone cuff (NB) surrounding a graft (G) that is essentially unchanged. Periosteal new bone (NB) on the left, graft (G) on the right.

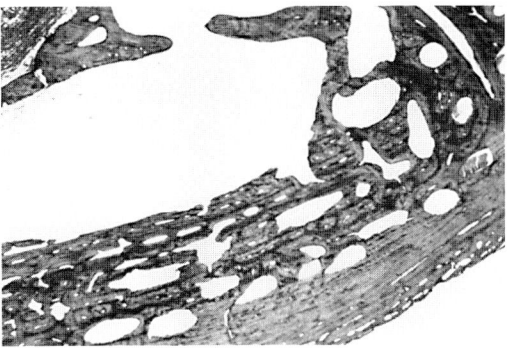

Fig. 14. Photomicrograph made at a cross-section of the cortex of a sheep tibia allograft that was partially demineralized. Graft retrieved at 9 mo postoperatively (Heidenheins Azan, ×4). Allograft remnant in the center (arrow). Note wide intratrabecular spaces in newly formed woven bone. Periosteal surface on the bottom, endosteal surface on the top.

transplanted with laser-perforated and partially demineralized allografts. In control allografts of group 1, an average 81 ± 9% of the original graft bone was found left intact; in partially demineralized bone allografts of group 2, this was 19 ± 21%.

6.2.2.2. HISTOLOGICAL ANALYSIS

Evaluation of serial undecalcified and decalcified histological sections and analysis of fluorochrome labeling corroborated radiographic findings. Control grafts showed little evidence of incorporation, and most of the original graft was essentially unchanged. Osteoclastic activity and revascularization was seen only at the periosteal surface, with little penetration into the graft. However, healing at the junction sites, with a sharp interface between the host and allograft bone, was frequently seen. Woven periosteal bone, forming a periosteal bone cuff around the graft, was consistently found on serial sections (Fig. 13).

Partially demineralized bone allografts were resorbed almost entirely. Only a few microscopic allogeneic bone fragments remained. These fragments either were found adjacent to a resorptive lacuna that was filled with fibrous tissue or were surrounded by loosely packed, new woven bone, similar in appearance to the periosteal woven bone originating from the host-bone–allograft junction sites. The newly formed woven bone was highly revascularized, very loosely packed with wide intratrabecular spaces (Fig. 14). No such vascular invasion was seen at the site of the bone allograft remnants.

In laser-perforated and partially demineralized bone allografts, healing at the junction site was evident by replacement of the graft cortex with newly formed woven bone. Some microscopic remnants of the allografts and the original sites of laser hole drilling were identified. Those laser holes seen were consistently filled with newly formed woven bone, and showed evidence of vascular invasion (Fig. 15). Holes were also found to be sites of advancing graft incorporation by resorption and new bone formation. Uniform and almost complete graft incorporation, with narrow intratrabecular spaces in the newly formed bone, was seen in all test bones of this group (Fig. 16).

6.2.3. BIOMECHANICAL TESTING

6.2.2.3.1. Method. Transplanted bones were subsequently tested using a nondestructive four-point bending test *(138)*. This test obtained a relative percentage rate measure of flexural rigidity by comparing the transplanted (left) tibia to the contralateral untreated control (right) tibia of the same animal.

6.2.2.3.2. Results. Test bones of group 1 were found to be stiffer than their untreated contra-

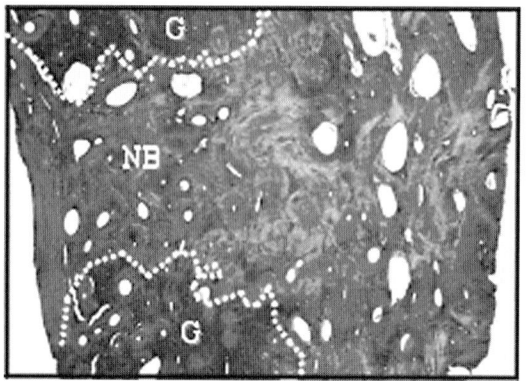

Fig. 15. Photomicrograph made from a cross-section of the cortex of a sheep tibia allograft that was laser-perforated and then partially demineralized. Graft retrieved at 9 mo postoperatively (Heidenheins Azan, ×4). Shown is an allograft remnant with original laser (outlined with dotted line). Hole is filled with new woven bone (NB); note allograft remnants (G) at the top and bottom. Periosteal surface on the right, endosteal surface on the left.

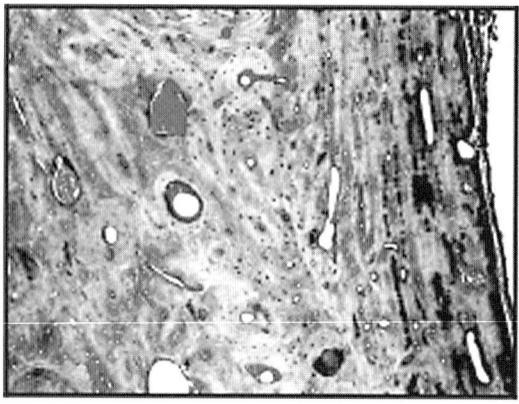

Fig. 16. Photomicrograph made at a cross-section of the cortex of a sheep tibia allograft that was partially demineralized. Graft retrieved at 9 mo postoperatively (Heidenheins Azan, ×4). Allograft incorporated. Cortex remodeled with mature new bone. Periosteal surface on the right.

lateral bones. Values for the SI ranged from 103 to 124% (112 ± 9%; mean ± standard deviation). Test bones of group 2 were transplanted with partially demineralized bone allografts. These test bones were the weakest of all the transplanted bones analyzed in this study. All test bones of group 2 were less stiff, compared to their untreated counterparts from the opposite hind leg. The average value attained for the SI was 69.3 ± 21%, with the SD being the largest in this group. Test bones of group 3 were transplanted with cortical bone allografts that were first laser-perforated and then partially demineralized. Even though test bones of this group did not reach the same stiffness as their contralateral control bones, they were consistently more rigid than group 2 test bones, resulting in the following: SI = 82.7 ± 7.6%, and area ratio = 83.7 ± 195%.

6.2.2.3.3. Conclusion. Processing of cortical bone allografts by laser perforation and partial demineralization resulted in superior healing, as evaluated by higher stiffness of the transplanted bones, compared to processing by partial demineralization alone.

6.2.2.4. IMMUNOLOGICAL STUDIES

6.2.2.4.1. Methods. All donor and recipient animals in the sheep study were tissue-typed by biochemical definition of the MHC-I molecules, using unidimensional isoelectric focusing and immunoblotting after detergent phase separation *(143–145).*

The relative positions of the bands were used for comparative analysis of sheep MHC-I Ags, because data on sheep MHC-I gene products were unavailable. Alleles were arbitrarily numbered and their frequency recorded. They are listed for each donor–recipient pair in Table 1–3. Mismatches were assessed by running samples of donor and recipient in parallel, and comparing specific bands (Fig. 17). All samples were run in duplicate. The authors were unable to evaluate cellular-mediated immune responses, because of methodological limitations.

Donor-specific allo-Abs were detected by cell-free enzyme-linked immunosorbent assay, in which donor MHC-I Ags were blotted as above, and reacted with recipient sera. Allo-Abs were stained with a peroxidase-tagged antisheep immunoglobulin G1 Ab.

6.2.2.4.2. Results. The immunological studies in sheep showed than only two donor–recipient pairs (S5/0901, Table 2; and 9/2101, Table 4) were perfectly matched for MHC-I Ags. Two

Table 2
Group 1 (Control Allografts) Donor–recipient Match and Donor-specific Allo-Abs

Donor	Donor MHC-I alleles	Recipient	Recipient MHC-I alleles	Mismatches	Ab response
6	18	0801	9, 16	1	
44	9	0104	3, 12	1	+
7	5	0401	17	1	
S4	7, 14	0301	12	2	
S2	9	0601	3, 12	1	
S3	4, 1	0701	11	2	
S5	20	0901	8, 20	0	
7	5	1001	8, 20	1	

Table 3
Group 2 (Partially Demineralized Allografts) Donor–recipient Match and Donor-specific Allo-Abs

Donor	Donor MHC-I alleles	Recipient	Recipient MHC-I alleles	Mismatches	Ab response
5	17	0801	9, 15	1	
5	17	1101	10, 14, 21	1	
44	9	1701	2, 10	1	
6	18	1201	10	1	
S5	20	1601	22	1	
6	15	1301	10, 17	1	
12	16	1801	2, 10, 17	1	
11	10, 16	2301	16, 19	1	

class I mismatches were observed in four donor–recipient pairs, and the remainder had one class I mismatch. Donor-specific Allo-Abs were detected in one animal receiving a control allograft (0104, Table 2), and in one animal receiving a laser-perforated and partially demineralized bone allograft (2501, Table 4). In these two recipient animals, Abs were detectable 3 mo after transplantation.

Despite the obvious limitations of the immunological studies in sheep, in which the authors have only been able to assess MHC-I histoincompatibility with humoral, but not cell-mediated, immune response, it appears noteworthy that the bone allografts used in this study showed little immunogenicity. This is supported by the fact that only two recipients demonstrated alloreactive Abs. Thus, development of Abs to donor MHC-I Ags was infrequent (at least within the time period studied), compared to studies in rodents *(81,86,88,90)*, dogs *(82)*, and humans *(101,102, 104,108,110–112)*. Grafts in these studies were not depleted of Ags by removal of the bone marrow or soft tissues, as was the case here. Also, in the two cases in which antidonor class I Abs were detected, their presence did not affect allograft outcome.

7. Discussion and Conclusions

The transplantation studies in rats and sheep have demonstrated that laser-perforated and partially demineralized cortical bone allografts showed the most promising results with respect to incorporation into host bone and mechanical strength of the allografted recipient bone. No pathological fractures were observed in either in vitro study, suggesting that the authors' mathematical models allow production of grafts strong enough to withstand skeletal forces, when used in long bone reconstruction. Cortical bone allografts used in the sheep study were poorly immunogenic, whether they were only fresh-frozen (as controls) or processed by additional laser drilling and/or partial demineralization. Compared to bone allografts in current clinical use, grafts in the authors

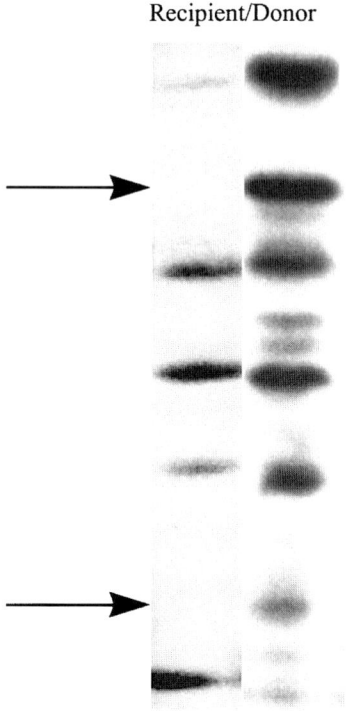

Fig. 17. Immunoblot of recipient (left, 0301, Table 1) and donor (right, s4, Table 1) MHC-I Ag gene products. Two MHC mismatches (alleles 7,14) as indicated by the arrows.

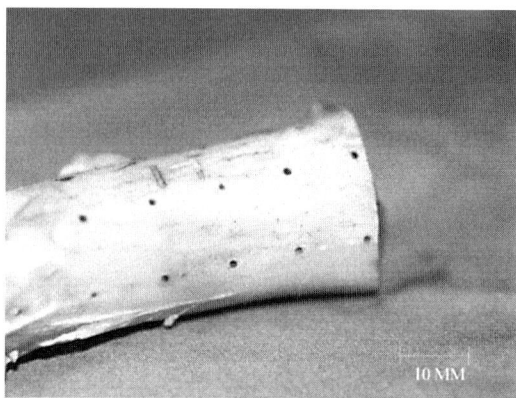

Fig. 18. Photograph of a clinical intercalary cortical bone allograft processed by laser perforation and subsequent partial demineralization.

animal studies were stripped of soft tissues, and the bone marrow was removed. Presumably, cellular sources of allostimulaton were largely eliminated *(146)*. In fact, it is possible that accelerated incorporation, with rapid resorption of the allograft, may have provided a sufficient antigenic stimulus to mount an Ab immune response in the animal that received a laser-perforated and partially demineralized bone allograft. Considering higher sensitization rates in rodent *(81,86, 88,90)*, canine *(82)*, and human *(101,102,104,108, 110–112)* studies, these findings suggest that immune responses to bone allografts may be drastically reduced, simply by removing the bone marrow and adjacent soft tissues. However, additional assessment of humoral responses to MHC-II Ags, and cellular responses to MHC-I and -II Ags, are necessary to further substantiate this statement.

On the basis of radiographic, histologic, and biomechanical observations, the authors are currently developing laser-perforated and partially demineralized bone allografts for clinical use (Fig. 18). If these findings can be reproduced in humans, this would represent a major advance in long bone reconstruction using cadaveric bone

Table 4
Group 3 (Laser-perforated and Partially Demineralized Allografts)
Donor–Recipient Match and Donor-specific Allo-Abs

Donor	Donor MHC-I alleles	Recipient	Recipient MHC-I alleles	Mismatches	Ab response
12	16	1501	2, 20	1	
9	8, 20	2101	8, 20	0	
11	10, 16	2001	6, 13, 22	2	
11	10, 16	0201	1, 10, 17	1	
9	8, 20	1901	10, 19	1	
S3	4, 1	2201	6, 13, 22	2	
44	9	2501	10, 15	1	+
12	16	2401	2, 10, 15	1	

allografts. Ultimately, it would allow the development of a new type of bone allograft, whose clinical application could extend beyond its use in tumor reconstruction.

Acknowledgments

This work was supported by National Institutes of Health (NIH) Grant AR-21896, NIH/NIAMS grant AR 45062, the Medical Free Electron Laser Program under Office of Naval Research contract N00014-91-C0084, and by DOE Grant DE-FG02-91 ER61228; in part, by a small grant (GGEST 355C-6) from the Going Global Program, Canadian Ministry of Foreign Affairs and International Trade, Ottawa, Ontario; by a grant (412.02-Knochentransplant) from the Hauptverband der gewerblichen Berufsgenossenschaften, St. Augustin, Germany; by a small grant (HMI) from the Science and Technology Cooperation, Germany/Canada; and in the form of donations by the AO-Research Institute, Davos, Switzerland, and by Synthes-Bochum, GmbH. No ownership or profit derived from this work. Furthermore, this project was supported by temporary and permanent loans by the AO-Research Institute, Davos, Switzerland, and Synthes-Bochum GmbH, Bochum, Germany.

For their continuous support of this work over the past 5 yr, and for their technical assistance, the authors are indebted to William W. Tomford, MD (Massachusetts General Hospital, Boston, MA), Henry J. Mankin, MD (Massachusetts General Hospital, Boston, MA), Hans K. Uhthoff, MD (Ottawa General Hospital, Ottawa, Ontario, Canada), Georg Schollmeier, MD PD (Potsdam, Germany), Axel Ekkernkamp, MD (Ruhr-University), Bergmannsheil Bochum, Germany), Prof. Gert Muhr, MD (Ruhr-University, Bergmannsheil Bochum, Germany), Wilson C. Hayes, PhD (Orthopaedic Biomechanics Laboratory, Beth Israel Deaconess Medical Center, Boston, MA), Thomas F. Deutsch, PhD (Wellman Laboratories of Photomedicine, Massachusetts General Hospital, Boston, MA), Kevin T. Schomacker, PhD (Wellman Laboratories of Photomedicine, Massachusetts General Hospital, Boston, MA), Thomas F. Flotte (Photopathology Laboratory, Massachusetts General Hospital, Boston, MA), Norman Michaud, MS (Photopathology Laboratory, Massachusetts General Hospital, Boston, MA), Vera Rebman, PhD (Institute of Immunology, University of Essen, Essen, Germany), Prof. P. Grosse-Wilde, MD (Institute of Immunology, University of Essen, Essen, Germany), Prof. Stephan Perren, MD (AO Research Institute, Davos, Switzerland), Prof. Baumgärtl (AO Research Institute, Davos, Switzerland), Ms. Brigitte Zimmerman (Ruhr-University, Bergmannsheil Bochum, Germany), Ms. Elvira Peter (Ruhr-University, Bergmannsheil Bochum, Germany), Ms. Monika Pässler (Institute of Immunology, University of Essen, Essen, Germany), Mr. Alan Yeadon (Ottawa General Hospital, Ottawa, Ontario, Canada), Mr. Roland Wieling (AO Research Institute, Davos, Switzerland), and Mr. Thesing (Synthes-Bochum GmbH, Bochum, Germany).

References

1. Mintzer CM, Robertson DD, Rackemann S, Ewald FC, Scott RD, and Spector M. Bone loss in the distal anterior femur after total knee arthroplasty. *Clin Orthop* 1990; 260: 135–143.
2. Thornhill TS, Ozuna RM, Shortkroff S, Keller K, Sledge CB, and Spectro M. Biochemical and histological evaluation of the synovial-like tissue around failed (loose) total joint replacement prostheses in human subjects and a canine model. *Biomaterials* 1990; 11: 69–72.
3. Hill GE and Droller DG. Acute and subacute deep infection after uncemented total hip replacement using antibacterial prophylaxis. *Orthop Rev* 1989; 18: 617–623.
4. Kim YH and Franks DJ. Cementless revision of cemented stem failures associated with massive femoral bone loss. A technical note. *Orthop Rev* 1992; 21: 375–380.
5. Spector M. Historical review of porous-coated implants. *J Arthroplasty* 1987; 2: 163–177.
6. Cara JA and Canadell J. Limb salvage for malignant bone tumors in young children. *J Pediatr Orthop* 1994; 14: 112–118.
7. Davis A, Bell RS, Allan DG, Langer F, Czitrom AA, and Gross AE. Fresh osteochondral transplants in the treatment of advanced giant cell tumors [in German]. *Orthopade* 1993; 22: 146–151.
8. Gebhardt MC, Roth YF, and Mankin HJ. Osteoarticular allografts for reconstruction in the proximal part of the humerus after excision of a musculo-

skeletal tumor. *J Bone Joint Surg Am* 1990; 72: 334–345.
9. Gitelis S and Piasecki P. Allograft prosthetic composite arthroplasty for osteosarcoma and other aggressive bone tumors. *Clin Orthop* 1991; 270: 197–201.
10. Koskinen EV. Wide resection of primary tumors of bone and replacement with massive bone grafts: an improved technique for transplanting allogeneic bone grafts. *Clin Orthop* 1978; 134: 302–319.
11. Mankin HJ, Doppelt SH, Sullivan TR, and Tomford WW. Osteoarticular and intercalary allograft transplantation in the management of malignant tumors of bone. *Cancer* 1982; 50: 613–630.
12. Mankin HJ, Fogelson FS, Thrasher AZ, and Jaffer F. Massive resection and allograft transplantation in the treatment of malignant bone tumors. *N Engl J Med* 1976; 294: 1247–1255.
13. Mankin HJ, Springfield DS, Gebhardt MC, and Tomford WW. Current status of allografting for bone tumors. *Orthopedics* 1992; 15: 1147–1154.
14. Mnaymneh W and Malinin T. Massive allografts in surgery of bone tumors. *Orthop Clin North Am* 1989; 20: 455–467.
15. Tomford WW, Bloem RM, and Mankin HJ. Osteoarticular allografts. *Acta Orthop Belg* 1992; 57 (Suppl 2): 98–102.
16. Wang JW and Shih CH. Allograft transplantation in aggressive or malignant bone tumors. *Clin Orthop* 1993; 203–209.
17. Jaffe KA, Morris SG, Sorrell RG, Gebhardt MC, and Mankin HJ. Massive bone allografts for traumatic skeletal defects. *South Med J* 1991; 84: 975–982.
18. Mahomed MN, Beaver RJ, and Gross AE. Long-term success of fresh, small fragment osteochondral allografts used for intraarticular post-traumatic defects in the knee joint. *Orthopedics* 1992; 15: 1191–1199.
19. Gitelis S, Heligman D, Quill G, and Piasecki P. Use of large allografts for tumor reconstruction and salvage of the failed total hip arthroplasty. *Clin Orthop* 1988; 231: 62–70.
20. Glowacki J. Cellular reactions to bone-derived material. *Clinical Orthop* 1996; 324: 47–54.
21. Kondo K and Nagaya I. Bone incorporation of frozen femoral head allograft in revision total hip replacement. *Nippon Seikeigeka Gakkai Zasshi* 1993; 67: 408–416.
22. Martin WR and Sutherland CJ. Complications of proximal femoral allografts in revision total hip anthroplasty. *Clin Orthop* 1993; 295: 161–167.
23. Pak JH, Paprosky WG, Jablonsky WS, and Lawrence JM. Femoral strut allografts in cementless revision total hip arthroplasty. *Clin Orthop* 1993; 295: 172–178.
24. Ries MD, Gomez MA, Eckhoff DG, Lewis DA, Brodie MR, and Wiedel JD. An in vitro study of proximal femoral allograft strains in revision hip arthroplasty. *Med Eng Phys* 1994; 16: 292–296.
25. Berrey BH Jr, Lord CF, Gebhardt MC, and Mankin HJ. Fractures of allografts. Frequency, treatment, and end results. *J Bone Joint Surg* 1990; 72: 825–833.
26. Berrey BHJ, Lord CF, Gebhardt MC, and Mankin HJ. Fractures of allografts. Frequency, treatment, and end results. *J Bone Joint Surg Am* 1990; 72: 825–833.
27. Enneking WF and Mindell ER. Observations on massive retrieved human allografts. *J Bone Joint Surg Am* 1991; 73: 1123–1142.
28. Mankin HJ, Doppelt S, and Tomford W. Clinical experience with allograft implantation. The first ten years. *Clin Orthop* 1983; 174: 69–86.
29. Gebhardt MC, Flugstad DI, Springfield DS, and Mankin HJ. The use of bone allografts for limb salvage in high-grade extremity osteosarcoma. *Clin Orthop* 1991; 270: 181–196.
30. Jofe MH, Gebhardt MC, Tomford WW, and Mankin HJ. Reconstruction for defects of the proximal part of the femur using allograft arthroplasty. *J Bone Joint Surg Am* 1988; 70: 507–516.
31. Johnson ME and Mankin HJ. Reconstructions after resections of tumors involving the proximal femur. *Orthop Clin North Am* 1991; 22: 87–103.
32. Power RA, Wood DJ, Tomford WW, and Mankin HJ. Revision osteoarticular allograft transplantation in weight-bearing joints. A clinical review. *J Bone Joint Surg Br* 1991; 73: 595–599.
33. Lord CF, Gebhardt MC, Tomford WW, and Mankin HJ. Infection in bone allografts. Incidence, nature, and treatment. *J Bone Joint Surg Am* 1988; 70: 369–376.
34. Tomford WW, Starkweather RJ, and Goldman MH. A study of the clinical incidence of infection in the use of banked allograft bone. *J Bone Joint Surg Am* 1981; 63: 244–248.
35. Tomford WW, Thongphasuk J, Mankin HJ, and Ferraro MJ. Frozen musculoskeletal allografts. A study of the clinical incidence and causes of infection associated with their use. *J Bone Joint Surg Am* 1990; 72: 1137–1143.
36. MacEwen W. Observations concerning transplantation of bone: illustrated by a case of inter-human osseous transplantation, whereby over two-thirds of the shaft of a humerus was restored. *Proc R Soc Lond* 1881; 32: 232–247.

37. Bauer H. Über Knochentransplantation. *Zentralbl Chir* 1910; 37: 20–21.
38. Tuffier T. Sur les graffes osteo-articulaires. *Bull Mem Soc Chir Paris* 1913; 39: 1078–1096.
39. Tuffier T. Des graffes de cartilage et d'os humain dans les resections articulaires. *Bull Mem Soc Chir Paris* 1911; 37: 278–286.
40. Carrel A. The preservation of tissues and its application in surgery. *JAMA* 1912; 59: 523–527.
41. Albee FH. Discussion of Carrell A: the preservation of tissues and its application in surgery. *JAMA* 1912; 59: 527–528.
42. Albee FH. The fundamental principles involved in the use of the bone graft in surgery. *Am J Med Sci* 1915; 149: 313–325.
43. Gallie WE. This history of a bone graft. *Am J Orthop Surg* 1914; 12: 201–212.
44. Gallie WE. The use of boiled bone in operative surgery. *Am J Orthop Surg* 1918; 16: 373–383.
45. Dobrowolskaja NA. On the regeneration of bone in its relation to the cultivation of bone tissue. *Br J Surg* 1916; 4: 332–335.
46. Lewis WH and McCoy CC. The survival of cells after the death of the organism. *Bull Johns Hopkins Hosp* 1922; 33: 284–289.
47. Webster JP. Refrigerated skin grafts. *Ann Surg* 1944; 120: 431–448.
48. Haas SL. A study of the viability of bone after removal from the body. *Arch Surg* 1923; 7: 213–226.
49. Haas SL. Further observations of the survival of bone after removal from the body. *Arch Surg* 1925; 10: 196–209.
50. Bush LF and Garber CZ. The bone bank. *JAMA* 1948; 137: 588–594.
51. Weaver JB. Experiences in the use of homogenous (bone-bank) bank. *J Bone Joint Surg Am* 1949; 31A: 778–792.
52. Hyatt GW. Fundamentals in the use and preservation of homogeneous bone. *US Armed Forces Med J* 1950; 1: 841–852.
53. Hyatt GW, Turner TC, Bassett CAL, Pate JW, and Sawyer PN. New methods for preserving bone, skin and blood vessels. *Postgrad Med* 1952; 12: 239–254.
54. Matthews DN. Storage of skin for autogenous grafts. *Lancet* 1945; 1: 775–776.
55. Flosdorf EW and Hyatt GW. The preservation of bone grafts by freeze-drying, *Surgery* 1952; 31: 716–719.
56. Flosdorf EW. *Freeze Drying,* 1949; Reinhold, New York.
57. Young MF, Kerr JM, Ibaraki K, Heegaard AM, and Robey PG. Structure, expression, and regulation of the major noncollagenous matrix proteins of bone. *Coin Orthop* 1992; 281: 275–294.
58. Celeste AJ, Iannazzi JA, Taylor RC, Hewick RM, Rosen V, Wang EA, and Wozney JM. Identification of transforming growth factor beta family members present in bone-inductive protein purified from bovine bone. *Proc Natl Acad Sci USA* 1990; 87: 9843–9847.
59. Centrella M, Horowitz MC, Wozney JM, and McCarthy TL. Transforming growth factor-beta gene family members and bone. *End Rev* 1994; 15: 27–39.
60. Wang EA, Rosen V, Cordes P, Hewick RM, Kriz MJ, Luxenberg DP, Sibley BS, and Wozney JM. Purification and characterization of other distinct bone-inducing factors. *Proc Natl Acad Sci USA* 1988; 85: 9484–9488.
61. Wozney JM. The bone morphogenetic protein family and osteogenesis. *Mol Reprod Dev* 1992; 32: 160–167.
62. Wozney JM, Rosen V, Byrne M, Celeste AJ, Moutsatsos I, and Wang EA. Growth factors influencing bone development. *J Cell Sci* 1990; 13 (Suppl): 149–156.
63. Wozney JM, Rosen V, Celeste AJ, Mitsock LM, Whitters MJ, Kriz RW, Hewick RM, and Wang EA. Novel regulators of bone formation: molecular clones and activities. *Science* 1988; 242: 1528–1534.
64. Chen J, Singh K, Mukherjee BB, and Sodek J. Developmental expression of osteopontin (OPN) mRNA in rat tissues: evidence for a role for OPN in bone formation and resorption. *Matrix* 1993; 13: 113–123.
65. Dohi Y, Ohgushi H, Tabata S, Yoshikawa T, Dohi K, and Moriyama T. Osteogenesis associated with bone gla protein gene expression in diffusion chambers by bone marrow cells with demineralized bone matrix. *J Bone Miner Res* 1992; 7: 1173–1180.
66. Heersche JN, Reimers SM, Wrana JL, Waye MM, and Gupta AK. Changes in expression of alpha 1 type 1 collagen and osteocalcin mRNA in osteoblasts and odontoblasts at different stages of maturity as shown by in situ hybridization. *Proc Finn Dent Soc* 1992; 88 (Suppl 1): 173–182.
67. Hinrichs B, Dreyer T, Battmann A, and Schulz A. Histomorphometry of active osteoblast surface labelled by antibodies against non-collagenous bone matrix proteins. *Bone* 1993; 14: 469–472.
68. Lian JB, McKee MD, Todd AM, and Gerstenfeld LC. Induction of bone-related proteins, osteocalcin and osteopontin, and their matrix ultrastructural localization with development of chondro-

cyte hypertrophy in vitro. *J Cell Biochem* 1993; 52: 206–219.
69. McKee MD, Glimcher MJ, and Nanci A. High-resolution immunolocalization of osteopontin and osteocalcin in bone and cartilage during endochondral ossification in the chicken tibia. *Anat Rec* 1992; 234: 479–492.
70. Glowacki J and Mulliken JB. Demineralized bone implants. *Clin Plast Surg* 1985; 12: 233–241.
71. Bos GD, Goldberg VM, Zika JM, Heiple KG, and Powell AE. Immune responses of rats to frozen bone allografts. *J Bone Joint Surg Am* 1983; 65: 239–246.
72. Daisaku H. Study on the immune response of mice receiving bone allografts. *Nippon Seikeigeka Gakkai Zasshi* 1988; 62: 71–83.
73. Friedlaender GE. Immune responses to osteochondral allografts. Current knowledge and future directions. *Clin Orthop* 1983; 174: 58–68.
74. Friedlaender GE, Strong DM, and Sell KW. Studies on the antigenicity of bone. I. Freeze-dried and deep-frozen bone allografts in rabbits. *J Bone Joint Surg Am* 1976; 58: 854–858.
75. Kaminska G, Kaminski M, and Komender A. Immunogenicity of fresh and preserved cortical and cancellous allogeneic bone grafts as tested by modified migration inhibition test in mice. *Arch Immunol Ther Exp Warsz* 1978; 26: 1053–1057.
76. Langer F, Czitrom A, Pritzker KP, and Gross AE. The immunogenicity of fresh and frozen allogeneic bone. *J Bone Joint Surg Am* 1975; 57: 216–220.
77. Nisbet NW. Antigenicity of bone. *J Bone Joint Surg Br* 1977; 59: 263–266.
78. Oda Y, Sato H, Kazama T, Ishii T, Sato M, Shirano T, Kudo I, Iwase T, and Moro I. A preliminary report on bone transplantation. 1. An immunohistochemical study on the distortion and proportions of lymphocyte subsets in lymphoid organs of normal rats. *J Nihon Univ Sch Dent* 1987; 29: 303–313.
79. Shigetomi M, Kawai S, and Fukumoto T. Studies of allotransplantation of bone using immunohistochemistry and radioimmunoassay in rats. *Clin Orthop* 1993; 292: 345–351.
80. Bos GD, Goldberg VM, Powell AE, Heiple KG, and Zika JM. The effect of histocompatibility matching on canine frozen bone allografts. *J Bone Joint Surg Am* 1983; 65: 89–96.
81. Musculo DL, Kawai S, and Ray RD. In vitro studies of transplantation antigens present on bone cells in the rat. *J Bone Joint Surg Br* 1977; 59: 342–348.
82. Stevenson S. The immune response to osteochondral allografts in dogs. *J Bone Joint Surg Am* 1987; 69: 573–582.
83. Czitrom AA, Langer F, McKee N, and Gross AE. Bone and cartilage allotransplantation. A review of 14 years of research and clinical studies. *Clin Orthop* 1986; 208: 141–145.
84. Esses S, Halloran P, Kliman M, and Langer F. Bone allografts in mice: determinants of immunogenicity and healing. *Transplant Proc* 1981; 13: 885–887.
85. Halloran PF, Lee E, Ziv I, and Langer F. Bone grafting in inbred mice: evidence for H-2K, H-2D, and non-H-2 antigens in bone. *Transplant Proc* 1979; 11: 1507–1509.
86. Halloran PF, Lee EH, Ziv I, Langer F, and Gross AE. Orthotopic bone transplantation in mice. II. Studies of the alloantibody response. *Transplantation* 1979; 27: 420–426.
87. Halloran PF, Ziv I, Lee EH, Langer F, Pritzker KP, and Gross AE. Orthotopic bone transplantation in mice. I. Technique and assessment of healing. *Transplantation* 1979; 27: 414–419.
88. Horowitz MC and Friedlaender GE. Induction of specific T-cell responsiveness to allogeneic bone. *J Bone Joint Surg Am* 1991; 73: 1157–1168.
89. Lipson RA, Halloran PF, Kawano H, and Langer F. A microsurgical model for vascularized bone and joint transplants in rats. *Transplant Proc* 1981; 13: 891–892.
90. Musculo DL, Kawai S, and Ray RD. Cellular and humoral immune response analysis of bone-allografted rats. *J Bone Joint Surg Am* 1976; 58: 826–832.
91. Stevenson S, Li XQ, Davy DT, Klein L, and Goldberg VM. Critical biological determinants of incorporation of non-vascularized cortical bone grafts. Quantification of a complex process and structure. *J Bone Joint Surg* 1997; 79-A: 1–16.
92. Stevenson S, Shaffer JW, and Goldberg VM. The humoral response to vascular and nonvascular allografts of bone. *Clin Orthop* 1996; 326: 86–95.
93. Li XQ, Stevenson S, Klein L, Davy DT, Shaffer JW, and Goldberg VM. Differential patterns of incorporation and remodeling among various types of bone grafts. *Acta Anat Basel* 1991; 140: 236–244.
94. Stevenson S, Shaffer JW, Davy D, Klein L, and Goldberg VM. Continuous high dose cyclosporin A maintains vascular potency and remodeling in canine fibular allografts. *trans. Orthop Res Soc 39th Meeting* 1993; p 537.
95. Weelter JF, Shaffer JW, Stevenson S, Davy DT, Field GA, Klein L, et al. Cyclosporin A and tissue antigen matching in bone transplantation. Fibular

allografts studied in the dog. *Acta Orthop Scand* 1990; 61: 517–527.

96. Zart DJ, Miya L, Wolff DA, Makley JT, and Stevenson S. The effects of cisplatin on the incorporation of fresh syngeneic and frozen cortical bone grafts. *J Orthop Res* 1993; 11: 240–249.

97. Friedlaender GE and Horowitz MC. Immune responses to osteochondral allografts: Nature and significance. *Orthopedics* 1992; 15: 1171–1175.

98. Stevenson S, Hohn RB, and Templeton JW. Effects of tissue antigen matching on the healing of fresh cancellous bone allografts in dogs. *Am J Vet Res* 1983; 44: 201–206.

99. Stevenson S and Horowitz M. The response to bone allografts. *J Bone Joint Surg Am* 1992; 74: 939–950.

100. Stevenson S, Li XQ, and Martin B. The fate of cancellous and cortical bone after transplantation of fresh and frozen tissue-antigen-matched and mismatched osteochondral allografts in dogs. *J Bone Joint Surg Am* 1991; 73: 1143–1156.

101. Langer F and Gross A. The clinical and immunological assessment of frozen bone allografts. *Acta Med Pol* 1978; 19: 271–275.

102. Friedlaender GE, Strong DM, and Sell KW. Studies on the antigenicity of bone. II. Donor-specific anti-HLA antibodies in human recipients of freeze-dried allografts. *J Bone Joint Surg Am* 1984; 66: 107–112.

103. Sepe WW, Bowers GM, Lawrence JJ, Friedlaender GE, and Koch RW. Clinical evaluation of freeze-dried bone allografts in periodontal osseous defects. Part II. *J Periodontal* 1978; 49: 9–14.

104. Rodrigo JJ, Fuller TC, and Mankin HJ. Cytotoxic HLA-antibodies in patients with bone and cartiage allografts. *Trans Orthop Res Soc* 1976; 1: 131.

105. Aho AJ, Eskola J, Ekfors T, Manner I, Kouri T, and Hollmen T. Immune responses and clinical outcome of massive human osteoarticular allografts. *Clin Orthop* 1998; 346: 196–206.

106. Lewandrowski KU, Ekkernkamp A, Tomford WW, and Muhr G. T-Zell Aktivierung nach allogener Knochentransplantation. *Langenbecks Arch Chir Suppl II* 1996; 1248.

107. Lewandrowski KU, Tomford WW, Springfield DS, and Mankin HJ. MHC-Restriktion zytotoxischer Antikörper nach Transplantation allogener Knochentransplantate. *Langenbecks Arch Chirurgie Suppl* 1996; 1: 157–162.

108. Muscolo DL, Caletti E, Schajowicz F, Araujo ES, and Makino A. Tissue-typing in human massive allografts of frozen bone. *J Bone Joint Surg Am* 1987; 69: 583–595.

109. Muscolo DL, Ayerza MA, Calabrese ME, Redal MA, and Santini Araujo E. Human leukocyte antigen matching, radiographic score, and histologic findings in massive frozen bone allografts. *Clin Orthop* 1996; 326: 115–126.

110. Strong DM, Friedlaender GE, Tomford WW, Springfield DS, Shives TC, Burchardt H, Enneking WF, and Mankin HJ. Immunologic responses in human recipients of osseous and osteochondral allografts. *Clinical Orthop* 1996; 326: 107–114.

111. Tomford WW, Schachar NS, Fuller TC, Henry WB, and Mankin HJ. Immunogenicity of frozen osteoarticular allografts. *Transplant Proc* 1981; 13: 888–890.

112. Tomford WW, Springfield DS, Mankin HJ, Hung HH, Lewandrowski KU, and Fuller TC. Immunology of large frozen bone allograft transplantation in humans. Antibody and T-Lymphocyte response and their effects on results. *Trans Orthop Res Soc* 1994; 39: 102.

113. Bernick S, Paule W, Ertl D, Nishimoto SK, and Nimni ME. Cellular events associated with the induction of bone by demineralized bone. *J Orthop Res* 1989; 7: 1–11.

114. Gendler E. Perforated demineralized bone matrix: a new form of osteoinductive biomaterial. *J Biomed Mater Res* 1986; 20: 687–697.

115. Gendler E. 1990; US Patent 4932973.

116. O'Donnell RJ, Deutsch TF, Flotte TJ, Lorente CA, Tomford WW, Mankin HJ, and Schomacker KT. Effect of Er:YAG laser holes on osteoinduction in demineralized rat calvarial allografts. *J Orthop Res* 1996; 14: 108–113.

117. Scanlon CE. *Analysis of laser-textured, demineralized bone allografts* 1991; Master's thesis. *Northwestern University, Biomedical Engineering Department*, Chicago.

118. Sires BS. 1992; US patent 5112354.

119. Nuss RC, Fabian RL, Sarkar R, and Puliafito CA. Infrared laser bone ablation. *Lasers Surg Med* 1988; 8: 381–391.

120. Walsh JT Jr, Flotte TJ, and Deutsch TF. Er:YAG laser ablation of tissue: effect of pulse duration and tissue type on thermal damage. *Lasers Surg Med* 1989; 9: 314–326.

121. Guo MZ, Xia ZS, and Lin LB. The mechanical and biological properties of demineralised cortical bone allografts in animals. *J Bone Joint Surg Br* 1991; 73: 791–794.

122. Hosny M and Sharawy M. Osteoinduction in rhesus monkeys using demineralized bone powder allografts. *J Oral Maxillofac Surg* 1985; 43: 837–844.

123. Hosny M and Sharawy M. Osteoinduction in young and old rats using demineralized bone

powder allografts. *J Oral Maxillofac Surg* 1985; 43: 925–931.

124. Narang R, Wells H, and Laskin DM. Experimental osteogenesis with demineralized allogeneic bone matrix in extraskeletal sites. *J Oral Maxillofac Surg* 1982; 40: 133–141.

125. Vandersteenhoven JJ and Spector M. Histological investigation of bone induction by demineralized allogeneic bone matrix: a natural biomaterial for osseous reconstruction. *J Biomed Mater Res* 1983; 17: 1003–1014.

126. Mulliken JB, Glowacki J, Kaban LB, Folkman J, and Murray JE. Use of demineralized allogeneic bone implants for the correction of maxillocraniofacial deformities. *Ann Surg* 1981; 194: 366–372.

127. Salyer KE, Gendler E, Menendez JL, Simon TR, Kelly KM, and Bardach J. Demineralized perforated bone implants in craniofacial surgery. *J Cranio Surg* 1992; 3: 55–62.

128. Sonis ST, Kaban LB, and Glowacki J. Clinical trial of demineralized bone powder in the treatment of periodontal defects. *J Oral Med* 1983; 38: 117–122.

129. Birkedal-Hansen H. Kinetics of acid demineralization in histologic technique. *J Histochem Cytochem* 1974; 22: 434–441.

130. Birkedal-Hansen H. Kinetics of acid demineralization in histologic technique. *J Histochem Cytochem* 1974; 22: 434–441.

131. Lewandrowski KU, Venugopalan V, Tomford WW, Schomacker KT, Mankin HJ, and Deutsch TF. Kinetics of cortical bone demineralization. A new method for modifying cortical bone allografts. *J Biomed Mater Res* 1996; 31: 365–372.

132. Levenspiel O. *Chemical Reaction Engineering* 1972; Wiley, New York.

133. Lewandrowski KU, Tomford WW, Michaud N, Flotte TF, Schomacker KT, and Deutsch TF. Electron microscopic studies on the process of cortical bone demineralization. *Calcif Tissue Int* 1997; 61: 294–297.

134. Lewandrowski KU, Tomford WW, Yeadon A, Deutsch TF, Mankin HJ, and Uhthoff HK. Flexural rigidity in partially demineralized diaphyseal bone grafts. *Clin Orthop* 1995; 317: 254–262.

135. Makarewicz PJ, Harasta L, and Webb SL. Kinetics of acid diffusion and demineralization of bone. *J Photogr Sci* 1980; 22: 148–159.

136. Lewandrowski KU, Ekkernkamp A, Muhr G, and Tomford WW. Osteoinduction in cortical bone grafts by controlled partial demineralization and laser-perforation. *Trans Eur Surg Res Soc* 1996; 1: 5.

137. Lewandrowski KU, Tomford WW, Mankin HJ, Schomacker KT, and Deutsch TF. Enhancement of incorporation of cortical bone grafts by partial demienralization and laser-perforation. *Trans Orthop Res Soc* 1995; 1: 87.

138. Lewandrowski KU, Schollmeier G, Uhthoff HK, and Tomford WW. Mechanical properties of laser-perforated and partially demineralized diaphyseal bone allografts. *Clin Orthop* 1998; 353: 238–246.

139. Lewandrowski KU, Tomford WW, Schomacker KT, Deutsch TF, and Mankin HJ. Enhancement of incorporation of cortical bone grafts by controlled partial demineralization and laser-perforation. *J Orthop Res* 1997; 15: 748–756.

140. Lewandrowski KU, Schollmeier G, Ekkernkamp A, Grosse-Wilde P, Rebmann V, and Tomford WW. Immune response to laser-perforated and partially demineralized cortical bone allografts. 1998; in preparation.

141. Lewandrowski KU, Schollmeier G, Ekkernkamp A, Muhr G, Uhthoff HK, and Tomford WW. Mechanical evaluation of incorporation of laser-perforated and partially demineralized cortical bone allografts. 1998; in preparation.

142. Lewandrowski KU, Schollmeier G, Ekkernkamp A, Uhthoff HK, Mankin HJ, and Tomford WW. Modification of cortical bone allografts by partial demineralization and laser perforation to enhance incorporation: a radiographic, histological and biomechanical study. *Trans Orthop Res Soc* 1998; 44: 1010.

143. Kubens BS, Arnett KL, Adams EJ, Parham P, and Grosse-Wilde H. Definition of a new HLA-B7 subtype (B0704) by isoelectric focusing, family studies and DNA sequence analysis. *Tissue Antigens* 1995; 45: 322–327.

144. Kubens BS, Krumbacher K, and Grosse-Wilde H. Biochemical definition of DLA-A and DLA-B gene products by one-dimensional isoelectric focusing and immunoblotting. *Eur J Immunogenet* 1995; 22: 199–207.

145. Rebmann V, Kubens BS, Ferencik S, and Grosse-Wilde H. Biochemical analysis of HLA-DP gene products by isoelectric focusing and comparison with cellular and molecular genetic typing results. *Exp Clin Immunogenet* 1995; 12: 36–47.

146. Rodrigo JJ, Heiden E, Hegyes M, and Sharkey NA. Immune response by irrigating subchondral bone with cytotoxic agents. *Clin Orthop* 1996; 326: 96–106.

8

Synthetic Osseous Grafting

A Necessary Component to Oral Reconstruction

Arthur Ashman and Jeffrey S. Gross

1. Introduction

Dental bone grafts (BGs) play an important role in situations in which structural or functional support, or both, is necessary. BGs are used to provide a scaffold for bone regeneration: promoting union of osteotomies and fractures; augmenting bony defects caused by trauma or surgery; restoring bone loss caused by dental disease; filling extraction sites to preserve the height and width of the alveolar ridge (ridge preservation); and augmenting and reconstructing the alveolar ridge *(1,2)*. In addition to alveolar ridge preservation and augmentation and repair of bony defects, grafting is being performed to improve the outcome of implant dentistry through sinus lift procedures of the maxillary sinus and to fill bony voids (e.g., in the immediate postextraction implant) and the osteotomy created during traditional implant surgery *(3)*.

Successful rehabilitation of a dental arch, with fixed prosthetic replacement of lost teeth, depends on the presence of stable abutment teeth *(4,5)*. Periodontal disease and surgical bone defects can compromise the reliability of these support structures. Resorption of the alveolar ridge following tooth extraction or surgery also can significantly affect the retention and stability of removable complete dentures, which are dependent on the size and shape of the residual alveolar ridge *(4,5)*.

In addition, the loss of alveolar bone, because of periodontal disease or secondary to surgery, is a source of numerous complications, including loss of the periodontal attachment, impaired restoration of the periodontium, and poor patient aesthetics *(4,5)*. Thus, a primary goal of treatment is repair and regeneration of the entire periodontal attachment complex which consists of cementum, periodontal ligament (PDL), and alveolar bone *(6)*.

Clinically, different substitute BGs have been utilized for ridge preservation postextraction; ridge augmentation; in periodontal bony defects; and in conjunction with the placement of dental implants *(7–9)*. The literature is replete with successful applications of BGs, both with or without membrane barriers. There is increasing evidence that most synthetic BG substitutes do not require the utilization of a membrane *(10)*.

2. Mechanisms of Bone Grafting

Bone grafting is accomplished through three different processes: osteogenesis, osteoinduction, and osteoconduction *(2,11–13)*. Osteogenesis is

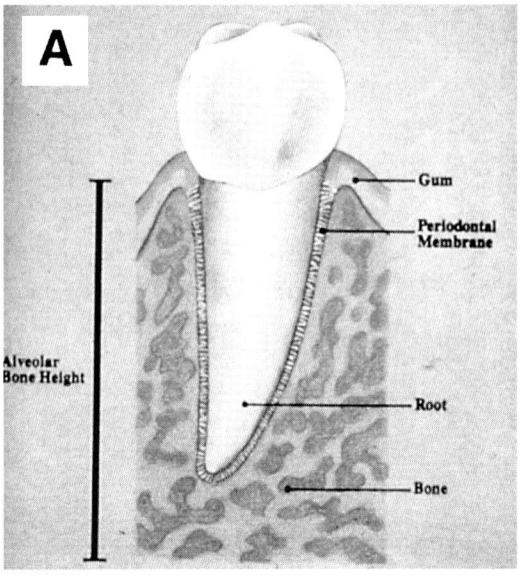

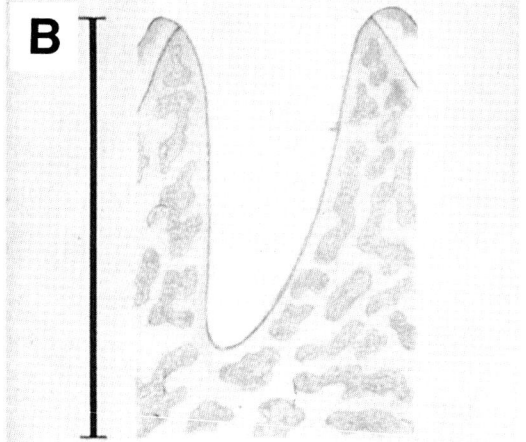

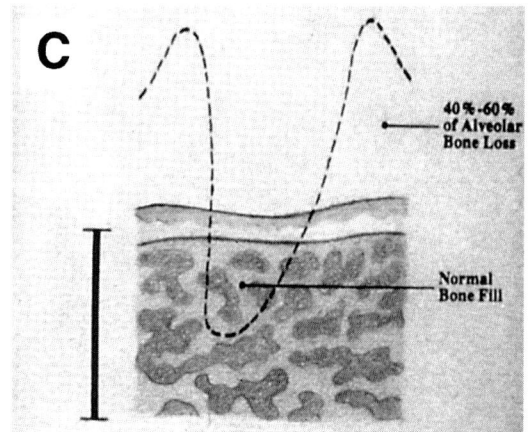

Fig. 1. (**A–C**) Diagrams demonstrating the normal bone repair response after tooth removal. Note the loss of 40–60% of bone 2–3 years after removal of teeth. (**A**) Normal, pre-extraction; (**B**) normal, immediate post-extraction; (**C**) normal, 2 yr post-extraction.

the formation and development of bone, even in the absence of local undifferentiated mesenchymal cells. An osteogenic graft is an organic material that is derived from or composed of living tissue that is involved with the growth or repair of bone. Osteogenic cells can differentiate and facilitate the different phases of bone regeneration, and encourage bone formation in soft tissues or activate quicker bone growth in bone sites. Osteoinduction is a process that brings about the transformation of undifferentiated mesenchymal cells into osteoblasts or chondroblasts through growth factors found only in living bone. By doing so, bone regeneration is enhanced, and bone may even extend or grow in places where it is not normally found. Osteoconduction provides a physical matrix that is, in essence, a bioinert scaffolding suitable for deposition of new bone. Osteoconductive graft materials are conducive to bone growth and allow bone apposition from existing bone, but they do not produce bone formation when placed within soft tissue. To encourage bone to grow across its surface, the osteoconductive materials (which are often inorganic)

Synthetic Osseous Grafting

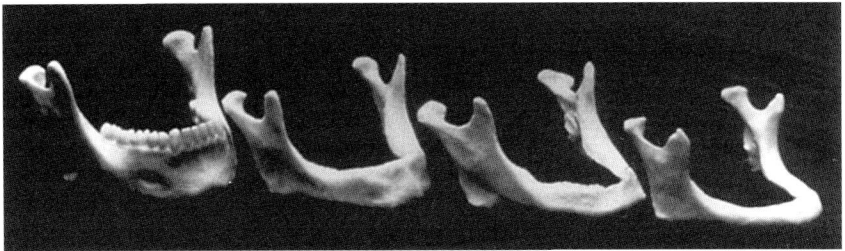

Fig. 2. Illustrates the three stages of bone destruction postextraction. Notice the atrophic jawbone on right. Bone continues to be lost from .25–.5%/yr until patients' death.

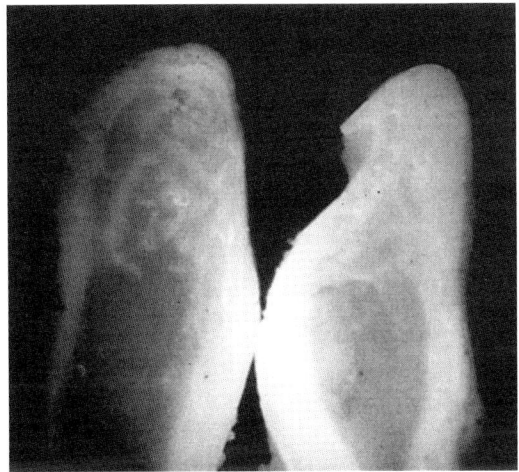

Fig. 3. Right side demonstrates loss of buccal plate of bone just 10 mo postextraction (monkey). Left side (tetracycline-staining bone regeneration shows grafted extraction socket (courtesy P. Boyne, Loma Linda University).

require the presence of existing bone or differentiated mesenchymal cells. All BG materials have one or more of these three modes of action.

3. Types of Graft Material

There are three primary forms of bone graft material: autogenous bone, allografts, and alloplasts. The origin and composition of the graft normally determine the mechanism by which they act (13,14). Autogenous bone, an organic autologous material, utilizes osteogenesis, osteoinduction, and osteoconduction in the formation of new bone. Allografts, which may be cortical or trabecular in nature, are osteoinductive and osteoconductive, but not osteogenetic. Alloplasts, which may be natural or synthetic materials, are typically only osteoconductive.

3.1. Autogenous Bone

Autogenous bone has long been considered the gold standard of grafting materials. Currently, it is the only osteogenic material available. Grafted autogenous bone heals into growing bone during the three processes of osteogenesis, osteoinduction, and osteoconduction. These stages are not separate and distinct: Instead, they overlap each other during the grafting process (13).

The organic component (i.e., collagen) of autogenous bone provides it with resilience, strength, and stability; the bone's inorganic property (a crystalline, ceramic-like material comprised primarily of hydroxylapatite [HA]) contributes to its firm, rigid qualities (13).

Grafted bone may be trabecular, corticotrabecular, or cortical (13). Trabecular bone provides osteogenic cells, and survives best when blood supply from the host bone is easily accessible. Corticotrabecular block grafts allow the dentist to shape and conform the graft to fit the recipient bed. The cortical aspect is placed on the surface of the graft; the trabecular segment is situated on the host bone. A cortical graft will stimulate osteogenesis only from surviving cells (which will be fewer in number than that of trabecular bone). However, cortical bone provides most of the bone morphogenetic protein (BMP), the chemical inductive agent essential during osteoinduction. BMP elicits the differentiation of host mesenchymal cells into osteoblasts. In addition, the cortical

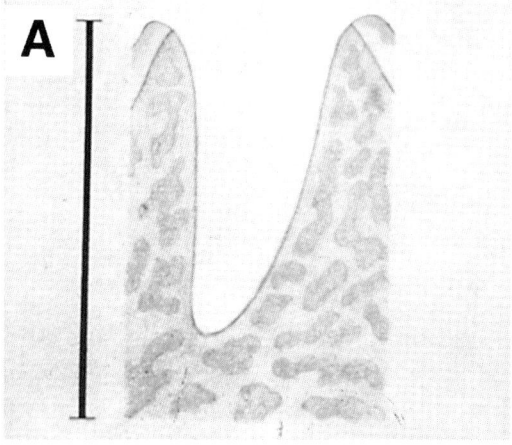
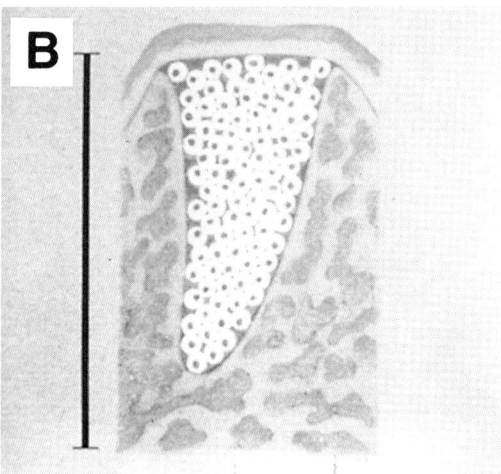
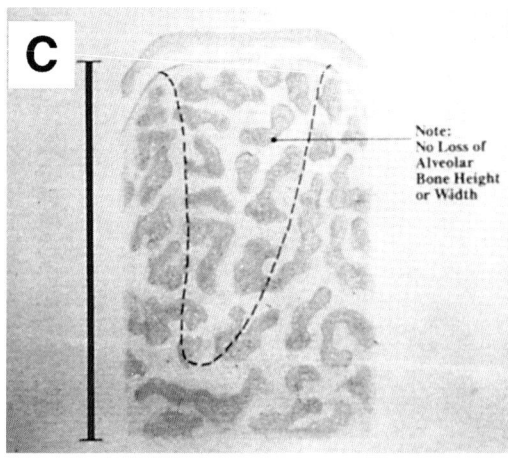

Fig. 4. **(A–C)** Demonstrates ridge preservation diagrams showing the filling of the extraction **(A)** socket with a synthetic graft **(B)** and bony regeneration maintaining the height and width of the jaw bone **(C)**.

portion provides a more resistant structure during osteoconduction, and may impede soft tissue invasion and prolong the time needed for blood vessels from the host bone to infiltrate the graft.

Autogenous bone can be harvested from the iliac crest or from intraoral sites, such as the mandibular symphysis, maxillary tuberosity, ramus, exostoses, and debris from an implant osteotomy *(13,15,16)*. Resorption of mandibular BGs following transplantation has been reported to be less, compared with that of iliac crest grafts *(15)*. In addition, intraorally obtained BGs result in less morbidity than that associated with iliac crest grafts. The procedure can be easily accomplished in an office setting, with the patient under parenteral sedation and local anesthesia *(16)*. Thus, there is no postoperative hospitalization, resulting in lower costs. A disadvantage, however, is that intraoral donor sites provide a smaller volume of bone than the iliac crest, but, in intraoral sites, the bony voids created at the donor areas can easily be grafted with a synthetic alloplast. The donor site is usually chosen according to the volume and type of bone desired.

Autogenous bone is highly osteogenic and best fulfills dental grafting requirements (i.e., providing a scaffold for bone regeneration, stimulating osteogenesis, promoting union of osteotomies and fractures, and preventing collapse of bony segments into iatrogenic defects) *(1)*. However, shortcomings, such as the requirement of a second operative site, the attendant patient morbidity, and the possibility of not being able to obtain sufficient material when there are extensive or multiple defects (especially from intraoral sites), have led to the development of allografts and alloplasts as alternative grafting materials *(1,2,6)*.

3.2. Allografts

Bone allografts are obtained from other individuals of the same species, but disparate genotypes. Donors include cadavers, living related persons, and living unrelated persons. Once procured, the allografts are processed under complete sterility and stored in bone banks. The primary forms of bone allografts are frozen, freeze-dried (lyophilized), demineralized freeze-dried bone, and irradiated bone.

Transplanted bone induces a host immune

Synthetic Osseous Grafting

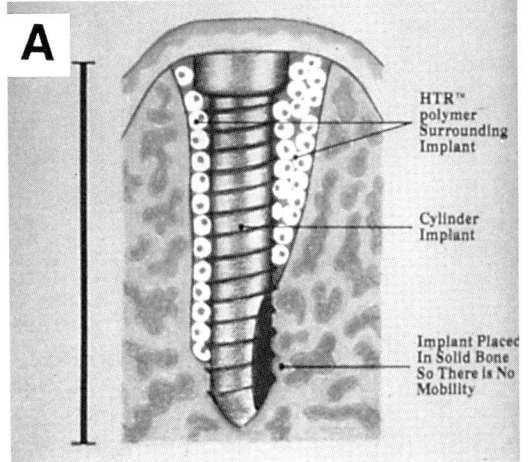

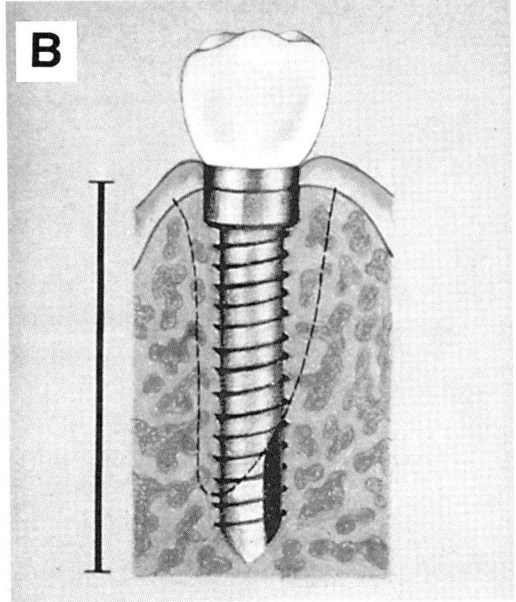

Fig. 5. (**A,B**) Also demonstrates ridge preservation and replacement therapy. With the immediate placement of a dental implant (**A**), osseointegration of regenerating bone around the implant (**B**).

response. Although fresh allografts are most antigenic, this can be reduced considerably by first freezing or freeze-drying the bone *(14)*. Freeze-dried bone allograft (FDBA) can be used in either a mineralized or demineralized form. Demineralization removes the mineral phase and exposes the underlying bone collagen and growth factors, in particular BMP *(2)*. Demineralizing cortical bone greatly enhances its osteogenic potential, by providing sufficient BMP to osteoinduce bone *(6,17)*. Without removal of the mineral phase, this bone induction process does not occur *(6)*.

Demineralized freeze-dried bone allograft (DFDBA) has been reported as having definite potential as a graft material in periodontal regenerative therapy *(17)*. However, when Rummelhart et al. *(6)* compared the efficacy of DFDBA with FDBA in promoting bone repair of human periodontal osseous defects, they did not find any significant differences for any clinical parameter 6 mo after surgery. Those authors felt there might be a number of reasons for this outcome. First, the small size of the defects may not have allowed for sufficient quantity of graft material, and the BMP of DFDBA, to be present in a biologically significant amount. Second, the fact that their study consisted primarily of one-wall defects may have contributed to a reduced clinical response. Finally, they concluded that 6 mo may not have been a sufficient time period for completion of bone deposition in severe defects.

DFDBA may form bone by osteoinduction, by its effect on surrounding undifferentiated mesenchymal cells in the soft tissue around the graft, as blood vessels penetrate the graft. DFDBA may also form bone by osteoconduction, when the host bone resorbs the material and forms a scaffold. However, because allografts are not osteogenic, bone formation takes longer and results in less volume, compared with autogenous grafts *(13)*.

Irradiated cancellous bone has also been used as a substitute graft material for autogenous bone *(18,19)*. During its initial use, the bone was exposed to 6–8 million rads of radiation. More recently, trabecular bone, obtained from the spinal column and treated with 2.5 million rads (Rocky Mountain Tissue Bank, Aurora, CO), has been utilized. Tatum et al. *(18)* reported that the expense and morbidity incurred in obtaining autogenous iliac bone made irradiated bone the most effective, readily available graft material that they have used, demonstrating rapid replacement and consistent establishment of a reasonable replacement ratio of new bone. Tatum *(19)* found the material provided a response closest to that achieved with autogenous bone.

The advantages of allografts include ready availability, elimination of the need to use a donor

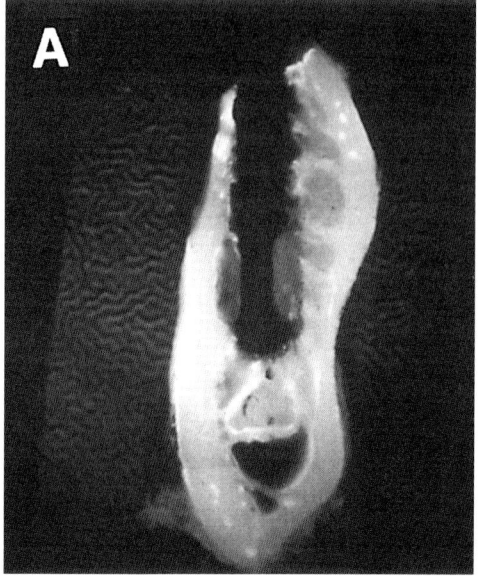
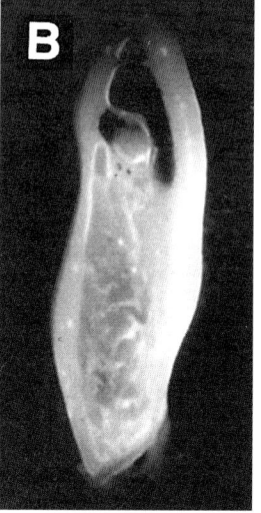

Fig. 6. (**A**) Radiograph immediate placement of dental implant 10 mo (monkey). Note osseointegration of the implant with new bone formation around it (tetracycline yellow stain). (**B**) Extraction socket radiograph with Bioplant HTR grafted in socket 10 mo (monkey). Note the preservation of the ridge and regeneration of bone.

site in the patient, reduced anesthesia and surgical time, decreased blood loss, and fewer complications *(13)*.

Disadvantages of allografts are primarily associated with the use of tissues from another individual. The quality of the BG and the subsequent health of the recipient depends on the donor not having a history of infections, malignant cancers, degenerative bone disease, hepatitis B or C, sexually transmitted diseases, autoimmune deficiency, and other medical problems *(2,5,13)*. Cadaver bone also may suffer the same rejection seen with other transplanted tissues or organs.

Problems reported with allografts include the considerable technical precision required to insert bulk allografts, the necessity for rigid fixation to the host bone to obtain successful union, and the high rate of infection, nonunion, and graft fracture *(2,14)*.

3.3. Synthetic Bone Substitutes: Alloplasts

Over the past two decades, ceramics, such as HA and tricalcium phosphate (TCP), and polymers (Bioplant hard tissue replacement [HTR]), have received the most attention as substitutes for autogenous bone. They have been found to be safe and well tolerated. However, ceramics, because they have minimal ability to encourage new attachment, are limited in effectively treating various osseous defects *(6)*. Recent advances in biomaterials, however, have greatly improved the use of synthetic bone substitutes in selected dental cases. These materials are being employed to eliminate periodontal pockets, replace bone lost to periodontal or other disease, regenerate new cementum, and form a normal PDL *(7–9)*. In addition, because of special characteristics and properties of some alloplasts, new philosophies and techniques, such as ridge preservation and advanced extraction therapy (AET), will prevent the collapse of the alveolar ridge in recent extraction sites. Dentists often encounter clinical situations in which teeth have been extracted in areas of aesthetic concern. Negative aesthetic results can be avoided by the use of ridge preservation techniques *(20)*. Augmentation materials can also be incorporated in the remodeling and healing processes of bone, to assist or stimulate bone growth in areas where resorption has occurred *(13)*.

Alloplastic materials are available in a variety of textures, sizes, and shapes (Table 1). They can be classified, based on their porosity, as dense, macroporous (pores usually between 100 and 350 μ in diameter), or microporous (pores about 1–5 μ in diameter). Alloplastics also may be either

Synthetic Osseous Grafting

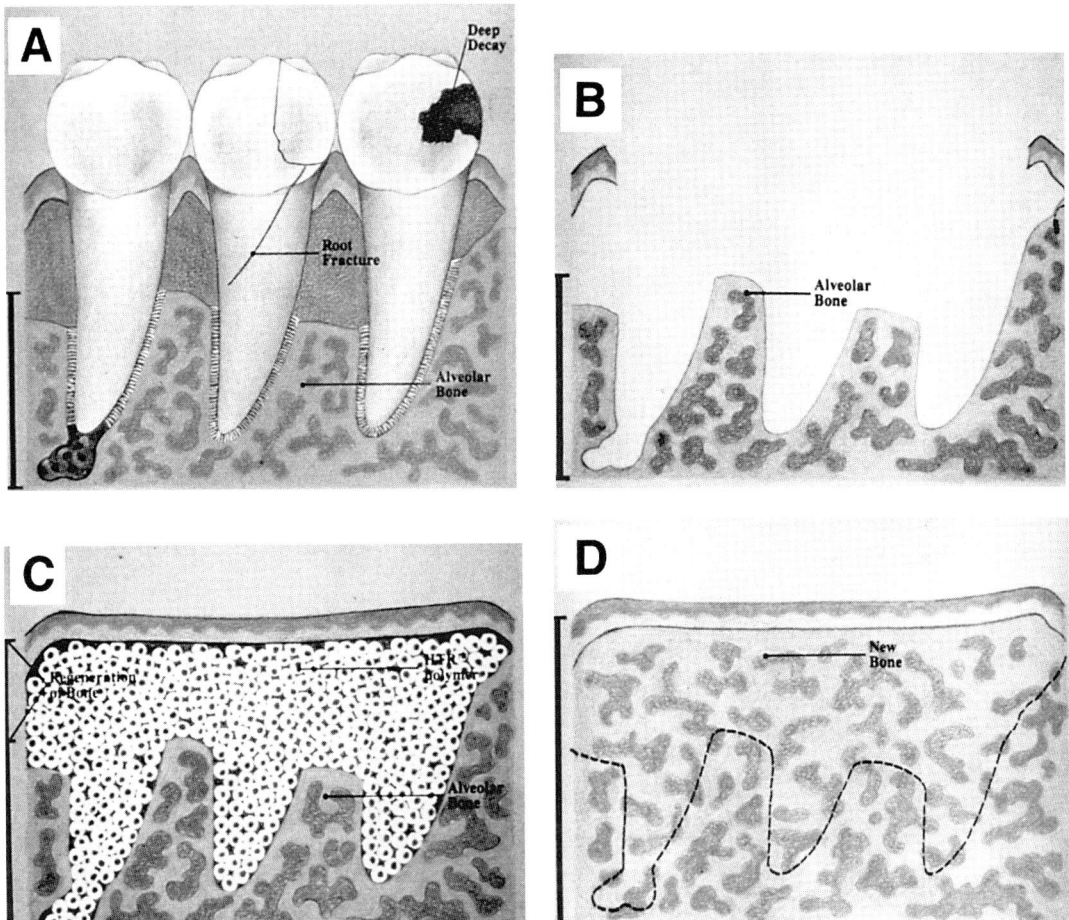

Fig. 7. (A–D) Diagrams of ridge augmentation procedure, which not only preserves the height and width of the ridge, but extends it with generated new bone. (A–B) Initial infection and extraction; (C) extraction socket filled with polymer; (D) polymer acts as scaffold for new bone regeneration.

crystalline or amorphous. They can be granular or molded in form. The different properties of these materials will determine which synthetic material is best for a specific application (7,13). Synthetic bone substitutes include calcium phosphate (CaP) ceramics (HA and TCP), calcium carbonate ($CaCO_3$), polymers, bioactive glass (BAG) ceramics, growth factors and cytokines, and BMPs. The characteristics of the ideal synthetic bone substitute, as defined by Ashman (7,8) are listed in Table 2.

The two primary applications of synthetic bone substitutes are prevention and restoration (7; Table 3). They should prevent postextraction alveolar bone loss, so that essential alveolar ridge is available for subsequent dentures or endosteal implants; postextraction osteitis (dry socket); loss of alveolar bone proximal to extraction sites; pocket formations secondary to extraction; proximal bone loss after anterior tooth extraction; alveolar bone loss following implant placement; and epithelium migration around the implant. They should restore alveolar bone atrophy (ridge augmentation) secondary to long-term tooth loss; bone lost to periodontal disease, while promoting formation of new bone, and acting as a scaffold for the new bone; bony defects, fracture areas, cysts, and granuloma sites with new bone; and

Table 1
Current Alloplastic BG Materials

Natural (from cows)	Interpore 200
	Osteograf N
	BioOss (deorganified)
Ceramics	
HA Synthetic	Calcitite
	Orthomatrix HA
	Osteogen
	Osteograf D
	Osteograf LD
TCP	Augmen
	CalciResorb
	SynthoGraf
Manmade Synthetics	
Calcium carbonate	BioCoral
Bioactive glass ceramics	Bioglass
	Biogran
	PerioGlas
Composite polymer	Bioplant HTR

Table 3
Alloplast Applications

Prevention
  Postextraction alveolar bone loss
  Postextraction osteitis
  Postoperative bleeding
  Pocket formation
  Shifting of teeth
  Soft-tissue ingrowth into bone void area
  Vulnerable maxillary sinus and/or mandibular nerve
Restoration
  Alveolar bone atrophy
  Periodontal pockets and bone loss
  Periodontal pocket ligament loss
  Bony defects and voids
  Cysts
  Granulomas
  Fractures
  Sinus bone architecture
  Hard and soft tissue aesthetics

Table 2
Characteristics of Ideal Alloplast BG Material

Biocompatible
Nonreactive (nontoxic, nonimmunogenic, noncarcinogenic)
Strong and porous
Viable
Ostenogenic potential
Serve as a scaffold for new bone
Radiopaque
Hydrophilic
Easy to manipulate
Not support growth of oral pathogens
Graftable surface (antibiotics, bone growth factors, and so on)
Intensively tested 10 or more years in varied applications
Well documented
Predictable results
Effectively treating various osseous defects
Sterile
Long shelf life
Readily available
Easily produced
Affordable
Nondisease transfer
Cell-attracting negative electric charge

partially atrophied jaw bones, when used in conjunction with dental implants.

3.3.1. Ceramics

In the past, the most commonly used alloplastics are bioactive ceramics, which includes synthetic CaP materials (HA and TCP) and those derived from natural sources (e.g., coralline or bovine bone). The mechanism of action for these ceramics is osteoconduction *(13,21)*. CaP ceramics act as filler materials, with new bone formation taking place along their surface *(4,5)*. These materials are used in the reconstruction of bony defects, and for the augmentation of resorbed alveolar ridges. The objective is to provide a scaffold for enhanced bone tissue repair and growth. In general, dense ceramics exhibit good compressive strength, but poor tensile strength (similar to bone). Although their biologic responses differ, all have been recommended for augmentation *(13)*.

However, ceramics do have disadvantages. After implantation, it has been reported *(11)* that particles at some distance from the pre-existing bone have been found to be encapsulated by fibrous tissue. Lack of particulate consolidation, dispersion of the particles into surrounding soft tissues (migration), exfoliation of the particles, and invagination of epithelial cells in periodontal pockets (resulting in long epithelial junction) also have been observed *(4,5,22)*. Synthesized ceramics (HA and TCP) have also been found to be brittle, lack direct porous connectivity, need bony ingrowth to improve their mechanical properties, and require either osteogenic cells or growth factors to succeed *(2)*.

3.3.1.1. HYDROXYAPATITE

HA is the primary inorganic, natural component of bone, comprising 60–70% of the calcified skeleton and 98% of dental enamel, with a Ca:P ratio of 10:6 *(11,13,21)*. HA is biocompatible and bonds readily to adjacent hard and soft tissues. The physical and chemical properties of HA will affect the rate of resorption and will determine the clinical applications of the graft *(13)*.

Physical properties include the surface area and the form of the product (block, particle), porosity (dense, macroporous, microporous), and crystallinity (crystalline or amorphous) *(25)*. Chemical properties are associated with the Ca:P ratio, elemental impurities, ionic substitution in HA, and the pH of the surrounding area. Larger crystalline particles take longer, and are called nonresorbable. Conversely, smaller-sized crystalline HA will resorb more rapidly. This is in addition to amorphous HA, which also breaks down quicker. Porosity will determine the extent of blood vessel ingrowth, but this may or may not affect remodeling of bone. Crystalline structure or the lack of it is the prime factor in determining resorbability *(23)*.

Solid, dense blocks have high compressive strengths, but are brittle. Although not considered suitable for load-bearing conditions, their mechanical strength is sufficient for alveolar ridge augmentation. Macroporous blocks vary in size, distribution, and extent of their interconnecting pores. Pores of 150–200 µ are reported to be optimal for ingrowth of mineralized bone *(11)*. A general disadvantage of porous ceramics is that their strength decreases exponentially with the increase in porosity. A strong, but porous, HA can be prepared, with compressive strength similar to bone. However, this material is difficult to contour, and is probably best used as an interpositional implant in the mandible, rather than as an onlay on the alveolar ridge. HA particles (about 1 mm in diameter) are often used for ridge augmentation, and conform well to the underlying bone structure. This approach minimizes the problems of brittleness of HA. However, implants cannot be placed in an HA-augmented ridge.

Porous HA blocks have been used as an alternative to HA particles *(11)*. In a dog study, Frame et al *(24)* reported greater bone ingrowth when they used porous HA particles for alveolar augmentation, compared with solid, dense HA. Boyne *(25)* noted a decreased use of nonresorbable, nonporous HA in alveolar ridge augmentation (which tends to lack cohesive strength, and migrates under stress during the healing period) and an increase in the use of a porous form of HA.

Currently available commercial HA graft materials include Calcitite HA 2040 and Calcitite 4060 (Calcitek, Carlsbad, CA), both of which are dense, nonresorbable, ceramic particulates; Osteo Graf/N (natural porous particles), OsteoGraf/LD (low density synthetic particles), and OsteoGraf/D (dense synthetic particles) (CeraMed, Lakewood, CO); OsteoGen (HA RESORB), highly porous, resorbable, crystalline, nonceramic particulates (Impladent, Holliswood, NY); Interpore 200 (a mixture of HA and TCP), natural, macroporous granules and blocks (Steri-Oss, Yorba Linda, CA); and Orthomatrix HA-1000 (420–840 µ) and Orthomatrix HA-500 (250–420 µ) (Lifecore Biomedical, Chaska, MN). Both products are dense, nonresorbable, synthetic particulates. Typically, when a manufacturer offers two sizes of an alloplast, the larger is recommended for ridge augmentation and preservation (AET); the smaller particles are used for periodontal and endodontic applications.

HA graft materials that appear in the literature, but have been discontinued and are no longer available, include PenoGraf, PerioGraf, and AlveolGraf. OstoMin (Pacific Coast Tissue Bank, Los Angeles, CA) is a natural byproduct of bone, which comes in particulate form. It is used primarily by orthopedic surgeons, and, although used by some dentists, is not directly marketed for dental applications.

In an effort to overcome some of the difficult handling and physical properties of HA (i.e., migration), a combination product was developed. Hapset (Lifecore Biomedical) is a synthetic composite bone grafting material that is 65% Orthomatrix HA-500 and 35% calcium sulfate ($CaSO_4$) hemihydrate (medical-grade plaster). The $CaSO_4$ acts as a bioresorbable binder, and helps to provide initial stabilization of the HA particles. It is recommended that the surgical site be free of bleeding, which promotes rapid hardening of the mass. The $CaSO_4$ resorbs within 1 mo leaving a scaffold of HA bone growth.

3.3.1.1.1. HA Summary:

- Natural component of bone
- 60–70% of the calcified skeleton
- 98% of dental enamel
- Ca:P ratio of 10:6
- Biocompatible
- Bonds readily to adjacent hard and soft tissues
- Porous or nonporous
- Resorbable or nonresorbable
- Blocks or particles
- Osteoconductive
- Strength decreases exponentially with increase in porosity
- Brittle
- Difficult to contour and control clinically
- Use with membrane desirable
- Difficult to handle
- Migrates under pressure stress during healing period
- Implants cannot be placed in a HA-treated ridge
- Moderate potential for infection
- Nonresorbable; in amorphous form, slowly resorbable.

3.3.1.2. TRICALCIUM PHOSPHATE

TCP is chemically similar to HA, but is not a natural component of bone mineral *(26)*. It has a Ca:P ratio of 3:2 *(13)*. TCP is converted in the body, in part, to HA *(2)*. The rate of TCP resorption is variable, and differs between soft tissue and bone implant sites *(11)*. Resorption appears to be very dependent on the material's chemical structure, porosity, and particle size. Heat and sterilization may change its chemical structure and alter its properties, including resorption rate *(13)*.

TCP is osteoconductive, and is intended to provide a physical matrix suitable for the initial deposition of new bone *(13)*. It is often considered desirable for repair of nonpathologic sites, where resorption of the implant graft, with concurrent bone replacement, might be expected *(26)*. TCP can also be used in combination with osteogenic (autogenous bone) or osteoinductive (allografts) materials, to improve the handling characteristics of the graft during placement *(13)*.

Commercially available TCP products include CalciResorb, a porous form (Ceraver Osteal, Paris, France), and SynthoGraf (dense and small particle size) and Augmen (dense and larger particle size) (Miter, Warsaw, IN).

3.3.1.2.1. TCP Summary:

- Chemically similar to HA
- Not a natural component of bone
- Ca:P ratio of 3:2
- Converts partially into HA in the body
- Osteoconductive
- Resorption rate is variable and unpredictable (very slow)
- Poor handling characteristics
- Only for nonpathologic sites
- High incidence of infection

3.3.1.3. CORALLINE

Coralline, a form of ceramic synthesized from the $CaCO_3$ skeleton of coral, has the three-dimensional (3-D) microstructure of bone and is available with average pore sizes of 500 and 200 μ *(2)*. One example of such a porous coralline HA is Interpore-200 (Interpore International, Irvine, CA) *(11,25)*. The material is essentially pure HA, with the balance consisting of TCP, and is osteoconductive in its mechanism of action.

Interpore-200 has an average pore diameter of 200 μ and consists of approx 60% void spaces. The bone substitute has a highly organized and permeable porous structure, with an interconnected 3-D porosity that is very uniform and consistent. The graft and its ingrown bone are remodeled in response to the same chemical and biomechanical forces that remodel normal bone. It has been reported *(11,27)* that its compressive strength increases following tissue ingrowth, and is sufficient to withstand the masticatory forces exerted by dentures.

Investigators have reported *(11,27)* that Interpore-200 (in blocks and granules) is an implant graft that provides an optimal matrix for bone ingrowth, as an onlay on the alveolar ridge, and as an interpositional implant in the mandible. The authors also found that the graft's properties allowed clinicians to readily modify its shape during surgery, to obtain an exact fit. Others *(19)*, however, have found the material to be brittle and difficult to use.

3.3.1.3.1. Coralline Summary:

- $CaCO_3$ skeleton of coral
- 3-D microstructure of bone
- Pores of 500 μm and 200 μm
- 60% void spaces
- Essentially pure HA and some TCP
- Provides an optimal matrix for bone ingrowth
- Osteoconductive
- Brittle, difficult to maintain micropores
- Difficult to use
- High potential for infection
- Poor handling characteristics
- Only for noninfectious sites
- Resorbability very slow or not at all

3.3.1.4. ANORGANIC BOVINE BONE

Bio-Oss (Osteohealth, Shirley, NY) is an anorganic bone (bovine) that is chemically treated to remove its organic components (Ca-deficient carbonate apatite). Although just like Osteograf/N, which comes from bovine bone, the end product is quite different, because of the low heat (300° C) chemical extraction process used by Bio-Oss. Osteograf/N uses a high heat (1100° C) sintering process. This high-heat process results in fusion of bone crystallites, which possesses a large, non-homogenous crystal morphology, with decreased porosity and surface area. The Bio-Oss process maintains the exact trabecular architecture and porosity of the original bone. Both human bone and Bio-Oss natural bone mineral have the same compact apatite crystalline structure. This similarity is important for remodeling (substitution of bone for bone as part of the natural growth and development process). Bone remodeling is needed for any graft to attain a degree of permanency. After the Ca is removed, it can be used as a graft without causing a host immune response *(1)*.

It has been stated that, although Bio-Oss has no osteoinductive or osteoconductive properties *(1,28)*, but its properties suggest that bone regeneration will occur *(1)*. The graft will undergo physiologic remodeling and become incorporated into bone over a period of time *(1)*. Bio-Oss is reportedly the most physiological bone substitute, with eventual complete integration into bone (unlike HA or TCP). Synthetic ceramics differ from this material in many features of chemical composition, structure, and mechanical and biologic properties. This is the rationale for an approach of deorganifying bone, to produce natural bone mineral as a graft substance *(20)*.

Bio-Oss has been reported to be effective as an interpositional graft in osteotomy sites, but its use in correcting posttraumatic deformities or hypoplastic areas is limited *(1)*. By itself, the anorganic bone should not be used for augmentation of the alveolar ridge; however, when combined with autogenous bone, it has been successful for this purpose *(1)*. The use of a titanium mesh, with a composite graft of autogenous bone and Bio-Oss, has been shown to be a viable alternative to the block-graft autogenous bone mentioned above. The mesh will dictate the area, size, and contour of the bone regenerated, and remodeling will occur at a rapid rate, compared to the block graft *(29)*.

3.3.1.4.1. Deorganified Bovine (Anorganic) Bone Summary:

- Anorganic bone from bovine origin (cows)
- Chemically treated to remove organic components by low heat (300°C) process
- Maintains the architecture of original bone
- Similar structure as human bone
- Undergoes physiologic remodeling
- Becomes incorporated into bone
- No osteoconductive properties
- Risk of host immune response
- Migrates easily
- Brittle
- Combination with autogenous bone recommended
- Use of a membrane always necessary
- Nonporous granules
- Moderate potential for infection
- Slow resorbability: usually not complete

3.3.1.5. CALCIUM CARBONATE

BioCoral (Inoteb, Saint Gonnery, France) is a slowly resorbing, porous, coralline, $CaCO_3$ graft material. It is a natural coral in the form of aragonite (>98% $CaCO_3$), which is not altered by processing. The material possesses a porosity of greater than 45%, with the average pore 150 μ in diameter, and good interconnectivity. For periodontal use, it is provided as granules 300–400 µ in diameter.

Yukna *(30)* recently evaluated the graft material in human periodontal osseous defects. In 1994, he reported that the clinical response, particularly related to osseous-defect fill, was essentially similar to, or slightly better than that of other grafting materials. The size and shape of the particles made handling and manipulation easy during surgery. It appeared to have good hemostatic properties, and was not readily displaced from the treatment site. He concluded that coralline $CaCO_3$ appeared safe and effective in treating periodontal osseous defects.

One potential advantage noted was the material's natural form, compared with other alloplastics, during initiation of bone formation. The other materials must undergo a surface transformation, from HA to carbonate, to start the formation cascade, but $CaCO_3$'s apparent elimination of this step may permit more rapid bone formation at the grafting site.

3.3.1.5.1. $CaCO_3$ Summary:

- Natural coral in the form of aragonite (>98% $CaCO_3$)
- Not altered by processing
- Porosity >45%
- Pores of 150 µ
- Granules of 300–400 µ
- No surface transformation necessary to start the bone formation cascade
- Resorbs slowly
- Hemostatic properties
- Easy handling and manipulation
- Brittle, but less so than porous HA
- Migrates under stress during healing period
- Only demonstrated effectiveness for periodontal defects
- Moderate potential for infection

3.3.1.6. BIOPLANT HTR SYNTHETIC BONE

Bioplant HTR Synthetic Bone Alloplast is one synthetic graft material that has been tested clinically for over 20 yr. It has served dentists well, as a safe, easy to handle, predictable bone substitute graft. Research has shown many desirable clinical and histological characteristics. HTR probably has the longest documented use in humans, and has over 200 publications (many of them international in scope, dating back to the early 1970s and 1980s). Successful grafting of up to 12 yr postgraft human bone biopsies have been reported *(31)*. Its ability to be used in the immediate postextraction implant, as well as in a grafted site for implant preparation, has been documented *(31–35)*.

Bioplant HTR Synthetic Bone is a microporous chemical mixture with a calcium hydroxide graft surface, which forms $CaCO_3$ apatite when introduced into the body, and interfaces with bleeding marrow *(7,8)*. A molded form was made available in 1968, and a particulate (granular) form in the mid-1970s. The synthetic is reported to be nonresorbable 1–4 yr after placement, but a recent study *(31)* indicated resorbability 12 yr postgrafting. Its unique, hollow, egg-shaped architecture, with a pore size of approx 350 µ in diameter, allows bone growth into and around the particles. Following healing of 10 mo and longer, only 10–12% of HTR particles have been observed in the total graft area. The balance of the graft is comprised of 88–90% regenerating, remodeling bone *(10)*. HTR also has the unique characteristic of a negative surface charge, which is believed to impede development of infection. HTR is neither bacteriostatic nor bactericidal, but, since both the material and bacteria have a negative surface charge, it is believed that bacteria do not easily colonize on the surface of the material. This negative charge also allows the material to adhere to bone, as well as to metal implants, which aids in placement of the graft into surgical sites, and serves to attract the pluripotential cells that will form osteoblasts to its surface *(10,35,36)*.

HTR interfaces with bone at its outermost Ca graft layers, where in vivo studies indicate the synthetic forms a strong surface bond with bone, and creates an environment that facilitates bone formation. The microporosity of HTR has demonstrated osteoconductive properties required to promote bone ingrowth through and around its own structure. Ashman *(7–9)* has reported that the HTR appears to meet all of the requirements of the ideal synthetic bone material (Table 1).

In a dog study *(7)* in which induced periodontal defects were eliminated completely, four important histologic observations were noted: New bone regenerated in and around the Bioplant HTR poly-

Synthetic Osseous Grafting

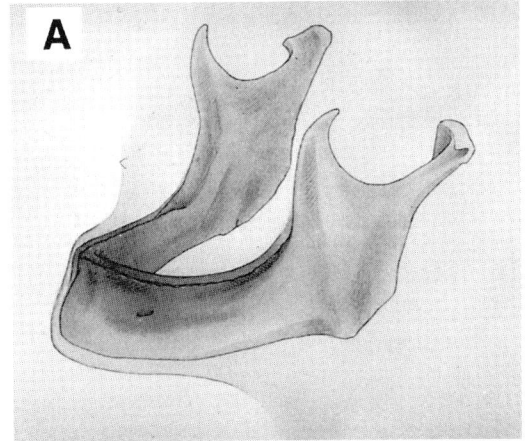

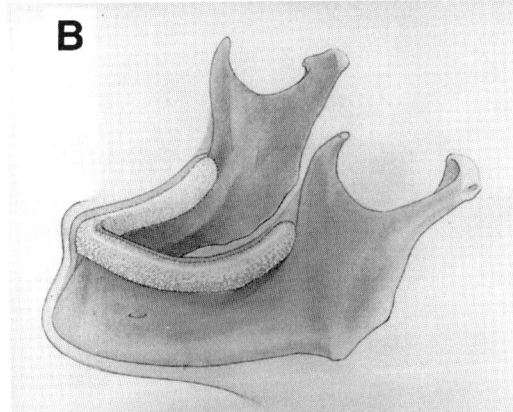

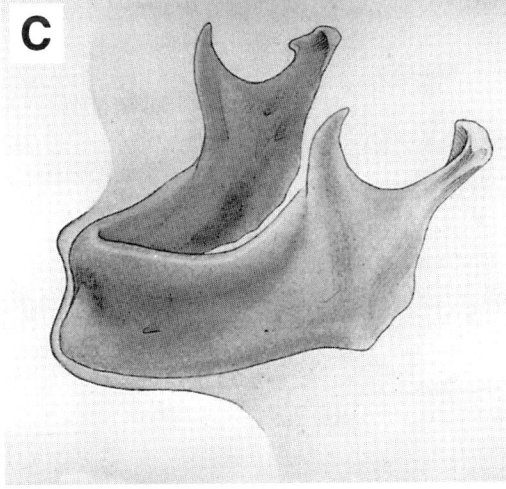

Fig. 8. (**A–C**) Diagrams represent a complete ridge augmentation with a synthetic graft material, HTR. The resulting jawbone will enable a prosthesis to function comfortably and the patient to chew. As an alternative treatment, implants can be placed into new graft regenerated bone complex after 12–15 mo.

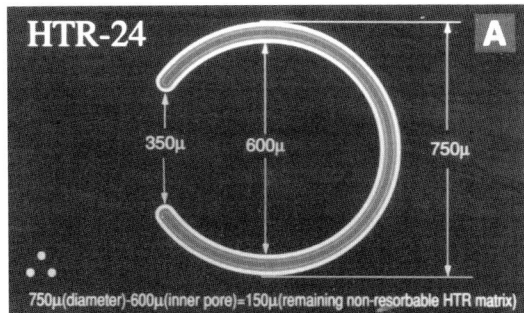

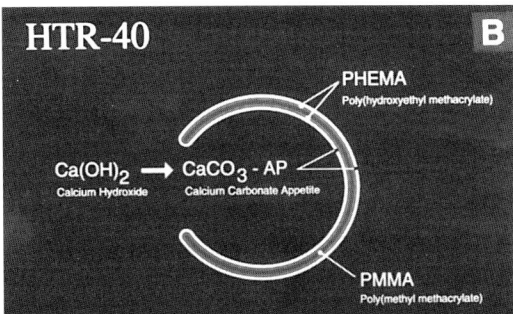

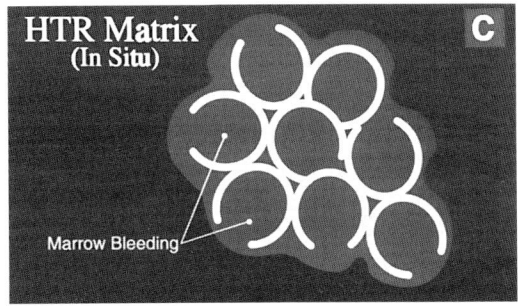

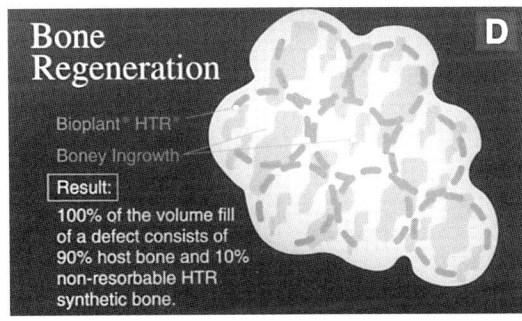

Fig. 9. (**A, B**) Characterization of one particulate of Bioplant HTR Synthetic Bone Alloplast. (**C**) Demonstrates the scaffold or matrix of HTR-graft material holding the blood clot for the normal regeneration of new bone. (**D**) Demonstrates 90% bone regeneration, with HTR acting as a scaffold for the new regenerating bone.

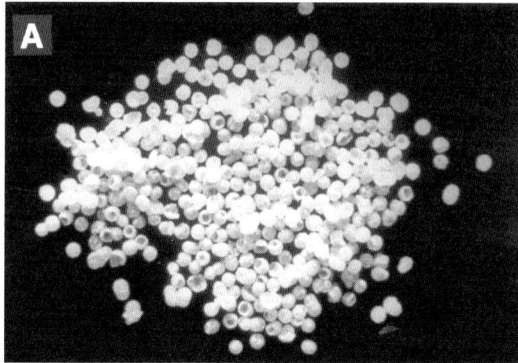

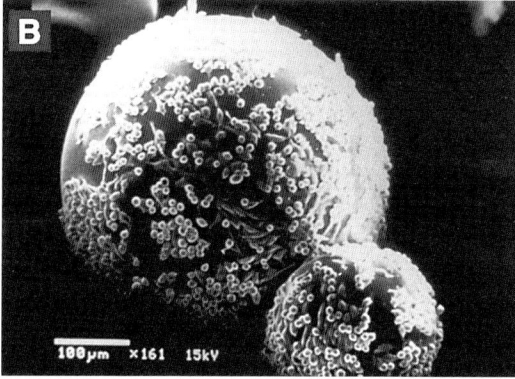

Fig. 10. (**A**) Particulate Bioplant HTR. Note the micropore on each individual sphere. (**B**) Shows bone precursor cells attracted to and growing on the surface of Bioplant HTR (courtesy P. Kamen, Columbia University).

mer, with no intervening fibrous tissue; no epithelial downgrowth was observed around tooth surfaces in the polymer-regenerated areas; new bone, formed around the HTR, was observed in apposition to a new PDL. A normal PDL was noted, together with new cementum, and Sharpey's fibers were observed without intervening fibrous connective tissue. This observation was confirmed in humans, with a 65% regeneration rate of new cementum, new bone, and a normal PDL. The fourth observation reported was complete bony regeneration, with no intervening connective tissue, when the HTR was placed immediately into extraction sockets *(8,33,34).*

HTR has been reported effective in a number of dental applications *(7–9).* In ridge preservation, HTR prevents the anticipated 50–60% loss of alveolar bone following extraction, and preserves the height and width of the alveolar ridge. For ridge augmentation, immediate use of particulate HTR following extractions increased the height and width of the alveolar ridge. In delayed augmentation (after extensive atrophy had already occurred), the particulate increased the dimensions of the alveolar ridge and corrected existing bony defects. In the repair of periodontal and other bony voids, the grafted periodontal bone defect stimulated regeneration of new bone, with subsequent reattachment of this bone to the tooth root *(39).* In a variety of bone defects, HTR grafting eliminated the periodontal defects, and bone has consistently regenerated. In apical lesions, cysts, and granulomas, and so on, Szabo *(36)* demonstrated, in human studies, the repair and elimination of bone destruction, all restored with the use of HTR 5 yr postgrafting. The material has also been used successfully, prior to dental implant placement: to build up the alveolar ridge, during implant placement to fill existing bony voids, or the osteotomy created during bone preparation. After implant placement, HTR has been used to repair the failing implant, for implant perforations, and in sinus lifts in combination with autogenous bone (50:50%) *(34,36).*

3.3.1.6.1. Bioplant HTR Summary:

- Chemically pure mixture of polymethylmethacrylate and polyhydroxyethylmethacrylate with an outer surface of calcium hydroxide, which converts to $CaCO_3$-apatite in body
- Unique, hollow, egg-shape architecture
- Spheres of 500–750 µ
- Pores of 250 and 350 µm
- Unique negative surface charge of −10mV
- Osteoinductive under conditions of attraction of body BMP
- Repels bacteria (because of negative charge)
- Adheres to bone, as well as to metal
- Regeneration of connective tissue (periodontal) ligament, up to 65%
- Hemostatic
- Strong and porous
- Easy to handle and to contour
- No migration
- No epithelial ingrowth (truly acts as a barrier)

Synthetic Osseous Grafting

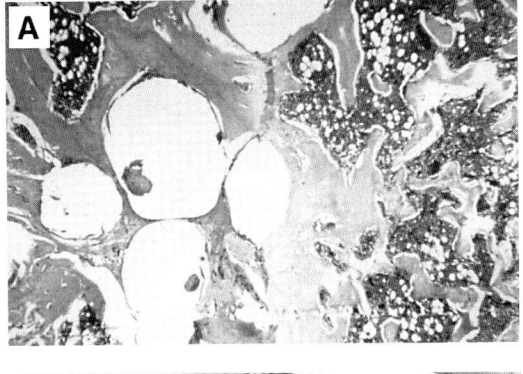
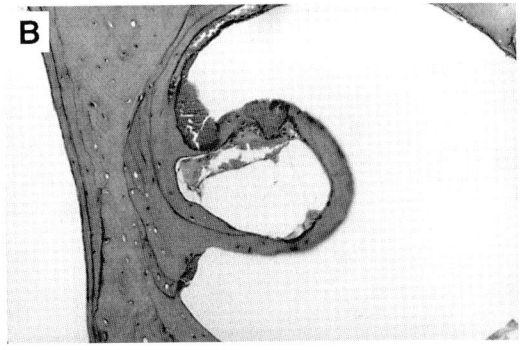
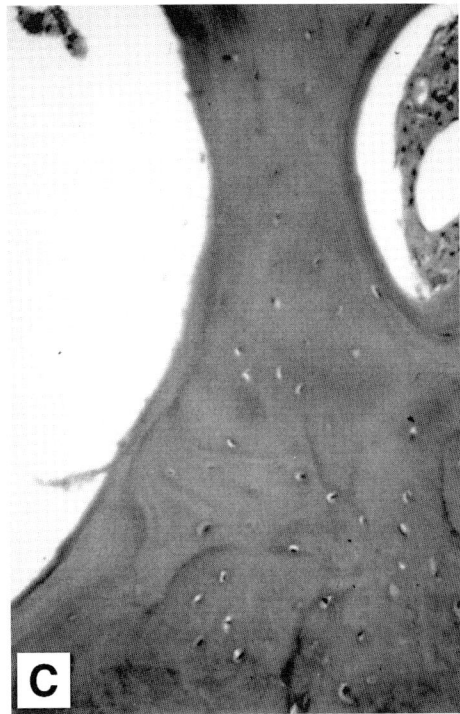

Fig. 11. (**A**) Healing of a non-union fracture 28 d. Note the new bone regenerating adjacent to the bioplant HTR. Rat model, 28 d (courtesy of I. Binderman, Tel Aviv University). (**B**) 12-yr human punch biopsy showing regenerating and remodeling bone around and into the micropore of one particle of bioplant HTR. (**C**) Demonstrates regenerating and remodeling of bone 12 yr post-graft. Note the dense lamina bone forming between the Bioplant HTR particulates.

- Has been shown to be effective in all dental applications in which a graft is used
- Regeneration of between 85 and 92% dense lamina bone, which is 2–3 times denser than normal alveolar bone
- Less than 1% infection, rejection (very low incidence of infection)
- User friendly; easy to handle

3.3.2. Bioactive Glass Ceramics

Until recently, FDBA, DFDBA, and ceramics, such as HA and TCP, were the primary allografts and alloplasts used for the restoration of osseous defects and promotion of periodontal attachment. Although these graft materials have been reported useful in rebuilding bone, none of them appear to encourage regeneration of connective tissue ligament *(40)*. As mentioned in subheading 3.3.1.6., one exception to this is Bioplant HTR. Other new materials, such as BAG ceramics, have become available, which purport to improve the practitioners' ability both to treat bony defects and to repair and restore the periodontium.

3.3.2.1. BIOGLASS

Bioglass (U.S. Biomaterials, Baltimore, MD) is made from Ca salts and phosphate (in the same proportions as in bone and teeth), sodium salts, and silicon (which is essential for bone to mineralize). This composition of silicon, sodium, Ca, and P is referred to as 45S5. Bioglass is an amorphous material, not available in a crystalline form (to strengthen the material), because its developers felt that degradation of the material by tissue fluids, and subsequent loss of the crystals, would cause the material to lose its integrity.

The material produces a compliant interface between bone and other tissue (100–300 µ), which

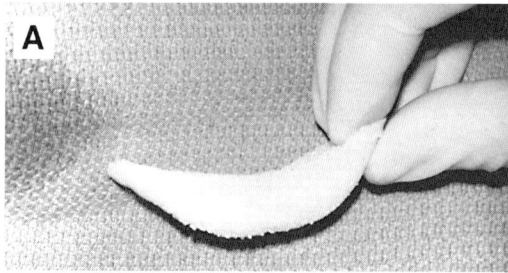
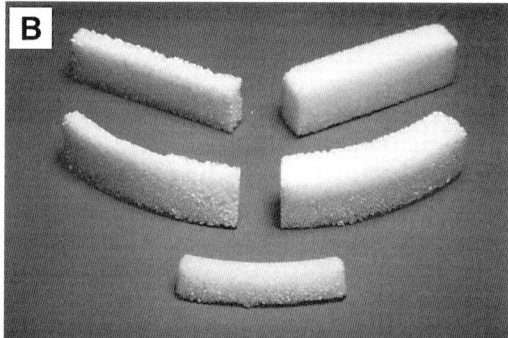
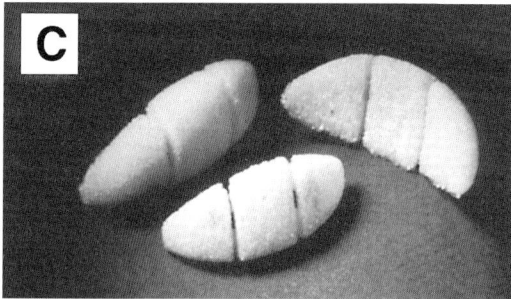

Fig. 12. (**A**) Chin implant custom formed, with CT scan and Bioplant HTR. (**B**) Various sizes and shapes of premolded Bioplant HTR used in orthomathic surgery. (**C**) Cheek, chin, and nose prosthesis fabricated from customized molded Bioplant HTR (courtesy of B. Eppley, University of Indiana).

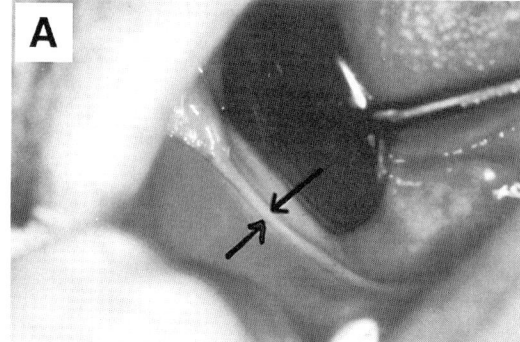
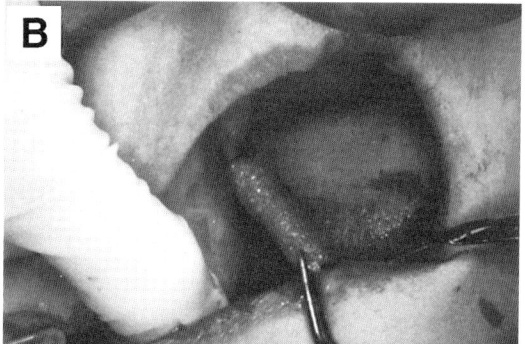
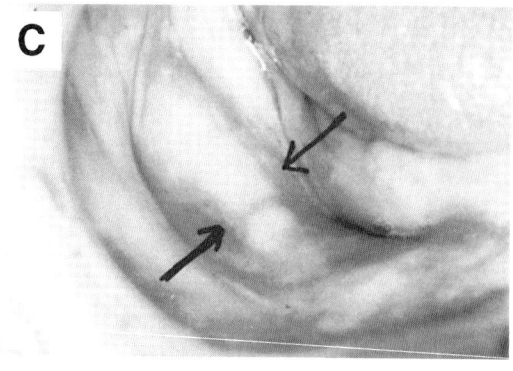

Fig. 13. (**A**) Preoperative atrophic ridge lower mandible. (**B**) Molded HTR piece being placed under the gingiva on mandible. (**C**) Three yr post-operative, demonstrating ridge augmentation with molded HTR, which enabled patient to function well with the prosthesis.

results in a normal stress transfer between Bioglass and the host tissue *(36)*. The material bonds to bone by forming a hydroxycarbonate apatite (HCA) layer on the surface of the glass *(37)*. In vivo, it has been theorized that the HCA layer closely imitates bone, as a result of the incorporation of host organic material *(38)*.

Bioglass bonds, not only to bone, but also to soft connective tissues *(35)*. A mechanically compliant layer, approx 0.3 μ in thickness, is created, which is very similar in dimensions to natural PDL *(40)*. This is how the material helps in the repair of connective tissue ligament.

It has been reported that the high degree of bioactivity of Bioglass can stimulate the reparative process and induce osteogenesis *(41)*. When the material is exposed to a mixture of osteogenic and nonosteogenic cells (e.g., fibroblasts), the bone-forming cells will spread and cover the surface area more rapidly than the others. If only nonosteogenic cells are present, the surface is covered more slowly. However, in both cases, collagen produced by the cells becomes embedded in the interfacial layer as it grows, and provides the compliant adherent interface with the Bioglass material. Osteoblasts then lay down bone mineral on top of the collagen.

The initial clinical use of Bioglass was to preserve the edentulous ridge, following tooth extraction. Clinical applications are now being expanded for more general grafting purposes, including the repair of osseous defects (in combination with autogenous bone), grafting for sinus lift procedures, and use around load-bearing dental implants *(41)*.

3.3.2.2. PERIOGLAS SYNTHETIC BG PARTICULATE

PerioGlas (Block Drug, Jersey City, NJ) is a recently developed particulate form of Bioglass, which is being used to fill intrabony defects secondary to periodontal disease *(41)*.

Within the limits of their animal study on PerioGlas, Fetner et al. *(40)* reported that the material appeared to partially repair intraosseous defects, by quickly filling the defects by osteoproduction; resulted in superior osseous and cementum repairs, compared with HA and TCP; initiated a rapid chemical bond that impeded epithelial downgrowth, which may contribute to the observed bone and cementum repair; and was easily mixed, transferred, packed, and well contained in the defect site (and may have hemostatic properties within intraosseous defects). Those authors concluded that, by bonding to both bone and connective tissues, PerioGlas showed improved results, compared with that of other ceramic graft materials.

3.3.2.3. BIOGRAN

BioGran (Orthovita, Malvern, PA) is a resorbable BG material consisting of 300–355 µ diameter bioactive glass granules, which have the same 45S5 composition as Bioglass.

Bone transformation and growth occur within each granule. This bone growth, guided by BAG particles, occurs at multiple sites, rapidly filling the osseous defect with new bone that continuously remodels in the normal physiological manner *(5,6,41)*.

This controlled bioactivity permits material and bone transformation to occur at the same time. Eventually, BioGran is resorbed, with animal studies *(4,37,41)* reporting that the material is replaced by new remodeling bone.

In an animal study, Schepers et al. *(4)* found the BAG granules to be easier to handle and pack into bony defects than HA granules, and did not show a tendency to disperse into the surrounding tissues. Osteoconduction, as well as aiding in differentiation of osteoprogenitor cells to osteoblasts, created a positive therapeutic response.

In a subsequent clinical study, Schepers et al. *(5)* reported that BioGran was an effective treatment for oral bone lesions, including periodontal defects and extraction sites. Restored bone was maintained over the full 3 yr of the study. In addition, those authors found the material easy to manipulate and pack during insertion (it formed a cohesive mass when contacting blood, and did not float with bleeding). However, Ashman and Gross have observed rapid breakdown and loss of the graft material when exposed to oral fluids. Studies are presently in progress to determine if regeneration of the PDL occurs when BioGran is used.

3.3.2.4. BAG CERAMICS SUMMARY

- Mixture of Ca salts, phosphate, sodium salts, and silicon (45S5)
- Forms: amorphous or 300–355-µ granules
- Formation of HCA on the surface
- Bonds to bone and soft connective tissues
- Formation of a 0.3-µ collagen layer
- Extensively osteoconductive
- Resorbable in amorphous form
- Easy to manipulate and pack
- Little migration
- Rapid breakdown and loss when exposed to oral fluids
- Very susceptible to infection

3.4. Growth Factors and Cytokines

Investigators are currently studying the potential therapeutic effects of growth factors and cytokines for regeneration of alveolar bone *(43)*. Many of these factors (including transforming growth factor β [TGF-β], platelet-derived growth factor, insulin-like growth factors I and II, and fibroblast growth factor) stimulate regeneration of bone and tissue, and influence bone growth and resorption. Thus, they may be of benefit in the regeneration process (44). However, these substances also affect many other tissues and cell types. Therefore, research must be directed toward developing site-specific effects.

3.5. Bone Morphogenetic Proteins

BMPs are osteoinductive compounds that induce new bone formation at the site of implantation, in contrast to growth factors and cytokines, which change the growth rate of pre-existing bone (43,44,45). The exact mechanism of action of BMPs is not completely understood, but it is believed that they stimulate the differentiation of mesenchymal cells into chondrocytes and osteoblasts (14). The subsequent process of endochondral bone differentiation may be regulated by growth factors such as TGF-β.

At least seven structurally unique BMPs have been identified, all of which can produce ectopic bone formation (14). Bone induced by BMPs has all the characteristics of normal bone, including cartilage formation followed by endochondral ossification. The genes that produce BMPs have been used to synthesize recombinant BMP: The protein that is produced is highly active and potentially available in larger quantities than was possible before.

Various animal studies have indicated that recombinant human BMP-2 (rhBMP-2) may have excellent therapeutic potential in dental and periodontal repair, i.e., replacement of lost alveolar bone and ridge augmentation (44). The use of rhBMP-2 may also help regenerate the periodontal attachment complex. Ridge augmentation or sinus lift procedures for dental implant placements may also benefit from implantation of rhBMP-2, along with accelerating the time of implant–bone integration. How to deliver this to the site still remains a question. Boyne (45,46) and Boyne and Scheer (46) have reported using Bioplant HTR as a vehicle or carrier for BMP, with good results. Boyne has also seen promising results with Bio-Oss. The full potential of BMP will require further clinical studies.

3.6. Composite Grafts

A number of authors have recommended combining different materials to improve the outcome of the grafting procedure. It has been suggested (47) that the addition of autogenous bone to HA particles could stimulate osteogenesis within the grafted area, rather than just the osteoconduction produced by HA. In addition, Garg (16) found that combining synthetic materials with autogenous bone decreased the amount of harvested bone necessary for procedures such as sinus lifts.

Kraut (48) used a composite graft system, consisting of allogeneic freeze-dried rib, autogenous cancellous bone and marrow, and HA, to augment atrophic mandibles in six patients. Marked improvement was reported in dental function, with 78% maintenance of the augmented height 1 yr later and 67% after 2 yr. Kent et al. (49) recommended mixing HA with autogenous cancellous bone and marrow, for patients with mandibles deficient in height and width (i.e., class IV). They suggessted that the mixture be composed of bone ground to a size similar to the HA particles, at a ratio of 1:1. Boyne (25) suggested mixing of the HA particles with the autogenous cancellous BG particles at the time of the initial surgical reconstruction. He found the optimal mixture to be 50% HA and 50% autogenous bone (the same as Kent et al.). A mixture containing more HA resulted in a decrease in osseous regeneration.

Other investigators, however, have not found any advantage in combining autogenous bone with alloplasts. Frame et al. (24) augmented the edentulous areas of dog jaws with HA particles alone, or combined with finely crushed autogenous bone. They reported that the addition of autogenous bone to the HA particles did not enhance bony deposition, and that none of the bone chips survived past 24 wk. Frame (11) also reported on other investigations, in which autogenous bone chips mixed with HA particles underwent resorption without enhancing new bone growth, and on an animal study in which autogenous bone chips, onlayed on alveolar ridges, resorbed after only 2 wk.

Finally, Pinholt et al. (12) implanted a combination of equal amounts of dense HA granules and an osteoinductive substrate (i.e., allogenic, demineralized, lyophilized dentin or bone), subperiosteally, for alveolar ridge augmentation.

They reported that bone incorporation was not enhanced around the HA granules, despite the presence of the osteoinductive material. However, those authors did acknowledge that positive results of increased incorporation of dense HA granules had been obtained using autogenous bone, but recommended against the use of the latter, to avoid the necessary harvesting procedure.

4. Selection of Graft Material Based on Degree of Defect

Deciding on the use of autogenous bone, allografts, or synthetic bone material, alone or in combination, can also be based on the degree of bony defect present *(13)*. The composition of the graft should correspond to the material's mechanism of action, and to the number of walls of host bone that remain in contact with the graft. In general, alloplasts, alone or in combination with allografts, can be used for small defects. Autogenous bone may need to be added to the graft for larger defects. It can also be used for smaller defects, if readily available. The larger the defect, the greater the amount of autogenous bone required.

5. Regenerative Therapy

Regenerative therapy refers to procedures used in the treatment of periodontal disease, to achieve replacement of lost periodontal tissue. Bone fill is defined as the clinical restoration of bone tissue in previously treated (grafted) periodontal defect. Some authors of case reports have presented histologic evidence of regeneration and new connective tissue attachment *(50)*; others state that there only exists the presence of a long junctional epithelium *(51)*. Therefore, it has been concluded that bone fill does not address the presence or absence of histologic evidence of new connective tissue attachment. Most of these reports are cases of autogenous grafts. Stahl et al. *(50)* demonstrated evidence that a limited amount of connective tissue attachment may be possible following use of a synthetic graft (Bioplant HTR) *(39,50)*.

Inorganic synthetic graft materials and allografts of various types have been used to correct periodontal defects. Their use leads to significant improvements in probing depth and clinical attachment levels. In controlled clinical trials treating furcation and intraosseous defects, graft materials have demonstrated clinical advantages beyond those achieved by debridement alone. Mean defect fills of 60–65% have been shown in a number of studies using DFDBA, and Bioplant HTR *(39,52)*.

It was suggested, in 1976, by Melcher *(51)* that cells that repopulate the root surface after periodontal surgery will determine the type of attachment that forms on the root surface during healing. This has been the basis for techniques using barrier membranes to allow selective cellular repopulation of the root surface. In theory, these membranes retard apical migration of the epithelium and exclude gingival tissue from the healing wound, which would favor healing directed by the PDL space and adjacent alveolar bone. The earliest barriers were nonresorbable. The most noted one is expanded polytetrafluoroethylene (Gore-Tex, W. L. Gore, Flagstaff, AZ), which has many years of clinical research behind it. The manufacturing process involves sintering the product, and creation of pores that are 5–30 µ. Another nonresorbable barrier similar to this is TefGen-GTR (Lifecore Biomedical). It differs from Gore-Tex in two major ways. The pore size is 0.2–0.3 µ, and thus the product is called nano-polytetrafluroethylene. The smaller particle size is believed to limit the amount of epithelial ingrowth and bacterial infiltration. The second difference is the elimination of the sintering process, which allows the material to be quite pliable, allowing easier tenting and adaptation.

One major drawback of a nonresorbable barrier is the need for a second surgical procedure to remove it. This, along with some other problems, has led to the development of resorbable barriers of various types. Examples of these are polylactic acid and citric acid ester (Guidor, Butler, Chicago, IL); lactide and glycolate polymers arranged in a random fiber, trilayer matrix lacking large holes (Resolut, Gore); collagen barrier from bovine Achilles tendon (Bio-Mend, Calcitek); a tightly woven mesh manufactured from a copolymer of glycolide and lactide (Vicryl Periodontal Mesh, Johnson & Johnson Ethicon, Somerville, NJ); and a slowly resorbing bilayer collagen membrane (BioGide, Geistlich, Wohlhusen, Switzerland). Products that degrade very slowly may be more ideal, for bone cell repopulation and ultimate bony growth, than other membranes that absorb in a more rapid fashion, although this may not be clinically significant when one is not trying to regenerate bone during specific periodontal soft tissue surgeries. Patient acceptance may be higher with the use of these resorbable membranes, because the need for a second surgery is obviated. It should be noted that it is believed that almost every alloplast (e.g., HTR) acts as its own membrane barrier by forming a layer of dense connective tissue under the soft-tissue flap (but over regenerating bone) *(10,45)*.

A new approach to bioresorbable membranes can be found in a synthetic liquid polymer. The material (Atrisorb, Block Drug) is a polymer of lactic acid, poly (DL-lactide, dissolved in N-methyl-2-pyrrolidone. The product is packaged as a liquid, which sets to a firm consistency on contact with water or other aqueous solutions. It can be shaped extraorally, and adheres to the defect without the use of sutures *(53)*. Degradation occurs, as with many other membranes, via hydrolysis, and is completely resorbed in 9–14 mo.

Another variation of free-form (moldable) resorbable barriers is $CaSO_4$ (plaster of Paris), which has been used safely in orthopedics for over 100 yr. Sottosanti *(53,54)* showed that, when mixed with DFDBA to form a composite graft, and when another mix placed over the composite graft as barrier, positive results were achieved in guilded tissue regeneration procedures. The composite graft is typically 75–80% DFDBA and 20–25% $CaSO_4$ binder. The $CaSO_4$ resorbs in approx 4 wk, and is well tolerated by oral tissues. The $CaSO_4$ barrier material, Capset (Lifecore Biomedical), is dispensed with an extra .25 g $CaSO_4$ to mix with the BG material. The majority of clinical documentation with this product has been done with DFDBA as the grafting material. Although it is now marketed also together with HA (Hapset), there is no documentation that this would be advantageous to other alloplastic materials.

6. Conclusion

Today's practitioner has a wide array of grafting materials available that can be used in a variety of dental applications in oral reconstruction. From a pure bone growth perspective, autogenous bone remains the best material, because of its osteogenic properties. This allows bone to form more rapidly and in conditions in which significant bone augmentation or repair is required. However, it has its shortcomings, and is not needed or indicated in every dental situation.

Thus, allografts and alloplasts have their appropriate place in dental applications. By knowing the physical and chemical properties of these materials, and their mechanism of action, the proper selection of a specific graft, or combination of grafts, can be made for treating the particular problem at hand. Examples of allografts are freeze-dried, demineralized freeze-dried, and irradiated bone. Alloplastic materials available today include CaP ceramics (HA and TCP), anorganic bone, $CaCO_3$, polymers (HTR), BAG ceramics, growth factors and cytokines, and BMPs. The use of these materials, as well as membranes, both nonresorbable and resorbable, have changed the scope and expectations of surgery, and will continue to so in the future. Research and clinical experience have shown that certain materials are better-suited for specific applications than others. In addition, certain products are much easier to handle than others. This must be kept in mind when evaluating a patient and a particular clinical situation, to aid in choosing the best material for the procedure.

References

1. Hislop WS, Finlay PM, and Moos KF. Preliminary study into the uses of anorganic bone in oral and maxillofacial surgery. *Br J Oral Maxillofac Surg* 1993; 31: 149–153.
2. Lane JM. Bone graft substitutes. *Western J Med* 1995; Dec: 565–567.
3. Gross J. Bone grafting materials for dental applications: a practical guide. *Compendium* 1997; 18: 1013–1036.
4. Schepers E, DeClerco M, Ducheyne P, and Kempeneers R. Bioactive glass particulate material as a filler for bone lesions. *J Oral Rehabil* 1991; 18: 439–452.
5. Schepers EJG, Ducheyne P, Barbier L, and Schepers S. Bioactive glass particles of narrow size range: a new material for the repair of bone defects. *Implant Dent* 1993; 2: 151–156.
6. Rummelhart JM, Mellonig JT, Gray JL, and Towle HJ. Comparison of freeze-dried bone allograft and

demineralized freeze-dried bone allograft in human periodontal osseous defects. *J Periodontal* 1989; 60: 655–663.

7. Ashman A. Use of synthetic bone materials in dentistry. *Compend Contin Educ Dent* 1984; 13: 1020–1034.

8. Ashman A. Clinical applications of synthetic bone in dentistry, part I. *Gen Dent* 1992; Nov/Dec: 481–487.

9. Ashman A. Clinical applications of synthetic bone in dentistry, Part II: periodontal and bony defects in conjunction with dental implants. *Gen Dent* 1993; Jan/Feb: 37–44.

10. Boyne P. Use of HTR in tooth extraction sockets to maintain the alveolar ridge height and increase concentration of alveolar bone matrix. *Gen Dent* 1995; 43: 470–473.

11. Frame JW. Hydroxyapatite as a biomaterial for alveolar ridge augmentation. *Int J Oral Maxillofac Surg* 1987; 16: 642–655.

12. Pinholt EM, Bang G, and Haanaes HR. Alveolar ridge augmentation in rats by combined hydroxylapatite and osteoconductive material. *Scand J Dent Res* 1991; 99: 64–74.

13. Misch CE and Dietsh F. Bone-grafting materials in implant dentistry. *Implant Dent* 1993; 2: 158–167.

14. Second-hand bones? (editorial) *Lancet* 1992; 340: 1443.

15. Koole R, Bosker H, and van der Dussen FN. Late secondary autogenous bone grafting in cleft patients comparing mandibular (ectomesenchymal) and iliac crest (mesenchymal) grafts. *J Cranio Max Fac Surg* 1989; 17: 28–30.

16. Garg AK. *Practical Implant Dentistry* 1996; Taylor, Houston, TX, 89–101.

17. Mellonig JT. Decalcified freeze-dried bone allograft as an implant material in human periodontal defects. *Int J Periodont Restorative Dent* 1984; 6: 41–55.

18. Tatum OJ Jr, Lebowitz MS, Tatum CA, and Borgner RA. Sinus augmentation: rationale, development, long-term results. *NY State Dent J* 1993; May: 43–48.

19. Tatum OJ Jr. Osseous grafts in intra-oral sites. *J Oral Implantol* 1996; 22: 51–52.

20. Christensen GJ. Ridge preservation: Why not? *JADA* 1996; 127: 669–670.

21. Meffert RM, Thomas JR, Hamilton KM, and Brownstein CN. Hydroxylapatite as an alloplastic graft in the treatment of human periodontal osseous defects. *J Periodontal* 1985; 56: 63–73.

22. Stahl SS and Froum SJ. Histologic and clinical responses to porous hydroxylapatite implants in human periodontal defects. *J Periodontal* 1987; 58: 689–695.

23. Boyle PJ. Personal communication.

24. Frame JW, Rout PG, and Browne RM. Ridge augmentation using solid and porous hydroxylapatite particles with and without autogenous bone or plaster. *J Oral Maxillofac Surg* 1987; 45: 771–777.

25. Boyne PJ. Advances in preprosthetic surgery and implantation. *Curr Opinion Dent* 1991; 1: 277–281.

26. Jarcho M. Biomaterial aspects of calcium phosphates. *Dent Clin North Am* 1986; 30: 25–47.

27. White E and Shors EC. Biomaterial aspects of Interpore-200 porous hydroxyapatite. *Dent Clin North Am* 1986; 30: 49–67.

28. Pinholt EM, Bang G, and Haanaes HR. Alveolar ridge augmentation in rats by BIO-OSS. *Scan J Dent Res* 1991; 99: 154–161.

29. Boyne PJ. *Osseous Reconstruction of the Maxilla and the Mandible: Surgical Techniques Using Titanium Mesh and Bone Mineral*, 1996; Quintessence.

30. Yukna RA. Clinical evaluation of coralline calcium carbonate as a bone replacement graft material in human periodontal osseous defects. *J Periodontal* 1994; 65: 177–185.

31. Froum S, et al. Treating fresh extraction sockets with an alloplast prior to implant placement: clinical and histological case reports. *Pract Perio Aesth Dent* (in press).

32. Schepers EJG and Pinruethai P. *Bioceramics*, vol. 6 1993; Butterworth-Heinemann, 113–116.

33. Rosenlicht J. Immediate postextraction placement of an alloplast and titanium screw implant: a seven-year case presentation. *Practical Periodont Aesthetic Dent* 1993; Dec.

34. Ashman A. Ridge preservation for immediate post-extraction implants: 8 yr study. *Pract Perio Aesth Dent* 7(2): 85–97.

35. Sarnachiaro O, et al. Immediate implantation of osseointegrated implants filled with Bioplant HTR Synthetic Bone into extraction sockets of Cynomolgus monkeys. (*Macaca fascicularis*): longitudinal study. Histologic observations. (in publication).

36. Szabo G, et al. HTR polymer and sinus elevation: a human histologic evaluation. *J Long-Term Effects Med Implants* 1992; 2: 81–92.

37. Wilson J and Low SB. Bioactive ceramics for periodontal treatment: comparative studies in the Patus monkey. *J Appl Biomater* 1992; 3: 123–129.

38. Wilson J, Clark AE, Hall M, and Hench LL. Tissue response to Bioglass endosseous ridge maintenance implants. *J Oral Implantol* 1993; 19: 295–302.

39. Yukna RA. Clinical evaluation of HTR polymer bone replacement grafts in human mandibular class II molar functions. *J Periodontol*, April 1994; 342–349.

40. Fetner AE, Hartigan MS, and Low SB. Periodontal

40. repair using PerioGlas in nonhuman primates: clinical and histologic observations. *Compend Contin Educ Dent* 15: 932–938.
41. Greenspan DC. Bioglass bioactivity and clinical use. Presented at the *Dent Implant Clin Res Group Annual Meeting* April 27–29, 1995; St. Thomas, VI.
42. Ducheyne P, Bianco P, Radin S, and Schepers E. *Bone-bonding biomaterials* 1992; Reed Healthcare Comm, The Netherlands, pp. 1–12.
43. Wozney JM. Potential role of bone morphogenetic proteins in periodontal reconstruction. *J Periodontal* 1995; 66: 506–510.
44. New bone? (bone grafts using bone morphogenetic proteins) *Lancet* 1992; 339: 463–465.
45. Boyne PJ. Bone induction and the use of HTR polymer as a vehicle of osseous inductor materials. *Compendium,* 1988; (Suppl 10): 337–341.
46. Boyne PJ and Scheer PM. Bone inductive effects of skeletal grown factor with hydroxylapatite and synthetic matrices. *J Oral and Maxillofac Surg* 1989; 10: 382–389.
47. Block MS and Kent JN. Healing of mandibular ridge augmentation using hydroxylapatite with and without autogenous bone in dogs. *J Oral Maxillofac Surg* 1985; 43: 3–7.
48. Kraut RA. Composite graft for mandibular alveolar ridge augmentation: a preliminary report. *J Oral Maxillofac Surg* 1985; 43: 856–859.
49. Kent JN, Finger IM, Quinn JH, and Guerra LR. Hydroxylapatite alveolar ridge reconstruction: clinical experiences, complications, and technical modifications. *J Oral Maxillofac Surg* 1986; 44: 37–49.
50. Stahl SS, Froum SJ, and Tarnow D. Human clinical and histologic responses to the placement of HTR polymer particles in 11 intrabony lesions. *J Periodontol* 1990; 61: 269–274.
51. Melcher AH. On the repair potential of periodontal tissues. *J Periodontol* 1976; 47: 256–260.
52. Polson AM, et al. Guided tissue regeneration in human furcation defects after using a biodegradable barrier: a multi-center feasibility study. *J Periodontol* May, 1995; 377–385.
53. Sottosanti J. Calcium sulfate: a biodegradable and biocompatible barrier for guided tissue regeneration. *Compend Cont Ed Dent* 1992; 13: 226.
54. Sottosanti J. Aesthetic extractions with calcium sulfate and the principles of guided tissue regeneration. *Pract Periodont Aesthet Dent* 1993; 5: 61.

9

HA-SAL2

Novel Bone Graft Substitute with Composition Mimicking Bone Mineral

Hannah Ben-Bassat, Benjamin Y. Klein, Isaac Leichter, Meir Liebergall, David Segal, Frigita Kahana, and Sara Sarig

1. Introduction

The advancement in orthopedic surgery is attributed, at least partially, to the continuous innovations in the field of implantable bioactive materials. Hydroxyapatite (HA) is the major inorganic component of calcified tissues in the human body *(1,2)*, is the end product of the biological mineralization process, and has high biocompatibility with living tissues *(3,4)*. HA and tricalcium phosphate (TCP) are regarded as bioactive implants, because of their chemical affinity, osteoconductivity, and connectivity with bone tissues. HA and TCP are the two calcium phosphates (CaPs) most commonly used in the clinic because of calcium:phosphate (Ca:P) ratios similar to those of natural bone *(5)*. CaP ceramics are also very useful as carriers, in bioengineering applications, for supporting growth of anchorage-dependent animal cells *(6)*. Sintered HA is also used to improve percutaneous implants, suggesting that this ceramic has also the potential to allow cell growth *(7)*. The nature and degree of tissue response to implants depend on the characteristics of the material: chemical composition, surface texture, porosity, density, shape, and size *(8–10)*. However, the bone and soft tissues around the implant can also be adversely affected by device-related factors, acting over a period of years *(11,12)*. Indeed, biocompatibility is evaluated by host tissue responses, assessed by morphological and histological examinations of the implant site *(12)*. Since it is difficult to examine the in vivo reactions of a specific cell type to the implant, because of various cell populations and biofactors present at the implantation site, in vitro models are also used *(13–16)*. Recently, it was suggested that the adhesiveness and growth of cells on ceramics are regulated by a time-dependent variation of the surface structure. To this point, cell functions are significantly affected by the surface structure and chemical composition of the ceramics *(9)*. Adhesiveness can be improved by modifying the surface, e.g., with serum proteins, fibronectin, or collagen *(17,18)*.

Screening for an ideal bioceramic as bone substitute is still a challenge for investigators of biomaterial and orthopedic research (extensively reviewed in ref. *19*). From the orthopedic point of view, mechanical integrity, time-controlled

From: *Biomaterials Engineering and Devices: Human Applications,* Volume 2
Edited by D. L. Wise, et al. © Humana Press, Inc., Totowa, NJ

degradation, and simultaneous replacement by newly formed bone comprise the ideal bone substitute (20–22).

Presently, attempts to improve the performance of bioactive implants are continuing, with the goal of achieving satisfactory rate, extent, and maintenance of bone tissues formed at the implant (19).

This chapter presents baseline studies on structural and biocompatible aspects of a novel composite HA, HA-SAL2, which is remarkably similar to bone mineral, is nontoxic, and supports bone growth.

2. HA-SAL2: New Upgraded HA Ceramic Incorporated with α-TCP

2.1. Preparation and Characterization of HA-SAL2 Powder and Disks

HA-SAL2 is a nonstoichiometric, Ca-deficient, and carbonate-containing HA powder. It has an X-ray diffraction (XRD) pattern remarkably similar to that of bone mineral, i.e., showing a broad peak at $2\Theta = 32.8°C$ (Fig. 1: Compare A to C). In Fig. 1C, note the lack of background, which may indicate the presence of amorphous CaP. In contrast, the XRD pattern of stoichiometric well-formed HA is shown in Fig. 1B. The Fourier transform infrared (FTIR) spectrum of HA-SAL2 powder shows phosphate, carbonate, and H_2O groups also similar to bone apatite (Fig. 2). The main peaks at 1035/cm and 565–633/cm are attributed to phosphate ions of apatite. The small split peaks 1418/ and 1454/cm are attributed to carbonate ions. The peak at 1628/cm indicates the presence of water molecules within the apatite structure (8). It must be stressed that the ceramic pellets contain significantly less water, and this is evidenced by weakening of the peak at 1628/cm in HA-SAL2 ceramics. This peak is also, as a rule, absent in all the commercial samples of pure apatite tested by the authors. Because human bone contains carbonate and water, it is conceivable that water-containing crystalline material will have improved biocompatible properties.

This apatite powder was precipitated from a dilute solution mixture of $CaCl_2$ and NaH_2PO_4 (Ca:PO_4 ratio of 5:3) irradiated by microwave (23). For the in vitro evaluation of cell attachment and growth, the HA-SAL2 powder was sintered into ceramic pellets (200 mg each) by mixing with ammonium hydrogen carbonate, (20% w/w), grinding the mixture, and compressing it under pressure of 4 t/cm^2 using a pellet dye (Graseby Specac). The XRD pattern of the powder, prepared according to the procedure, is similar to that of bone mineral (compare Fig. 1A to 1C). When heated to 500°C, the special crystallinity did not change (Fig. 1D). Only when heated to 700°C, transition to β-TCP and HA took place. The most interesting feature of this transition was the appearance of α-TCP, as evidenced by the peak of 30.7°C. It was further sustained by two smaller characteristic peaks at 24.1 and 12.1°C (24) (Fig. 3). The advantage of the authors' method is in obtaining α-TCP at temperatures much lower than the expected 1125°C, according to phase diagram. Compared to β-TCP, α-TCP has a looser structure, higher internal energy, and, therefore, a faster resorbability than β-TCP.

2.2. Scanning Electron Microscopy of HA-SAL2

HA-SAL2 particles are mostly spherical agglomerates 2–4 μm closely linked with a particularly homogeneous distribution of sizes (Fig. 4A). The small portion of submicron particles cannot be detected by volume-based measurements. Figure 4B illustrates an important phenomenal aspect of HA-SAL2, consistent with one of bone properties: The individual particles comprising the powder are tiny (approx 300 nm long), flat crystallites, distinctively similar to bone mineral apatite. Thus, the particularly well-adjusted rate of biological interaction of the authors' implant material with the body fluid as a result of its similarity to the bone mineral XRD pattern, is strengthened by the geometrical similarity. This similarity implies an almost equal surface area, and therefore a close rate of dissolution, i.e., resorbability. In sharp contrast, the particles of a commercial chemical exhibit a very different morphology, mean size, and size distribution (Fig. 4C). Here, the majority of the particles are large, some of them approx 10 μm. They are accompanied by many tiny irregular crystallites. This array is definitely different from the apatite of bone mineral, and may serve to emphasize the unique similarity between HA-SAL2 and the morphology of bone mineral.

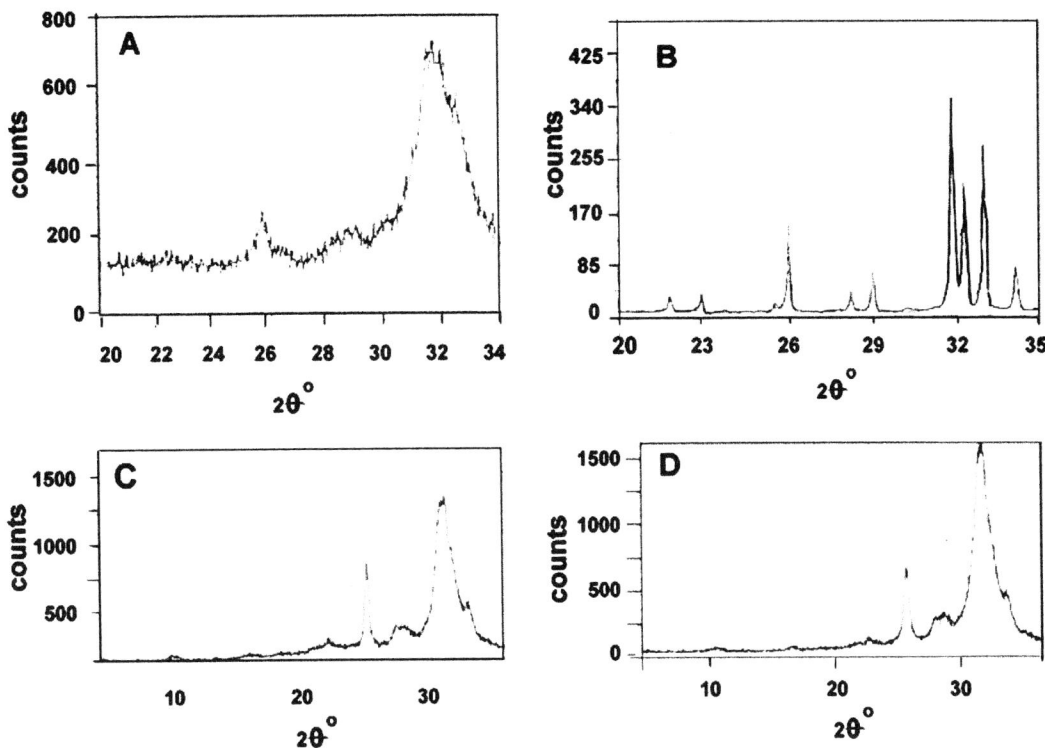

Fig. 1. (**A**) XRD pattern of human bone mineral. (**B**) XRD pattern of well-crystallized sintered HA. (**C**) XRD pattern of powder form HA-SAL2. This pattern is similar to the XRD of bone mineral. (**D**) XRD pattern of the ceramic sintered from powder in (**C**) at 500°C.

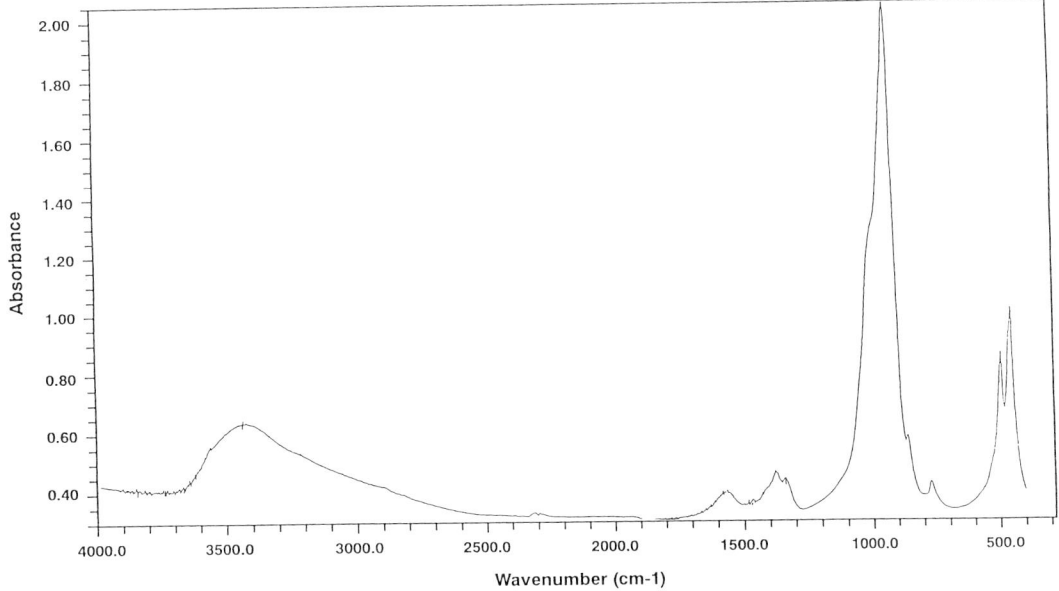

Fig. 2. FTIR spectrum of HA-SAL2 powder. The 1628/cm peak indicates the presence of water.

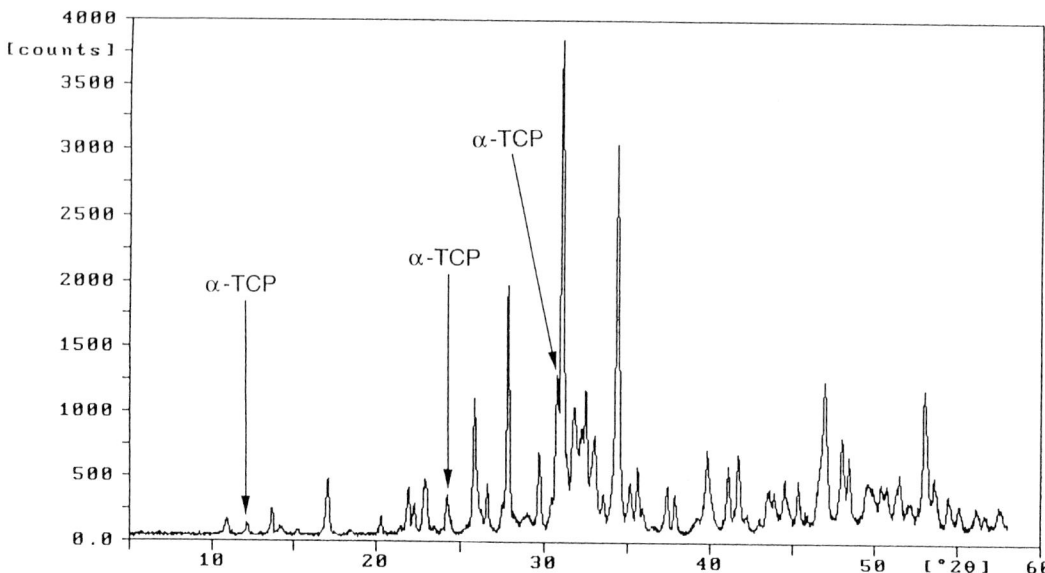

Fig. 3. XRD pattern of ceramic from microwave-precipitated HA-SAL2, sintered at 700°C. Note the differentiation of the 31.77, 32.2, and 32.9°C peaks of apatite and the appearance 30.7, 24.1, and 12.1°C peaks characteristic of α-TCP.

3. Biocompatibility of HA-SAL2

HA ceramics seem particularly suitable as bone graft (BG) substitutes, because their chemical composition is similar to the mineral nature of bone (4,20,21). Bioactive substrates have been shown to establish a direct biological bond with the surface of the implant (25–28). The interfacial bond that is formed by bioactive materials and adjacent tissue is time-dependent, and its strength, mechanism, and thickness of the bonding zone differ for the various materials (8,25,27,28). Although the mechanisms of these bonding phenomena are not fully understood, they imply cellular, molecular, and ionic activity between tissue and surface (8,10,20,28). An important observation in this connection is that many cells fail to proliferate, grow, and differentiate if they cannot adhere to the substrate (6,14–18). This anchorage dependence seems to be a prerequisite for bone formation in vitro and in vivo (14,20,30–33). Anchorage, attachment adhesion, and spreading of cells, as well as formation and deposition of bone directly on the implant, requires a surface that is not only non toxic, but also allows and favors this cell behavior (10,28,30,35). Recently, it was suggested that the intensive negative charge of the surface of HA/TCP carriers increases the adhesion strength of the cells on the ceramic (9). It was also found that the wettability of the ceramic is related to the ionic density within the surface layer (9,34,35). The production of extracellular matrix (ECM) by the cells, and the formation of interface between the cells and materials through collagen bonding, are also crucial for the development of bone bond (36–39). Indeed, cell adhesion on ceramics is enhanced by modifying the surface with serum proteins, fibronectin, or collagen (6,18,26). Thus, a satisfactory experimental application of an implant will be primarily result from its speed of incorporation into host tissue and its vascularization, followed by ingrowth of new bone (20).

Biocompatibility is defined as "the ability of a material to perform with an appropriate host response in a specific application" (11). Host response is a principal issue in the complex set of phenomena that comprise biocompatibility. Since the responses of individual cell types are difficult to assess in animal models, because of the numerous and complex events that occur at the grafted site, in vitro models are useful in this respect

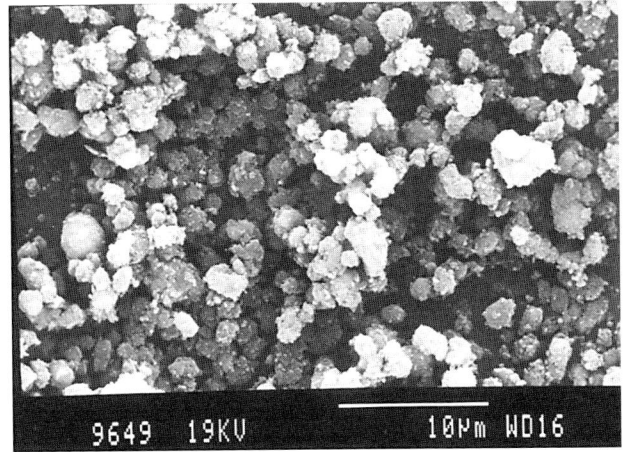

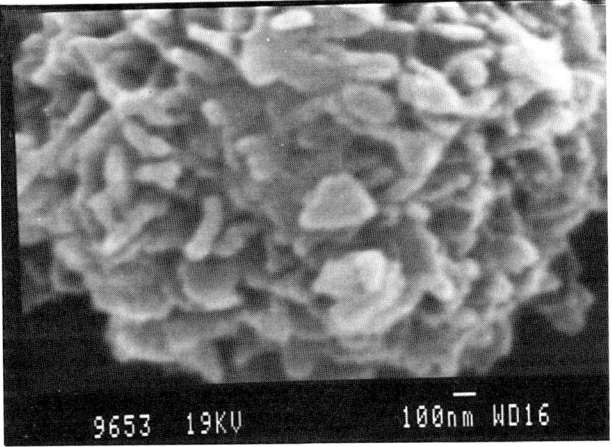

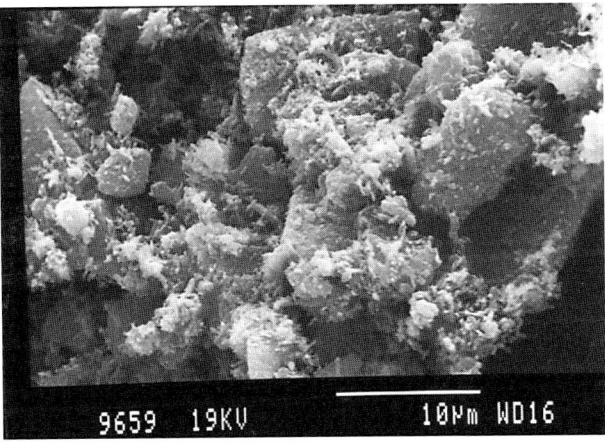

Fig. 4. **(A)** SEM appearance of HA-SAL2 (×300). **(B)** Individual crystals, which comprise the aggregates of HA-SAL2, are approx 300 nm (×50,000). **(C)** Apatite crystallites manufactured by Sigma (×300).

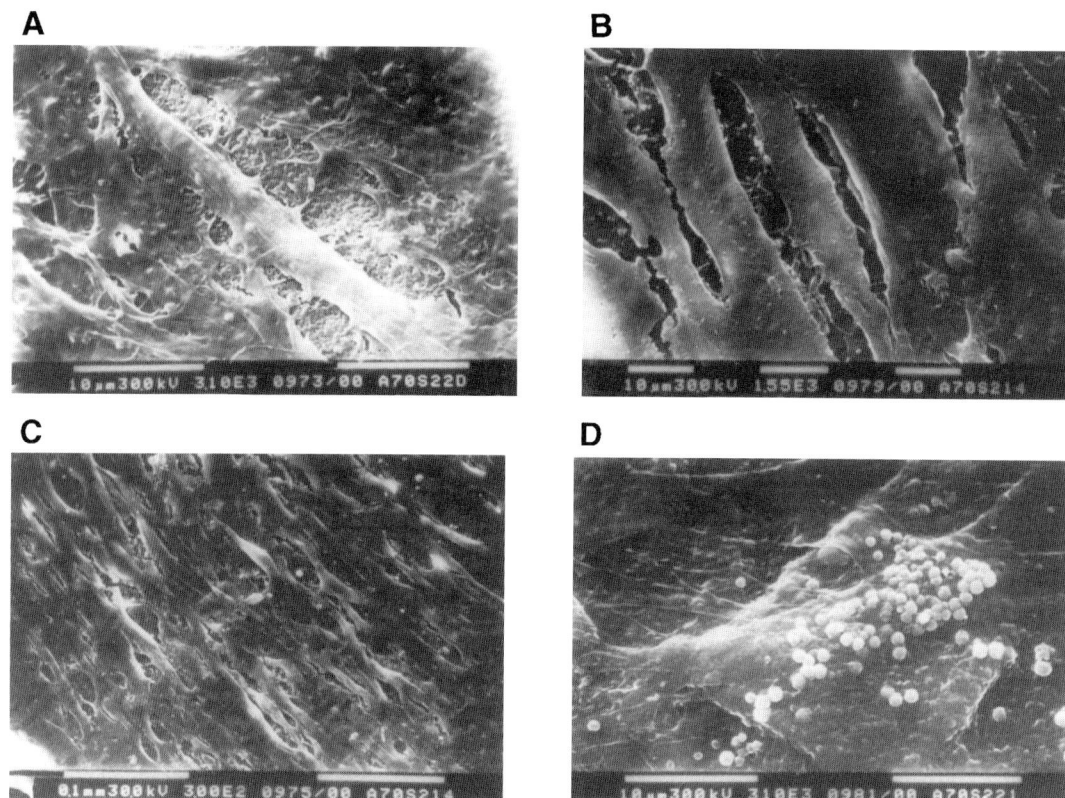

Fig. 5. Human-bone-derived cells cultures on HA-SAL2. (**A**) 2 d after seeding. The cells have anchored, attached, and are well spread on the disk (×3100). (**B**) and (**C**) 14 d in culture. The cells formed a multilayered sheet. They retained their typical broad and flattened morphology, and exhibited good culture organization (×1550 and ×600, respectively). (**D**) 21 d in culture. Globular masses on the surface of some bone cells in culture (×3100).

(13–16). In developing in vitro models for screening materials, it is recommended to use human cell lines relevant to the material application *(13,16,40,41)*.

3.1. Biocompatibility In Vitro of HA-SAL2

The biocompatibility in vitro of HA-SAL2 was evaluated with cells relevant to osteogenesis: human bone cells *(14)* and cells from a permanent line with osteoblastic properties (Saos2) *(14,42, 43)*.

Human-bone-derived cells were seeded on HA-SAL2 disks and examined by scanning electron microscopy (SEM) after 2, 14, and 21 d of culture. Ultrastructural observation indicated that the cells had anchored, attached, and spread onto the disks within 2 d after seeding (Fig. 5A). The cells were well spread, displaying a flat configuration, and in contract with neighboring cells (Fig. 5B). Within 14 d after seeding, the cells had colonized large areas of the substrate surface (Fig. 5C). They maintained physical contact with one another through multiple extensions, and formed a multilayer sheet. They overlapped and superimposed, making it difficult to distinguish the borders of the individual cells (Fig. 5C). Cells seeded at higher density took less time to cover the apatite surface, although there were variations from one culture batch to another. No signs of cytotoxicity or cell degeneration were evident throughout the experiment. The cells retained their typical broad and flattened morphology, and exhibited good culture organization.

Concurrent with continuous cultivation of

Table 1
Quantitative Release of Cytokines by Peripheral Blood Monocytes Incubated with HA-SAL2

Sample	24 h; (pg/mL)			48 h; (pg/mL)		
	IL-1β	IL-6	TNF-α	IL-1β	IL-6	TNF-α
HA-SAL2	5.2	<8	13.6	4.8	<8	28.8
Commercial-HA	5.0	<8	8.8	2.8	<8	10.2
Control PBL-M	3.2	<8	<8	2.6	<8	2.8
Medium only	0.8	<8	<8	0.2	<8	<0.8

human-bone-derived cells, formation of ECM like material, and ECM-containing fibrous material secreted by the osteoblasts, could be observed (Fig. 5B). The authors have also observed globular masses on the cell surface of bone cells in culture (Fig. 5D). It has been suggested that mineralization begins with matrix vesicles, and is followed by additional mineral deposition on collagen fibrils *(36,44)*.

Ceramic surfaces of HA-SAL2 did not show microscopic degeneration or altered surface morphology resulting from interaction with the cultured cells, and/or incubation in protein-containing medium, for the duration of the experiments.

Light microscopy and SEM examination of the periphery of the specimen and the outgrowth of the cells on the culture dishes showed no signs of toxicity within the rest period. The cells were well spread, looked healthy, maintained contact with neighboring cells, and formed a well-organized monolayer (not shown).

3.2. Effect of HA-SAL2 Powder on Release of Proinflammatory Products

One significant disadvantage of the use of HA or HA/TCP coating on implant devices is their tendency to fragment and generate particulate wear debris, which could produce adverse tissue reactions *(9,45)*. The change in physical form or in crystalline structure may be critical for the biological responses to HA or HA/TCP *(45)*. Several reports indicate that HA or HA/TCP have significant proinflammatory effects on target cells, when transformed from intact surface coating to particulate form *(47,48)*.

To address this issue, the authors examined the effect of HA-SAL2 powder granules on the capacity of human peripheral blood monocytes (PBL-M) to release proinflammatory products: interleukin (IL)-1β, IL-6, and tumor necrosis factor (TNF-α) *(45)*. Implant granules 0.03% (w/v) in medium were incubated with PBL-M for 24 and 48 h, according to Harada et al. *(45)*. IL-1β, IL-6, and TNF-α were assayed by enzyme-linked immunabsorbent assay (ELISA; R&D Systems), carried out routinely at the Oncology Laboratories of Hadassah *(49)*.

Results (Table 1) indicate that incubation of HA-SAL2 particles with PBL-M for 24 and 48 h did not significantly effect the release of IL-1β, compared to another commercial HA (Com-HA); IL-6 release was unaffected, and similar to control PBL-M; the release of TNF-α after 48-h incubation with HA-SAL2 was higher than that of the Com-HA (28.8 pg/mL and 10.2 pg/mL, respectively).

3.3. Local Tissue Effects After Implantation of HA-SAL2

Assessment of the local effects of HA-SAL2 powder on living tissues at the microscopic level was carried out: Samples of HA-SAL2 and of a Com-HA, 12 mg/sample, were implanted subcutaneously onto white female Sabra rats (200–300 g). Histological evaluation at 2, 4, and 6 wk post-implantation was carried out by scoring, according to predetermined histologic criteria (Table 2). The results indicate that there was no difference in the histological score between the HA-SAL2 and the Com-HA implanted sites (Fig. 6). No adverse toxic effects, e.g., inflammation, degeneration, and/or changes in tissue morphology, were observed at the implantation site of HA-SAL2 or Com-HA.

Table 2
Microscopic Criteria for Evaluation and Scoring of Subcutaneous Tissues Implanted with HA-SAL2

Criterion	Score		
	0	1	2
Leukocyte infiltration	Prominent	Partial	Very few
Vascularity	Not observed	Partial	Normal
Necrosis	Prominent	Partial	Not observed
Giant cells[a]	>10	Very few	Not observed
Fibrosis (capsule)	Thin	Intermediate	Thick

[a]Per field (×400 magnification).

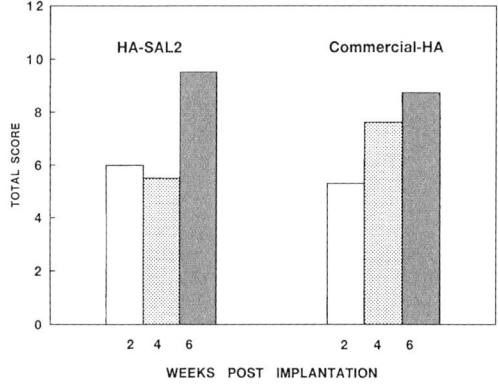

Fig. 6. Histological total score of subcutaneous tissues implanted with HA-SAL2 and a commercial HA, 2, 4, and 6 wk after implantation. Maximal score of 10.

4. Mineralization of Small HA-SAL2 Implants in Bone

4.1. Dual Energy X-Ray Absorptiometry: Noninvasive Measurement of Mineral Content at Site of Implantation

To date, surgeons note no available means of assessing bone ingrowth into porous mineral, and find it difficult to compare ingrowth rate into CaP ceramics and other bone substitutes (50,51). Conventional imaging techniques do not reflect these properties, yet specialized noninvasive methods are routinely used to measure bone density and skeletal mineral content (MC) in the assessment of osteoporosis (53). This worldwide common skeletal disorder is characterized by a decrease in bone mass per unit volume (density), and early detection of bone loss is the key to its treatment (1,2).

Accurate and quantitative monitoring of minute changes in MC at the site of implantation gages the degree of bioceramic implant integration, and markedly enhances its clinical evaluation. The mineral content, which can be measured noninvasively, refers to the minerals in both the bioceramics and host bone. Sequential measurements of bone MC at the site of implantation reflects the current rate of remodeling (51–53).

Previously, the authors proposed two suitable techniques for such noninvasive sequential analysis of the ceramic implant and host bone: dual energy X-ray absorptiometry (DEXA) and the Compton densitometry (51,52). DEXA, which is more suitable for small animals, relies on the attenuation of a collimated X-ray photon beam as it passes through the examined bone. The degree of beam attenuation is related to the mineral content in the bone cross-section. The photons so transmitted are detected by a collimated scintillation counter, moved back and forth on the other side of the region under investigation.

The device uses an X-ray tube with two filters, to provide two photon beams of discrete energies, distinguishable on the basis of their attenuation by bone and soft tissue. One energy serves as a reference for soft tissue thickness, and the attenuation of the other reflects the bone mineral content (53). Measurements are thus enabled in skeletal regions heavily surrounded by soft tissues, such as hip or spine. Findings are expressed as mass of bone mineral per unit area of the bone scanned (g/cm^2). The scanning of several cross-sections at different levels, and averaging the results, reduces

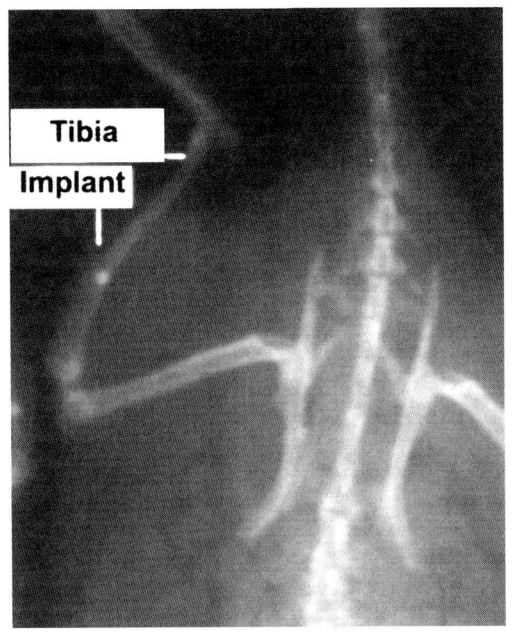

Fig. 7. X-ray of HA implant in the right tibia of a rat.

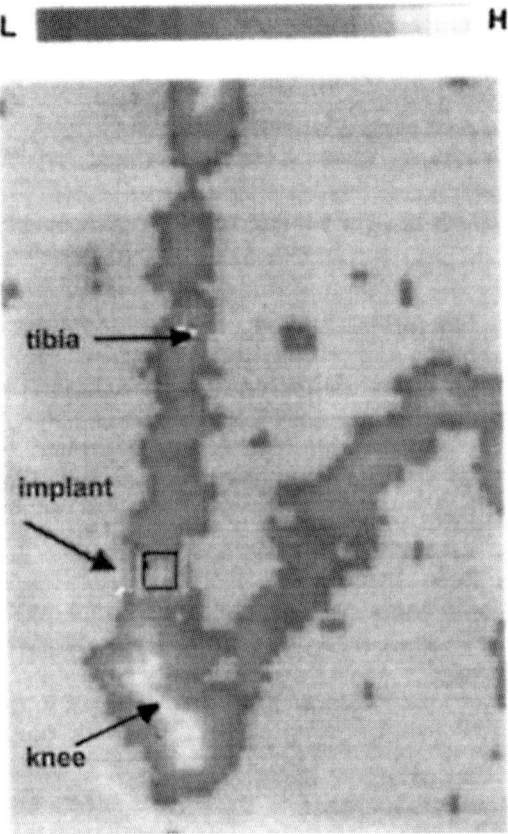

Fig. 8. DEXA mineral image of HA implant in rat tibia. Image resolution is 0.5 × 0.5 mm.

positioning errors at sequential examinations. The degree of mineralization at each measuring point is displayed, either in varying shades of gray or in color, thus, a mineral image of the scanned site is depicted (Figs. 7 and 8). The implant can be identified on the image, and its MC calculated independently of surrounding tissue.

In the present studies, XR-26 model (Norland Instruments, Weesp, The Netherlands) was used. This model contains software that enables calculation of MC at any desired region within the image. The dimensions of such a region can be predetermined with an accuracy of 0.5 mm. Such resolution is essential for the accurate measurement of changes in the implant MC.

4.2. Surgical Model to Follow MC Changes in Small Ceramic Implants in Rat Tibia

HA ceramics have been used for filling bone defects in tibial plateau fractures, and in bone tumor surgery (4,19–21,54–58,60). However, it is still difficult to follow healing progression in these patients. Previously, the authors demonstrated the use of DEXA in vivo for detecting small changes of mineral content (MC) within a ceramic implant in a surgical model the authors have developed (51,52,55): HA cylinders were implanted in rat proximal tibiae, and followed periodically. Although the ceramic implant presents a high mineral background, the precision of the in vivo DEXA measurements at the implant site in the rat tibiae was found to be very reliable, and the deviation in measurement is only 1%. Previous results clearly indicated that DEXA imaging is useful in measuring bone ingrowth in small ceramic HA implants in vivo (51,52,55).

4.3. Mineralization of HA-SAL2 Implants in Rat Tibiae

HA-SAL2 powder, washed extensively with distilled water, and autoclaved, as previously described (52), was implanted in bone defects created in rat proximal tibiae, and its mineralization was followed for 7 wk by the DEXA tech-

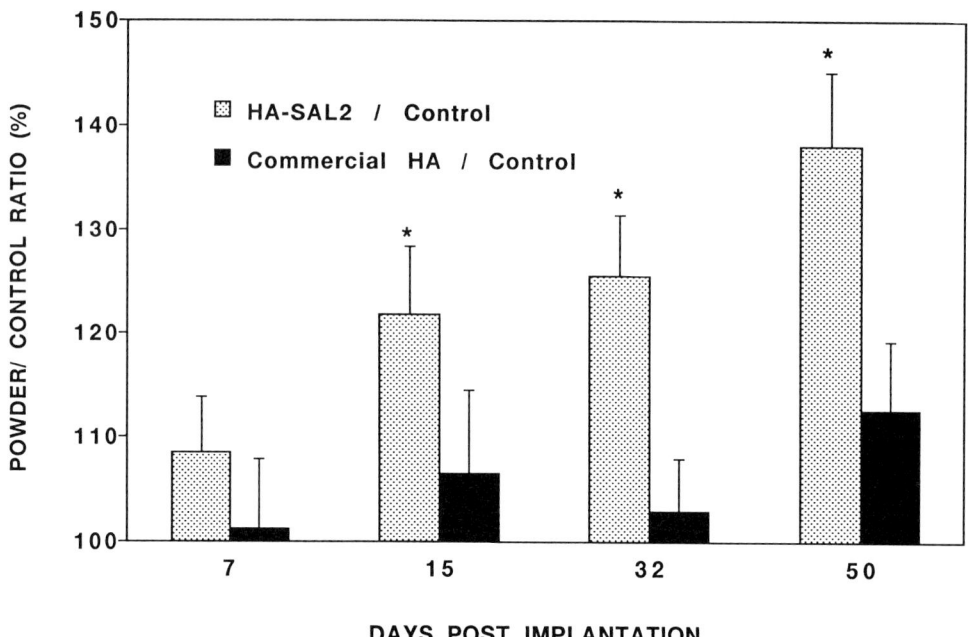

Fig. 9. MCC of HA-SAL2 powder implants as a function of postimplantation period. The implants were inserted in the right proximal tibia of rats. MCC was measured in a 3 × 3 mm region of interest around the mplant. Increment in the mineral content is expressed as the percentage change of the initial postoperative mineral content. Asterisks denote significant difference from controls, ($p < 0.05$).

nique. The defects were created in the right tibial methaphyses, 3–4 mm below the collateral ligament insertion, by drilling a hole of 2 mm diameter. In one group, the bone defects were filled with the autoclaved HA-SAL2 powder, and the contralateral tibia remained intact and served as a control. In the second group, the bone defects were filled with autoclaved Com-HA powder.

The implant filled the entire bone defect, and its inherent mineral content provided a baseline value for measuring the MC changes within the bone defects. The MC in the bone defects was determined, using the DEXA technique, for a region of 2.5 × 2.5 mm, which included the lateral cross-section image of the implant (Fig. 8). The MC in the bone defects was measured at d 1, 7, 15, 32, and 50 postimplantation, and the results were used to calculate the mineralization change of each implant. The mineral content change (MCC) was expressed as an index describing the ratio between the MC value obtained at each time-point and the value obtained on d 1 postimplantation. In addition, mineralization in the bone defect at each time-point was expressed as an index relative to the control MC at the contralateral intact tibia.

The Mann-Whitney U test for small samples *(59)* was used to determine the significance of differences between the MCC values obtained in the controls (nonimplanted contralateral sites) and in each of the implant groups (HA-SAL2 and commercial HA). This nonparametric test was used, because the distribution of the variables in each group was not normal, and the assumptions of Student's *t*-test did not apply. The MC increase at each time-point was analyzed both for the implants and for the control nonimplanted bone sites. Therefore, MC measurement at each time-point served as a separate result in the statistical analysis.

When the MC of each implant was compared with that of the intact contralateral tibia, and expressed relative to its own control, it was found that the implant:control ratio was significantly higher for HA-SAL2 implants than for commercial HA implants on d 15, 32, and 50 post-implantation (Fig. 9).

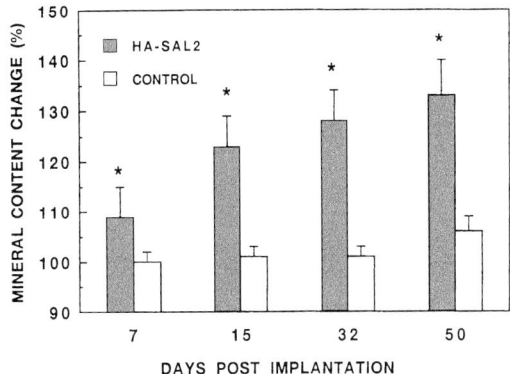

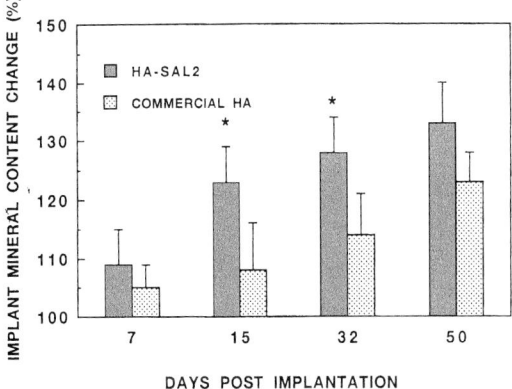

Fig. 10. (Top) MCC of HA-SAL2 implants, compared to controls, as a function of postimplantation period. (Bottom) MCC of HA-SAL2 implants, compared to commercial HA implants, as a function of postimplantation period. Asterisks denote significant difference from controls ($p < 0.05$).

The MCC in HA-SAL2 implants augmented significantly, up to a 33% increase on d 50 postimplantation (Fig. 10, top). The MC of the contralateral proximal tibiae did not augment significantly. At each time-point, the MCC in HA-SAL2 implants was significantly higher than that in the control contralateral tibiae (Fig. 10, top). The MC in the commercial powdered implants augmented significantly, as well, showing an increase of 23% on d 50 postimplantation (Fig. 10, bottom). The difference between the MCC in the commercial implants and the control (contralateral tibiae) was not significant.

The MCC in the bone defects filled with HA-SAL2 powder was higher than the MCC in those filled with the commercial HA powder during the entire follow-up period (Fig. 10, bottom). The difference between the two implants was statistically significant on d 15 and 32 postimplantation (Fig. 10, bottom).

Previous and present results demonstrate that the noninvasive DEXA technique for measuring bone mass is useful for the follow-up of mineralization status in and around small bioceramic implants (51,52,55). The high resolution of the mineralization image obtained with the DEXA device enables the evaluation of even such small implants. For economic and ethical reasons, screening experiments should be in small animals, in which repeated measurements are possible without sacrifice of animals at each step during the follow-up. The MCCs determined by the noninvasive DEXA imaging reflect the mineralization process occurring during callus formation in ceramic implanted in bone defects. The mineral background contributed by the implant itself did not obscure the small changes in MC values caused by callus formation. The curve obtained by sequential DEXA measurements demonstrated a steady increase in MC during the first 7 wk after implantation, which reflects the massive mineralization of soft callus in the healing bone.

4.4. Histology

After the rats were sacrificed, samples of tibiae, including the implants, were excised, to evaluate histological differences in bone ingrowth. The bone fragments were fixed with 4% formaldehyde in saline decalcified in a 10% formic acid aqueous solution. Samples were embedded in paraffin wax, sectioned at 5 μm thickness, and stained by hematoxylin and eosin. The gross cell morphology, cell abundance, and appearance of extracellular material were examined.

Figure 11 shows histological sections of implants 100 d postimplantation. In the section of HA-SAL2 (Fig. 11A,B), bone growth is reflected by osteoblast-containing osteoid surrounding cavities previously occupied by the implant granules. These granules were dissolved upon decalcification of the sections, leaving empty spaces. A similar bone ingrowth is seen in a section of a commercial HA implant (Fig. 11C).

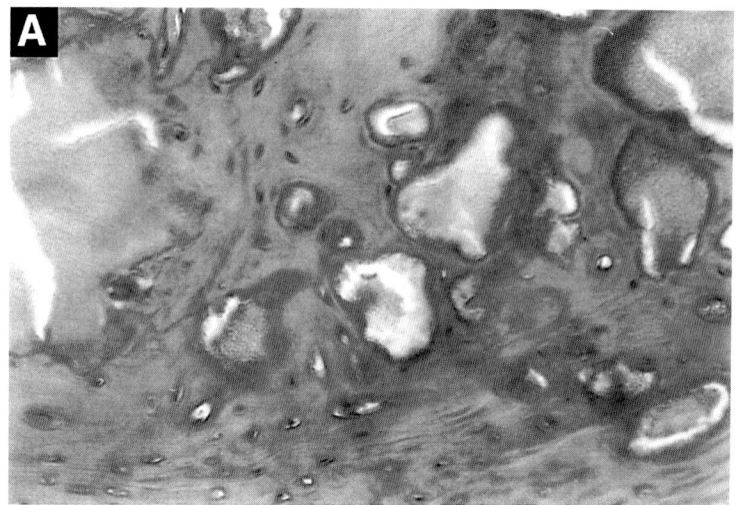
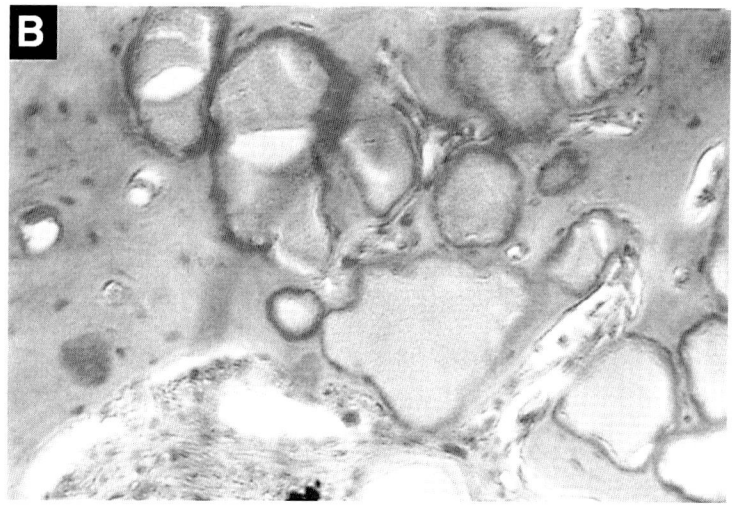
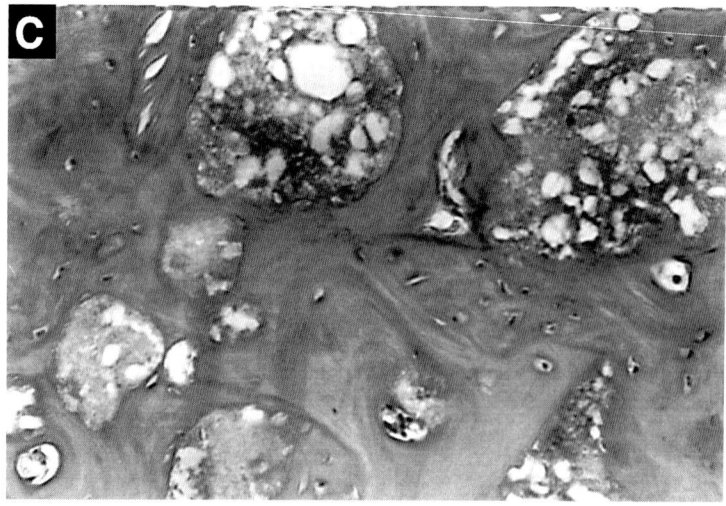

Fig. 11. Histological sections of implants 3 mo postimplantation. (**A**) and (**B**) HA-SAL2 implants. (**C**) Commercial HA implants.

5. Conclusions

HA-SAL2 is a nonstoichiometric, Ca-deficient and carbonate-containing HA. In its ceramic form, it is a novel composite containing HA, β-TCP, and α-TCP. The CaP powder is precipitated from dilute solutions irradiated by microwave. The X-ray diffraction patterns are remarkably similar to those of bone mineral (Fig. 1). α-TCP was detected in the ceramic sintered from this powder at 700°C (Fig. 3).

HA ceramic is preferable as BG substitute, because of its similarity to the chemical composition and the crystal structure of bone mineral (Figs. 1–4), thus exhibiting lack of toxicity and biocompatibility. In addition, HA, in a solid or particulate form, is conductive for bone growth. These characteristics form the basis for the use of HA as BG substitutes. Generally, CaP materials are devoid of intrinsic osteoinductive properties. Recently, it was shown that ceramics containing α-TCP induced bone formation in the pores of the ceramic.

The definition of degrees of HA crystallinity differs markedly when applied by crystallographers, compared to the definition by biologists, especially with reference to bone and dental deposits. The exact stoichiometry of bone apatite depends on age, isomorphous substitution, and other factors. Bone material is a microcrystalline-imperfect HA; the ceramics available for implantation are usually produced from pure, well-crystallized apatite powders, considerably different from bone mineral.

The authors have shown that apatite of a desired degree of crystallinity, with incorporation of accompanying compounds, can be produced quickly, using simple and inexpensive procedures. Microwave energy adsorption during precipitation of CaP species can change the degree of hydration of Ca in the formed crystals, thus modifying their crystallographic structure. HA crystals have lattice defects that cause the release of Ca^{2+} ions in aqueous media. Ca^{2+} and $magnesium^{2+}$ enhance cell adhesion; lack of these cations prevents cell spreading, but not cell attachment. Fibronectin has specific binding sites for Ca^{2+}, thus increasing adhesion.

The authors' results demonstrate the biocompatibility of the new material, HA-SAL2. The experiments demonstrate bone regeneration on the HA-SAL2 implants *in vivo*, and they prove the applicability of DEXA to follow-up mineralization changes in small implants *in vivo*. Apatite grafting with biomaterials, such as HA-SAL2, offer several advantages compared to alternative modalities. HA-SAL2 has a faster mineralization rate than a comparable commercial apatite. By using HA implants, the problem of rejection by the patient's immunosystem and the risk of disease transmission are eliminated. There is no need for a second surgery at another site of the skeleton, and thus recovery time is reduced and medical care costs are significantly lowered.

Acknowledgments

The authors gratefully acknowledge the support of Hadassit–Hadassah Medical Research Services Development Company Limited, the MJF Foundation (Exp. Surg.) and the Yeshaya Horowitz Association Grant-Yissum Ltd., the Hebrew University of Jerusalem. The excellent assistance of E. Rahamim with the SEM photography is gratefully acknowledged.

References

1. Posner AS. Bone mineral and the mineralization process. *Bone Mineral Res* 1987; 5: 65–116.
2. Posner AS. Mineralization of bone. *Clin Orthop* 1985; 200: 87–99.
3. Ohtsuka S. Basic and clinical study of HA. *J Jpn Soc Biomater* 1989; 7: 59–72.
4. Bucholz RW, Carlton A, and Holmes RE. Hydroxyapatite and tricalcium phosphate as bone graft substitutes. *Orthop Clin North Am* 1987; 18: 323–334.
5. Kitsugi T, Yamanuro T, Nakamura S, Kotani T, Kokubo T, and Takenachi H. Four calcium phosphate ceramics as bone substitutes for non-weight-bearing. *Biomaterials* 1993; 14: 216–224.
6. Suzuki T, Toriyoma M, Kawamoto Y, Yokogawa Y, and Kawamura S. Adhesiveness and growth of anchorage-dependent animal cells on biocompatible ceramic culture carriers. *J Fermet Bioenz* 1991; 72: 450–456.
7. Niohihara K. Studies on artificial root therapeutics with new tailored hydroxyapatite root. *J Jpn Soc Biomat* 1993; 11: 135–152.
8. Yubao L, Klein CPAT, Xingdong Z, and De Groot K. Formation of a bone apatite-like layer on the

surface of porous hydroxyapatite ceramics. *Biomaterials* 1994; 15: 835–841.

9 Suzuki T, Yamamoto T, Toriyama M, Nishizawa K, Yokogawa Y, Mucalo M, et al. Surface instability of calcium phosphate ceramics in tissue culture medium and the effect on adhesion and growth of anchorage-dependent animal cells. *J Biomed Mater Res* 1997; 34: 507–517.

10 Ducheyne P. Bioceramics: material characteristics versus *in-vivo* behavior. *J Biomed Mater Res Appl Biomater* 1987; 21A: 219–236.

11 Remes A and Williams DF. Immune response in biocompatibility. *Biomaterials* 1992; 13: 731–743.

12 Amstutz HC, Campbell P, Kossovsky N, and Clarke IC. Mechanism and clinical significance of wear debris-induced osteolysis. *Clin Orthop* 1992; 276: 7–18.

13 Sgouras D and Duncan S. Methods for the evaluation of biocompatibility of soluble synthetic polymers which have potential biomedical use. 1. Use of the MTT colorimetric assay as a preliminary screen for the evaluation of in-vitro cytotoxicity. *J Mater Sci Mater Med* 1990; 1: 61–68.

14 Ben-Bassat H, Klein BY, Lerner E, Azoury R, Rahamim E, Shlomai Z and Sarig S. In-vitro biocompatibility study of a new hydroxyapatite ceramic HA-SAL1: comparison to bioactive bone substitute ceramics. *Cell Mater* 1994; 4: 37–50.

15 Sautier JM, Nefussi JR, and Forest N. Surface reactive biomaterials in osteoblast cultures: an ultrastructure study. *Biomaterials* 1993; 13: 400–402.

16 Sun JS, Tsuang YH, Liao CJ, Liu HC, Hang YS, and Lin FH. Effect of calcium phosphate particles on the growth of osteoblasts. *J Biomed Mater Res* 1997; 37: 324–334.

17 Grinell F. Serum dependence of baby hamster kidney attachment to a substratum. *Exp Cell Res* 1976; 97: 265–274.

18 Amphlett GW and Hrinda ME. Binding of calcium to human fibronectin. *Biochem Biophys Res Commun* 1983; 111: 1045–1452.

19 Wise DL, Trantolo DJ, Altobelli DE, Yaszemski MJ, Gresser JD, and Schwartz ER. (eds) *Encyclopedic Handbook of Biomaterials and Bioengineering. Part A: Materials;* Part B: *Applications* 1995; M Dekker, New York.

20 Hench LL. Bioceramics: from concept to clinic. *J Am Ceramics Soc* 1991; 74: 1487–1510.

21 De Groot K. Bioceramics of calcium phosphate: preparation and properties, in *Bioceramics of Calcium Phosphates* 1983; CRC, Boca Raton, FL pp. 99–114.

22 Gao TY, Tuominen TK, Lindholm TS, Kommonen B, and Lindholm TC. Morphological and biomechanical difference in healing segmental tibial defects implanted with Biocoral® or tricalcium phosphate cylinders. *Biomaterials* 1997; 18: 219–223.

23 Lerner E, Sarig S, and Azoury R. Enhanced maturation of hydroxyapatite from aqueous solutions using microwave irradiation. *J Miner Sci* 1991; 2: 44–47.

24 Sarig S, Apfelbaum F, and Kahana F. Upgrading of hydroxyapatite ceramic biocompatibility by incorporation of α-tricalcium phosphate. *Bioceramics* 1997; 10: 397–400.

25 Hench LL and Ethridge EC. Biomaterials: an intrafacial approach. *Biophys Bioeng Series* 1982; 4: 279–288.

26 Davies JE and Matsuda T. Extracellular matrix production by Osteoblasts on bioactive substrata *in vitro. Scan Microsc* 1988; 2: 1445–1452.

27 Ito G, Matsuda T, Inoue N, and Kamegan T. Biologic comparison of the tissue interface to bioglass. *J Biomed Mater Res* 1987; 21: 585–497.

28 Bruijn JD, Klein CPAT, De Groot K, and Van Blitterswijk CA. Ultrastructure of the bone-hydroxyapatite interface *in vitro. J Biomed Mater Res* 1992; 26: 1362–1382.

29 Taylor SE and Gibbons DF. Effect of surface texture on the soft tissue response to polymer implants. *J Biomed Mater Res* 1983; 17: 205–227.

30 Bagambisa FB and Joos U. Preliminary studies on the phenomenological behavior of osteoblasts cultures on the hydroxyapatite ceramics. *Biomaterials* 1990; 11: 50–56.

31 Davies JE, Causton B, Bovell Y, Davy K, and Sturt CS. Migration of osteoblasts over substrata of discrete surface change. *Biomaterials* 1986; 7: 231–233.

32 Shimazaki K and Mooney V. Comparative study of porous hydroxyapatit and tricalcium phosphate as bone sunstitute. *J Orthop Res* 1985; 3: 301–310.

33 Malick MA, Puelo DA, Bizios R, and Doremus RH. Osteoblasts on hydroxyapatite, alumina and bone surface in vitro: morphology during the first 2 hours of attachment. *Biomaterials* 1992; 13: 123–128.

34 Nishizana K, Toriyama M, Suzuki T, Kawamoto Y, and Yokogawa Y. Effects of surface wettability and zeta potential of bioceramics on the adhesiveness and anchorage-dependent animal cells. *J Ferment Bioeng* 1993; 75: 435–437.

35 Toriyama M, Kawamoto Y, Suzuki T, Yokogawa Y, Nishizawa K, and Nagata F. Wettability of calcium phosphate ceramics by water. *J Ceramics Soc Jpn* 1995; 103: 46–49.

36 Anderson HC. Matrix vesicle calcification: review

and update. *Bone and Mineral Res* 1985; 3: 109–149.
37 Boskey AL. Current concepts of physiology and biochemistry of calcification. *Clin Orthop Res* 1981; 157: 225–257.
38 Nao M, Kotani S, and Fujita Y. Differences in ceramic-bone interface between surface-active ceramics and resorbable ceramics: a study by scanning and transmission electron microscopy. *J Biomed Mater Res* 1992; 26: 255–267.
39 Niki M. Comparative study of the histological, physical and chemical properties of bone-biomaterial interface. *J Jap Soc Biomater* 1994; 12: 5–21.
40 Villanueva JE and Nimmi ME. Modulation of osteogenesis by isolated calvaria cells: a model for tissue interactions. *Biomaterials* 1990; 11: 13–15.
41 Brook IM, Craig GT, and Lamb DJ. In-vitro interaction between primary bone organ culture, glass-ionomer cements and hydroxyapatite/tricalcium phosphate ceramics. *Biomaterials* 1991; 12: 179–186.
42 Farley JR, Hall SL, Herring S, Tarbauz NM, Matsuyama T, and Wergedal JE. Skeletal alkaline phosphatase specific activity ia an index of the osteoblastic phenotype in subpopulations of the human osteosarcoma cell line Saos-2. *Metabolism* 1991; 40: 664–671.
43 Rodan SB, Imai Y, Thiede MA, Wesolowski G, Thompson D, Bar-Shavit Z, et al. Characterization of a human osteosarcoma cell line (Saos-2) with osteoblastic properties. *Cancer Res* 1987; 47: 4961–4966.
44 Weiss RE and Reddi AH. Synthesis and localization of fibronectin during collagenous matrix mesenchymal cell interaction and differentiation of cartilage and bone in-vitro. *Proc Natl Acad Sci USA* 1980; 77: 2074–2078.
45 Harada Y, Wang JT, Doppalapudi VA, Willis AA, Jasty M, Harris WH, Nagase M, and Goldring SR. Differential effects of different forms of hydroxyapatite/tricalcium phosphate particulates on human monocyte/macrophage, in vitro. *J Biomed Mater Res* 1996; 31: 19–26.
46 Cheung HS, Story MT, and McCarty DJ. Mitogenic effects of hydroxyapatite and calcium phosphate dihydrate crystals on cultured mammalian cells. *Arthritis Rheum* 1984; 27: 668–674.
47 Nagase M, Barker DG, and Schumacher R Jr. Prolonged inflammatory reactions induced by artificial ceramics in the rat air pouch model. *J Rheumatol* 1988; 15: 1334–1338.
48 Ross L, Benghuzzi H, Tucci M, Callender M, Cason Z, and Spence L. Effect of HA, TCP and ALCAP bioceramic capsules on the viability of human monocyte and monocyte derived macrophages. *Biomed Sci Instrum* 1996; 32: 71–79.
49 Abramov Y, Schenber JG, Lewin A, Friedler S, Nisman B, and Barak V. Plasma inflammatory cytokines correlate to the ovarian hyperstimulation syndrome. *Hum Reprod* 1996; 11: 1381–1386.
50 Pleilschrifter J and Mundy GR. Modulation of TGF-? activity in bone cultures by osteotropic hormones. *Proc Natl Acad Sci USA* 1987; 84: 2024–2028.
51 Leichter I and Bloch B. Evaluation of calcium phosphate ceramic implant by non-invasive techniques. *Biomaterials* 1992; 13: 478–482.
52 Moshieff R, Klein BY, Leichter I, Chaimsky G, Nyska A, Peyser A, and Segal D. Use of dual-energy X-ray absorptiometry (DEXA) to follow mineral content changes in small ceramic implants in rats. *Biomaterials* 1992; 13: 462–466.
53 Wilson CR and Madsen M. Dichromatic absorptiometry of vertebrate bone mineral content. *Invest Radiol* 1977; 12: 180–184.
54 Uchida A, Araki N, Shinto Y, Yoshikawa H, and Ono K. Use of calcium ceramic hydroxyapatite in bone tumor surgery. *J Bone Joint Surg* 1990; 72B: 298–302.
55 Ben-Bassat H, Klein BY, and Leichter I. Biocompatibility of a new apatite (HA-SAL1) as a bone graft substitute, in *Encyclopedic Handbook of Biomaterials and Bioengineering*, Part A, vol. 2, 1995; (Wise DL, et al., eds), M. Dekker, New York, pp. 1545–1563.
56 Giannini S, Moroni A, Pompilli M, Cerccarelli F, Cantagalli S, Pezzuto V, et al. Bioceramics in orthopedic surgery: state of the art and preliminary results. *Ital Orthop Traumatol* 1992; 18: 431–441.
57 Einhorn TA. Enhancement of fracture healing. *J Bone Joint Surg Am* 1995; 77: 940–956.
58 Klein C, De Groot K, Weigum C, Yubao L, and Xingdong Z. Osseous substance formation inducedin porous calcium phosphate ceramics in soft tissues. *Biomaterials* 1994; 15: 31–34.
59 Mann HB and Whitney DR. On a test of whether one of two random variables is stochastically larger than the other. *Ann Math Stat* 1947; 18: 50–60.
60 Matsuda T, Yliheikkila PK, Felton DA, and Cooper LF. Generalizations regarding the process and phenomenon of osseointegration. Part I: in-vivo studies. *Inter J Oral Maxillofac Implants* 1998; 13: 17–29.

10

Soluble Calcium Salts in Bioresorbable Bone Grafts

Joseph D. Gresser, Kai-Uwe Lewandrowski, Debra J. Trantolo, Donald L. Wise, and Yung-Yueh Hsu

1. Introduction

Bone is the second most implanted material in the body, after blood. There are over 450,000 bone graft (BG) procedures annually in the United States (2.2 million worldwide), with a market potential of $400–600 million. Autografts and allografts are used in current BG procedures to repair defects caused by surgery, tumors, trauma, implant revisions, and infections, and also for joint fusion. However, drawbacks, such as the need for a second surgery to retrieve the graft (autograft), or the risk of viral infection, contamination, and long-term complications (allografts), make bioresorbable BG substitutes viable alternatives to autografts and allografts. Only 10% of these procedures use synthetic materials, because the currently approved synthetic grafts are considered to be inferior to the use of autograft or allograft. Significant problems include lack of resorbability, inclusion of animal- or marine-derived components, and poor handling characteristics.

Therefore, development of bioresorbable BG substitutes seems eminently worthwhile. They could serve immediately as an osteoconductive path to bone reconstruction. Ultimately, one could incorporate an osteoinductive growth factor, such as a bone morphogenic protein (BMP) to accelerate healing. The developmental goals of a biodegradable for void filling should address degradation *(1)*, porosity *(2)*, *in situ* curing properties, and the ultimate flexibility in formulation, to permit use in reconstructive situations calling for varying rates of degradation and bony recovery.

Currently approved synthetic products have significant disadvantages. The authors have developed a BG substitute that does not contain biological material, either collagen or protein, and does not stay in the bone after the healing process has occurred. This bioresorbable BG substitute is made from the unsaturated polyester, poly(propylene glycol-co-fumaric acid) (PPF), which can be crosslinked in the presence of soluble and insoluble calcium (Ca) filler salts, and grouted directly in the void created by removal of a cyst or infected bone, or from trauma. The graft material could provide an osteoconductive pathway by which bone will grow in faster. Several clinical indications would benefit from such a bioresorbable osteoconductive BG substitute.

2. Clinical Indications for Bioresorbable BG Substitutes

Immediate applicability may be for reconstruction of defects caused by surgical debridement of infections, previous surgery, tumor removal, trauma, and implant revisions, and for joint fusion.

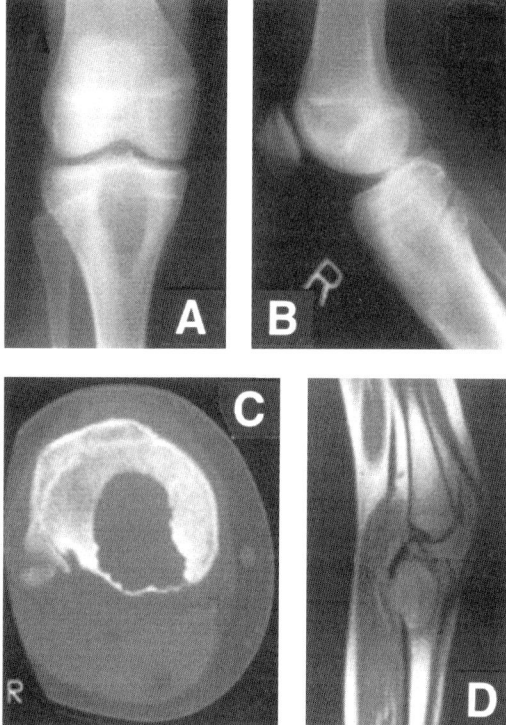

Fig. 1. (**A**) AP and (**B**) lateral radiographs of the right knee. (**C**) axial cut and (**D**) sagittal MRIs (tl-weighted) of the right knee, showing osteomyelitis in the proximal tibial plateau.

2.1. Surgical Debridement of Osteolysis

In osteomyelitis (OM), pathogenic microorganisms can invade bone by hematogenous spread, direct extension from a contiguous site of infection, and direct introduction. Acute hematogenous OM occurs predominantly in children, and before the age of epiphysial closure. It typically originates in the metaphysis of long bones in the region of most rapid growth and greatest vascularity (Fig. 1). The bloodborne bacteria are carried to the marrow space by way of the nutrient artery. The initial site of infection within a particular bone is determined by the vascular anatomy as related to the epiphysial growth plate. Hematogenous OM in adults rarely involves the long bones, but usually occurs in the vertebrae, which are generally highly vascular. The hematogenous spread of infection can occur by way of the nutrient branches of the spinal artery or by flow from the pelvic veins to the lumbar veins, and, under conditions of increased abdominal pressure, retrograde flow through the paravertebral venous plexus of Batson. The complications of vertebral OM include extension of the infection to the adjacent disk space, and extension to retropharyngeal, mediastinal, peritoneal, and meningeal sites, depending on the vertebrae involved. In general, the clinical course of OM will depend on the characteristics of the causative organism, the route of the infection, and the age of the patient.

With continuation of the bone infection, chronic inflammatory cells (lymphocytes, histiocytes, plasma cells), proliferating fibroblasts, and reactive new bone formation contribute to the microscopic picture of chronic OM. Reactive new bone formation occurs. The elevated periosteum is stimulated to form new bone, which surrounds the underlying infected and inflamed bone with a bony envelope, termed an "involucrum." If chronic OM is undiagnosed or inadequately treated, the avascular dead tissue, pus, and bacteria may remain isolated within an area of bone fibrosis and sclerosis, and give rise to recurrent episodes of acute OM. The treatment of these chronic bone infections usually requires, in addition to antimicrobial therapy, surgical intervention to drain abscesses and remove necrotic tissue. Reconstruction of the surgical defect can be accomplished with the authors' bioresorbable BG substitute filler. In fact, it may prove to be particularly suitable for this application, because it is bioresorbable.

2.2. Treatment of Solitary Lucent Bone Lesions

Another potential application of a bioresorbable BG substitute is in the reconstruction of defects created during the surgical treatment of solitary lucent bone lesions. The differential diagnosis includes fibrous dysplasia, osteoblastoma, giant cell tumor, metastasis/myeloma, aneurysmal bone cyst, chondroblastoma/chondromyxoid fibroma, hyperparathyroidism (brown tumors)/ hemangioma, nonossifying fibroma, eosinophilic granuloma/enchondroma, and solitary bone cyst (Fig. 2). Most expansile, lucent lesions are located in the medullary space of the bone and tend to occur in a "favorite" part of the bone.

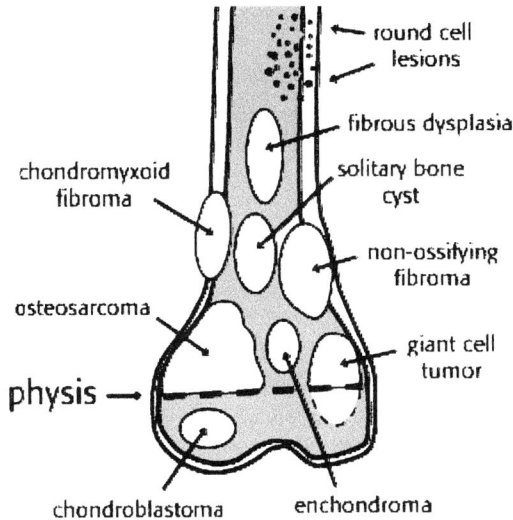

Fig. 2. Radiologic and pathologic analysis of solitary bone lesions. Part I: Internal margins. Reproduced with permission from ref.

2.3. Failed Total Hip Arthroplasties with Acetabular Osteolysis

A further potential application of the bioresorbable BG substitute is in reconstruction of osteolytic acetabular defects in patients in whom revision of a total hip arthroplasty became necessary. Typically, these implants begin to loosen, or otherwise fail, after 10–15 yr, at which point the implant needs to be surgically replaced. This procedure is known as revision total hip replacement surgery (RTHR). In this surgery, the failing orthopedic hip implant is replaced with a new one by removing the old implant, removing the bone cement, enlarging the implant cavity, and inserting the new implant. Therefore, RTHR is more complex than PTHR. After removal of the old implant and the old cement, before cutting the new canal cavity, one must be prepared to fill or pack skeletal defects in the acetabulum, so that the new implant socket can be held in place. Although it is generally accepted that acetabular osteolysis is less common than osteolysis around femoral components, where debris and wear can cause inflammatory responses (3–5), it is not infrequent (Fig. 3A,B).

As noted by Devane et al. (6), osteolysis was associated with an increased rate of polyethylene wear only in hips that were inserted without cement. In a study by Maloney et al. (7), 35 THR patients with porous acetabular components demonstrated acetabular osteolysis.

These observations were confirmed by Zicat et al. (8), who have recently investigated patterns of osteolysis around total hip components inserted with and without cement. They reviewed the radiographs of 137 patients (137 hips) who had been managed with a total hip arthroplasty, with insertion of an extensively porous-coated femoral component without cement, because of osteoarthrosis or avascular necrosis. A porous-coated acetabular component had been inserted with cement in 63 of these patients (group A) and without cement in 74 patients (group B). The radiographs were examined for osteolysis, either directly adjacent to the joint or at locations remote from the joint. The mean duration of follow-up was 105 mo (range 54–142 mo). The rate of osteolysis of the acetabulum in the unrevised hips, in which the acetabular component had been inserted with cement, was 37% (19/51). The osteolysis was most frequently of the linear type, a pattern that was associated with a high prevalence of loosening in the hips that had a cemented cup (30%). The rate of acetabular osteolysis (18%) in the patients who had a cup that had not been inserted with cement, and that had not been revised, was not as high as that associated with the surviving cups that had been inserted with cement ($p < 0.05$). The osteolysis associated with the cups that had not been inserted with cement was localized and expansile, and it was not associated with loosening of the component. However, it produced more loss of bone than did the linear pattern of osteolysis around the cemented cups.

The patients of Maloney et al. (7) were managed by liner removal, debridement of the osteolytic defect, and BG, followed by liner exchange. After an average of 3 yr, the BGs had appeared to consolidate, and no progressive bone erosion was seen. Instead of using autologous or allogeneic BGs (with their associated risks of donor-site morbidity or disease transmission), or even bone cement such as polymethylmethacrylate, this clinical problem could be developed into an indication for the authors' bioresorbable PPF-based bone grout.

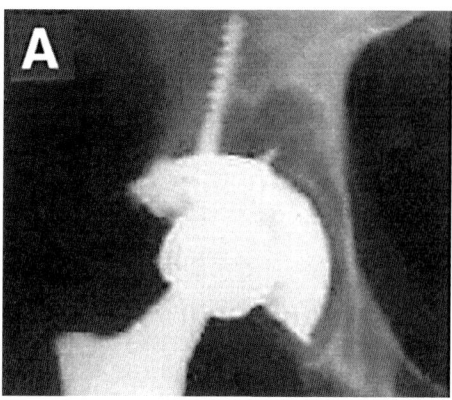 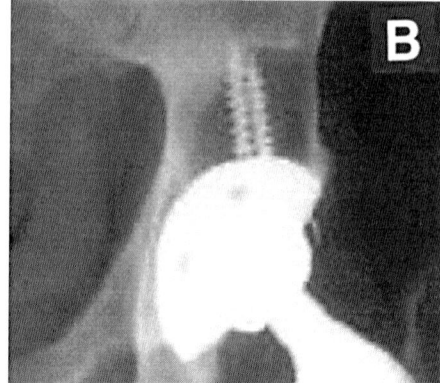

Fig. 3A,B. 50-yr-old patient with a well-placed acetabular cup (against the tear drop) and well-placed femoral stem. After 7 yr, the patient has developed extensive osteolysis.

3. Comparison to Other Bone Void Fillers/BG Substitutes

There are several bone void fillers/BG substitutes, some of which are hydroxyapatite (HA)-based, with and without various collagen extracts. Some are now undergoing clinical testing. The materials currently available or under development are summarized in Tables 1 and 2. They are reviewed here in brief, to compare with the authors' bioresorbable bone void filler with respect to its composition and potential clinical applications.

3.1. Interpore 200

Interpore 200 (Steri-Oss) is a porous coralline HA bone void filler for repairing periodontal defects. Interpore 200 is similar to human cortical bone in both structure and chemical composition. Its porous structure comes from the mineral skeleton of specific corals. These corals are converted to HA (essentially $Ca_{10}[PO_4]_6[OH]_2$).

3.2. Osteoset

Osteoset is an extremity HA-based BG substitute, which is offered in a 3-mm pellet size designed to be packed into bony voids or gaps of the skeletal system, e.g., distal radius fractures, fusions of the hand or foot, fracture gaps, filling voids resulting from benign bone cysts, backfilling biopsy and autograft harvest sites, and filling voids left behind by removal of orthopedic hardware. Osteoset is resorbable and biocompatible, and may be used in the presence of infection.

3.3. Skeletal Repair System (SRS)

The Skeletal Repair System (SRS) (Norian) is an injectable cement that consists of a unique formulation of Ca carbonate and calcium triphosphate salts that undergo continuous mineralization once mixed in a solution, and form dahllites of low crystallinity and small grain size. The injectable cement cures within 10 min, and reaches its full mechanical strength within 12 h. This material resembles the structure of HA found in bone, and in fact was found to stimulate bone ingrowth. The Norian cement relies on the body's ability to incorporate it by ongoing resorption and concomitant new bone formation. The Norian cement is one of the few bone substitute materials that are now undergoing multicenter clinical trials for approval by the U.S. Food and Drug Administration (FDA).

According to the results of a study presented at the 1996 annual meeting of the American Academy of Orthopaedic Surgeons (9) at Massachusetts General Hospital, researchers have found that a bone paste compound, injected through the skin into a wrist fracture, will heal bones faster than traditional methods. The Norian SRS bone paste was found to provide internal stabilization of the fracture, with little morbidity. Fracture healing and functional restoration were evaluated among women age 49–57 yr who had fractured their

Table 1
New Bone Grafts

PRO OSTEON	• Interpore International • Type: BG substitute • Composition: Sea coral converted by hydrothermal exchange reaction into coralline HA • Action: Acts as lattice for new bone formation • Indications (approved): Metaphyseal fractures of long bones • Trials: Being evaluated in cervical spine fusions
BIOGLASS	• US Biomaterials • Type: Bioactive glass implant • Action: Reacts with body fluid, causing bone-like pores to evolve on the implant surface; collagen bonds to the surface and new bone forms and fills the space between the implant, collagen fibers, and bone • Indications (approved): Only for grafting facial bones, replacing bones in the middle ear, and repairing periodontal defects • Trials: Long bone fracture fixation, spinal fusions
COLLAGRAFT	• Zimmer • Type: Synthetic BG substitute • Composition: HA/tricalcium phosphate (TCP) and pure bovine fibrillar collagen • Action: Mix with autogenous bone marrow to produce an osteoconductive and osteoinductive substance that acts as a matrix for repair process • Indications (approved): Repair of diaphyseal/metaphyseal fxs • Note: fx should be stabilized with skeletal fixation and recommended maximum defect site of 30 cc • Risk: Immunologic risk secondary to bovine collagen (no reported serious cases)
GRAFTON	• Osteotech • Type: Banked human tissue • Composition: Demineralized bone matrix glycerol suspension • Action: Elicits new bone formation by osteoconduction and osteoinduction • Indications (approved): As adjunctive to spinal and joint fusions, repair of osseous defects, and arthroplasties • Risk: Possible disease transmission • Note: Processing of Grafton has been shown to inactivate HIV, hepatitis B and C, cytomegalovirus, and polio
OSTEOSET	• Wright Bio-Orthopaedics • Type: Synthetic BG substitute • Composition: HA/TCP • Action: Extremity BG substitute is offered in a 3-mm pellet size • Indications (approved): Designed to be packed into bony voids or gaps of the skeletal system
INTERPORE	• Type: Synthetic bone void filler • Composition: HA/TCP • Action: Extremity BG substitute is offered in a 3-mm pellet size • Indications (approved): Designed to be packed into bony voids or gaps of the skeletal system

wrist. At 1-yr follow-up, the grip strength in a hand that was conventionally treated ranged between 60 and 85% that of the other hand. The grip strength of a hand that had the bone paste treatment was about 98% that of the other hand. Three, 6, and 12 mo after surgery, manual dexterity was normal for all patients who received the bone paste treatment. These patients lost about 1 mm radial bone length, compared to length losses of up to 10 mm with conventional treatment. X-rays of patient wrists were taken throughout the year. Range of motion improved by 50% at

Table 2
Experimental Products (Awaiting FDA Approval)

Norian Skeletal Repair System (SRS)	• Type: Bone mineral substitute • Composition: Monocalcium and TCP, Ca carbonate, and liquid sodium phosphate • Action: Paste that hardens to turn into the mineral phase of bone (osteoconductive). Is replaced by bone; maximum comp, strength greater than cancellous bone
Bone Source HA Cement (Developmental)	• Type: HA bone substitute • Composition: Nonceramic HA • Action: Initially formed into a paste that hardens over 20–30 min and converts to HA in 4 h. Eventually replaced by new bone.
Transforming Growth Factor-β1	• Type: Osteoinductive protein • Action: awaiting FDA approval on its effects on bone tissue growth and regeneration • Note: No humans studies yet • Future applications: Nonunions, bone defects, and revision • Implant surgery
OP-1 (currently in clinical trials)	• Type: Morphogenic protein • Action: Stimulates bone formation by causing precursor stem cells to differentiate into bone-forming cells
BMP-2 (human clinical trials)	• Type: Bone growth protein • Action: Induces bone growth and repair when mixed with carrier and implanted into site of fracture • Future applications: Trauma, AVN, bone loss from tumor, and spinal reconstruction

3 mo, and further improved through 12 mo. Bone-paste-treated patients had a mean pronation of 100%; a mean supination of 93%; a mean wrist extension of 95%; a mean flexion of 85%, a radial deviation mean of 88%; and an ulnar deviation mean of 89%. There were no side effects or complications.

3.4. Bioglass

Bioglass has been known for almost 20 yr, and has been proven to allow excellent osseointegration. It allows more freedom in the composition, so that the dissolution rate can be controlled. However, despite good biocompatibility, very few applications are implemented in biomedical devices. A major drawback is production cost. However, a single process was developed by which bioglass is synthesized and applied by plasma spraying. Therefore, a free-flowing powder is prepared from the basic chemical compounds, ordinarily used for synthesis of the glass. The chief components are the oxides of silicon, Ca, sodium, phosphorus, and Ca fluoride. If the plasma spraying is performed in a closed vessel, the powder can be collected and used as such. Exposing a metal substrate to the plasma allows the production of coatings, which were obtained with adhesion strengths over 30 MPa. In vivo behavior is currently under investigation. A patent has been allowed for the process, not only for bioglass, but also, in general, for other glasses containing no phosphates. In 1985, the FDA cleared Bioglass for use in repairing tiny inner ear bones to restore conductive hearing loss. In 1994, the manufacturer, US Biomaterials, received FDA clearance to market PerioGlas for repairing bone lost to periodontal disease.

3.5. Collagraft

Collagraft consists of a mixture of porous beads composed of 60% HA and 40% tricalcium phosphate (TCP) ceramic and fibrillar bovine collagen. The HA has mineral resorbancy, and acts as a long-term scaffold for bony ingrowth by providing a fixed structure for calcification. The TCP has an increased bioactivity for more rapid resorption, thus allowing for the early release of Ca and phosphate ions, which may be used in the natural process of bone mineralization. The different resorption rates for these two granules provide a diminishing scaffold for bone formation and an orderly remodeling over time. When mixed with autogenous bone marrow, it serves as an effective BG substitute, because the bovine fibrillar cartilage provides an extracellular matrix, a favorable environment for cell growth and sites for mineral deposit during the repair process, enhancing bone formation and revascularization.

Since January 1987, this material has been used in a multiclinic prospective trial, randomized against cancellous iliac crest autograft in treatment of severe long bone fractures. To date, 232 patients have entered this study, 117 receiving cancellous autograft and 115 receiving Collagraft and autogenous marrow. At 6- and 12-mo follow-up, Collagraft appeared to function as well as autogenous graft when used in the treatment of acute long bone fractures. Collagraft was approved by the FDA for use in the treatment of acute long bone fractures (metaphyseal and diaphyseal) and traumatic osseous defects.

4. Biodegradable PPF-Based BG Substitutes and Cements

PPF has a long and active history as a bone repair material (10). The authors development of a biodegradable BG substitute stems from earlier experiments with a bioresorbable cement carried out by Wise et al. (11), who used PPF with vinyl pyrrolidone (VP) as a crosslinking agent, rather than methylmethacrylate. The authors have extended this work, noting the minimum amounts of VP necessary for the crosslinking (10).

In a study of the affect of the PPF:VP ratio on the structure of the crosslinked network, they showed that 94.76.2% of the PPF was crosslinked at PPF:VP ratios ranging from 0.33 to 1.00, but that the fraction of VP included in the network increased with increasing PPF:VP ratio and that, at a PPF:VP of 2.0, about 73% of the VP is incorporated into the crosslinked network. It should also be pointed out that both VP and PVP were observed in the in vitro supernatants. The very low accelerator concentrations (0–0.0007% w/w) account for much of the unpolymerized VP, and, with higher accelerator concentrations, virtually all of the VP will either be crosslinked with the PPF or will have formed polyvinyl pyrrolidone (PVP).

**Table 3
Phases of Bone Healing**

Phase	Duration
Induction	0› n2 d
Inflammation	2–14 d
Soft callus	2–8 wk
Hard callus	2–12 mo
Remodeling	1 or more yr

5. Bone Healing and Degradable BG Substitutes

In the design of a degradable BG substitute for applications to bone healing, one must take into account the function of the cement, as well as the normal healing process of bone defects. An immediate function of the BG substitute is osteoconduction, i.e., provision of a framework or scaffolding for vascular ingress, cellular infiltration and attachment, cartilage formation, and calcified tissue deposition. This function requires rapid development of porosity after placement of the cement. The bone-healing sequence for fractures can be divided into five major phases, as indicated in Table 3. This serves as a reference also for defect filling and bony recovery.

Cartilage calcification occurs during the hard callus phase. It seems reasonable to assume that similar periods of time are required for cystic bony defects to heal and to consolidate. Thus, the formulation of a BG substitute for healing of bony voids should be completely resorbed during this period. As indicated by Kenley et al. (1), it is now believed that osseous regeneration can be promoted by combining osteoconductive materials (the bioresorbable BG substitute) with osteogenic and/or osteoinductive materials. On this basis, a longer-range goal of the authors' development work is promotion of the healing process by incorporation of an osteoinductive material into the BG substitute.

In light of these considerations, the authors reasoned that degradation of a bioresorbable, PPF-based BG substitute by polymer hydrolysis could be supported by dissolution of the Ca filler salts, upon ingress of biological fluids. Therefore, the rate of degradation is determined by its composition, and, thus, is independent of the recipient bed. The authors anticipated resorption times for the PPF-based BG substitute faster than those reportedly seen with the Norian cement or with Collagraft materials.

6. Design of Biodegradable BGs

The authors have demonstrated the feasibility of a bioresorbable BG substitute. A high-viscosity, biodegradable putty has been formulated that can be directly grouted into a bony defect with *in situ* curing. The cure reaction is based of the crosslinking of the unsaturated polyester, PPF, with the vinyl monomer, VP. Fillers include both soluble and insoluble components, which control the rate of degradation, as well as the development of porosity and osteoconductivity to facilitate bony ingrowth. Further degradation depends on hydrolysis of the polymer bonds.

7. Formulations

This subheading summarizes studies of four formulations. The grout formulations all varied with respect to the solubilities of the filler. The fillers were HA, a filler designed to support osteoconduction, and 1:3 ratios of HA to the following soluble fillers: calcium gluconate (CG), calcium propionate (CP), or calcium acetate (CA). The rapid leaching of the soluble fillers led to a porous scaffold, which facilitated bony ingrowth commensurate with degradation. Of the various formulations, the one containing the CA–HA filler combination will serve as the basis for further development, based on experimental indications for favorable in vitro physiochemical and mechanical properties and encouraging early-stage in vivo activity, reported herein.

Cement formulations were prepared containing both HA (solubility = 0.002 g/100 mL) and CA, CP, or CG. In addition, a control formulation was prepared containing only HA. The solubilities of these salts, given in Table 4 at 0°C (or 15°C) and

Table 4
Phases of Bone Healing

Temperature (°C)	Solubility (g/100 mL)			
	0	15	37	100
Ca propionate	49.0	–	51.0	55.8
Ca acetate	37.4	–	34.5	29.7
Ca gluconate	–	3.3	7.0	20.0

100°C are reported values *(12)*; those at 37°C are estimated by linear interpolation. The composition of each formulation is summarized in Table 5.

In vivo and in vitro samples were prepared. All in vivo samples exploited a low PPF:VP ratio to accelerate the solubility. The in vitro samples included an HA–CG formulation at the preferred higher PPF:VP ratio for practical material comparisons. These variations allowed us to evaluate, semiquantitatively and separately, weight loss caused by dissolution of the soluble salt and weight loss caused by formation of the water-soluble homopolymer, PVP.

In the short term, the HA-only formulation can lose only PVP, because there is no very soluble salt. PVP formation is greater at low PPF:VP ratios *(10)*. The higher PPF:VP ratio of the HA–CG in vitro formulation significantly depresses PVP formation, and thus weight loss primarily results from loss of soluble salt. Weight loss of the other formulations is caused by loss of both PVP and the salt. This experimental design allowed estimation of the loss of each component. All formulations were tested with fillers in two particle size ranges, 45–125 μm and 125–180 μm.

8. Evaluation

After mixing, the grouts were injected into a Teflon-lined multiple-well cylindrical mold (each well measuring 2.5 mm diameter × 10 mm length), and allowed to cure at 37°C. Multiple samples were prepared for in vitro and in vivo testing. In vitro analyses included mechanical testing for compressive strength and modulus, weight loss, porosity, and scanning electron microscopy (SEM). In vivo analyses included histological and histomorphological evaluation in rat tibial defects.

Table 5
BG Composition (Wt%)

Component	Evaluation				Evaluation in vivo only
	HA only	HA + CG	HA + CP	HA + CA	HA + CG
PPF	15.58	40.58	15.58	15.58	15.58
VP	41.56	34.78	41.56	41.56	41.56
HA	41.56	5.80	10.39	10.39	10.39
CG		17.39			31.17
CP			31.17		
CA				31.17	
BP	1.30	1.45	1.30	1.30	1.30
PPF:VP[a]	0.375	1.167	0.375	0.375	0.375

[a]Weight ratio of PPF to VP.
BP, benzoyl peroxide.

8.1. In Vitro Evaluation

Individual rods were incubated at 37°C in 4 mL phosphate-buffered saline (PBS). Rods were withdrawn periodically and rinsed in distilled water to remove buffer salts. Dimensions (diameter, length) were measured before and on removal from the bath, while still wet. Following these wet measurements, some samples were maintained hydrated in saline-soaked gauze for mechanical testing; others were dried to constant weight for weight loss and microstructure studies.

8.1.1. In Vitro Weight Loss

Although the mean weight loss at comparable time-points for rods containing the larger particle-size filler was slightly greater, the differences were not significant. All samples rapidly lost weight during the first 24 h; thereafter weights remained fairly constant, allowing choice of a time-point (d 7) at which to compare the in vitro weight loss. Formulations containing CP and CA lost approx 50% of their weight during the first day in vitro; this had not changed significantly by d 7. Thus, by d 7, it can be assumed that the soluble components had had sufficient time to diffuse out, but that all other components were still present. Table 6 gives relevant formulation data, the PPF:VP weight ratio, and the 7-d weight loss. The column heading "%Sol." indicates the content of the soluble salts, CG, CA, or CP. Formulations are identified by filler composition: Thus HA + CG refers to the formulation containing both salts.

The PPF:VP ratio is significant. Low value (indicating an excess of VP over PPF) favors PVP formation at the expense of crosslinking. As the PPF increases relative to the VP, the probability of reaction of the VP with the PPF unsaturation increases. The HA + CG formulation has a relatively high PPF:VP ratio (1.167), which favors VP participation in crosslink formation. The 15.5% weight loss is thus mostly caused by loss of CG, and corresponds closely to the initial CG content of 17.4%. The formulation with HA as the single filler has a low PPF:VP ratio (0.375) and no soluble salt to lose. Its 7-d weight loss was 15.8%, which is therefore mostly PVP.

Formulations HA + CP and HA + CA both have low PPF:VP ratios (0.375), and both contain 31.2% of soluble filler. It is likely that the PVP loss from these samples is similar to that from the HA formulation; thus, one can estimate the soluble salt loss at d 7, and compare the estimated loss with the initial content, as shown in Table 7.

The fairly good correspondence between the estimated soluble salt loss and the original soluble salt content lends credence to this analysis, and is in accord with the results of Gresser (10).

8.1.2. In Vitro Density Changes

Evidence for development of porosity was obtained by measurement of densities. Dimensions (rod length and diameter) and dry weights were recorded before and after incubation. Densities were computed from the formula $\rho = 4w / \pi d^2 l$, where w = weight in mg (or grams), d = diameter in mm (or cm), and l = rod length in cm. The density is then reportable as grams per

Table 6
Formulation Data and 7-D Weight Loss

Formulation	%PPF	%VP	%Sol.	%HA	PPF:VP	Wt. loss	Origin of wt loss
HA only	15.6	41.6	0.0	41.6	0.375	15.8	Mostly PVP
HA + CG	40.6	34.8	17.4	5.8	1.167	15.5	Mostly CG
HA + CP	15.6	41.6	31.2	10.4	0.375	53.0	Both PVP and CP
HA + CA	15.6	41.6	31.2	10.4	0.375	50.2	Both PVP and CA

Table 7
Soluble Salt Loss vs Initial Content

Formulation	Total weight loss (%)	–	Weight loss caused by PVP (assumed)	=	Weight loss caused by soluble salt (estimated)	Original soluble salt content
HA + CP	53.0	–	15.8	=	37.2	CP = 31.2
HA + CA	50.2	–	15.8	=	34.4	CA = 31.2

cubic centimeter. From these data, porosities can be computed at each time-point from the relationship $P_t = (\rho_0 \rho_t)^{-1}$ where P_t = porosity at time, t, and ρ_0, ρ_t = initial density and densities at time t.

As shown Fig. 4, for the larger particle sizes, by d 40, the formulations had all developed porosities between 49 and 56%. The porosity measurements for the smaller particle sizes (not shown here) were similar. Porosities of the HA–CP and HA–CA developed rapidly, as expected, from their rapid weight loss.

The HA–CG formulation developed porosity more slowly, although it remained fairly low (approx 15%) from d 1 to d 14, after which it rose linearly, to approx 50% by d 35. The development of porosity is rapid for both HA–CP and HA–CA: by d 1 in vitro, each had developed essentially their maximum porosities, and, further, these porosities are independent of particle size. The HA-only and HA–CG formulations show a similar pattern in porosity development. The porosity developed by d 1 remains fairly constant to d 14, after which loss of CG is accompanied by increasing porosity. Porosity of the HA–CG system is also independent of particle size. Judging from the HA-only pattern of weight loss and porosity development, PVP loss is a slower process than loss of soluble salt. This is reasonable, because the long PVP chains diffuse more slowly than the smaller soluble salt molecules.

8.1.3. In Vitro Mechanical Testing: Compressive Strength and Modulus

Compressive strength and moduli were measured. All measurements were conducted at room temperature, using either an Instron 8511 (Instron, Canton, MA) Servo-hydraulic materials test system equipped with a 2500 lb load cell, and operating at a displacement rate of 0.1 mm/s until failure with load, and displacement data collected using LabView (Version 3.01, National Instruments, Austin, TX), or a TA-XT2 Texture Analyzer (Texture Technologies, Scarsdale, NY, US distributors for Stable Micro Systems, Surrey, UK), equipped with a 5-kg load cell operating at a displacement rate of 0.1 mm/s, with load and displacement data recorded using Stable Micro Systems XTRA-Dimensions (Version 3.7J).

As seen in Fig. 4, the initial compressive modulus and strength of the HA and HA + CA formulations are significantly greater than those of the HA + CP and HA + CA formulations. The values of these parameters for the HA and HA + CG formulations decrease over time in similar fashions, and it is only on d 36 that the HA + CG parameter values approach those of the HA + CP and HA + CA materials. The HA + CP and HA + CA strength and modulus remain fairly constant over time, but are lower than values for HA and HA + CP.

The similar mechanical properties over time

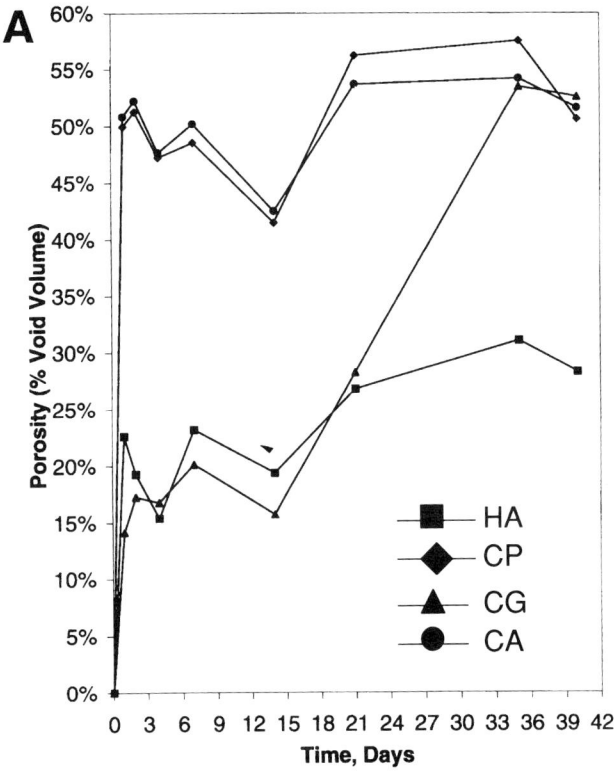
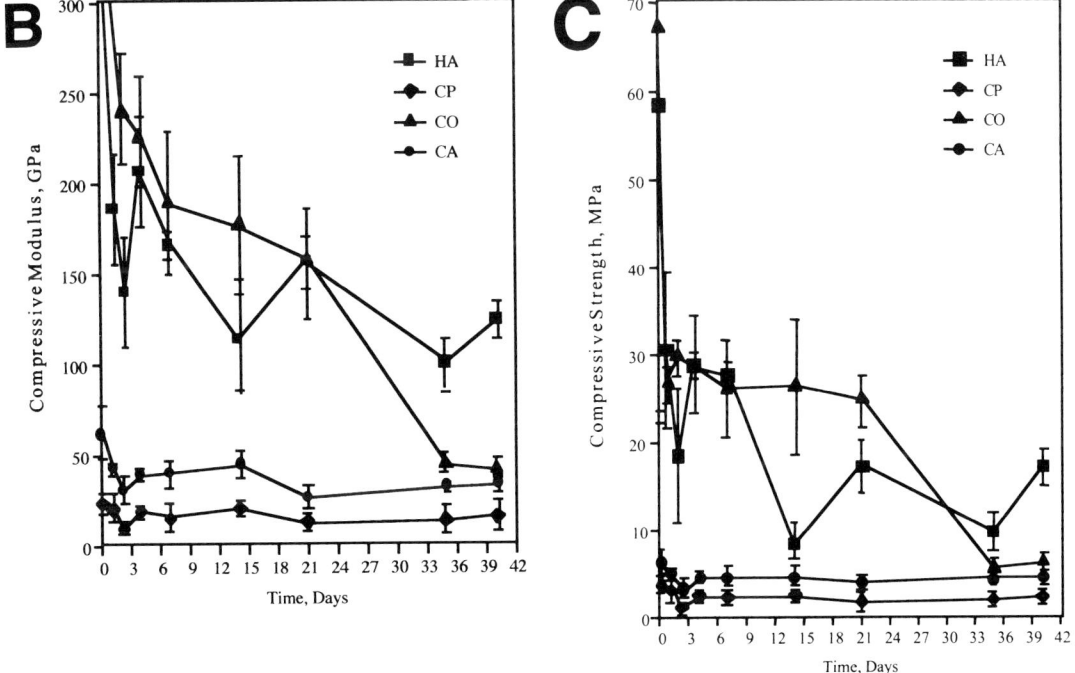

Fig. 4 (**A**) Porosity (% Void volume) vs time for 125–180mm. (**B**) Compressive modulus vs time for 125–180 mm. (**C**) Compressive strength vs time for 125–180mm.

Table 8
Formulation Comparisons

Formulation	HA	HA + CG	HA + CA	HA + CP
PPF + VP, %(w/w)	57.2	75.4	57.2	57.2
PPF:VP ratio	0.375	1.167	0.375	0.375
Sol Salt + HA, %(w/w)	41.6	23.2	41.6	41.6
Sol Salt:HA ratio	0	3.00	3.00	3.00

of the HA and HA + CG systems are reflections of their similar compositions. Although the compositions of the HA and HA + CG formulations are similar with respect to the PPF:VP ratio, total polymer (PPF + VP), and total salt (filler), the absence of a soluble salt in the former (the soluble salt being replaced with HA) contributes to its strength and modulus (Table 8). The HA + CG system has both lower total filler and less HA than the other three formulations. Its high compressive strength and modulus appear to result from both the high total polymer content (PPF + VP = 75.4%) and the high PPF:VP ratio, which results in a strong, extensively crosslinked network. These results suggest that the HA + CP or HA + CA cements could be reformulated with compositions similar to the HA + CG cement, in order to develop similar mechanical properties.

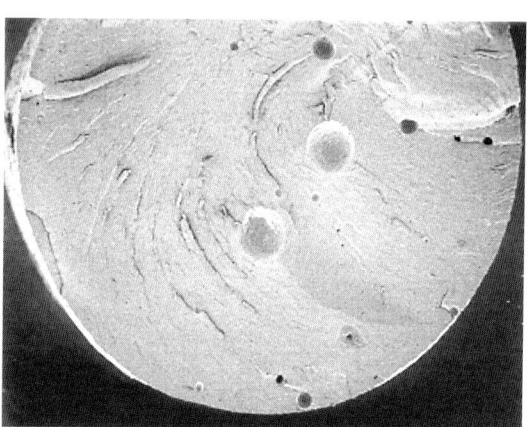

Fig. 5. Scanning electron micrograph of a HA grout (7 d in vitro).

8.1.4. In Vitro Microstructure Analyses: Scanning Electron Microscopy

(SEMs) were taken on an Amray AMR-1000 scanning electron microscope (Amray), and examined qualitatively for progressive degradation at various times of in vitro incubation. The d-7 SEMs are most indicative of the pattern of progressive disintegration observed at later timepoints, and thus were used to evaluate the several formulations. Comparisons of the formulations containing the soluble salts in both particle-size ranges, with the formulation containing only HA, showed the development of pores. Supporting SEM evidence is provided in Fig. 5.

Examination of the SEMs indicated that, of the three formulations including soluble salts, the formulation including CA shows least damage over time on in vitro incubation in PBS at 37°C. In the group containing the soluble salts, more spallation was evident with the smaller particle size than with the larger, although no spallation

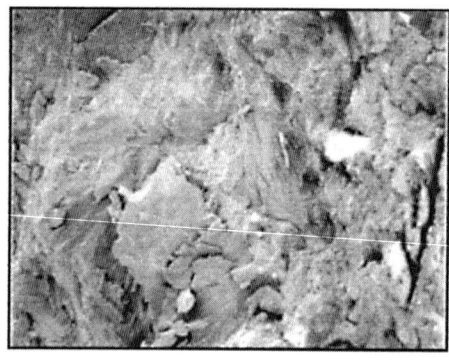

Fig. 6. Scanning electron micrograph of a HA–CA grout (7 d in vitro).

was observed with either particle size of CA as shown. SEMs of the d-7 HA-only and HA + CA formulations are shown in Figs. 5 and 6.

8.2. In Vivo Evaluation

The biocompatibility of the BG substitutes was evaluated in male Sprague-Dawley rats (Charles

River Breeding Laboratories) weighing approx 200 g. Rats were anesthetized with 0.3 mL 10 mg/mL ketamine (Fort Dodge NDA Laboratory) and 0.15 mL 20 mg/mL xylazine (Gemeni). The left rear leg was shaved with an electric clipper, and swabbed with betadine. An incision (approx 1.5 cm in length) was made in the lower ventral portion of the leg, parallel to, and exposing, the tibia. A hole was drilled into the ventral cortex of the tibia with a 75K surgical drill (Walter Lorenz) equipped with a sterile drill bit (1.06 × 5.5 mm). Cured grout pellets, sterilized by 2.75 Mrad irradiation, were inserted into the tibial defect, after which the wound was closed with prolene 5.0 sutures.

8.2.1. In Vivo Study Design

As indicated in subheading, BG substitutes with various soluble Ca salts were implanted into a rat tibia defect model. Four sets of fillers, each having three groups of eight animals each, were included in this study. Thus, a total of 96 animals were included in this study. Each of the four sets was designated to test one of four different formulations. Formulations varied as to the type of soluble salt filler used in combination with the HA (set 1—CA, set 2—CG, set 3—CP, and set 4—control with HA only). Animals were sacrificed in groups of eight, with groups 1 through 4 of each set being sacrificed at po wk 1, 3, 7.

The most promising results were obtained in the CA group, in which the implant remained structurally stable, and did not disintegrate either by dissolution or active resorption from the recipient site. Although there was some moderate infiltration with polymorphonuclear cells (PMNs) at 1 wk postoperatively, this seemed consistent with early postoperative (po) inflammatory changes. In addition, there was increasing new bone formation around the implant, which, at 7 wk postoperatively, was very tight, without any interposition of fibrous or inflammatory tissue. There was osteoclastic and osteoblastic activity at the surface of the implant, suggesting that it was undergoing active remodeling, which seemed to have originated from the bone surrounding the implant, rather than by inflammation or foreign body responses. There were no macrophages present that would indicate implant breakdown or failure by sequestration. Although undergoing active remodeling, the implant remained structurally intact (Figs. 7A–D).

In the CG group, the implant surface was found to be eroded as early as in the first po week. There were multiple areas of implant breakdown, with the surrounding soft tissues being infiltrated by PMNs. There was very little newly formed woven bone in close proximity to the implant, and this remained as such throughout the remainder of the po follow-up period. Moreover, the implant was found to be further disintegrated, and in part replaced by newly formed woven bone at 3 wk postoperatively. There was some new bone formation around the implant, and there were multiple implant remnants between the newly formed woven bone trabeculae, with an accompanying inflammatory component. At 7 wk postoperatively, the implant continued to dissolve. If present, there was a thin, newly formed bone cuff around the implant. In other areas, the implant remnants were increasingly taken up by macrophages. There is some reactive bone formation at the former implantation site (Fig. 8A–F).

In the CP group, there was significant surface erosion, with sequestration of implant material into the surrounding soft tissues at 1 wk postoperatively. In addition, there were multiple areas of implant breakdown, with infiltration by PMNs, with almost no newly formed woven bone in close proximity to the implant. At 3 wk postoperatively, there were large areas of implant disintegration, with multiple implant sequester and some reactive new bone formation. There were also multiple macrophages around these implant sequestrations. At 7 wk postoperatively, there was progression of implant breakdown, with large areas of the implant being dissolved. If present, there was a thin, newly formed bone cuff around the implant. However, there was no intimate contact. In addition, there was less infiltration by PMNs and macrophages suggestive of a chronic inflammation (Fig. 9a–f).

In the control group, containing no soluble Ca salt, but only 40% HA, the implant remained intact throughout the entire po follow-up period. There was no surface erosion, nor did the implant fail in any other way. At 1 wk postoperatively, there was very little accompanying infiltration with PMNs, consistent with early po changes. Additionally, there was vigorous new woven bone for-

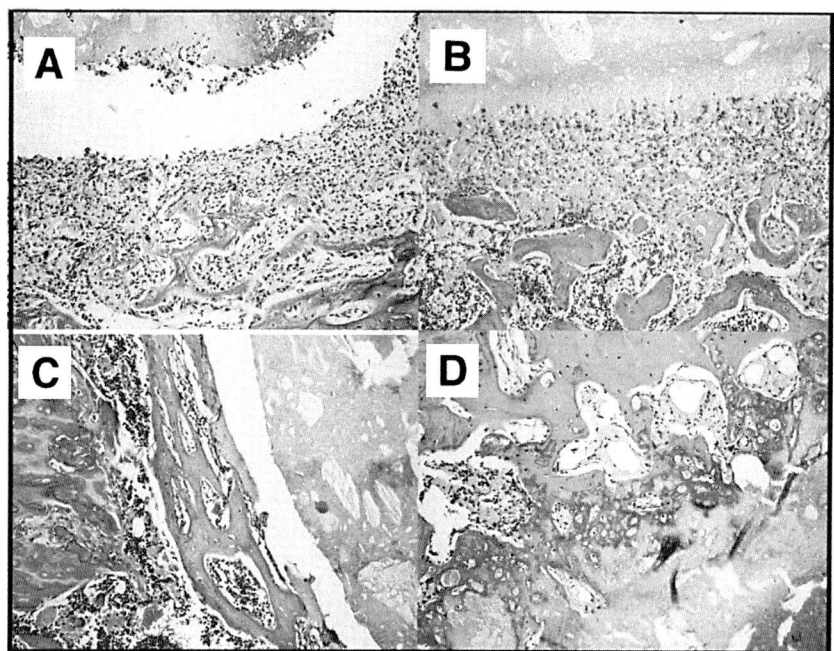

Fig. 7. Photomicrograph of a longitudinal section (H&E) of rat tibia in which a PPF-based bone void filler containing 10.4% HA and 31.2% CA was injected. Plates A–D represent the following different po time intervals: (**A**) 1 wk postoperatively (×10). The implant surface is relatively intact. There is moderate infiltration with PMNs consistent with early po changes. Additionally, there is some newly formed woven bone in close proximity to the implant. (**B**) 3 wk postoperatively (×10). There is intimate contact between the implant and the surrounding reactive soft tissue cuff. There is an increasing amount of newly formed woven bone adjacent to the implant. (**C** and **D**) 7 wk postoperatively (×20). There is intimate contact between the implant and the new woven bone cuff that has formed around it. As shown in fig. 5D, newly formed bone around the implant grew onto the implant in an interdigitating manner, generating a tight interface with active remodeling. However, the implant itself remained structurally intact.

mation in close proximity to the implant. An intimate contact between the implant and a surrounding newly formed bone cuff without any interposition of fibrous tissues had formed at 3 wk postoperatively. Overall, there was an increased amount of newly formed woven bone adjacent to the implant. At 7 wk postoperatively, this continued to form an intimate contact between the entirely intact implant and the new woven bone cuff that has formed around it. Occasionally, there is bone marrow between the newly formed bone traculae. However, most of the implant was surrounded by a dense new bone cuff at the end of the follow-up period (Fig. 10A–D).

These initial in vivo results suggested that the osteoconductive properties of a 85:15-PPF-based BG substitute, containing nominally 10% HA and 30% of a soluble salt filler, can be modulated by the type of Ca salt used. In controls, in which HA only was used, with no additional soluble salt filler, it was clearly evident that PPF-based bone implants containing HA are osteoconductive, and that they can retain the structural integrity for a long period of time. At least for the time-period analyzed in this rodent study (7 wk), there was no evidence of implant failure or disintegration.

By using calcium salts of different solubilities, it appears possible to influence the temporal development of implant porosity in vivo. Together with physicochemical properties of the implant, such as compressive strength or density, implant porosity seemed to be the key factor determining the in vivo performance of the BG substitute. In fact, it seemed important at which time-point after

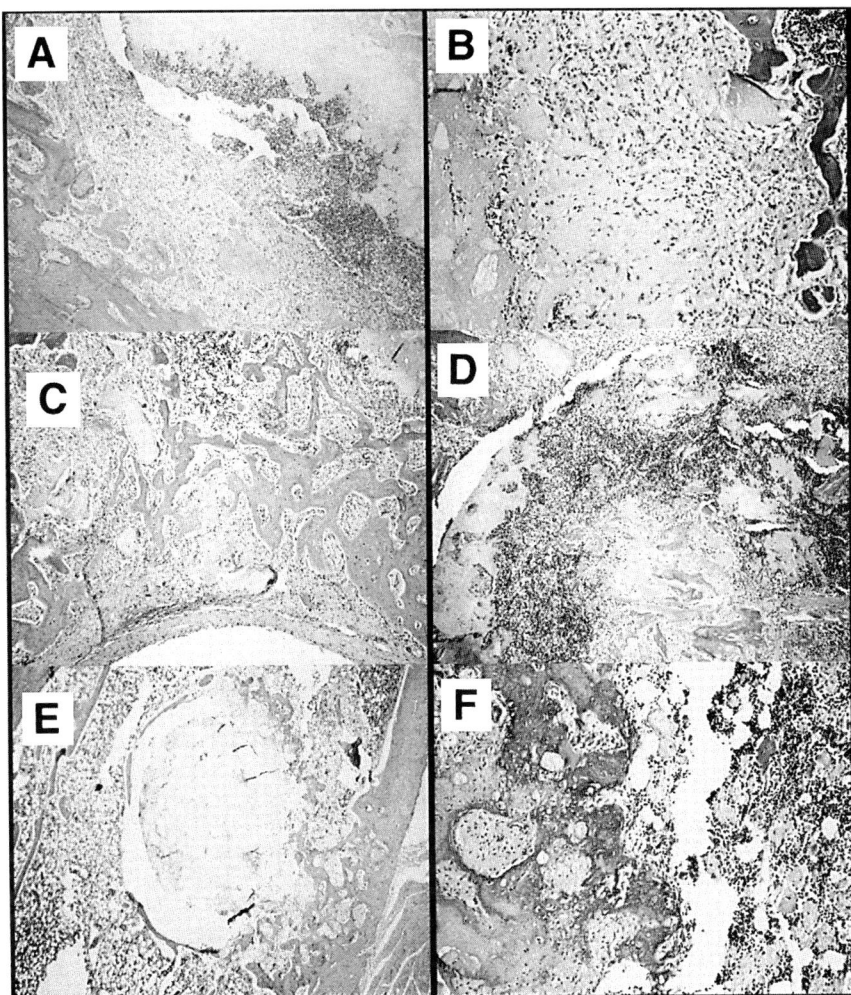

Fig. 8. Photomicrograph of a longitudinal sections (H&E) of rat tibias, in which a PPF-based bone void filler containing 10.4% HA and 31.2% CG was injected. Plates A–F represent the following different po time intervals: (**A** and **B**) 1 wk postoperatively, (×10 and ×20). The implant surface is eroded, and there are multiple areas of implant breakdown with infiltration by PMNs. There is little newly formed woven bone in close proximity to the implant. (**C** and **D**) 3 wk postoperatively (×5). The implant has further disintegrated, and is in part replaced by newly formed woven bone. Between the newly formed woven bone trabeculae, there are multiple remnants of the implant, with an accompanying inflammatory component. (**E** and **F**) 7 wk postoperatively. There is no further change. The implant continued to dissolve. If present, there is a thin, newly formed bone cuff around the implant. In other areas, the implant remnants are increasingly taken up by macrophages. There is some reactive bone formation at the former implantation site.

implantation maximum porosity developed in vivo. In turn, this seemed to correspond with good osteoconductive properties. But, if porosity developed too early after implantation, before sufficient bone material had grown onto the implant, implant failure may ensue by surface erosion, which also could evoke an accompanying inflammatory response. This seemed to have been the case with the CG and CP. However, the best in vivo results were seen with the CA, with which excellent osteoconductive properties between wk 1 and 3 have led to an exceptional osteointegration of the

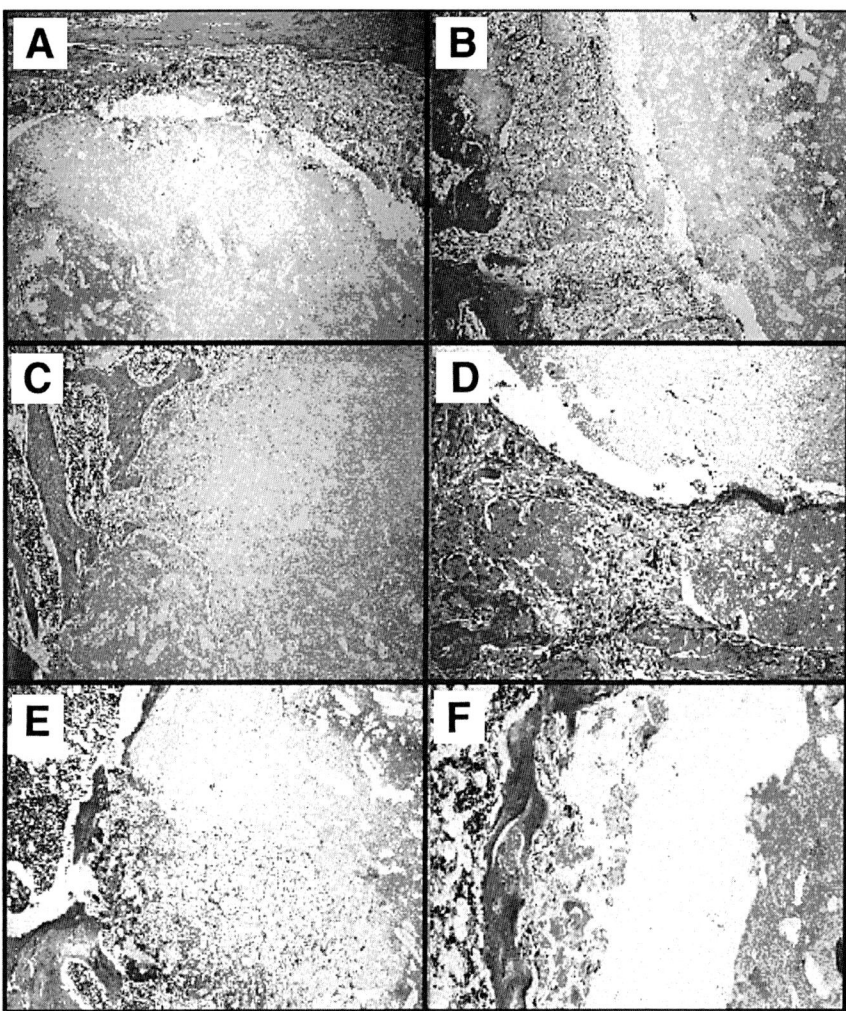

Fig. 9. Photomicrograph of a longitudinal section (H&E) of rat tibia, in which a PPF-based bone void filler containing 10.4% HA and 31.2% CP was injected. Plates A–F represent the following different po time intervals: (**A** and **B**) 1 wk postoperatively, (×10 and ×10). There is surface erosion of the implant with sequestration of implant material into the surrounding soft tissues. There are multiple areas of implant breakdown, with infiltration by PMNs. There is almost no newly formed woven bone in close proximity to the implant. (**C** and **D**) 3 wk postoperatively (×10 and ×20). There are large areas of implant disintegration with multiple implant sequester and some reactive new bone formation. There are multiple macrophages around these implant sequestrations. (**E** and **F**) 7 wk postoperatively (×10 and ×20). There is progression of implant breakdown, with large areas of the implant being dissolved. If present, there is a thin, newly formed bone cuff around the implant. However, there is no intimate contact between the implant and the surrounding bone cuff. There is less infiltration by PMNs and macrophages suggestive of a chronic inflammation.

BG substitute at 7 wk postoperatively. This was unparalleled by the other implant combinations.

This initial study in rats has indicated that optimized modulation of developing porosity after implantation is critical. It needs to be further studied to determine formulations that are structurally stable, yet are capable of developing initial in vivo porosities that are synchronized with the sequence of histologic events of the bone-healing process in the defect sites where they are being implanted.

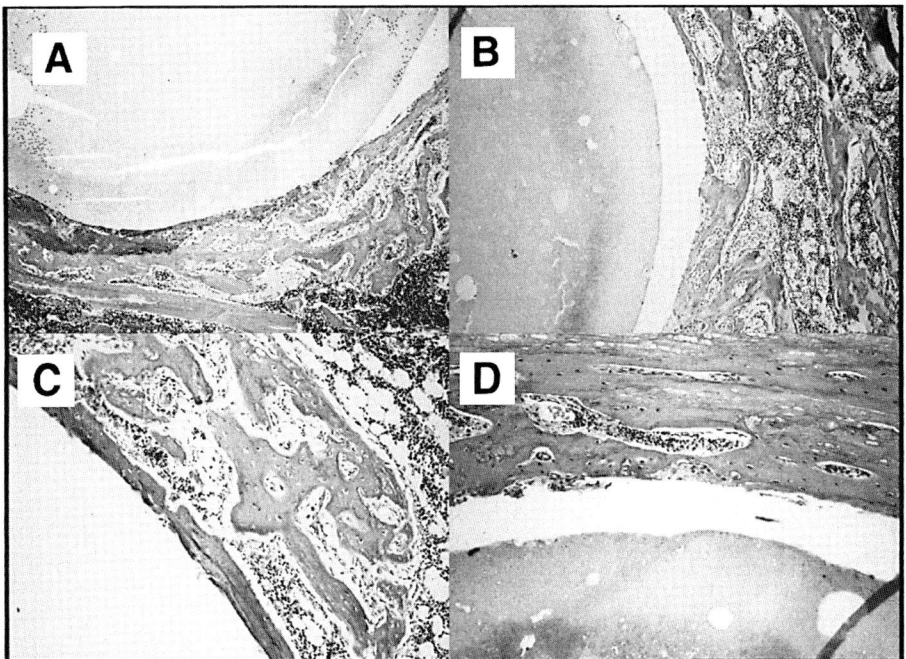

Fig. 10. Photomicrograph of a longitudinal section (H&E) of rat tibia, in which a PPF-based bone void filler containing only 41.6% HA, and no soluble Ca salt (control), was injected. Plates A–D represent the following different po time intervals: (**A**) 1 wk postoperatively, (×10). The implant surface is intact. There is little accompanying infiltration with PMNs, consistent with early postoperatively changes. Additionally, there is vigorous, newly formed woven bone in close proximity to the implant. (**B**) 3 wk postoperatively (×10). There is intimate contact between the implant and a surrounding newly formed bone cuff, without any interposition of fibrous tissues. There is an increasing amount of newly formed woven bone adjacent to the implant. (**C** and **D**) 7 wk postoperatively (×20). There is intimate contact between the entirely intact implant and the new woven bone cuff that has formed around it. Occasionally, there is bone marrow between the newly formed bone traculae. However, most of the implant was surrounded by a dense new bone cuff.

9. Summary and Conclusions

Three types of soluble HA–salt BG substitute formulations were investigated in vivo, all varying with respect to the solubility of the filler composition in combination with the insoluble, but osteoconductive, HA filler. The soluble fillers were CA, CG, and CP, all filler combinations designed to support bony ingrowth, using concepts of both developing porosity and osteoconduction. Of those formulations investigated, that including the HA–CA filler combination showed best results, in terms of bony ingrowth. On the basis of these observations, the HA–CA filler combination will serve as the basis for further development, given its amenability to the design of a degradable (based on its solubility properties) and osteoconductive (based on the inclusion of HA) BG substitute. In vivo biocompatibility and histomorphology studies showed that the cured cement caused little or no inflammatory reaction, and that the inclusion of the osteoconductive HA filler at a 10% filler loading was sufficient for osteoconductivity.

10. Further Developmental Goals

This initial study in rats has indicated that optimized modulation of developing porosity after implantation is critical. It needs to be further studied to determine formulations that are structurally stable, yet are capable of developing initial in vivo porosities that are synchronized with the sequence of histologic events of the bone-healing process in the defect sites where they are being implanted. The ultimate objective of further animal studies should be the development of a designed BG substitute acting as bone filling grout that initially provides space filling with dimensional stability in a bony defect, then an osteoconductive network that degrades at a rate commensurate with bone recovery.

Therefore, further screening studies employing the rat tibial defect model should focus on HA + CA formulations that vary with respect to the HA + CA ratio and content, as well as the PPF:VP ratio. Optimization in rats should be followed by testing and further optimization testing in a large animal model. The purpose of large-animal studies should be the testing of the final candidate formulations employing a cystic defect model of a long weight-bearing bone. Large-animal testing appears necessary, because the amount of BG substitute used is substantially larger. Hence, the contributions of the host bed at the implantation site to the osteointegration of the bioresorbable BG substitute may prove more critical in large animals, and later in humans, than in small animals because, in addition, these types of studies could comprehensively determine the in vivo performance of the BG substitute with use of a comparative mechanical evaluation before its clinical application in humans.

Acknowledgments

The authors wish to thank Dr. Joseph Alroy, DVM, Associate Professor in Pathology, Tufts University Schools of Medicine and Veterinary Medicine, for his assistance in the histologic analysis of this study. Furthermore, the authors are indebted to Shrikar Bondre and Eric Gusek for their assistance with animal care. This work was supported in part by National Institutes of Health (NIH)/National Institute of Dental Research grant no. 1 R43 DE 12290-01A1 (to D.J.T.), and NIH/National Institute of Arthritis, Musculoskeletal and Skin Diseases grant AR 45062 (K.-U.L.).

References

1. Kenley RA, Yim K, Abrams J, Ron E, Turek T, Marden LJ, and Hollinger JO. Biotechnology and bone graft substitutes. *Pharm Res* 1993; 10: 1393–1401.
2. Gazdag AR, Lane JM, Galser D, and Forster RA. Alternatives to autogenous bone graft: efficacy and indications. *J Am Acad Orthop Surg* 1995; 3: 1–8.
3. Lombardi AV Jr, et al. Aseptic loosening in total hip arthroplasty secondary to osteolysis induced by wear debris from titanium alloy modular femoral heads. *J Bone Joint Surg* 1989; 71: 1337–1342.
4. Agins HJ. "Metallic wear in failed titanium alloy total hip replacements: A histological and quantitative analysis". *J Bone Joint Surg* 1988; 70: 347–356.
5. Horowitz SM. "Studies of the mechanism by which the mechanical failure of polymethylmethacrylate leads to bone resorption". *J Bone Joint Surg* 1993; 75: 802–813.
6. Devane PA, et al. "Measurement of polyethylene wear in acetabular components inserted with and without cement. A randomized trial. *J Bone Joint Surg* 1997; 79: 682.
7. Maloney WJ, et al. "Treatment of pelvic osteolysis associated with a stable acetabular component inserted with cement as part of a total hip replacement". *J Bone Joint Surg* 1997; 79: 1628.
8. Zicat B, Engh CA, and Gokcen E. Anderson Orthopaedic Research Institute, Arlington, Virginia. *J Bone Joint Surg Am* 1995; 77: 432–439.
9. American Academy of Orthopaedic Surgeons, Annual Meeting, Feb 22–26, 1996; GA.
10. Gresser JD, Hsu S-H, Nagaoka H, Lyons CM, Nieratko DP, Wise DL, Barabino GA, and Trantolo DJ. "Analysis of a vinyl pyrrolidone/poly(propylene fumarate) resorbable bone cement". *J Biomed Mater Res* 1995; 29: 1241–1247.
11. Wise DL, Wentworth RL, Sanderson JE, and Crooker SC. Evaluation of repair materials for avulsive combat-type maxillofacial injuries, in *Biopolymeric Controlled Release Systems* 1984; (Wise DL, ed), CRC, Boca Raton, FL.
12. Weast RC, ed. *Handbook of Chemistry and Physics*, 54th ed., 1974; CRC, Cleveland.

PART 3
ORTHOPEDIC FIXTURES AND CEMENT

11

Surface Hardening of Orthopedic Implants

Ravi H. Shetty

1. Introduction

Implanted biomedical prosthetic devices are intended to perform safely, reliably, and effectively in the human body for prolonged periods of time. Stability under the imposition of repetitive loading in a hostile environment places unique demands on the materials, designs, and manufacturing methods used to create the implant. Materials used for orthopedic devices should possess good biocompatibility, adequate mechanical properties, and sufficient wear and corrosion resistance, and they should be manufacturable at a reasonable cost. Titanium-aluminum-vanadium (Ti-Al-V) and cobalt-chromium-molybdenum (Co-Cr-Mo) alloys possess these unique requirements, and have found successful applications in the field of orthopedics as prosthetic and fracture fixation devices. These alloys are used extensively in hip and knee implants as an articular surface sliding against ultra-high molecular-weight polyethylene (UHMWPE). The presence of abrasive particles, such as bone, bone cement, or other foreign materials, can substantially increase wear and debris generation rates of the articulating surfaces *(1)*. By increasing the alloy's resistance to scratching, surface-hardened alloys can assist in reducing polymer wear.

In the past, surface hardening of Ti-Al-V and Co-Cr-Mo orthopedic implants have been achieved by the ion implantation and Ti nitride ceramic-coating processes *(2–9)*. Other known surface-hardening processes, used to harden metal surfaces, are gas nitriding, chemical salt-bath nitriding, and plasma nitriding. Of these processes, the gas nitriding process exhibits advantages over other processes, in terms of cost and ease of manufacture. For example, gas nitriding permits efficient batch processing of many parts concurrently in a furnace chamber; the ion implantation process requires line-of-sight bombardment of the work piece with ions, thereby limiting the dose uniformity and number of parts that may be processed concurrently.

It is well known that Ti-Al-V and Co-Cr-Mo alloys can be strengthened by adding nitrogen (N) into the alloy in the molten state. However, this process will change the bulk chemistry of the alloy. It has been also found that, when N is added in this manner, the fracture toughness of the alloy will be reduced significantly, because of change in the chemistry and microstructure of the alloy.

This chapter describes the application of the nitrogen diffusion hardening (NDH) process to harden the surfaces of Ti-6Al-4V and Co-Cr-Mo alloys *(10,11)*, and its effect on the mechanical, fatigue, corrosion, and wear properties of surface-hardened Ti-6Al-4V and Co-Cr-Mo alloy components for implant application.

2. Materials

Wrought Ti-6Al-4V (ELI) alloy (American Society for Testing and Materials [ASTM] F-136), cast Ti-6Al-4V Alloy (ASTM-F1108), cast Co-Cr-Mo alloy (ASTM F-75), and UHMWPE (ASTM F-648) have been used in this investigation.

3. Methods

3.1. NDH Process

Ti-6Al-4V and Co-Cr-Mo alloys are hardened by NDH processes called Ti-Nidium (Zimmer, Warsaw, IN) and Co-Nidium surface-hardening processes, respectively. The Ti-6Al-4V alloy surface is hardened by exposing the surface to an atmosphere of N gas at a process temperature of 566°C for 8 h, while the Co-Cr-Mo alloy is hardened by exposing the surface to a N gas atmosphere at 1093°C for 2 h. The process produces a N-rich region on the alloy surface. N reacts with Ti and Co-Cr-Mo alloy, and forms Ti nitrides and Cr nitrides and solid solutions of N in Ti and Co-Cr-Mo alloy.

3.2. Surface Analysis

The chemical composition and depth to which N has penetrated the surface of NDH specimens were determined by electron spectroscopy for chemical analysis (ESCA), which was performed on NDH Ti-6Al-4V and Co-Cr-Mo alloy specimens by Surface Science, Mountain View, CA. All surface scans and depth profiles were performed on an SSX-100 ESCA spectrometer equipped with a Leybold Heraeus ion etching system and an argon gas source. The surface of each specimen was analyzed in the as-received condition, and then repeatedly ion-etched and analyzed for preset lengths of time, until the desired depth of 2000 Å (angstrom units) was reached. The resulting profile data show the chemical composition of the surface and the underlying substrate as a function of depth.

3.3. Hardness Measurement

Microhardness measurement was made on NDH Ti-6Al-4V and Co-Cr-Mo alloy specimens using Buhler Ultralight Micromet-II digital Microhardness Tester. Microhardness was also measured on N-ion-implanted Ti-6Al-4V alloy, untreated Ti-6Al-4V alloy, and cast Co-Cr-Mo alloy specimens. A 10-g load was used to make microhardness measurements on these alloys. Three specimens were used in each group, and three microhardness readings were taken from each specimen. Mean microhardness and standard deviation from each group were calculated.

Microhardness measurements on NDH cast Co-Cr-Mo alloy specimens were made at 2 g load. Five NDH cast Co-Cr-Mo alloy knees were used for this measurement. The mean microhardness and standard deviation for this group were calculated. Microhardness was also measured from the surface to center of cross-sections of these knees, to measure the thickness of the hardened layer.

3.4. Fatigue Test

Fatigue testing was performed on 33 NDH constant surface stress Ti-6Al-4V alloy specimens from 11 different furnace loads and six control specimens, using MTS servohydraulic machines. All tests were conducted in air, at a stress ratio of 0.1 and frequency of 30 Hz. Tests were run to 10 million cycles (Mcs) or fracture of the specimen, whichever occurred earlier. The 10-Mc median fatigue endurance limit was calculated for each group of these specimens.

Fatigue testing was performed on six NDH cast Co-Cr-Mo alloy NexGen Complete Knee Solution and six control knees. The test method is designed to determine the maximum strength of a single condyle, when oriented at 60-degree flexion. Both medial and lateral condyles were tested under this condition. All tests were run in air, at a stress ratio of 0.1 and frequency of 30 Hz. Tests were run to 10 Mcs or fracture of the specimen, whichever occurred first. The 10-Mc median fatigue endurance limit was calculated for each group of specimens.

3.5. Wear Test

3.5.1. Pin-on-Flat Wear Test

Three groups of metallographically polished disks (measuring 5.1 cm diameter and 0.64 cm thickness), three fabricated from Ti-6Al-4V alloy with the NDH process, three from Ti-6Al-4V alloy, and three from cast Co-Cr-Mo alloy, were evaluated using the pin-on-flat test. The bovine cortical bone and acrylic bone cement pins of diameter 0.90 cm were used in the study. All tests were conducted at 1Hz, using distilled water as lubricant. The tests with bovine pins were carried out at 50-lb load for 700 cycles; tests with bone cement pins were performed at 10 lb, for 350 cycles. The average surface roughness, R_a has been measured across segments of the wear tracks produced on all these disks.

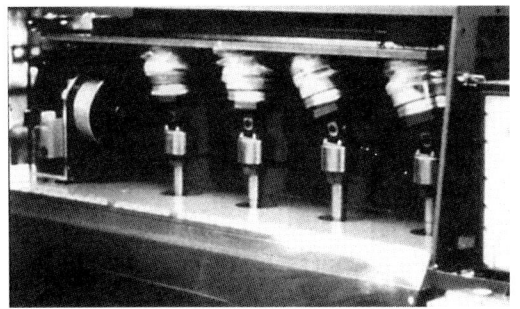

Fig. 1. Knee simulator.

3.5.2. Knee Simulator Wear Test

Wear properties of NDH Ti-6Al-4V and cast Co-Cr-Mo alloy knees have been evaluated in this laboratory using two four-station knee simulators (Fig. 1). The knee simulator cycled through 36 degrees of flexion at 1 Hz, with an articular surface-loading range of 135–600 lb. The prostheses were free to rotate internally and externally throughout the full range of flexion. Each knee test station was maintained near body temperature (37 ± 3°C) and lubricated with bovine calf serum containing 3 g/L sodium azide (bactericide) and 8 g/L disodium ethylenediamine tetra acetic acid (chelating agent for calcium [Ca] ion). The knee joint was environmentally sealed to minimize airborne contamination, which could cause third-body wear. The test specimens were removed from the knee simulator at intervals of .5 Mc, for cleaning, visual assessment, and to weigh the inserts. The insert weights were recorded to 0.01 mg, after correcting for fluid uptake and air buoyancy *(12–14)*. The test was resumed at each interval with fresh serum lubricant.

Two groups of Ti-6Al-4V alloy MG II Total Knee System femoral prostheses (Zimmer): seven fabricated with the application of the NDH process, and four with the N-ion implantation process, were evaluated against UHMWPE articulating surfaces.

Four direct-compression-molded UHMWPE inserts from UHMWPE flakes and four machined inserts from extruded UHMWPE bar were wear-tested against four NDH and four control cast Co-Cr-Mo femoral components. All these polyethylene (PE) inserts have been γ-sterilized to 3.7 Mrad per Zimmer's standard. The inserts and femoral components were paired to yield all the possible combinations (molded UHMWPE against NDH Co-Cr-Mo, and so on) in equal numbers, resulting in a two-level, two-factor, two-replicated experiment. One molded-inserts-against-control Co-Cr-Mo knee (KSB7), briefly ran dry at 1.8 Mc, because of a fixture failure, but its wear behavior did not seem to be adversely affected, except for a one-time small increase (<3.2 mg) in the total PE wear during the incident. Knee KSB7 was excluded from the PE wear data analysis.

The inserts were weighed before the start of the wear test and at 0.5 Mc intervals thereafter. The knee components, their fixtures, and the reservoir were cleaned at 0.5 Mc intervals. Each 0.5 Mc run was started with fresh serum.

To compensate for fluid absorption by the UHMWPE, load-soak samples were run, along with the wear samples. The load-soak samples were loaded like the wear samples, but without the flexion–extension motion of the femoral component. The gain in weight of the load-soak samples was taken to be the amount of fluid absorbed by the wear samples.

The surface roughness measurements and profilometry were performed using a Perthometer S8P Surface Measuring Instrument (Feinpruf Perthen, Gottingen, Germany) equipped with a Focodyn noncontact optical probe. The surface roughness values in the text refer to the arithmetic average value R_a.

The surface roughness measured here is referred to as "microroughness," because it involves an effective tracing length of only 0.40 mm, the minimum length possible with the S8P Perthometer. A small area, typically 0.40 × 0.56 mm, was scanned and chosen to be as free as possible of coarse scratches. The purpose of the microroughness measurement is to determine the local roughness of the articulating surfaces. It may be more significant than roughness on a larger scale (macroroughness) in determining the wear mechanism and wear rates. Macroroughness is dominated by scratches in the sliding direction, which do not seem to affect the wear rate markedly, i.e., even though the number of scratches increases with the number of cycles, the UHMWPE wear rate remains approximately linear. The macroroughness includes the visible and coarse scratches, and gives an indication of the resistance to scratching or abrasion.

The serum analysis for Ti and Co content was performed by Sherry Laboratories (Muncie, IN). Each serum specimen consisted of the serum lubricant charge used for the particular 0.5 Mc interval, because, as mentioned earlier, the serum lubricant was changed every 0.5 Mc. In preparation for the analysis, the serum specimen was agitated on a shaker for at least 24 h, to suspend solid matter and make the specimen quasihomogeneous. An approx 30-mL aliquot of the specimen was then digested with nitric acid, diluted to 50 mL with water, and the metal content determined by inductively coupled plasma (ICP) spectroscopy. The Co analysis was performed on every serum specimen, for a total of 157 specimens (three were unavailable).

3.6. Corrosion Test

The electrochemical corrosion test was performed on NDH wrought Ti-6Al-4V, cast Co-Cr-Mo alloy, and control specimens, using a potentiodynamic anodic and cathodic polarization method described in ASTM G5. A cylindrical specimen of 3 cm^2 surface area was used in the test. EG&G/Princeton Applied Research Potentiostat/Galvanostat Model 273, IBM Personal System Model 70-386 with EG&G/Princeton Applied Research Corrosion Measurement Software Model 342; and Epson FX-850 printer were used in the test. All tests were conducted in oxygen (O)-aerated Ringer's solution (8.6 g sodium chloride, 0.3 g potassium chloride, and 0.33 g Ca chloride dissolved in 1000 mL deionized water) at 37°C. The specimens were allowed to equilibrate in the electrolyte for 1 h. The potential sweep was then carried out, from approx 200 mV negative to the rest potential. At this point, the anodic polarization sweep was started at a sweep rate of 10 mV/min. This was continued until the corrosion current density reached at least 10 µA/cm^2. The direction of the potential sweep was then reversed to the active (negative) direction. The active sweep was continued until the protection potential was reached, when the corrosion current density equaled the value obtained in the passive region of the noble polarization sweep. The corrosion potential, the breakdown potential, and corrosion current density of the specimens were determined from these

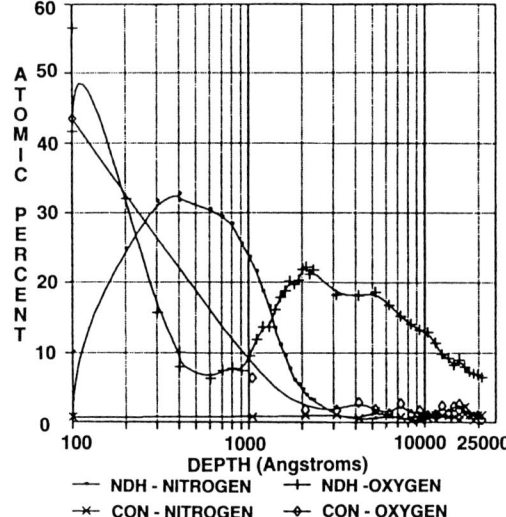

Fig. 2. ESCA analysis of N and O concentrations in NDH and control Ti-6Al-4V alloy specimens.

plots. The Tafel extrapolation method was used to determine corrosion potential and corrosion current density.

For long-term soak test, NDH and control Co-Cr-Mo alloy NexGen knee femoral components were used in this study. Each knee was immersed in a beaker containing 3500 mL Ringer's solution. The temperature of the solution was maintained at 37°C, and the test solution was aerated during the course of experiment. The test was run for 10 mo.

After completing the test, the samples were removed from the electrolyte, cleaned in deionized water, and examined visually, in optical and scanning electron microscope, to evaluate any corrosion attack on the surfaces of these knees.

Atomic absorption spectroscopy and inductively coupled Argon plasma emission spectrometry were used to analyze the Ringer's solution before and after the corrosion test.

4. Results and Discussion

4.1. NDH Ti-6Al-4V Alloy

N and O concentrations on the surface of Ti-6Al-4V alloy are indicators of hardening of the alloy. Figure 2 displays concentrations of N and

Surface Hardening of Orthopedic Implants

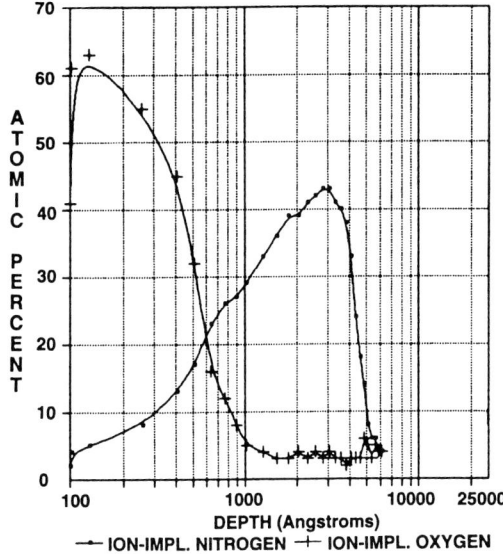

ION-IMPL = ION-IMPLANTED

Fig. 3. ESCA analysis of N and O concentrations in N-ion-implanted Ti-6Al-4V alloy specimen.

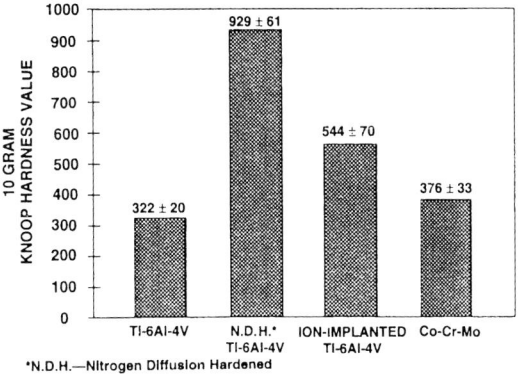

Fig. 4. Comparison of microhardness.

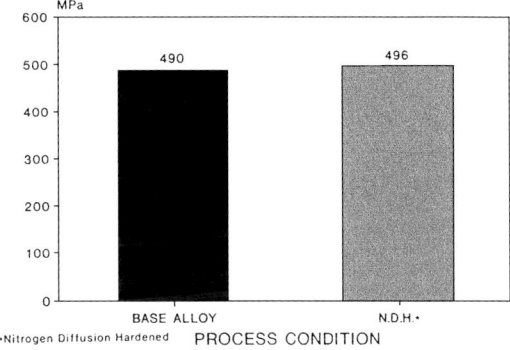

Fig. 5. Fatigue strength of base material and NDH Ti-6Al-4V alloy.

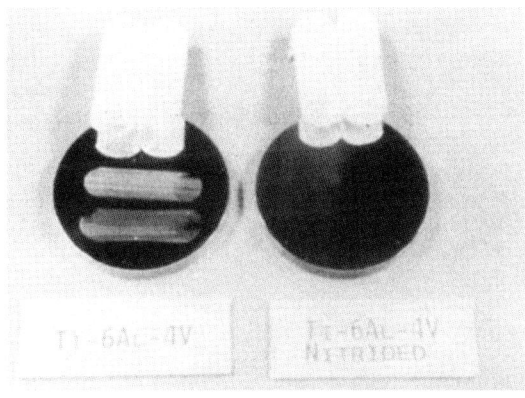

Fig. 6. Pin-on-flat wear results: Ti-6Al-4V (left) and NDH Ti-6Al-4V.

O on the surface of NDH Ti-6Al-4V alloy and control Ti-6Al-4V alloy specimens. Also shown here (Fig. 3) are concentrations of N and O on the surface of a N-ion-implanted Ti-6Al-4V alloy specimen. It is evident from these data that the NDH Ti-6Al-4V alloy exhibits hardening effect beyond 2 µm from the surface, the ion implanted specimen exhibited hardening no further than 0.5 µm. The deep hardening that can be achieved with the NDH process is a clear advantage over the ion-implantation process.

Microhardness ranges determined for NDH Ti-6Al-4V alloy, N-ion-implanted Ti-6Al-4V alloy, untreated Ti-6Al-4V alloy, and Co-Cr-Mo alloy are given in Fig. 4. The NDH Ti-6Al-4V alloy surface exhibited the highest microhardness of these materials. The 10-g microhardness of NDH alloy is 3 × that of untreated alloy, 2.5 × that of Co-Cr-Mo alloy, and 1.7 × that of N-ion-implanted Ti-6Al-4V alloy.

The fatigue strength of NDH Ti-6Al-4V alloy together with the fatigue strength of control Ti-6Al-4V alloy, are shown in Fig. 5. The results indicate there is no loss in fatigue strength of the alloy because of the NDH treatment.

Pin-on-flat wear test results (Fig. 6) demon-

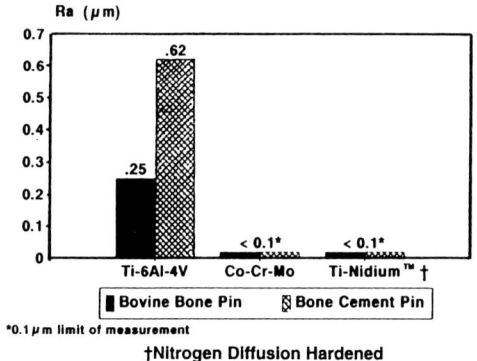

Fig. 7. Ti-6Al-4V alloy surface roughness after pin-on-flat wear test.

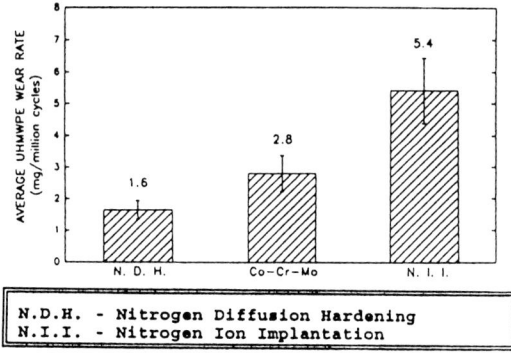

Fig. 8. Knee simulator wear test data for MGII knees.

strated substantially reduced abrasion with NDH Ti-6Al-4V alloy specimen, compared to control Ti-6Al-4V alloy specimen. The wear performance of NDH Ti-6Al-4V and polished Co-Cr-Mo alloy are not distinguishable, based on surface roughness value R_a of the disk (Fig. 7). Both NDH Ti-6Al-4V alloy and polished Co-Cr-Mo alloy surfaces are superior to untreated Ti-6Al-4V alloy surface.

The average UHMWPE wear rates for NDH Ti-6Al-4V alloy and MGII Total Knee System knees and N-ion-implanted MGII knees are shown in Fig. 8. Also shown for comparison, average UHMWPE wear rates (1.6 mg/Mcs for NDH knees, 2.8 mg/Mcs for Co-Cr-Mo alloy knees, and 5.4 mg/Mcs for ion-implanted knees) and their variance are smaller for NDH knees than for ion-implanted knees and Co-Cr-Mo alloy knees. Comparing the NDH knees and the ion-implanted knees, a statistically significant ($p < 0.05$) difference was found, both in the wear rates (2-tailed t-test, log-transformed data) and their variances (F-test). The difference is less significant between NDH Ti-6Al-4V alloy knees and Co-Cr-Mo alloy knees.

Ti content in the serum samples, measured at different intervals in the test, is given in Table 1. The average Ti content of NDH knees is approx 29% lower than that of ion-implanted knees. Lower metal wear is consistent with higher surface hardness and lower serum surface contact angle of NDH knees than ion-implanted knees. Visual examination and side-by-side comparison indicates NDH MG II Ti-6Al-4V alloy knees exhibited fewer and less severe scratches than both the ion-implanted MGII Ti-6Al-4V alloy and MGII Co-Cr-Mo alloy knees (Fig. 9).

The results of anodic and cathodic polarization test on NDH Ti-6Al-4V alloy and control specimens are given in Table 2. The data showed no significant difference in corrosion properties between the two groups.

Table 1
Ti Content in Serum

	Metal content (µg)							
	NDH knees				Ion implanted knees			
Wear cycles (Mcs)	KS89	KS91	Average	Group Average	KS88	KS90	Average	Group Average
0–0.5	28	58	43	—	70	62	66	—
2–2.5	38	36	37	32.3	58	52	55	45.3
5–5.5	18	16	17	—	16	15	15	—

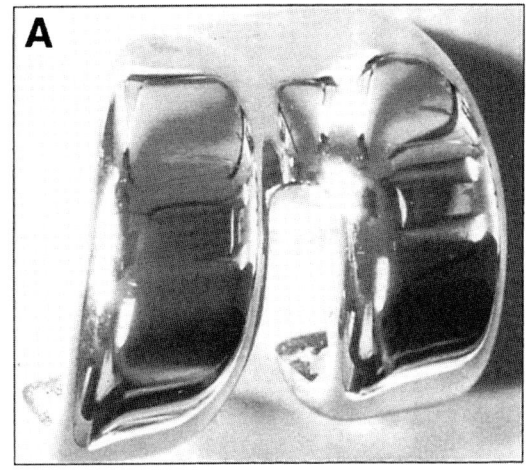

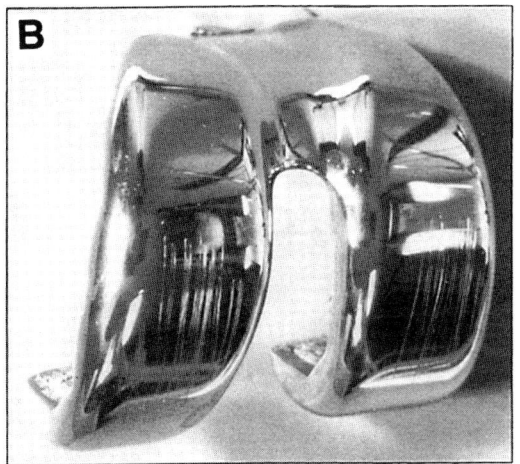

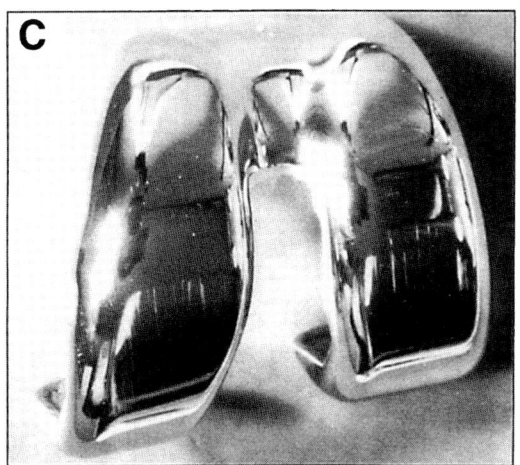

Fig. 9. Femoral knee components after simulator wear testing. (**A**) NDH Ti-6Al-4V at 3–5 Mc; (**B**) N-ion-implanted Ti-6Al-4V at 2–7 Mc; (**C**) Cast Co-Cr-Mo at 3–5 Mc.

4.2. NDH Cast Co-Cr-Mo Alloy

N concentration on the surface of Co-Cr-Mo alloy is a good indicator of hardening of the alloy. Figure 10 displays concentration of N on the surface of NDH Co-Cr-Mo alloy. It is evident from this data that the NDH Co-Cr-Mo alloy exhibits hardening effects beyond 2000 Å.

Microhardness data, determined for NDH Co-Cr-Mo alloy and control Co-Cr-Mo alloy, are given in Table 3. The data indicate that a significant level of hardening has been achieved by the NDH process. The thickness of NDH layer extended to approx 45 µm from the surface. The deep hardening that can be achieved with the NDH process is a clear advantage over other commercially available surface-hardening processes.

Data from the knee fatigue tests are given in Fig. 11. The authors' estimate of the conservative fatigue strength is 600 Mpa (87 ksi) for both NDH and control groups. Data from the lateral condyles indicated a slightly higher strength than the medial condyle. This is because the stress calculations are sensitive to small errors in determining orientation and the exact load point on the knee. There may also be some geometric reasons for the difference in the lateral condyle values. In either case, the comparison of fatigue test data on NDH and control groups showed no significant difference.

Graphs of the group-averaged wear values vs cycles for NDH and control knees are shown in Fig. 12. The overall performance of the NDH knees is clearly superior to that of the control knees.

The group-averaged total wear values and wear rates are compared by means of bar graphs in Fig. 13. An analysis of variance of the total wear values at 10 Mc, using a two-factor, two-level model, indicates that surface treatment is highly significant, but that the PE type is not. No significant interaction was found between the metal and the PE type, i.e., the reduction in PE wear with the NDH femoral components is similar for both types of PE.

The average PE wear rate and total wear were found to be lower for a group of four NDH knees than for a group of three control knees tested concurrently. The average wear rates were 2.08 ± 0.32 mg/Mc for the control vs 1.35 ± 0.14 mg/Mc for the NDH knees; the corresponding total wear values at 10 Mc were 20.9 ± 3.4 and

Table 2
Corrosion Properties of NDH Ti-6Al-4V Alloy

Alloy condition	Corrosion potential E_c (mV)	Corrosion current density, I_c (μA/cm^2)	Breakdown potential E_b (mV)
Hardened alloy	−19	0.0168	932
control	−209	0.0223	930

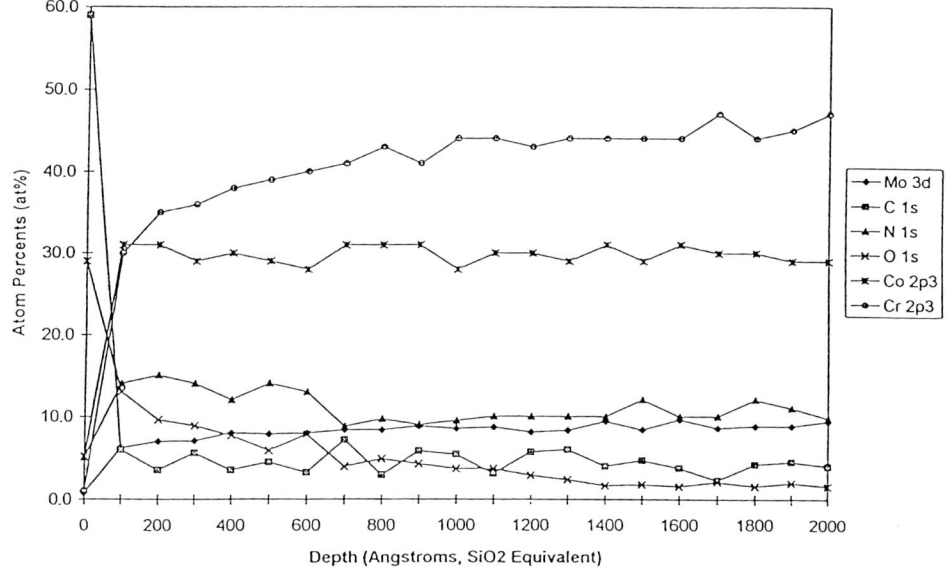

Fig. 10. ESCA depth profile plot for a NDH cast Co-Cr-Mo alloy knee specimen.

Table 3
Microhardness Depth Profile Data for NDH Cast Co-Cr-Mo Alloy Knees[a]

Surface hardness[b] (KHN$_2$g)	SD	Core hardness[c] (KHN$_2$g)	SD	Hardness traverse from surface to core[d]	
				Distance (μm)	Hardness (KHN$_2$g)
853.12	162.23	565.20	43.10	5	991.46
				10	778.70
				15	706.62
				20	691.34
				25	674.76
				30	664.56
				35	671.20
				40	580.02
				45	572.04
				50	564.62

[a]Average of five knees.
[b]Five readings are taken on each knee.
[c]Three readings are taken on each knee.
[d]One reading on each knee.

Surface Hardening of Orthopedic Implants

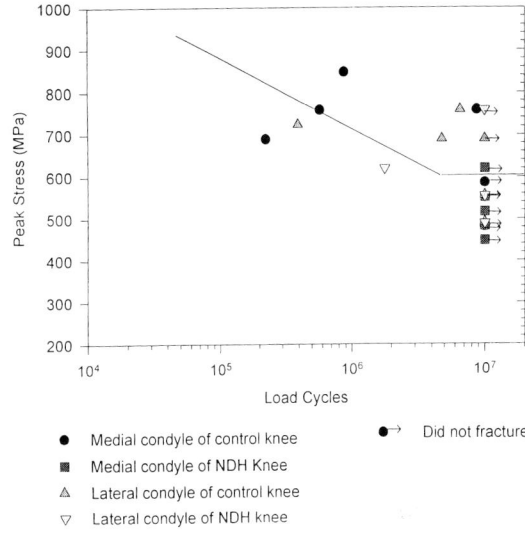

- ● Medial condyle of control knee
- ■ Medial condyle of NDH Knee
- △ Lateral condyle of control knee
- ▽ Lateral condyle of NDH knee
- ●→ Did not fracture

Fig. 11. Fatigue properties of NDH NexGen complete knee solution.

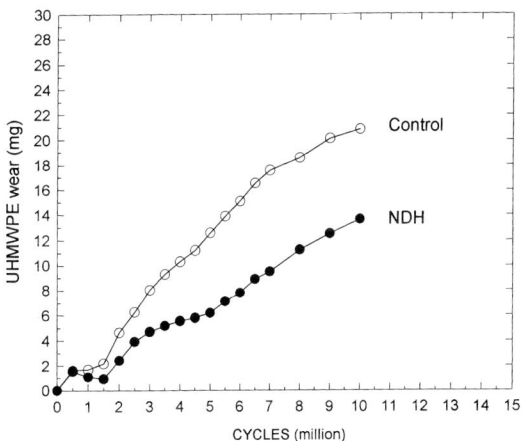

Fig. 12. Average PE wear data for NDH and control groups.

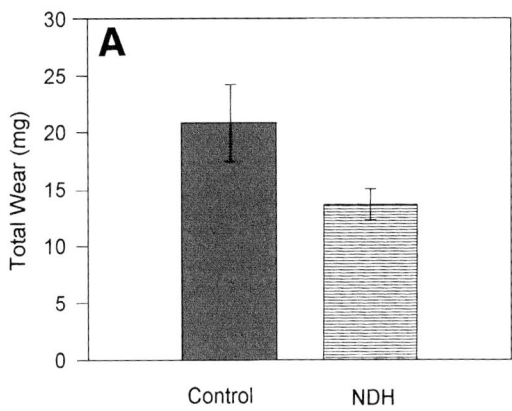

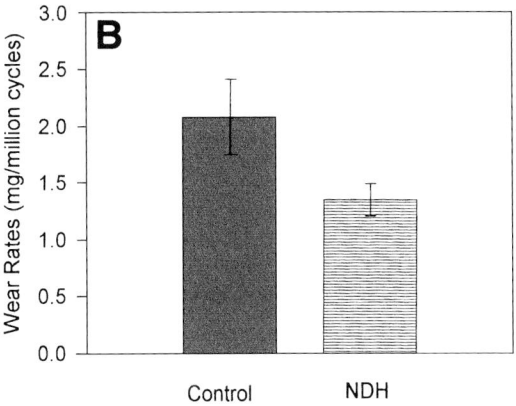

Fig. 13. Total PE wear and wear rate data for NDH and control groups.

13.6 ± 1.4 mg, respectively (the ± value is the standard error of the respective average). These are statistically significant results.

A repeated-measures ANOVA of the wear data indicates a high significance level ($p = 0.024$) for the metal effect (NDH vs control knees). The improvement in wear was similar for both types of PE ($p = 0.50$). The KSB7 knee was included in this analysis. The mechanism by which the NDH knees produces less PE wear remains to be elucidated.

The Co contents of serum samples collected at intervals of 0.5 Mc are given in Table 4. Each value is the metal lost by the femoral component over the 0.5 Mc run, ending at the indicated number of cycles. It is therefore not the cumulative metal loss, but is proportional to the average metal wear rate over the 0.5 Mc interval.

Analysis of the serum lubricant for Co content revealed that the two groups of knees performed comparably, except for one knee, a control component against a molded insert, which had a total Co loss 2–4 × greater than that of the other knees. Although the difference in Co loss between the two groups, NDH and control knees, is not found to be statistically significant ($p = 0.43$), the total amount of metal released per knee after 10 Mc was lower for the NDH knees (0.5–0.9 mg) than the control knees (0.5–1.8 mg).

Table 4
NexGen 10 Mc Wear Test: Serum Analysis for Co

	Group averages and totals	
Mc	Control	NDH
0.5	31.5	20.1
1.0	17.5	9.2
1.5	18.2	20.7
2.0	47.9	23.1
2.5	31.3	22.7
3.0	38.5	24.1
3.5	10.2	10.0
4.0	25.1	13.0
4.5	30.9	6.0
5.0	34.0	15.6
5.5	48.2	33.3
6.0	25.0	26.8
6.5	28.5	11.5
7.0	13.0	17.5
7.5	43.8	30.8
8.0	39.5	44.0
8.5	40.9	24.7
9.0	35.5	23.7
9.5	15.5	21.8
10.0	26.5	26.6
Total Co	**602**	**425**
Total metal	**936**	**664**

NOTE: Each value in the "Totals" tables is the amount of Co lost by the knee to the serum in the interval beginning at the previous Mc and ending at the Mc for that row. The first number in bold at the bottom of each column is the total Co lost (0–10 Mc), and it is therefore the sum of the numbers above it.

Mc, millions of cycles.

All metal content values are in micrograms.

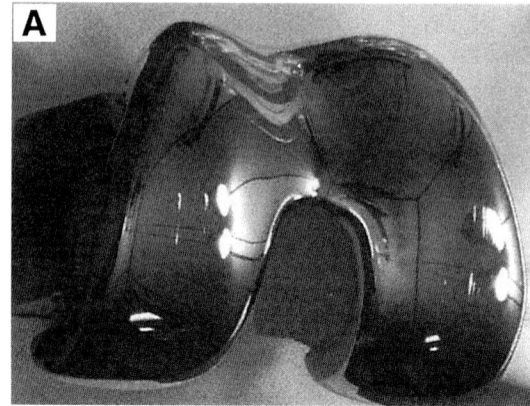

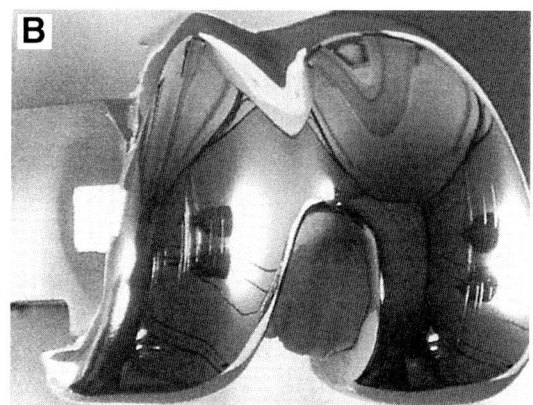

Fig. 14. Photographs of NexGen knee femoral components after 10 Mcs. (**A**) NDH knee; (**B**) control knee.

Visual examination of the femoral components, in the course of the wear test, revealed that the NDH-treated femoral components tended to have fewer scratches than the control components. This is reflected in the average R_{max} values at the end of the test: 111 μin for the NDH components vs 182 μin for the controls. The individual R_{max} values are given in Table 5. Both groups exhibited some deep scratches, many of which appeared during the first 0.5 Mc. Representative photographs of NDH and control femoral components after 10 Mc wear tests are given in Fig. 14.

The initial average microroughness of the NDH femoral components was somewhat lower than that of the control components, 2.36 vs 2.72 μin R_a. However, the average microroughness of the NDH femoral components became somewhat larger than that of the controls during the course of the test. The greatest measured difference occurred at 8 Mc, with average R_a values of 3.42 and 2.31 μin, respectively. The greater roughening of the NDH surface is surprising, because this surface has a much higher hardness than the untreated surface. It suggests that the NDH microstructure is different from that of the untreated surface. Both metal surfaces seem to undergo polishing during wear, as suggested by the final average R_a values at 10 Mc of 2.31 μin (NDH femoral components) and 1.91 μin (controls).

Potentiodynamic anodic and cathodic polarization of data for NDH and control cast Co-Cr-Mo alloy specimens are given in Table 6. The results

Table 5
R_{max} Microroughness Values for Virgin and Worn Areas of the Knee Femoral Components After 10 Mc

Femoral Comp. Test Code	R_{max} (μin)					
	Virgin areas			Worn areas (10 Mc)		
	Left condyle	Right condyle	Knee average	Left condyle	Right condyle	Knee average
Controls						
KSB5	71	60	66	371	127	249
KSB7	32	77	54	137	168	152
KSC6	45	112	78	87	217	152
KSC8	49	35	42	122	231	176
			60 ± 4			182 ± 23
NDH						
KSB6	59	71	65	70	187	128
KSB8	70	56	63	135	109	122
KSC5	35	63	49	76	172	124
KSC7	54	55	54	68	71	70
			58 ± 4			111 ± 14

R_{max} is the largest of the five roughness depths determined for the corresponding five successive sample lengths composing the evaluation length. The ± value following each average value is the standard error. Measurement parameters:

trace length = 0.224 in.; evaluation length = 0.160 in.; cutoff length = 0.032 in.; filter: Gaussian; probe: Focodyn Optical Probe (1 μm).

Values for the virgin areas may be viewed as before test values.

Table 6
Potential and Current Density Values for NDH Cast Co-Cr-Mo Alloy Specimens

Specimen no.	Specimen description	Corrosion potential (E_c) (MV)		Corrosion current density (I_c) (μA/cm²)		Breakdown potential (E_b) (MV)	
		Individual specimen	Average	Individual specimen	Average	Individual specimen	Average
1	Cast Co-Cr-Mo alloy: NDH, color buffed, passivated	−158		4.50 × 10⁻³		621.1	
2	Same	−207	−97	4.61 × 10⁻³		568.4	569.8
3	Same	158		1.75 × 10⁻³	2.9 × 10⁻³	584.2	
4	Same	−179		0.75 × 10⁻³		505.3	
5	Cast Co-Cr-Mo alloy: color buffed, passivated (controls)	−220		1.70 × 10⁻³		562.3	
6	Same	−212	−207	2.05 × 10⁻³	2.18 × 10⁻³	526.3	545.9
7	Same	−194		2.83 × 10⁻³		547.4	
8	Same	−200		2.14 × 10⁻³		547.4	

showed no significant difference in the corrosion current density and breakdown potential (the potential required to produce 10 µA/cm^2 current density on the specimen was taken as breakdown potential of the specimen) between the control and NDH groups. The immersion test results did not show any sign of corrosion on the surface of NDH knees, and there is also no significant increase in the concentration of metal ions in the Ringer's solution after corrosion testing.

5. Conclusion

The application of the NDH process to Ti-6Al-4V and cast Co-Cr-Mo alloy increased the alloy's surface hardness and wear resistance, without compromising other desirable properties of the implants. Therefore, the NDH process can be used to surface-harden Ti-6Al-4V and Co-Cr-Mo alloy implants.

Acknowledgments

The author wishes to thank Dr. Michel Laurent, Steve Humphrey, Frank Jones, Vicky Long, Mike Hawley, Rick Compton, Bill Deerwester, Monna Baum, Dr. Sushil Bhambri, Les Gilbertson, and Dr. Steve Lin for their assistance in this study.

References

1. Davidson JA, Poggie RA, and Mishra AK. Abrasive wear of ceramic, metal, and UHMWPE bearing surfaces from third-body bone, PMMA bone cement, and Titanium debris. *Bio-med Mater Eng* 1994; 4: 213–229.
2. Sioshansi P. Improving the properties of titanium alloys by ion implantation. *JOM* 1990; 42: 30–31.
3. Buchanan RA, Rigney ED Jr, and Williams JM. Ion implantation of surfical Ti-6Al-4V for improving resistance to wear-accelerated corrosion. *J Biomed Mater Res* 1987; 21: 355–366.
4. Martinella R, Giovanardi S, Chevallard V, and Villani V. Wear behavior of nitrogen-implanted and nitrided Ti-6Al-4V alloy. *Mater Sci Eng* 1985; 69: 247–252.
5. Rolinski e. Surface properties of plasma-nitrided titanium alloys. *Mater Sci and Eng* 1989; A108: 37–44.
6. Conrad JR, Radke JL, Dodd KA, Worzala FJ, and Tran NC. Plasma source ion-implantation techniques for surface modification of materials. *J Appl Phys* 1987; 62: 4591–4596.
7. Chen A, Conrad JR, Dodd RA, Worzala F, and Blanchard J. Wear behavior of surgical Ti-6Al-4V alloy by plasma source ion implantation, in *Wear of Materials* 1991; (Ludema KC and Bayer RG, eds), pp. 667–670.
8. Sioshansi P. Ion implantation of cobalt-chromium prosthetic components to reduce polyethylene wear. *Orthop Today* 1991; 11: 24–25.
9. Pappas MJ, Makris G, and Buechel FF. Titanium nitride ceramic film against polyethylene. *Clin Orthop Related Res* 1995; 317: 64–70.
10. Shetty RH, Ottersberg WH, Parr JE, and Crowninshield RD. 1993; US Patent 5192323, and 1994; US Patent 5326362.
11. Shetty RH and Ottersberg WH. 1994; US Patent 5308412.
12. Dumbleton JH. *Tribology of Natural and Artificial Joints* 1981; Elsevier, New York, pp. 283–284.
13. Clarke IC. Fluid absorption phenomenon in sterilized polyethylene acetabular prostheses. *Biomaterials* 1985; 6: 184–186.
14. Lower JL and Price HC. Weight loss technique for measurement of wear of polymeric orthopaedic implants, in *Factors that Affect the Precision of Mechanical Tests* 1989; (Papirno R and Weiss HC, eds), ASTM STP 1025, American Society for Testing and Materials, Philadelphia, PA, pp. 233–239.

12

Orthopedic Applications of Carbon Fiber Composites

Joseph A. Longo III and James B. Koeneman

1. Introduction

Carbon fiber (CF) composite materials have unique advantages for use in orthopedic surgery, because of their excellent fatigue characteristics, radiolucency, and high strength: weight ratios. The materials can be easily manipulated into complex composite designs, to take advantage of each material's biomechanical and biocompatible properties, and minimize their weaknesses in the overall composite design. By allowing individual material properties, mechanical properties, and geometrical design considerations to blend into an overall composite design, composite materials of CF exhibit remarkable versatility for orthopedic applications. This versatility is enhanced by the ability of complex designs or shapes to be manufactured by injection- or compression-molding techniques, to modify the biologic and/or biomechanical composite properties. Surface topography and coatings can be easily applied to permanent CF–thermoplastic composites for use as implant devices, to modify interface conditions with host tissue. The ability to vary stiffness within the composite material allows for matching the biomechanical requirements necessary for long-term periprosthetic implantation, as well as fracture fixation with short-term devices, such as external fixators and plates. Orthopedic radiographic imaging techniques are enhanced because of the relative radiolucency of the CF composites, which also allows for in vitro and in vivo implant imaging analysis, to monitor the structural integrity of the device itself. To enhance their clinical utility, the CF composites can be sterilized by standard techniques; customized to size, shape, and appearance; adjusted to weight requirements; and maintained at reasonable shelf lives. In this chapter the versatility of CF composites is illustrated in a joint reconstructive femoral hip implant and acetabular component, as well as in a unique external fixator device for use in orthopedic trauma fracture care.

2. Femoral Hip Component

Long-term function of current femoral total hip components depends on implant stability, which is a consequence of implant design, implant material properties, and type of interface or fixation. These key factors determine not only initial implant stability, but also long-term effective stress transfer across the hip joint. The ideal implant would allow for anatomic restoration of hip anatomy for joint and gait stability, minimize resection of bone in the proximal femur for maintaining vascular supply and bone stock, and restore the normal strain to the proximal femur in a manner to effect positive bone remodeling and maintenance. Current human design femoral stems composed of metallic materials (cobalt-chromium [CoCr], and titanium [Ti] alloys), and utilizing different interface boundary conditions, fall short of this ideal femoral component in the clinical arena *(1)*. Proximal femoral strain is usually not restored effectively, leading to proximal bone resorption, which is often compounded by techniques used to enhance fixation at the interface, such as porous coating and bioactive hydroxyapatite (HA) coating *(2)*. Current metallic stem designs necessitate an increase in girth in the proximal femur, to optimize canal fit and fill, in order to minimize micromotion. This necessarily increases their overall structural rigidity, compared with the normal femoral cortical bone, thus also adversely affecting femoral remodeling. Straight stem designs require a generous proximal femur resection, in order to fit into the canal, and subsequently have increased micromotion with gait and hip flexion, compared with anatomic design stems *(3–5)*.

In an attempt to circumvent these current clinical problems in human metallic femoral hip components, a CF/polysulfone (CF/PSF) composite femoral hip implant has been investigated in a long-term canine hip hemiarthroplasty model *(6)*. This CF/PSF artificial hip implant design and material analysis has been discussed previously *(7)*. The greyhound was felt to be an effective animal model regarding predictive behavior of bone remodeling, adaptive stress transfer, restoration of anatomical structures and stability, and biocompatibility with long-term performance. Concerning anatomy, the canine has been shown to have proximal metaphyseal region and cortical bone structure comparable to humans *(8)*.

Anteversion of the greyhound femoral neck is similar to humans (12:15 degrees), based on measurement from the central axis of the femoral shaft. Loading conditions are felt to be similar, based on strain gage analysis *(9,10)*. Cortical bone remodeling in the greyhound is essentially 3 × faster than in comparably aged humans (sigma of 60 d vs 140 d) *(11)*, which allows for a more rapid prediction of long-term bone remodeling with a femoral component.

Serial sections of cadaver greyhound femurs were radiographed and compared with computed tomography (CT) scan data of intact femora, to construct an finite element model (FEM). A detailed anatomical study was performed in order to delineate the internal bony architecture of the proximal femur, in order to define the extent of the laminated structures of the calcar femoralis and the greater trochanter. The internal canal, so defined, correlated well with predicted FEM results based on CT scan data, and appeared to define the neutral axis of the proximal canine femur. A gently curved, tapered, antetorted stem was designed to fill the internal support structure of the femur anatomically, thus filling its own envelope upon insertion. This necessitates right and left stems, in order to comply with the internal structural restraints of each femur.

A basic philosophy of bone preservation was followed, and a subcapital neck cut was utilized. This was approx 15 mm proximal to the lesser trochanter in the canine, and would simulate a 25-mm neck cut in humans. The high neck cut allowed for preservation of some of the vascular supply entering the femoral neck through the retinacular vessels and the piriformis fossa, which, in most standard neck-level cuts, are sacrificed. The mechanical advantages of the high neck cut are that it allows for a natural bony restraint to torsional moments applied to the hip with gait, particularly retroversional with hip flexion, such as rising from a chair or climbing stairs *(3,12)*. It also allows for a continued support of the curved implant to varus loading through the compression-aligned trabecular walls of the medial neck and calcar femoralis. The rotation of elliptical cross-sections of the implant increases from the distal tip of the stem to the proximal region. This tapered surface twist of the prosthesis allows for a twist-type, multiple-contact interlock between the stem and the complementary-shaped internal canal of the proximal femur. This allows for utilization of the internal support geometry of the proximal femur, to dissipate the loads in a more natural manner. By retaining the proximal femoral neck region and anatomic anteversion, a derotational or antirotational buttress to out-of-plane forces across the hip joint is maintained. The corkscrew effect of loading the anatomic prosthetic stem actually increases the hoop strain and dissipates the out-of-plane forces. The long-term remodeling response is not subsidence, but, instead, a normalization of the strain of the proximal femur, with a resultant increase in corticocancellous structural support bone. This is demonstrated by the mainte-

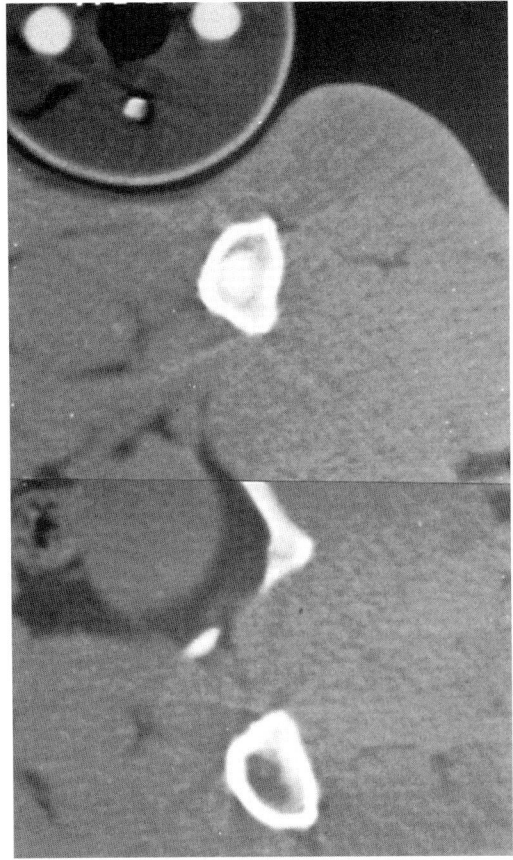

Fig. 1. CT scan of right implanted proximal femur (top) and left control proximal femur (bottom) at 4 yr. Note the maintenance of cortical bone.

nance of bone along the proximal femoral cross-sections on CT scans and contact radiographs at long-term follow-up (Fig. 1).

The proximal taper to the stem allows wedging at the proximal femoral neck cut surface, and interface wedging at the prosthesis–endosteal surface. This accomplishes a biologic barrier to penetration of any debris, by essentially limiting access to the canal. However, this is probably not as effective as a biologic interactive interface, such as with a bioactive coating or surface porous coating. The biomechanical benefits of the proximal wedge are that, with hip loading, an increase in hoop strain occurs. This enhances a continued loading at the neck cut or collar region, which limits resorption of the bone because of disuse. In fact, maintenance of the bone is observed, and actual increase of the cortical thickness is seen as early as 6 mo postoperatively, and maintained at 6.5 y (Fig. 2).

The interface itself is essentially a functionally loaded fibrous tissue membrane, buffering to a circumferential inner wall of surrounding layered trabecular bone resembling a neocortex around the implant. Radially directed trabecular bone patterns emanate to the surrounding corticocancellous endosteal surface, or to the cortex directly (Fig. 3). This is apparent at nearly every section, from the neck to the tip of the implant distally.

A similar soft tissue buffer from implant to a neocortex bone shell is seen around retrievals of long-term, functioning smooth metal implants, such as seen around Austin-Moore prostheses (13), as well as around the smooth portion of most current porous-coated implants.

By maximizing the stem geometry to fit the natural inner-support bone structures in the proximal femur, this stress-transfer technique can be fully utilized. If the stem geometry does not fulfill the internal geometry, i.e., the stem is too small or too large, then this transfer technique is wasted. In the case of a markedly undersized stem (whether a straight or anatomic design), too much of the load may be transferred to cancellous structures that lack proximity to inner (endosteal) corticocancellous strut-support structures. Without proximity to support structures, the cancellous trabecula would be unable to support the load, and stress transfer would occur through the distal stem, with resultant pedestal formation.

In an oversized stem, the internal supporting bony structures are necessarily sacrificed, in order to fit the implant in the cortical shell of the proximal femur. A straight stem would necessarily wedge in three-point fixation, with resultant remodeling, such as distal lateral cortical hypertrophy.

3. Clinical Imaging

The use of composite femoral hip prosthesis allows for improved radiological assessment of the implant–bone interface, and for adaptive bone remodeling. Edge effects caused by the relative radio density of metallic implants hamper the ability to determine changes in the immediate interface of the implant and bond on routine X-rays,

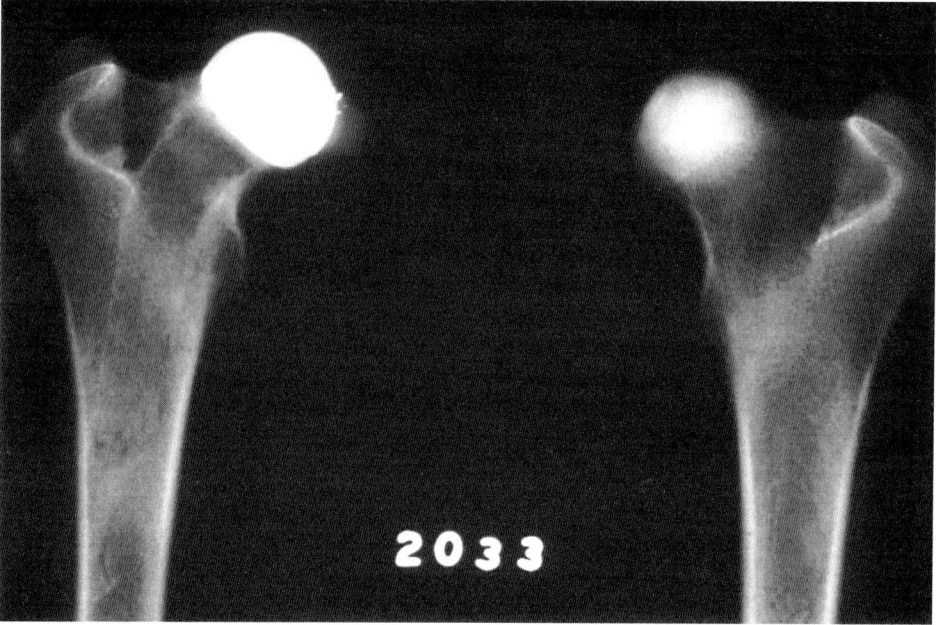

Fig. 2. Explanted femora at 6.5 yr. Note the thickening of the medial cortical bone of the implanted femur (left), compared to the control (right).

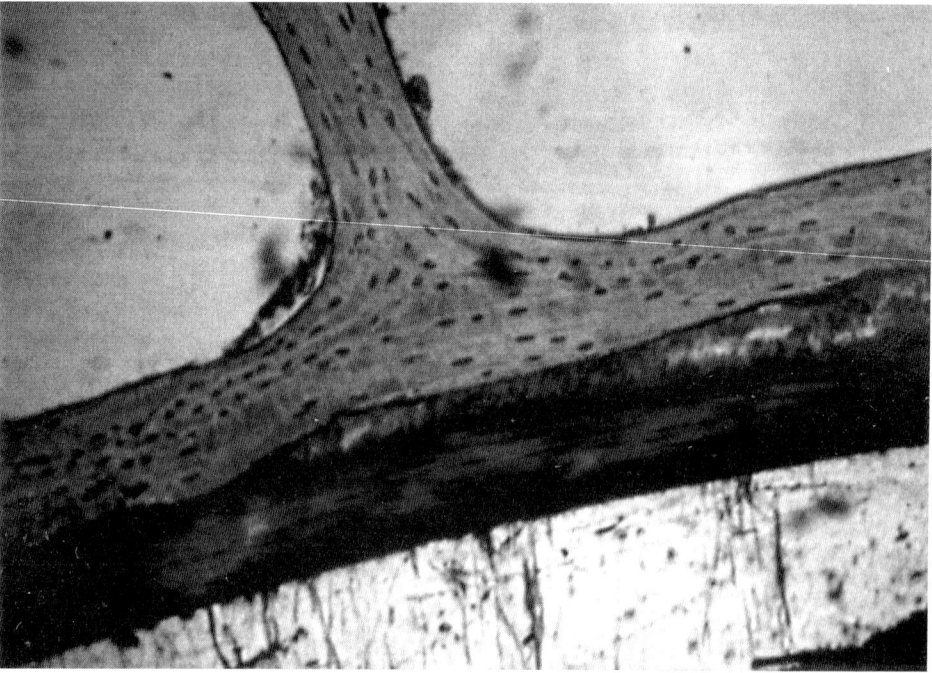

Fig. 3. Neocortex with radially oriented trabecula surrounding the implant (bottom) and a circumferential fibrous tissue interface (ground section histology).

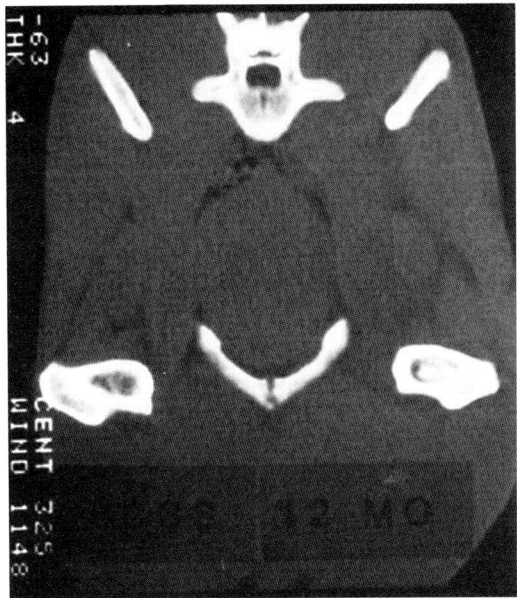

Fig. 4. CT scan of proximal femora at 12 mo. The implanted (right) fills the internal canal, which corresponds to the neutral axis of the proximal femur.

cross-sectional images. Postimplantation monitoring can detect early stress fractures related to material voids or fatigue of the implant, and allow for early clinical modifications to prevent ultimate failure. Fit and fill of the composite implant in the proximal femur can be determined much more accurately than with metallic stems and routine X-ray examination. Quantitative CT scans can be preformed sequentially, to determine changes in bone density with time around the composite femoral stems.

As the quality of X-ray and CT scan images is improved with composite materials, changes in the interface conditions between the implant and bone can be detected and evaluated much earlier with composite implants than with those made of metal alloys. In the canine model, bone changes, such as the identification of a radiodense line at the interface, were seen as early as 4 wk on both X-ray and CT scan images (Fig. 5). Clinical monitoring of the adaptive bony remodeling and stress-transfer changes is facilitated by the use of CT scans (17). Potentially, even magnetic resonance scanning techniques may be utilized to evaluate marrow or soft tissue changes around the composite material implant, without the scatter artifacts associated with metal implants (18).

4. HA-Coated Composite Femoral Component

Early comparisons were made between a group of six greyhounds, each with an uncoated CF/PSF hip hemiarthroplasty, and six with an HA-coated CF/PSF total hip arthroplasty, at up to 14 mo (19,20). Both components in the total hip group were coated with particulate HA, in order to enhance bone–prosthesis fixation. The particulate HA (150–300 µm in diameter) was airbrushed onto the proximal half of the femoral hip component after the PSF surface was softened with methylene chloride. The implant was then oven-dried at 130°F for 24 h, to remove any remaining solvent. This coating technique provided a durable embedded-particulate HA coating in the thermoplastic, much like pebble aggregate surfacing on concrete (Fig. 6). Histological analysis showed the implants to be intact, without evidence of wear, particulate debris, delamination or separation of the HA, or PSF coating at 14 mo (Fig.

short of monumental gross changes of 30–40% density. Image scatter and artifacts caused by large metallic implants effectively reduce the use of CT scans in total hip arthroplasty to gross determinations of implant position or orientation relative to gross anatomical landmarks (14,15). The lower attenuation coefficient of composite materials, compared with CoCr or Ti alloys, allows for improved X-ray beam penetration, thus significantly increasing the quality of CT and X-ray images (16). The ability to image with CT scans allows for the confirmation of achieving the desired implant position and fit in proximal femur. Preoperative CT scans demonstrate the femoral intramedullary void or pseudocanal, corresponding to the FEM-predicted neutral axis of the femur. Postoperative CT scans show the fulfillment of the design criteria, with the carbon composite stem filling the neutral axis canal, with preservation of the internal bony support structures such as the calcar femoralis (Fig. 4).

CT scan imaging can be used to detect gross changes in the structural integrity of the complex composite design in vivo. Early delamination or debonding of the material can be seen on the

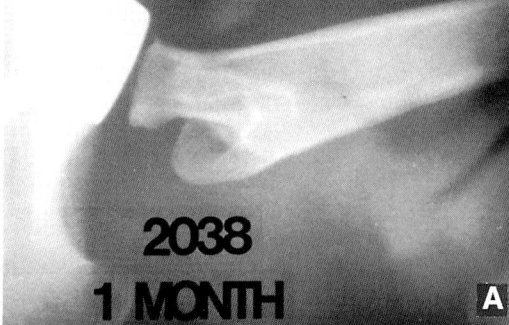
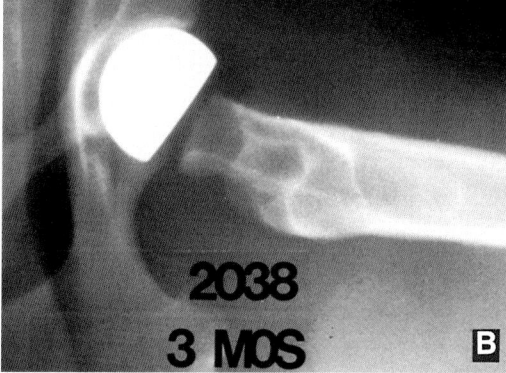
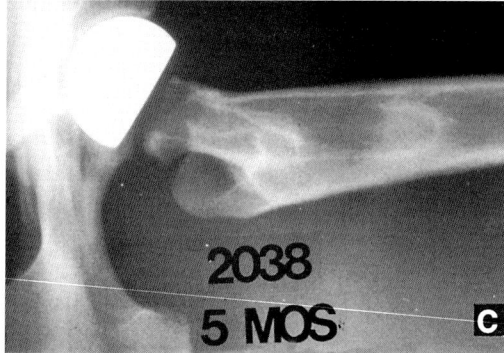
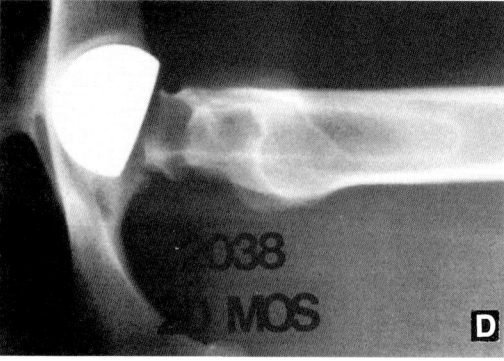

Fig. 5. Lateral radiographs with a progression of the radio-dense line surrounding the implant from 1 to 20 mo postoperatively. (A, B, C, D)

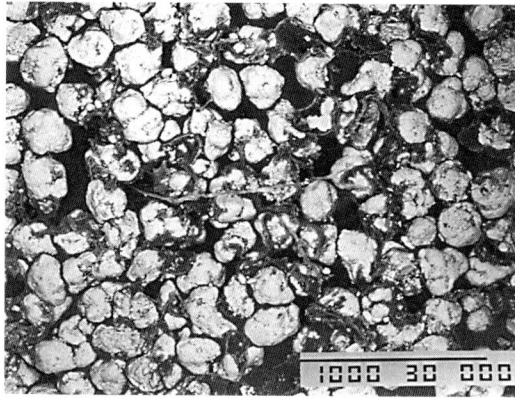

Fig. 6. Back-scattered electron micrograph of particulate HA coating on PSF ($\times$ 35).

7). A slight increase in cortical porosity in the endosteal surface surrounding the HA-coated implants proximally, compared with the press-fit composite components, was evident. A radiodense line of bone was seen around both types of implants at 6 wk, but appeared more dense and pronounced around the HA-coated implants. However, both types of implants were functionally and clinically indistinguishable at 14 mo. A lamellar-type fibrous tissue membrane, with a circumferential orientation, developed around the smooth portions of all the stems. This fibrous tissue membrane remained stable, with little if any change in thickness or appearance, from 14 mo to 6.5 yr, around the press-fit stem types. There is a concern with the eventual disposition of the HA coating, regarding long-term stability, possible resorption, and osteolysis, effecting the interface.

Long-term artificial joint performance is also dependent on limiting particulate debris, which contributes to wear at the articulating joint surface. There has been maintenance of a normal-appearing joint capsule and synovial fluid after 6.5 yr postimplantation with the press-fit stems. Porous PSF coatings have previously demonstrated excellent biocompatibility (21). In the author's femoral prosthesis, the thermoplastic (PSF) effectively encased the CF portion of the composite stem, so that CF exposure at the interface or joint was eliminated. In addition, the unidirectional CF/PSF core Morse taper lock, with the

Orthopedic CF Composites

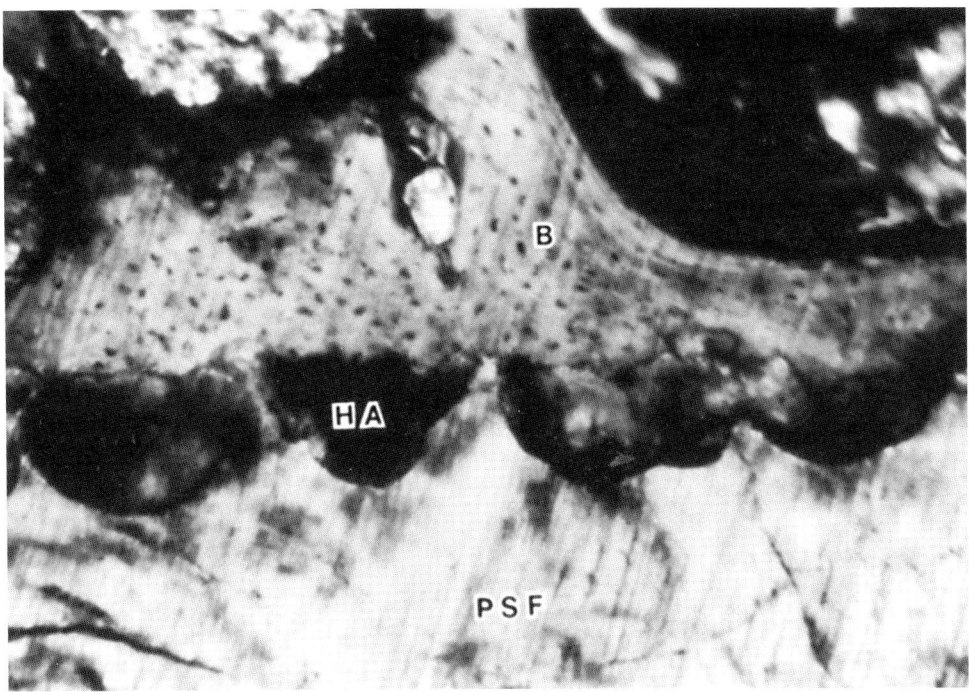

Fig. 7. Apposition of trabecular bone (B) to HA Coating (HA), with the HA/PSF interface intact (ground section histology).

polished Ti head, remained intact and stable at 6.5 yr.

5. Acetabular Component

A hemispherical acetabular component, with diameter (od) of 30 mm (id 18 mm) and a fixation peg 6.4 mm in diameter and 15 mm in length, was designed for canine implantation. Chopped CF/PSF composite was injection-molded around an ultra-high-molecular weight-polyethylene-bearing surface (3 mm thick), with a stainless steel wire placed at the opening of the hemisphere as a radiographic marker for determining position (Fig. 8). Particulate HA coating was airbrushed on the entire convex surface and fixation peg of the implant in a fashion similar to the femoral component. An 18-mm polished Ti femoral head was used on the Morse taper neck of the CF/PSF HA-coated femoral stems for the total hip group. A craniolateral hip approach was used for total group, so that the acetabulum could be reamed to subchondral bone with a cheese-grater type reamer. A custom drill hole was made for the

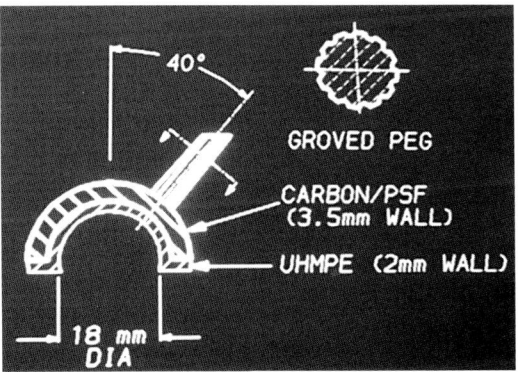

Fig. 8. Canine composite acetabular component design.

fixation peg in the quadrilateral space of the ileum, and the implant seated using mallet impaction. CT scan imaging demonstrated a radiodense line around the acetabular components, at 2 mo postoperatively. Bone remained in intimate contact with the implant throughout the 14-mo follow-up period, with eventual hypertrophy of the subchon-

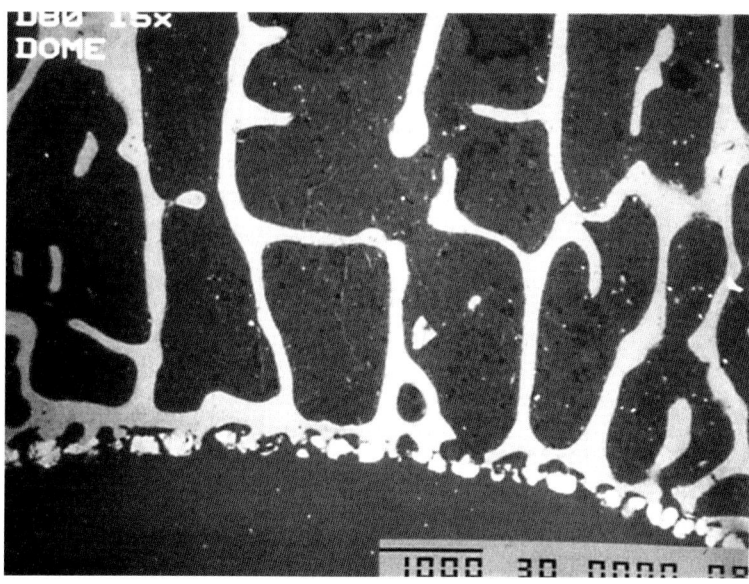

Fig. 9. Back-scattered electron micrograph of HA-coated acetabular dome (bottom) and bone apposition at 14 mo.

dral plate, particularly along the medial wall of the acetabulum (22). Histological analysis demonstrated the composite material to have remained intact, with no evidence of delamination of the implant or HA coating. Back-scattered electron microscopy demonstrated excellent trabecular bone apposition to the exposed HA granules (Fig. 9). A compression trabecular pattern, emanating from the HA-coated surface of the dome, was observed, suggesting physiologic stable-load transfer.

6. Composite External Fixator Fracture Frame

External fixation techniques are currently employed in the management of severe soft tissue injuries associated with unstable long bone fractures or significant joint injuries. They are commonly used for multiple fractures in pediatric trauma or burn victims, and for stabilizing pelvis diastasis or fractures. Current external fixation systems require the use of multiple metallic (primarily stainless steel, Ti alloy or high-strength aluminum) bars and clamps and pin blocks to be built around a reduced fracture, in order to maintain the reduction. The resulting metallic construct is heavy, reduces the surgeon's ability to visualize the fracture by X-rays, and limits the ability to fine-tune reduce the limb alignment. The lack of versatility of these frames increases hospital inventory, because multiple size/length of bars, clamps, and pins are used for specific skeletal locations.

Composite materials have unique advantages for use in external fixation of fractures because of their excellent fatigue characteristics, high stiffness and strength: weight ratios, radiolucency, and ability to be molded into various shapes. A composite external fixator frame (OrthoFrame, Ortho-logic, Tempe, AZ) has been designed utilizing continuous CF graphite-in-epoxy matrix, in order to address concerns with current metallic external fixator frames. The frame is designed with two graphite bars (0.5 in. diameter), octagonal in cross-section, and jointed together by an articulating double-spoon hinge that can be centered over a fracture site or joint. Crossed slots in the central spoon hinge allow for a direct reduction of a fracture of joint, by allowing translation longitudinally, transversely, or in bending, and can be locked in position by a locking nut. The octagonal bar allows for placement of a pin clamp, which can be mechanically locked in 45-degree rotations to accommodate different-size limbs. The pin clamps of the OrthoFrame are molded woven graphite fiber–epoxy composite, and contain a spherical pin holder at one end. The spherical pin holder allows for an additional arc of rotation for a 5.0-mm Ti pin, and can be separately locked, thus enhancing pin placement around a fracture. The frame configuration can be adjusted through the central spoon hinge, from a straight position in varying degrees to an L or V configuration, to improve position across a joint, such as an ankle (Fig. 10).

In a straight-frame configuration, the pin blocks can be offset on each side of the central bar, creating triangular arch between the pins. Thus, a unilateral frame can easily be converted to a Δ-frame configuration, enhancing the fracture stability to out-of-plane and rotational forces (Fig. 11). Other frames must use additional longitudinal bars, connecting bars, and additional pins, to convert from a unilateral to a Δ-frame configuration, which significantly increases the size and weight of the metallic fixator configurations. The graphite bars of the OrthoFrame can be easily cut with a cast saw or reciprocating saw, to customize the frame to the body contour, resulting in a low profile, cosmetically acceptable, lightweight fracture fixation frame. This composite external fixator frame has been used clinically for treating multiple trauma patients with pelvic diastasis, in order to reduce the intrapelvic volume and stabilize the pelvis. Imaging studies, such as CT scans of the abdomen/pelvis, or cystograms, can be performed with the frame on, because it is relatively transparent to X-rays (Fig. 12). Metallic construct frames must be removed, in order to obtain optimal X-ray studies of the pelvis or abdomen.

A downsized wrist fixator, with injection-molded chopped CF pin clamps, was also produced for use in the treatment of distal radius (Colles-type) fractures (Fig. 13). The carbon composite material in a wrist fixator design allows for sufficient strength to maintain and control the reduction of the fracture, without adding detrimental weight to the extremity. The current frame weight is only 85 g. The relatively low-profile, lightweight design allows for an improved patient perception of their use of the extremity. Heavier fixators or designs that are lightweight, but much more bulky in appearance, are a deterrent to nor-

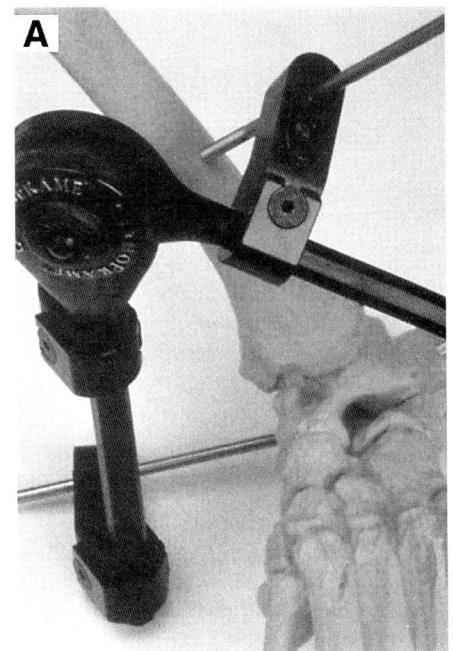

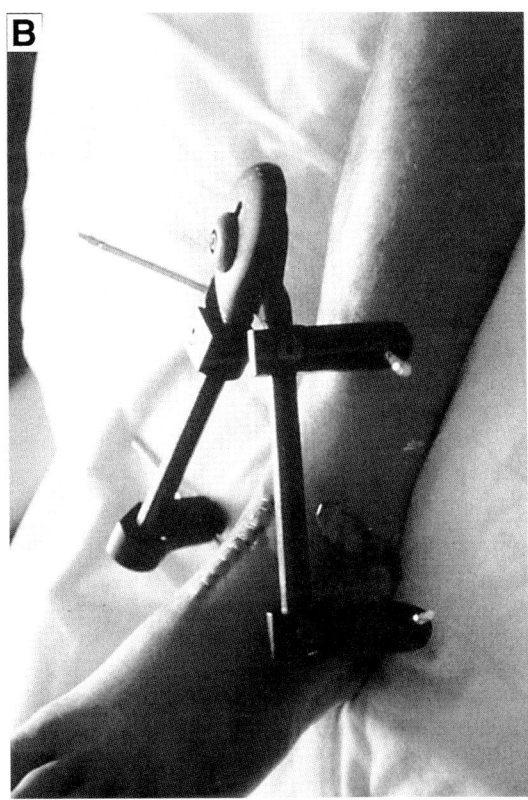

Fig. 10. Application of carbon composite external fixator (OrthoFrame) in V configuration across the ankle, on a model (A) and usual clinical position (B).

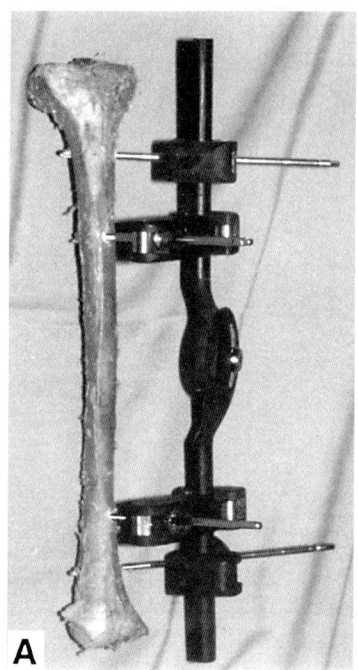
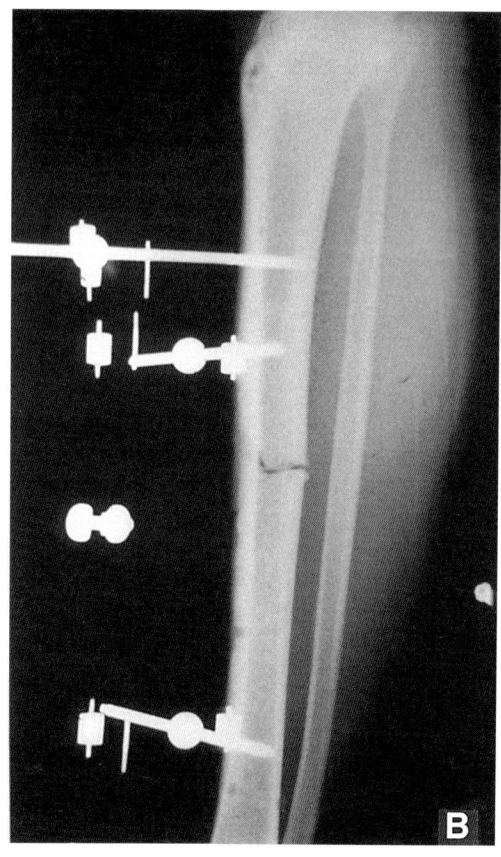

Fig. 11. Illustration (A) and lateral radiograph (B) of OrthoFrame applied to a midshaft tibia fracture. Note the radiolucency of the frame. Pins are in a Δ configuration, with almost 85-degree angulation between the pin placements.

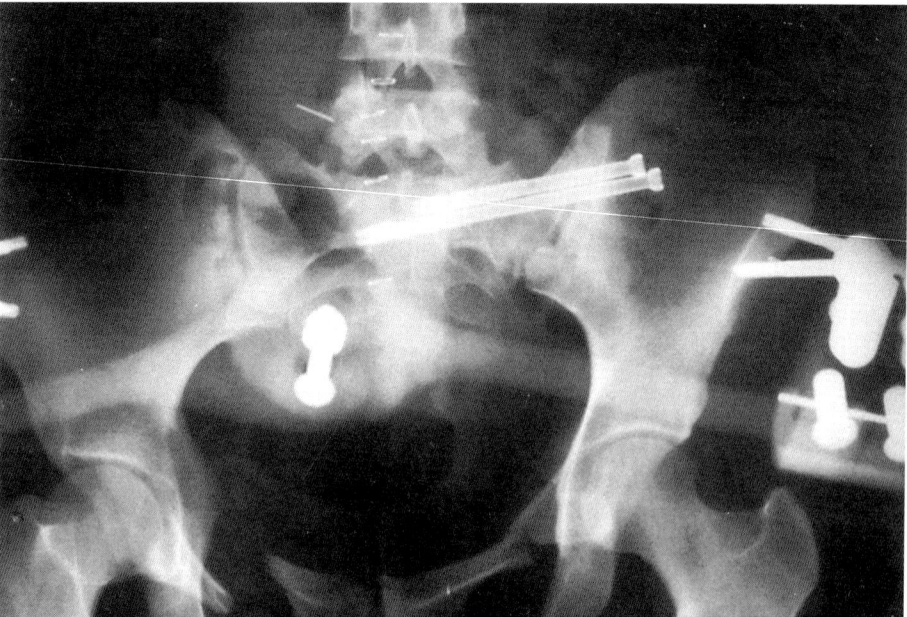

Fig. 12. AP radiograph of a pelvis with an anterior OrthoFrame applied. Additional Ti cannulated screws are utilized to stabilize the unstable posterior sacroiliac joint disruption.

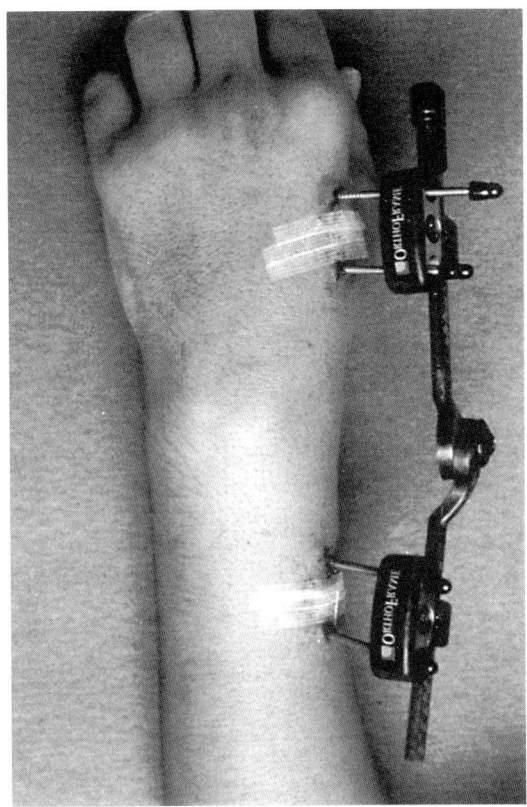

Fig. 13. Smaller version of the carbon composite external fixator used to stabilize and maintain reduction of a distal radius fracture.

malizing function and use of the hand and wrist during active movement. This may lead to an increased incidence of treatment disuse atrophy, swelling, and reflex sympathetic dystrophy complications. This is particularly true in the elderly population, in whom these types of wrist fractures and complications are common. In addition, the size, weight, and design of this frame allows for its use in small-bone and joint reductions, such as pediatric orthopedic trauma of the foot, ankle, and elbow.

7. Conclusion

CF composite materials have been effectively utilized in long-term hip implantation, as well as in short-term clinical fracture fixation. Their use in the formation of a complex composite design allows for the complementary use of each material's properties, to minimize the influence of each single material's deficiencies. For instance, the authors have shown, in this CF/PSF hip design, that the CFs provide structural support to bending forces; the braid provides structural support to rotational forces; and the PSF thermoplastic prevents any adverse biologic contact with the CFs. The thermoplastic coating surface can also be modified from a smooth surface to a micro- or macrotextured surface, or enhanced by a bioactive coating. Because of the relative radiolucency of CF composites, clinical imaging and evaluation by either radiographic or CT scan techniques of long-term prosthesis or short-term fracture fixation performance of CF composite devices is enhanced. The exceptional versatility of CF composite materials for orthopedic applications has been demonstrated in a long-term canine hip arthroplasty model, as well as in a unique external fixator for use in fracture care.

Acknowledgments

The authors wish to recognize and thank the following people for their significant technical expertise and contributions to this work: Allan Weinstein, Frank Magee, Robert Poser, Ron Yapp, Tom Hansen, Mark Phillips, Roger Johnson, Steven Mather, Thomas Lee, Debbie Lumbardo, Mary Overland, Roy Gealer, Janson Emmanuel, Tom Murray, Anthony Villanueva, Ed Koeneman, and Dave Derminio.

References

1. Callaghan JJ. Current concept review: the clinical results and basic science of total hip arthroplasty with porous-coated prostheses. *J Bone Joint Surg* 1993; 75: 299–310.
2. Poser RD, Magee FP, Longo JA, Koeneman JB, and Hedley AK. In-vivo evaluation of four stem interface conditions in a canine hemiarthroplasty. *Trans 38th Orthopaedic Research Society* 1992; 385.
3. Andriacchi T. Personal communication, 1993.
4. Longo JA, McTighe T, Koeneman JB, and Gealer RL. Torsional stability of uncemented revision hip stems. *Trans 38th Orthopaedic Research Society* 1992; p 308.
5. Sugiyama M, Whiteside LA, and Kaiser AD. Examination of rotational fixation of the femoral

component in total hip replacement: a mechanical study of micromovement and acoustic emission. *Clin Orth Rel Res* 1989; 249: 122.

6 Magee FP, Weinstein AM, Longo JA, Koeneman JB, and Yapp RA. Canine composite femoral stem: an in-vivo study. *Clin Orth Rel Res* 1988; 235: 237.

7 Koeneman JB, Overland MK, and Longo JA III. Design, analysis, and material considerations of a composite material artificial hip implant, in *Encyclopedic Handbook of Biomaterials and Engineering*, Part B: Applications. 1995; vol. 1 (Wise DL, et al., eds.), Dekker, New York, pp 171–187.

8 Goel VK, Drinker H, Panjobi MM, and Strongwater A. Selection of an animal model for implant fixation studies: anatomical aspects, *Yale J Bio Med* 1982; 55:113–122.

9 Arnoczky SP and Torzilli PA. Biomechanical analysis of forces acting about the canine hip. *Am J Vet Res* 1981; 42: 1581–1585.

10 Bergmann G, Siraky J, Rohlmann A, and Koelbel R. Comparison of hip joint forces in sheep, dog, and man. *J Biotech* 1984; 17: 907–921.

11 Villanueva AR. Personal communication, 1989.

12 Braud P and Freeman MAR. Effect of retention of the femoral neck and of cement upon the stability of a proximal femoral prosthesis. *J Arthroplasty* 1990; 5: S5–S10.

13 Kozinn SC, Johanson NA, and Bullough PG. Biologic interface between bone and cementless femoral endoprostheses. *J Arthroplasty* 1986; 1: 249.

14 Fishman EK, Magid D, Robertson DD, Brooker AF, Weiss MS, and Siegelman SS. Metallic hip implants: CT with multiplanar reconstruction. *Radiology* 1986; 160: 675–681.

15 Robertson DD, Weiss PJ, Fishman EK, Magid D, and Walker PS. Evaluation of CT techniques for reducing artifacts in the presence of metallic orthopedic implants. *J Comput Assisted Tomogr* 1988; 12: 23–24.

16 Ebraheim NA, Coombs R, Rusin JJ, and Jackson WT. Reduction of postoperative CT artifacts of pelvic fractures by use of titanium implants. *Orthopedics* 1990; 13: 1357.

17 Smith HW, De Smet AA, and Levine E. Measurement of cortical thickness in a human cadaver femur: conventional roentgenography versus computed tomography. *Clin Orthop Related Res* 1982; 169: 269–274.

18 Bassett LW and Gold RH. Magnetic imaging of the musculoskeletal system: an overview. *Clin Orthop Related Res* 1989; 244: 17–28.

19 Longo JA, Magee FP, Mather SE, Emmanuel JE, Koeneman JB, and Weinstein AM. Interface comparison between a press-fit and HA-coated composite hip prosthesis. *Interfaces 90*, September 1990; Bologna, Italy.

20 Longo JA, Magee FP, Mather SE, Yapp RA, Koeneman JB, and Weinstein AM. Comparison of HA and non-HA-coated carbon composite femoral stems. *Trans 35th ORS* 1989; p. 384.

21 Spector M, Davis RJ, Lunceford EM, and Harmon SL. Porous polysulfone coatings for fixation of femoral stems by bony ingrowth. *Clin Orth Rel Res* 1983; 176: 34–41.

22 Magee FP, Longo JA, Mather SE, Yapp RA, Koeneman JB, and Weinstein AM. One year performance of an HA-coated composite acetabular component. *Trans 15th Soc Biomater* 1989; 15: 206.

13

Development of a Bioresorbable Interbody Fusion Device

Kai-Uwe Lewandrowski, Joseph D. Gresser, Debra J. Trantolo, Georg Schollmeier, Frank Kandziora, and Donald L. Wise

1. Introduction

Although low back pain is the most common cause of disability in the adult, Hult *(1)* recognized that neck, shoulder, and arm pain affected 51% of the adult population. This is most commonly caused by cervical spondylosis, with degeneration of the intervertebral disk, hypertrophy of the vertebral joints, and narrowing of the neuroforamen (Fig. 1). It commonly produces neck pain and referred pain to the shoulder and medial border of the scapula. It is commonly responsible for headaches, and produces pain radiating below the elbow, numbness and tingling in the fingers, weakness and loss of coordination in the upper extremities, and, in advanced cases, may result in compressive lesions of the spinal cord, resulting in spastic paraplegia. Usually, this is a self-limited process that can be treated with conservative measures, such as home traction, exercise, anti-inflammatory medication, or a soft cervical collar. For more recalcitrant cases, chiropractic or physical therapy are valuable adjuncts. Occasionally, however, the symptoms do not respond to conservative measures.

The diagnosis and treatment of neck disorders is easy, once it is remembered that the spine has two basic functions. First, it serves as a series of articulated joints that allows positioning of eyes and ears in space, and allows optimal locomotor function of legs and prehensile function of arms. Each motor segment consists of a disk and two facet joints, which are subject to the same degenerative changes that affect hips, knees, and other joints. In some circumstances, when the disk collapses, movements of the affected segment are altered and initiate an inflammatory process in the spinal joint, which can cause headache, shoulder

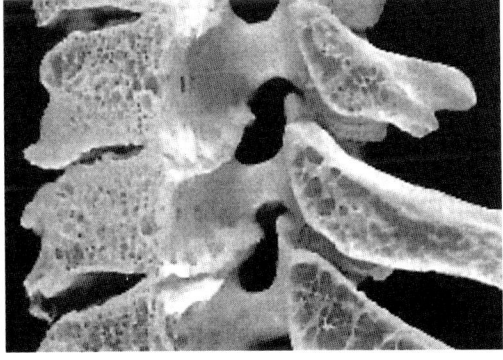

Fig. 1. Photograph of a severely arthritic cervical motion segment caused by collapse of the disk, with growth of marginal osteopophytes, enlargement of unconvertebral joints, narrowing of the nerve root canals, and overriding of the facet joints, which can result in a variety of cervical pain syndromes.

From: *Biomaterials Engineering and Devices: Human Applications,* Volume 2
Edited by D. L. Wise, et al. © Humana Press, Inc., Totowa, NJ

pain, pain referred to the medial border of the scapula, and neck pain. This commonly occurs in the absence of a herniated disk.

The second basic function is that the spine serves as a scaffold for the nervous system. With advanced degenerative conditions, herniated disks, tumors, trauma, or infections, the scaffolding can compress or destroy the spinal cord or spinal segmental nerve, producing radicular pain, spastic quadriplegia, or paralysis. Neck, shoulder, upper arm, and scapular symptoms usually occur as a result of referred pain from compromised spinal joints, not from herniated disks, and compressed nerves. Conversely, pain that commonly travels below the elbow, and produces numbness and weakness in the forearm and hand, is usually caused by a compressed spinal nerve and a herniated disk. Removal of a compromised disk that causes one of the referred pain syndromes will commonly make the condition worse, because further disk space collapse and joint dysfunction ensues. Furthermore, denying the patient with a severely degenerative spinal joint treatment leads to a very unhappy patient, and to a failure as well.

In the past 10 yr, fusions of the cervical spine have been increasingly performed. Fusion of the cervical spine can be done with posterior or anterior instrumentation. However, the anterior approach has been favored, because of the relative ease of the surgical exposure, compared to the posterior approach (2). The anterior approach allows good exposure of the cervical spine from C1 to C7.

2. Techniques of Anterior Fusion

Taylor and Collier (3) were among the first to recommend laminectomy and a transdural approach for excision of a ventral extradural chondroma. Scoville (4) modified this approach for removal of herniated disks, but such procedures were unsatisfactory in bringing about permanent and lasting relief of pain. Adequate exposure of the midline was impossible, and there was a risk of damaging the spinal cord. Postoperative morbidity was prolonged, and, with the exception of the patient with a lateral disk extrusion, few patients improved. Furthermore, narrowing of the disk, compromise of the neuroforamen, and pain

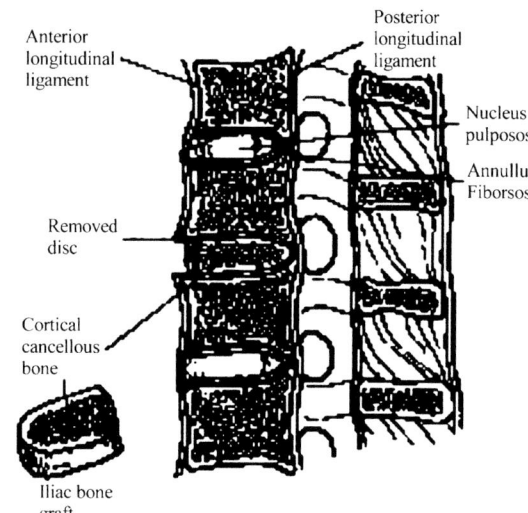

Fig. 2. Smith-Robinson anterior discectomy and fusion with horseshoe-shaped graft, as originally described.

emanating from the arthritic spinal joint, which worsened as a result of the surgery, continued.

Robinson and Smith popularized the fact that "disc degeneration with or without osteophyte formation, subluxations, instability of one cervical vertebra on another, or intervertebral disc protrusions are the pathologic changes usually associated with neck, shoulder arm, and hand pain." They published their results on anterior discectomy and fusion in 1958. Nine of 14 patients had complete relief of symptoms, which correlated with solid fusion of the spine; problems occurred when the small horseshoe-shaped graft collapsed and failed to heal (Fig. 2).

Cloward (2) obtained excellent results in 42/47 patients with anterior discectomy and fusion, using the drill-and-dowel technique. Problems included paralysis in several patients from drilling into the spinal cord. Symmetrical drilling of adjacent vertebrae was technically difficult, making fusion less predictable. The dowel was not an inherently stable structure, and could not maintain fixed distraction. Spontaneous extrusion of the graft was also common, making reoperation necessary (Fig. 3).

Simmons (6) published results on 84 patients undergoing anterior cervical discectomy and

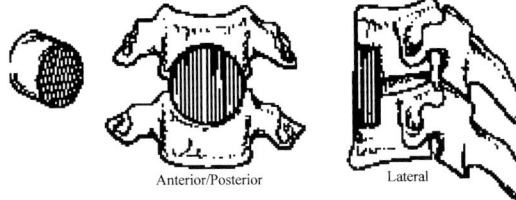

Fig. 3. Cloward cylindrical dowel cannot maintain fixed distraction, and is prone to spontaneous extrusion. Asymmetrical drilling can also lead to nonunion.

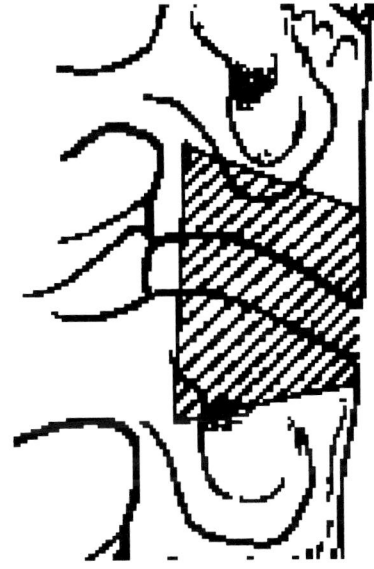

Fig. 4. The Keystone graft which is larger post disk. The graft provides instant biologic fixator.

fusion, using the Keystone technique. Good results were obtained in 80.8% of patients. No patient had a nonunion, and only one graft was ejected. When compared with a cylindrical graft, a one-level Keystone has 30%, and a two-level Keystone 70%, more surface area available for fusion. The Keystone itself is an inherently stable structure, and resists extrusion and lateral bend. Biomechanical tests have shown that the dowel extrudes at 20–25 degrees of extension; the Keystone graft does not extrude until the posterior elements are either fractured or disrupted (Fig. 4).

The Simmons Keystone anterior cervical discectomy and fusion has evolved as an effective surgical procedure in the treatment of these more difficult cases. During this procedure, the intervertebral disk is resected, and the defect is filled with an autologous bone graft. This technique allows excellent exposure of the spine for excision of disk, tumor, osteophytes, or fracture fragments, if necessary. The nerve root or spinal cord can be decompressed under direct vision. It provides instant rigid immobilization of the painful arthritic spinal segment in distraction, which effectively enlarges the nerve root canal and eliminates pain. It results in a high rate of fusion, even with prior surgery, and is associated with minimal postoperative morbidity and few complications. Healing is usually complete in 12 wk, and return to normal activity occurs a short time thereafter. Others report solid spinal fusion between the adjacent vertebral bodies to be achieved within 3–6 mo.

3. Clinical Considerations for Spinal Fusion

Clinically, surgery should only be considered for severe and disabling pain syndromes that have failed an intensive course of conservative treatment. If a patient has struggled with severe pain for an extended period, and chiropractic or physical therapy has not improved the situation, it is unlikely that continuation of the same treatment will be helpful, and surgery may be a consideration. If the pain is less severe, and can be controlled with conservative modalities, then surgery is not indicated.

4. Available Interbody Fusion Devices (IFDs)

Several devices are available for stabilization of vertebrae during spinal fusion that have been developed for replacement of the intervertebral disk (Harm's cage, or hydroxyapatite (HA) and polymethylmethacrylate [7]). Migration of the intervertebral disk implant is a common problem, because of poor fixation of the implant against the adjacent vertebral bodies. Those investigators concluded that anterior instability of the cervical spine, as is the case after anterior resection of the intervertebral disk, requires additional fixation, using a plate (i.e., an Orozco plate). Additional use of fixation material is required to achieve stable osteosynthesis, allowing the spine to withstand skeletal forces under load-bearing conditions. With the objective of minimizing surgical exposure by avoiding additional use of plates, fusion cages were developed for the lumbar spine. These threaded cages provide a stable osteosynthesis between the endplates of vertebral bodies after anterior discectomy.

Other similar implants include the Ray Threaded Fusion Cage (U.S. Surgical) and the BAK Interbody Fusion System (Spine-Tech, Minneapolis, MN). The Moss Cage System is a titanium support that has been used in conjunction with iliac crest autografts; however, complications have encouraged investigators to substitute it with ProOsteon 500, a coralline HA with a mean pore size of 500 μ (8). Thalgott et al. (9) have also reported on a titanium interbody fusion device (IFD). This is a perforated titanium ring, serrated on both upper and lower edges, surrounding a ProOsteon 500 core. The investigators implanted 103 devices in 76 patients (L1–2 to L5–S1). In follow-ups ranging from 11 to 37 mo, no devices had migrated, no evidence of pseudoarthrosis was observed, and no device-related complications were reported. Radiographic evaluation was indistinct, making fusion difficult to prove, probably because of the presence of the HA core.

5. Resorbable Polymers for IFDs

Biopolymers, including poly lactic acid (PLA), poly glycolic acid (PGA), and poly(PL-lactide-co-glycolide (PLGA), appear suitable for development of a biodegradable interbody fusion device. The process by which α-polyesters, such as PLA, PGA, and PLGA, biodegrade is primarily by nonspecific hydrolytic scission of the ester bonds. The lactic acid that is generated when PLA or PLGA degrades becomes incorporated into the tricarboxylic acid (TCA) cycle, and is excreted from the lungs as carbon dioxide and water. Glycolic acid, produced both by random hydrolytic scission and by enzymatically mediated hydrolysis, may be excreted in the urine, and also can enter the TCA cycle and eventually be oxidized to carbon dioxide and water (10). It has been postulated that the mechanical characteristics of such implant materials should at least match the properties of the cancellous bone of vertebrae, as in Table 1 (11).

**Table 1
Compressive Strength Properties of Cancellous Bone of Vertebrae**

Physical property	Magnitude
Proportional limit stress	1.37–4.0 MPa
Compression at proportional limit	6.0–6.7%
Modulus of elasticity	22.8–55.6 MPa
Failure stress	1.55–4.6 MPa
Compression at failure	7.4–9.5%

White and Panjabi (11) also summarize data on the vertebral compression strengths for C3–L5. Of interest are the data for cervical vertebrae, because most spinal fusions are performed between C4–C5, C5–C6, and C6–C7. For C3–C7, compressive strengths are 1400–1680 N (11), although estimates are also reported as high as 2800–4200 N (11). Approximating the load-bearing area of a cervical disk by about 100 mm^2 (1 cm^2), these compressive forces (strengths) translate into 14–42 MPa, significantly higher than failure stress reported above.

Although mechanical properties of PLGAs and the homopolymers of lactic or glycolic acids have been reported, the interest has centered mostly on tensile, shear, and flexural behavior, rather than on compressive properties. One study investigated compressive properties of several fiber-reinforced copolymers of caprolactone and dilactide on exposure to phosphate-buffered saline at pH 7.4 and 37°C. The copolymer of interest contained only 10% of the caprolactone and 90% lactic acid, and therefore was similar to PLA. The initial compressive strength and modulus were, respectively, 21 MPa and 0.44 GPa (440 MPa). After 40, 84, and 180 d in vitro, the strength had fallen to 6, 4, and 2 MPa, and the modulus had declined to approx 60, 50, and 40 MPa (12). However, even though ultimate tensile and compressive strengths may significantly differ, Young's modulus will usually be similar in both tension and compression. Daniels et al. (13) have reviewed much of the mechanical data of PGA, PLA, and PLGA. The tensile modulus of PGA is about 6.5 GPa, and that of copolymers of PLLA/PDLLA vary from approx 2.8 to 5.1 GPa.

6. Spinal Fusion Animal Models

Several animal models have been used to study spinal fusion. Boden et al. *(14)* developed a rabbit model for studying radiographic, histologic, and biomechanical healing characteristics in an experimental lumbar intertransverse spinal fusion model. The cervical spine of the sheep appears suitable as an experimental model, because of accessibility, technical considerations, and the upright position of this part of the animal's spine, warranting sufficient compressive loads. Guigui et al. *(15)* used sheep as an experimental model of posterolateral spinal arthodesis. These investigators evaluated two bone substitutes: coral porites (99% calcium carbonate) and a biphasic ceramic (65% HA, 35% tricalcium phosphate). Both materials functioned well, even though pore sizes differed: The coral had a total porosity of 49%, with a mean pore size of 250 µm (range 150–400 µm); the phosphate ceramic had a mean pore size of 400 µm, with a range of 100–1000 µm. Posterolateral (transverse process) spinal fusion has also been evaluated in dogs, using an open cell PLA (93% void volume) as a carrier for recombinant human bone morphogenetic protein-2. (rhBMP-2), which was applied as a solution to the PLA strips prior to surgery. At 3 mo, 100% of the rhBMP-2 implanted sites had solid transverse process fusion; none of the autografted sites had fused by that time *(16)*.

A viable model for testing graft materials in the cervical spine is the in vivo goat model. Pintar et al. *(7)* compared fusion rates and biomechanical stiffness of dense, nonbioresorbable HA, and autogenous bone grafts for anterior discectomy in 56 spinal units from 14 goats. Autogenous tricortical grafts were taken from the iliac crest. Fusion rates were 55% for the bone preparation and 50% for the HA blocks at 12 and 24 wk, but the blocks were superior at maintaining disk space height. The goat model has also been used by Zdeblick et al. *(17)* to compare allograft bone vs autogenous bone for vertebral fusion.

To assure optimum fit of an biodegradable IFD, the authors studied the anatomy of the sheep's cervical spine. Figures 5–8 show the anatomical situs of the sheep cervical spine and the placement of the IFD. On the basis of these anatomical considerations in the sheep animal model, the authors

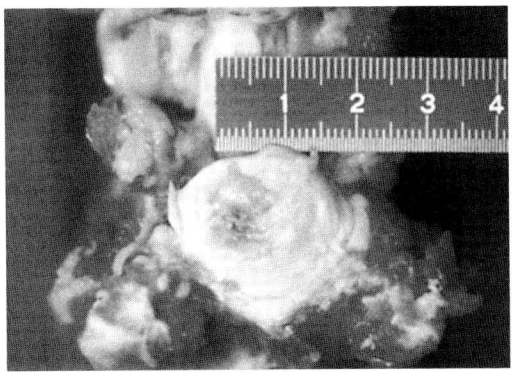

Fig. 5. Anatomical situs after dissection of the C5–C6 segment, showing the intervertebral disk.

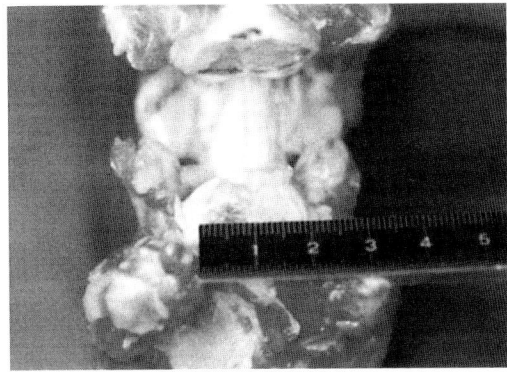

Fig. 6. Anatomical situs after dissection of the C5–C6 segment, showing the adjacent endplates at the top and bottom, the spinal cord (middle), and the facet joints (left and right).

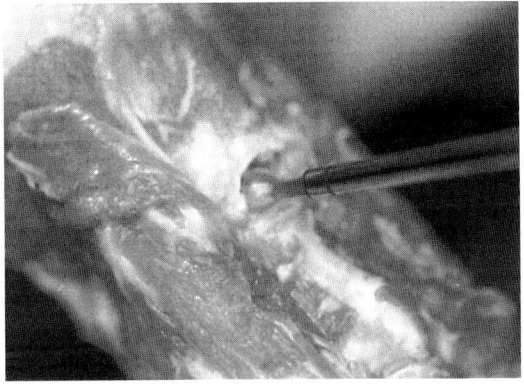

Fig. 7. Placement of an IFD at the C5–C6 level.

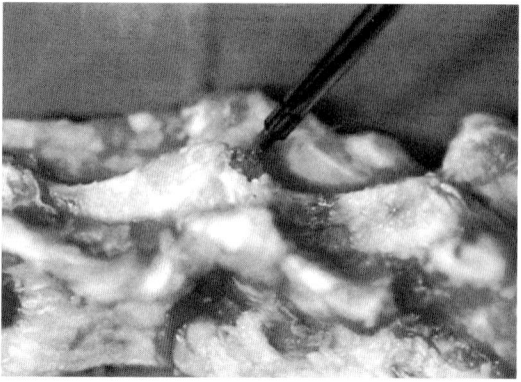

Fig. 8. Placement of an IFD at the C5–C6 level. Lateral view showing the oblique orientation of the fusion device.

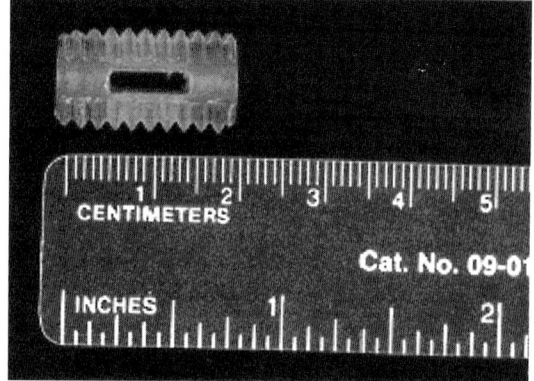

Fig. 9. Resorbable spinal cage.

designed a suitable IFD resembling a self-tapering hollow screw with longitudinal and perpendicular perforations.

This device is described in the following in more detail.

7. Fabrication and Preliminary Characterization of a Resorbable Spinal Implant

The practicability of designing and fabricating a spinal implant from a biocompatible and biodegradable polyester was investigated. One design is an adaptation of that described in US patent 5609636 (18) assigned to Spine-Tech. This device, referred to as a spinal cage, is described, as quoted here: "An implant for use in spinal stabilization includes four generally linear thread segments. The thread segments are maintained and spaced apart alignment by rigid supports. The thread segments include a plurality of individual threads with the individual threads of the segments defining a thread pattern. The supports and the thread segments define a hollow implant interior exposed to an exterior of the implant" (18). A photograph of a resorbable fabricated cage is shown in Fig. 9. The purpose of preparing this device was to establish that complex geometries could be prepared easily by machining a molded rod from PLGA-85:15 material, and that fabrication could be accomplished with or without

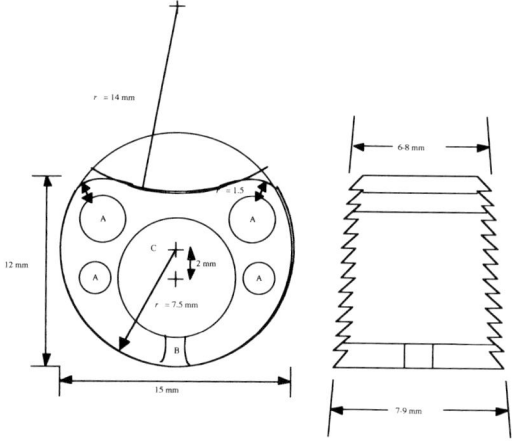

Fig. 10. Design of the proposed IFD. A, holes of arbitrary diameter may be drilled through the device to facilitate resorption; B, channel or port for introduction of autologous bone; C, large center hole for autologous bone.

including extraneous materials, such as plasticizers or other machining aids, in the polymer.

The authors' fabrication of one wedge-type IFD, PLGA-85:15 (Resomer RG 506, Boehringer-Ingelheim, Germany, mol wt = 98,000) was molded at 57°C at a pressure of 135 MPa (19,500 psi) to form a clear cylindrical rod with a 1.3-cm diameter. The device was then machined to the dimensions shown in Fig. 10. Figure 11 is a photograph of the device.

Cylinders of this polymer, measuring 5.96 ± 0.08 mm in diameter by 10.26 ± 0.28 in length, were molded under the same conditions. Com-

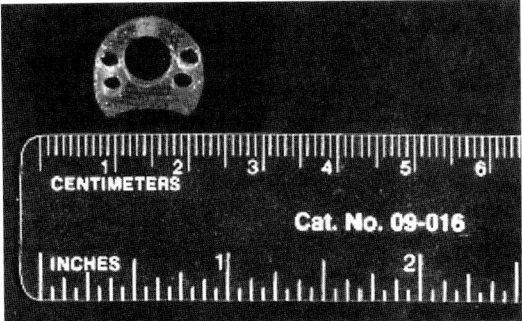

Fig. 11. Resorbable IFD.

pressive strength and modulus, measured in triplicate, were, respectively, 66.0 ± 2.6 Mpa and 1.24 ± 0.20 Gpa. The compressive strength may be compared with values reported by Carter and Hayes, who measured this property as a function of strain rate and density. The relationship between these parameters is $S = 68\ \varepsilon^{0.06}\rho^2$, where S is the compressive strength (MPa); ε, the strain rate (s^{-1}); and ρ, the density (g/cm^3). At a strain rate of 0.01/s, the compressive strength of trabecular bone ($\rho = 0.31$ g/cm^3) is 5.0 MPa, and for cortical bone ($\rho = 2.0$ g/cm^3) is 200 MPa. White and Panjabi *(11)* report dimensions and stresses to which thoracic vertebrae are subject. The average area of the upper and lower endplates of T1 is about 340 mm^2, and is subject to a loading force of about 2000 N; thus, the compressive pressure is about 6 MPa. Thus, the initial strength of the PLGA-85:15 is in excess of the stress to which cervical vertebrae will be subject.

8. Discussion

The technical objectives of this project were directed toward the evaluation of a biocompatible, resorbable IFD for maintaining spacing and alignment of cervical vertebrae during the process of spinal fusion. The IFD is fabricated from PLGA, a polyester that, on contact with body fluids, hydrolyzes slowly to lactic and glycolic acids. The design of the IFD and the PLGA co-monomer ratio (i.e., lactide:glycolide ratio) should enable the device to function through the four stages of healing, with progressive loss of mass and strength. Based on reported degradation rates and the size of the implant, the authors estimate that, in clinically stable situations, at the end of stage I of fusion healing (approx 6 wk), the device should retain 70–80% of its mechanical strength, and at the end of stage II of fusion healing (after approx 12 wk), 50% of its strength should be retained. During stages III and IV, further slow degradation should occur, with complete resorption by 1 yr.

A prototype device was prepared that will be used for future in vitro determination of weight loss and failure strength as a function of time. Because of the asymmetric design of the IFD, it is not feasible to measure the compressive modulus of the in vitro prototypes over time. This parameter, as well as failure and ultimate strength over time in vitro, should therefore be measured on cylindrical disks of the same overall dimensions. In vitro experiments will also allow monitoring of the change in mol wt in time for correlation to the mechanical measurements.

Prototype devices will also be prepared for feasibility trials, using the sheep cervical spine as the animal model. In this planned large-animal study, the fusion rate and biomechanical stiffness will be evaluated for fused spinal segments. In addition, radiographic and biomechanical assessment of fusion, including a histological analysis, will be performed. The results will be compared to conventional autologous bone grafts; the goal of the proposed device to establish superior union and eliminate fusion nonunions.

Acknowledgments

This work was supported in part by an internal research project of Cambridge Scientific, and National Institutes of Health/National Institute of Arthritis, Musculoskeletal and Skin Diseases Grant AR 45062 (to K.-U. L.).

References

1 Hult L. Munkfors investigation. *Acta Orthop Scand* 1954; 16 (Suppl): 1.
2 Cloward RB. Anterior approach for removal of ruptured cervical discs. *J Neurosurg* 1958; 15: 602.
3 Taylor R and Collier J. Occurrence of optic neuritis in lesions of the spinal cord injury, tumor, myelitis. *Brain* 1901; 24: 532.

4. Scoville WB. Types of cervical disc lesions and their surgical approaches. *JAMA* 1966; 196: 479.
5. Robinson PA and Smith GW. Treatment of certain cervical spine disorders by the anterior removal of the intervertebral disc and interbody fusion. *J Bone Joint Surg* 1958; 40A: 607.
6. Simmons EH and Bhalla SK. Anterior cervical discectomy and fusion: a clinical and biomechanical study with a year follow-up. *J Bone Joint Surg* 1969; 51B: 225.
7. Pintar FA, Maiman DJ, Hollowell JP, Yoganandan N, Droese KW, Reinartz JM, and Cuddy B. Fusion rate and biomechanical stiffness of hydroxylapatite versus autogenous bone grafts for anterior discectomy. *Spine* 1994; 19: 2524–2528.
8. Thalgott JS, Kabins MB, Fritts K, and Guiffre JM. Anterior interbody fusion of the lumbar spine with MOSS titanium cages and coralline hydroxyapatite, presented at *North American Spine Society*, October 1995; Washington, DC, and at *International Intradiscal Therapy Society*, May 1996; Amsterdam, Holland.
9. Thalgott JS, Abei M, Fritts K, and Guiffre JM. Preliminary report on the new AO titanium interbody fusion device (TIS): a non-articulating disc replacement, presented at *International Intradiscal Therapy Society,* May 1996; Amsterdam, Holland, and at *American Spinal Injury Assoc,* March 1997; Houston, Texas.
10. Hollinger JO and Battistone GC. Biodegradable bone repair materials. *Clin Orthop* 1986; 207: 290.
11. White AA III and Panjabi MM. *Clinical Biomechanics of the Spine* 2nd ed, 1990; Lippincott, Philadelphia.
12. Andriano KP, Daniels AU, Smutz WP, Wyatt RWB, and Heller J. Initial histological and mechanical comparison of several fiber reinforced polymers. *Trans Soc Biomater* 1989; 12: 74.
13. Daniels AU, Chang MKO, Andriano KP, and Heller J. Mechanical properties of biodegradable polymers and composites proposed for internal fixation of bone. *J Appl Biomater* 1990; 1: 58.
14. Boden SD, Schimandle JH, and Hutton WC. Experimental lumbar intertransverse process spinal fusion model. *Spine* 1995; 20: 412–420.
15. Guigui P, Plais PY, Flautre B, Viguier E, Blary MC, Chopin D, Lavaste F, and Hardouin P. Experimental model of postlateral spinal arthrodesis in sheep. Part 2. *Spine* 1994; 19: 2798–2803.
16. Sandhu HS, Kanin LEA, Kabo JM, Toth JM, Zeegen EN, Liu D, Seager LL, and Dawson EG. Evaluation of rhBMP-2 with an OPLA carrier in a canine postlateral (transverse process) spinal fusion model. *Spine* 1995; 20: 2669–2682.
17. Zdeblick TA, Wilson D, Cooke ME, Kunz DN, McCabe R, Ulm MJ, and Vanderby R. "Anterior cervical disectomy and fusion: a comparison of techniques in an animal model." *Spine* 1992; 17(10S): S418–S426.
18. 1997; US Patent 5609636.

14

Follow-up-Study–Based Wear Debris Reduction with Ceramic–Metal–Modular Hip Replacements

Günther Heimke and Gerd Willmann

1. Introduction

Total hip replacements (THRs) have reached higher levels of reliability during the past three decades. Recently, some clinics reported success rates of well above 90% after 10 yr, and more than 80% after 15 yr *(1,2)*. The chief cause of the remaining failures after mid- and long-term service times, nearly independent of the implant material and design, is late aseptic loosening *(3)*.

Loosenings are generally assumed to follow the appearance of radiolucencies along extended portions of the bone–cement or bone–implant interfaces. They are believed to result from soft tissue interlayers separating the implant from its bony bed. Such layers were first observed and described in detail for the bone–cement interfaces in the early 1970s *(4)*. Their composition was found to closely resemble the seams of pseudarthroses seen in cases of failed fracture healing, the nonunion cases. This similarity immediately indicates one of the primary causes of the appearance of these soft tissue interlayers: interfacial movements (for details on this phenomenon, *see* e.g., ref. 5).

The other cause of these soft tissue separations between implants and the surrounding bony bed was demonstrated by the disaster of the so-called Weber-Huggler total hip system *(6)* in Europe, in the late 1960s and early 1970s, with its 50% severe aseptic loosenings within less than 27 mo *(7)*, and nearly 100% after less than 5 yr: The wear particles of their polyester, separately rotating femoral heads migrated into the anchorage portions of the cemented sockets, and caused a massive transformation of the adjacent bony into granulation tissue.

It was this event that drew the attention of all concerned again to the wear-and-tear phenomenon in total joint arthroplasty, after the introduction of the so-called low-friction combination of the polyethylene (PE) against stainless steel by Charnley *(8)* in 1960. It stimulated the teams exploring the potential of ceramics for improving bone replacements to not only study the tissue compatibility of these alumina ceramics as bulk materials *(9–11)*, but also its tribological properties *(12)*, and, simultaneously, the eventual hazards of their wear particles. First results *(13)* confirmed the high biocompatibility of this material "without foreign body reaction or progressive fibrosis" *(13)*.

The results of the first generations of THRs with alumina ceramic sockets and balls confirmed expectations regarding frictional and wear behavior. The few cases that demanded reoperations allowed for detailed studies on the retrieved components *(14)*. Most of them showed the expected behavior of wear phenomenon, and some gave new insights that could be used for further

From: *Biomaterials Engineering and Devices: Human Applications,* Volume 2
Edited by D. L. Wise, et al. © Humana Press, Inc., Totowa, NJ

Table 1
Survey of Experiences with Different Material Combinations for Articulating Surfaces in Hip Arthroplasty

Wear couple		
Acetabular socket	Femoral head	Comment
Metal	Teflon	Withdrawn
Metal	Polyethylene	Satisfactory, presently still widely used
Polyester	Metal	Withdrawn
Metal	Metal	First generation with considerable metallosis; present new generation regarded with caution because of possible long-term systemic effects.
Alumina ceramic	Polyethylene	Improvement by at least a factor of 2, compared to metal/PE
Zirconia ceramic	Polyethylene	Caution, controversial
Alumina ceramic	Alumina ceramic	Combination with by far lowest wear

improvements (15). In one of the earliest follow-up studies of one of those new THRs with ceramic–ceramic articulation, a comparison with one of the standard PE–metal systems of that time was included. Both systems had the same cemented femoral components, and were inserted by the same teams under identical conditions as far as possible. Radiographically, clearly less-calcar resorptions were seen in the ceramic–ceramic cases, and were at that time tentatively ascribed to the reduced incidence of wear particles (16).

Now, 20 yr later, long-term follow-up studies of those early systems (17–20), as well as midterm follow-up studies of new generations of total hip implants with metal-backed ceramic sockets articulating against ceramic balls, confirm those early expectations (21–23).

Their potential of a nearly complete avoidance of any wear debris was confirmed. Thus, large-scale introduction of this kind of articulation provides the most promising tool for a further reduction of the remaining few percent of failures in total hip arthroplasty. Table 1 summarizes the accumulated experiences with different material combinations for the articulating surfaces in total hip arthroplasty.

2. Tissue Compatibility of Alumina Ceramics

2.1. Materials

Ceramics are nonmetallic, inorganic materials. They consist of closely packed, tiny crystals of metal oxides, in which the bonds between oxygen (O) and metal are ionic, resulting, in contrast to metals, in a strong localization of electrical charges. The classical ceramics, such as pottery, earthen and stone ware, and porcelain, are characterized by high percentages of crystallized silicates, with some glassy components between. Glasses are noncrystallized silicates: In a sense, they are undercooled liquids. In glass ceramics, small oxide particles had been precipitated into a glassy matrix. The bioactive glasses (for definitions, see Table 2) belong to this group (24,25). Glazes are glass or glass ceramic layers on a ceramic substrate: In enamels, they are on a metal substrate. Particular properties can be achieved with nonoxide materials, such as silicon nitride-, boron carbide-, and silicon carbide-ceramics, the special ceramics. Bioactive hydroxyapatite (HA) and tricalcium phosphate (TCP) ceramics can be regarded as another special group.

Ceramics containing more than 85% Al_2O_3 are called aluminum (Al) oxide, alumina, or corundum ceramics. Corundum is the crystallographic name of the high-purity, colorless version of ruby and sapphire. In the ceramic version, the material consists of micrometer-size, closely packed, single crystals. This ceramic is the chief representative of the oxide ceramics, consisting of the oxides of the least noble metals, the metals with the highest energy of oxide formation. They have a relatively high chemical and thermal stability (melting temperature 2050°C), and have been used in heavy-duty applications in mechanical and

Table 2
Grouping of Materials for Skeletal Reconstruction According to Their Compatibility in Bony Tissue

Degree of compatibility	Typical reactions of bony tissue	Materials
Biotolerant	Implants separated from adjacent bone by a soft tissue layer along most of the interface: distant osteogenesis.	Stainless steels; PMMA bone cements and Co-based alloys.
Bioinert	Direct contact to bone tissue: contact osseogenesis.	Alumina ceramics; zirconia ceramics, Ti, Ta, Nb.
Bioactive	Bonding to bony tissue in the sense of a gluing effect: bonding osteogenesis.	Ca-phosphate containing glasses and glass ceramics; HA and TCP ceramics; Ti (?).

Table 3
Specifications of Medical Grade Alumina Ceramics

Property[a]	Unit	Specification according to Standards (ASTM F603-83; ISO 6474, 2nd edition, 1994, Type A)	Commercially realized, e.g., (BIOLOX forte**).[b] Typical values
Density	g/cm^3	>3.94	>3.98
Alumina content	%	>99.5	>99.7
Impurities $SiO_2 + CaO + Na_2O$	%	<0.1	<0.05
Additives (MgO)	%	<0.3	<0.25
Porosity	%	[c]	0
Microstructure, mean grain size	μm	<4.5	<1.8
Hardness	HV	[c]	2300
Average biaxial flexural strength	MPa	>250	580[d]
Elastic modulus	GPa	[c]	>380
Fracture toughness	MPa/m	[c]	4

[a]For test methods, *see*, e.g., ISO 6474:1994 (E).
[b]Biolox is the trade name for medical-grade alumina ceramic products of CeramTec.
[c]No values mentioned in the standard.
[d]Four-point bending test.

chemical engineering during the past 70 yr. The strong bond of the Al to the O ions, and thus the extreme localization of all electrical charges, makes this material one of the best electrical insulators. Details about the structural particularities and unique property combinations of ceramic materials have been described elsewhere with particular emphasis on medical applications (26,27). Table 3 summarizes most of the biomedically important specifications of this material. The high performance values presented in the right column are the third step in continuous improvements of this material, since its introduction into orthopedic surgery in 1974 (28,29).

2.2. Compatibility Studies of Bulk Ceramics

One of the first compatibility studies on dense alumina ceramics, with Al_2O_3 contents of more than 85%, had shown that high-purity versions of this material, with purities well above 99%, can be used for implant purposes only (30). Thus, all future evaluations could be confined to this kind of ceramic.

In the early stages of the evaluation of possible advantages of alumina ceramics as a material for bone replacements, the biocompatibility of these materials was tested by several teams. The original work of Hulbert et al. (9) was immediately followed by the first implantations of ceramic hip joint components by Boutin in 1970 *(31)*. Other teams chose to first study in more detail the tissue responses that this material provokes before applying it in joint replacements for humans.

The remodeling process of the bony tissue adjacent to alumina ceramic implants could be disclosed and compared with stainless steel and cobalt-chromium-molybdenum (Co-Cr-Mo) alloy implants *(11,18,32)*. The results of these extended studies showed that dense alumina ceramics are contacted faster by newly formed woven bone than those metal implants. This behavior was ascribed to the chemical inertness of this ceramic, and, thus, to the absence of anything going into solution and disturbing the activity of adjacent cells chemically. The term "bioinertness" was chosen to describe this aspect. A further feature was soon realized *(33)*. The steps and time sequences of bony regeneration along bioinert implants are identical with the processes and timescales necessary for successful fracture healing. These observations led to the schematic scaling of implant materials given in Table 4 (modified from Osborn's original scheme) *(34)*. Definitions of the concepts used in Table 4 are explained in Table 5 (*see* p. 231).

The coating of the surfaces of samples of alumina ceramics mentioned in Table 4 is a consequence of the high surface tension of this material, and resulting wetting behavior. Within less than 1 min after contact with body fluids, the surface of the ceramic is densely covered with the body's own molecules *(35)*. This phenomenon is not only an important contribution to the bioinertness of this material, but it is also a major requirement for its tribological and wear behavior *(36,37)*. It can be assumed that the articulating surfaces are mostly separated from each other by such adsorbed layers.

It was the chemical inertness of alumina ceramic that, for the first time, allowed study of all interfacial tissue reactions without influences of anything going into solution from the implant surface, such as ions or monomers. There were no biochemical influences on the cell activities around such implants. This facilitated the interpretation of the observation of interfacial areas showing close bone contact after adequate times for fracture healing, and sometimes neighboring areas with soft tissue interlayers. The compositional similarity of the soft tissue portions with the pseudarthrosis seams mentioned above, and their location at portions of the interface, along which, during implantation, tangentially oriented forces had been acting, allowed to correlate them with relative movements *(38)*. Thus, the design of such ceramic or generally bioinert implants, intended for direct, cement-free anchorage in bony tissue, could rely only on interfaces, along which the forces resulting from functional loading meet these interfaces perpendicularly, or nearly so. All tangentially loaded interfaces cannot contribute to their reliable fixation. The design of some of the first-generation ceramic sockets for direct, cement-free fixation had been based on these conclusions *(39)*. They were fully confirmed in many follow-up studies of these hip implants *(40)*, and also of similarly designed dental implants *(41)*.

The observation of interfacial portions with different kinds of adjacent tissues, with either direct bone contact or a soft tissue interlayer, around the same bioinert implant, demonstrated that any interpretation of histological results of compatibility studies in bony tissue can be completely obscured by biomechanical effect, as just described. Any results presented about histological observations along implants in a bony bed must be accompanied by a clear statement about the loading conditions during implantation at the location from which the sample was taken; otherwise, they are meaningless *(42–44)*.

2.3. Compatibility of Alumina Ceramic Wear Particles

Compatibility tests of alumina ceramic powders simulating the effects of ceramic wear particles commenced simultaneously with the studies on bulk samples of the same material by Griss et al. *(13)*. In this early study, artificially produced powder in a ball mill, with an alumina content of 99.7%, the rest magnesium oxide (MgO), and a grain-size distribution from 0.5 to 5 µm, with the majority below 2 µm, was suspended in a physiological saline solution. 150 SPF Swiss mice were divided into three groups, which received this suspension subcutaneously, into the hind pads, and into both knees, respectively. After 1, 3, 7, 15, 30, 60, 120, and 150 d, four animals of each group were sacrificed, and the three injec-

Table 4
Definitions of Terms Used for Compatibility Rating of Bone Replacement Materials

Degree of compatibility	Material influences on adjacent bony tissue	Result	Typical materials
Biotolerance (distance osteogenesis)	Components of the material, e.g., ions or monomers are leaching into the surrounding tissue	Irritation of the differentiation of precursor cells into osteoblasts, formation of a collagen rich interlayer.	PMMA, Co Cr Mo alloys, stainless steels
Bioinert (contact osteogenesis)	Nothing goes into solution, leaching ions and other matter below detectability of adjacent tissue. Fast absorption of molecules from body fluent; (coating).	No biochemical influences on cell activities, no biochemical information about presence of implant. No enzyme controlled foreign body reactions, implant camouflaged against host's immune system.	Alumina and some zirconia ceramics, Ti, Ta, Nb, because of their oxide surfaces.
Bioactive (bonding osteogenesis)	Deposition of collagen and/or HA from the surrounding tissue onto the surface of the implant.	Bond formation in the sense of a gluing effect.	HA[a] and TCP[b] ceramics, bioactive glasses and glass ceramics.

[a]hydroxylapatite
[b]tricalciumphosphate

tion site were evaluated morphologically. All three injection sites did not show any differing tissue reaction. Initial tissue edema and granulocytic infiltrations were soon replaced by monohistocytic cells, which started with crystal phagocytosis. Simultaneously, a moderate fibroblast activity surrounded the crystal depositions, resulting in a discrete connective tissue encapsulation. About 30 d after injection, the tissue reaction described above became stationary, until the end of the experimental period. The crystals, mostly deposited in macrophages, were then tolerated without signs of further inflammatory reactions. Propagation of crystals into the lymphatics and blood vessels revealed a short time deposition in the RES of the lymphatics, the liver, the spleen, and the lung, without foreign body reactions or progressive fibrosis in these organs. It was concluded that alumina ceramic particles appeared to be inert, atoxic, and well tolerated by the organism.

This early study was supplemented by Harms and Mäusle *(45)*, who tested two different-size fractions of alumina powders of similar composition (0–5 µm and 5–10 µm) by means of macrophage cultures, intraperitoneal and intramuscular, and found no acute cytotoxicity. In the cell culture, the ceramic particles were partly absorbed by macrophages at the cell membrane and partly free in the medium. With the lymphocyte transformation test, no decrease of the synthesis rate, under the influence of the supernatant macrophages treated with powdered particles, could be stated. The intraperitoneal and intramuscular applications also did not show any particle-size-controlled difference after 1 d. Four wk later, in the mesenterium, they found, in addition to small groups, several separate, large, focuslike concentrations of powder particles interdispersed with mononuclear cells. The leukocytes had almost completely disappeared. For some of the particles a beginning of fiber formation was noticed. In the spleen and liver, only a few powder-loaded macrophages could be found. The foci at 10 µm particles show a wall of lymphocytes and many large macrophages around the particles.

Together with the first study, Griss et al. *(46)* initiated an investigation on possible nonspecific foreign body sarcoma induced by alumina ceramics. In this extended test (the animals had to be maintained until their natural death), solid and porous disks were subcutaneously implanted in 150 male Sprague-Dawley rats. The dimensions and configuration of the samples, as well as the experimental conditions, were chosen according to Nothdurft *(47,48)* and Ott *(49)*. Solid and porous disks produced a sarcoma rate of 17.4 and 18% respectively; perforated disks initiated sarcomas at the rate of 25.4%. These values were lower than comparative values reported in the literature for samples of different metals and medical-grade plastics. Powdered alumina ceramic deposits did not produce any sarcoma. This latter result could be used for prognostic assumptions concerning the clinical application of this ceramic, and indicated that the tested material may not possess any significant sarcoma potency. With this study, alumina ceramic was the first implant material for which the evaluation of its sarcoma potential was initiated, several years before these teams started its clinical applications.

The results of these sarcoma rate studies have gained an unexpected importance recently in the analysis of the New Zealand Cancer Registry: Observations by Gillepsie et al. *(50)* of an increased incidence of tumors at remote sites following THRs raised the question of possible causes. In a careful review, Black *(50)* drew attention to the probable influence of dissolution products from metal implants, such as stainless steels and Co-based alloys. With concentrations of 2.6–248 µg/g of dry tissue, with an average of 35 µg/g, and the extension of the survival times of hip implants to 15, 20, and even more years, information from the epidemiology of human workplace exposure to metal-bearing chemicals and other possible carcinogens, with latencies in this order of magnitude, must be considered *(52)*. An extended animal study, initiated in order to find more details about the processes concerned, led to the conclusion that "early intervention in the removal of loose metal devices is warranted to mitigate against foreign body-induced carcinogenesis" *(53)*. It is this kind of problem that cautions against the use of any metal–metal combination for articulating components in joint replacements, as was suggested recently *(54)*. The tiny Co-, Cr-, Mo-, and nickel-containing wear

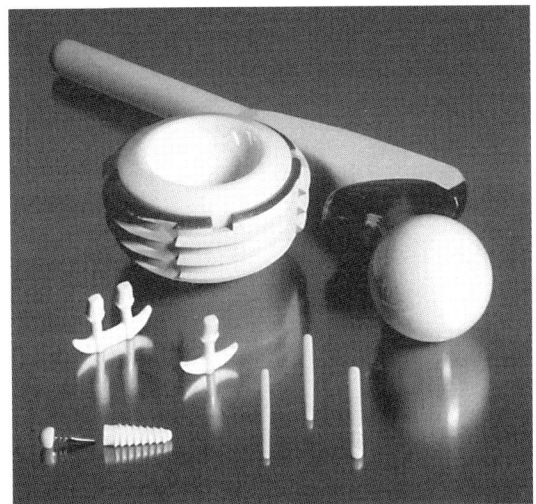

Fig. 1. In the foreground, screw and anchor type dental implants and transdental fixation pins of Biolox alumina ceramic, and, in the rear, a Furlong hip prosthesis with an alumina ceramic (Biolox) femoral head and insert into a HA-coated metal backing.

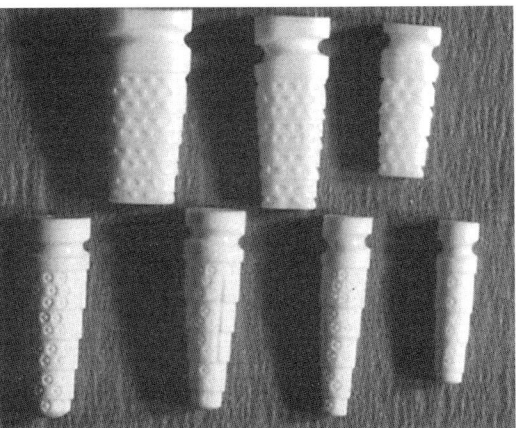

Fig. 2. Tübingen dental implants of alumina ceramic (Frialiti Friatec AG, Mannheim, Germany) with steps and lacunae allowing for osseointegration after an adequate healing phase.

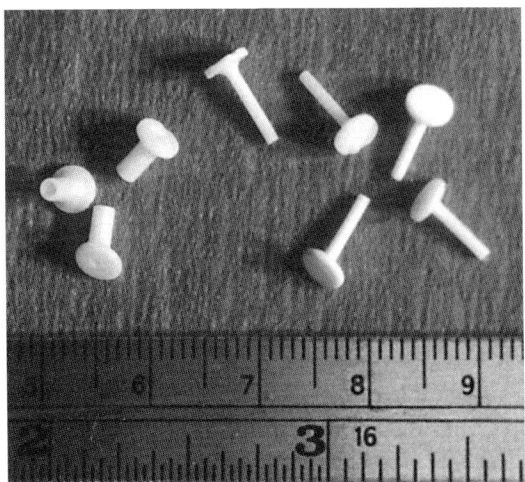

Fig. 3. Frialit middle ear implants.

particles produced in such cases must be regarded as a particularly effective source of those metal ions in body fluids.

2.4. Alumina Ceramic, Prototype of a Bioinert Material, in Other Fields of Reconstructive Surgery

Initiated by, and based on, the results of early compatibility studies, several teams from other branches of reconstructive surgery studied the possibility of improvements by the application of alumina ceramic. Most of them have stood the test of time, and have become either standard treatments in their field or the nucleus of even further improvements (for a short survey, *see* ref. 55).

In dentistry, the inertness of the alumina ceramics was well confirmed with implants, as shown in the lower portion of Fig. 1 *(56)*, and the application of the aforementioned design criteria allowed achievement of a fully reliable osseointegration of the implants presented in Fig. 2 *(57–59)*. In addition, long-term follow-up studies revealed that this material is particularly beneficial for the most critical part of any oral implant; its pergingival portion. Careful measurements of sulcus fluid flow rates and pocket depths, including comparisons of these alumina ceramic implants with natural teeth of the same patients over more than 10 yr, resulted in equal or even slightly better values for the implant *(60–62)*.

The application of the bioinert ceramic in ear, nose, and throat surgery also contributed to improved success rates. Besides middle ear implants *(63;* Fig. 3), trachea-supporting rings

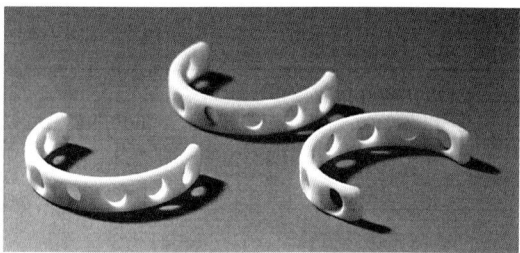

Fig. 4. Frialit trachea-supporting ring.

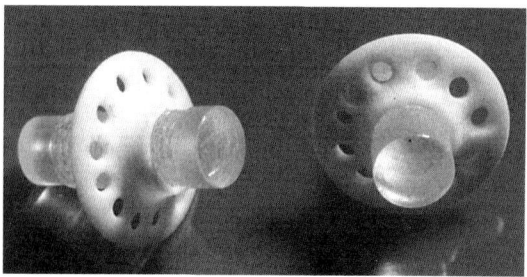

Fig. 6. Keratoprosthesis consisting of an alumina ceramic (Frialit) supporting ring, for insertion into the cornea, and a corundum single-crystal optical component.

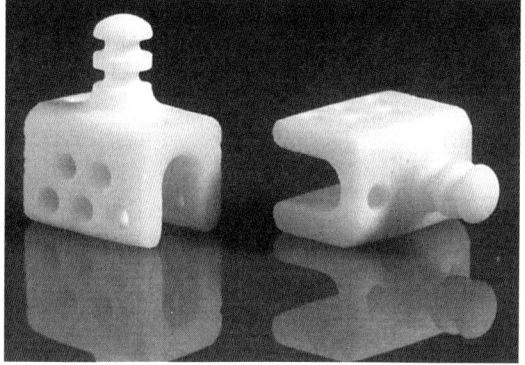

Fig. 5. Frialit septum support.

(64; Fig. 4) and a septum support *(65;* Fig. 5) were tested and clinically applied, with favorable results.

After the confirmation of the bioinertness of alumina ceramics in the eyes of rabbits, keratoprostheses, consisting of supporting rings of this material carrying optical cylinders of corundum single crystals, as shown in Fig. 6, were successfully introduced clinically *(66,67).*

The results of early compatibility studies, and on fully functional THRs with solid ceramic sockets in sheep and dogs, together with equivalent experiments with ceramic dental implants, have allowed for the summary of the interfacial remodeling reactions of the bony tissue adjacent to bioinert implants presented in Table 5. Midterm follow-up evaluations of subsequently developed human hip and dental implants completely confirmed these statements.

Generally, all these clinical applications of the dense, high-purity alumina ceramic, which, by now, have *in situ* times of up to more than 20 yr, have firmly established the predicted bioinertness, according to the definition given in Table 4.

3. Experiences with First-generation Ceramic Acetabular Sockets and Femoral Heads

As briefly mentioned in subheading 2.2., the first alumina ceramic components of THRs were implanted by Boutin *(31)* in 1970. His foregoing compatibility test was a self experiment about which he reported more than 15 yr later *(68).* His alumina ceramic acetabular components essentially followed the shape of PE sockets. The ceramic balls were provided with cylindrical holes into which metal bushings were glued. These bushings had threaded bores, by which the balls were to be screwed onto the threaded ends of the neck portions of the metal femoral stems. In the first series, sockets and stems were fixed via a polymethylmethacrylate (PMMA) bone cement. Many of these implants had to be removed, because either the ball unscrewed or the bushings loosened because the glue had deteriorated during steam sterilization *(69).* In later series, the essentially hemispherical sockets were provided with parallel studs for rotational stabilization, if implanted cement-free *(70).* Different designs were used for the connection of the ceramic balls onto the metal stems, until the French team finally also adopted the conical fixation *(71),* which had been introduced for this purpose by the two German teams. The long-term evaluation of these prostheses, which were used mostly in France and

Table 5
Survey of Sequence of Interface Reactions of Bony Tissue Adjacent to Bioinert Implant

Cause	Reaction
Trauma or surgical intervention	Bleeding, stimulation of the immune system by cell and other debris; thus, activated cells start to remove remainders of disrupted tissues and cells.
Insertion of implant	Nutrition of tissue layer in contact with implant is severely reduced (one-half space is no longer contributing) and openings of blood vessels blocked by clotting, resulting in predominantly osteoclastic activity; surface layer of bone loses much of its mechanical strength.
Motionlessness at interface and absence of chemical influences	Osteoblastic activity increases, first contact of bony tissue with implant surface where softened interlayer is thinnest (in most cases at corners and edges).
Blood clot formation in spaces between implant surface and tissue and inside surface undulations like lacunae	If dimensions of clot are small enough, either osteoblasts or the precursor cells migrate into the clot along fibrinogen fibers and start bone formation.
Load application	Along interfaces without tangential movements (essentially loaded by pure pressure): further bone deposition until bone contact area has become large enough for stress, reaching the optimum of Wolff's law; along interfaces with shear motion: formation of a pseudarthrosis seam.

Canada, showed excellent results, with, minimal wear, if any (72).

The first alumina ceramic sockets, particularly designed for direct, cement-free anchorage, were implanted in September (33) and October (73) 1974, by two teams in Germany. Examples of these two systems are given in Figs. 7 and 8. Evidently, the shapes of these sockets had been especially chosen accounting for the property combination of alumina ceramics and its bioinertness to achieve a stable initial press-fit, and allowing for interfacial remodeling and ingrowth of bony tissue into the grooves. Other teams in Vienna and Bologna tried to reach a bony fixation of ceramic sockets (74), with modifications of hemispherical sockets similar to those originally introduced by Boutin (31).

For some time, the Bologna group used, besides alumina ceramic sockets and balls, Co-Cr-Mo stems carrying a flame-strayed coating of alumina. In some of the few reoperation cases, a severe osteolysis of the femoral cortical bone was found around these shafts. Histologically, alumina ceramic particles were found, which could be identified as crystallographically belonging to the alumina γ-phase by Toni et al. (75). In this phase, the Al ions are much less strongly bound, and, therefore, can go into solution in aqueous environments. Their presence results from the flame-sprayed alumina coating: Even if the initial alumina powder consists of nothing but α-phase particles, after spraying, the coating contains about 70% γ-phase particles. In contrast to α-alumina, the γ-phase alumina is not stable in body environment.

Generally, the analysis of the midterm follow-up studies of these systems showed overall success rates in the range of 75% and more (14,76). This was in accordance with the overall survival rates of hip replacements fixed with PMMA, with what is now called the first generation of cementing techniques (77), but it was not better. Thus, many clinics turned back to the cementing techniques, which, at that time (around 1980), had reached a higher level of success by using, e.g., more careful mixing procedures and pressurization in the application of the cements (78).

However, the analysis of retrieved alumina ceramic sockets and balls and capsular tissue (18–21), which could be harvested on some occasions, allowed for additional insights: The few cases of severe wear were found to be associated almost always with abnormal or pathological situations, such as loosenings of sockets and stems, or with subluxations of balls and general inflammations.

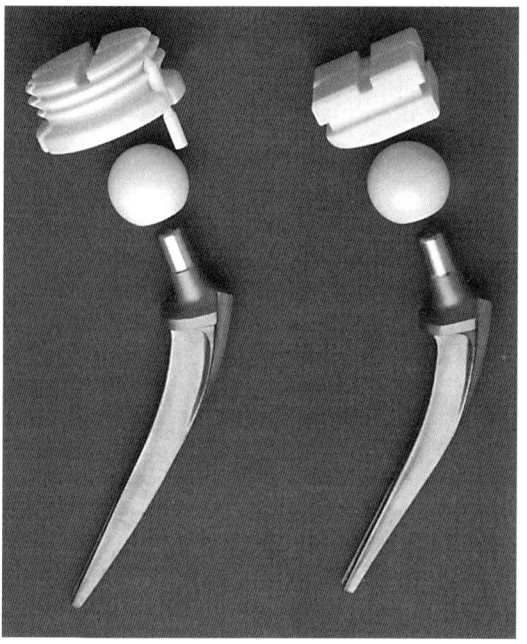

Fig. 7. First-generation Lindenhof THR system with a cylindrical and a rectangular socket of alumina ceramic (Frialit). Note the asymmetrical cross-section of the threads of the cylindrical socket, intended for the largest possible interfacial area for pressure transmission (forces meet the interface perpendicularly), and the marked grooves for additional stabilization by ingrown bony tissue. The pin was to be inserted for additional rotational stabilization. The specially designed shafts (Griss) were for cement fixation.

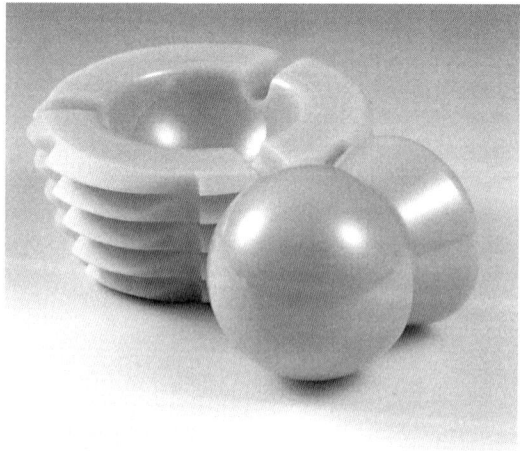

Fig. 8. Threaded conical socket and femoral head with sleeve (Mittelmeier) of alumina ceramic (Biolox).

Histologically, the crystalline alumina wear particles were always seen in different amounts, predominantly in the surface layers of the capsule. They were stored either interstitially or intracellularly within macrophages, or partly concentrated in perivascular spaces or in perivascular lymphatic vessels ready for removal. Accompanying inflammatory reactions could only be found in remarkably small numbers around or between clusters of ceramic wear particles. Round cells and foreign body giant cells could be seen only if the ceramic wear particles were accompanied by metal wear debris or fragments of bone cement. Although most of the small crystals (approx 2 µm or less) were stored in macrophages, single larger particles (up to 20 µm) could be found mostly between the fibers of the scar tissue, without any cellular reaction (18).

These results correspond to early observations in animal experiments with artificially produced alumina particles (13,45). In cases of high concentrations of large alumina ceramic particles, Willert et al. (79) observed the formation of granulation tissue within and around such agglomerations, and, considering previous results with wear particles of other materials, came to the conclusion that such densely packed, large, stable particles initiate the formation of granulation tissue in any case, independent of their chemical and crystallographic nature.

About 5 yr later, however, nearly all long-term follow-ups of these first-generation ceramic–ceramic combinations almost completely agreed on one issue: the minimal wear found in retrieved samples (71,80–83 with comments in ref. 84), or deduced from a well-preserved cement to bone interfaces along the femoral components (16,17).

3.1. Prerequisites for Low Wear and Their Realization

The results of the mid- and long-term follow-up studies of the solid alumina ceramic acetabular components had not confirmed expectations regarding an increase of safety and the survival rates, which had been the motivation for their development and clinical application. For this application, obviously, bioinertness, in the sense outlined in Table 4, is not a sufficient requirement. In order to achieve a reliable, direct, cement-free anchorage of the acetabular components, the material facing the bone tissue, such as titanium (Ti), must have properties resembling most of the features of bioactivity. However, all the previously discussed studies repeatedly confirm the considerable advantage of alumina ceramic sockets and balls for all aspects of tear and wear. Because this property of the material is the central motivation for its application in joint replacements, the most important requirements for the realization and maintenance of the low wear rates are presented in more detail.

There are different aspects to the problem: One is the surgical technique; others are the material itself, the kind of surface treatment, and design considerations regarding the artificial joint gap and related tolerances.

3.1.1. Surgical Aspects

The aforementioned wetting property of the alumina ceramic, and its ability to adsorb a dense layer of body molecules within less than a minute after contact with body fluids, must be regarded as an essential contribution to its high wear resistance *(32,85)*. Thus, any disturbance or destruction of this absorption layer will severely impair wear resistance. The requirement for the reliable maintenance of the stability of this layer implies that concentrations of forces on small areas, in other words, high pressures at the articulating surfaces, must be avoided strictly. Such peak stresses will be created if, e.g., the ceramic ball articulates against the edge of a ceramic socket. This requires strict avoidance of any kind of subluxation, and, consequently, the implantation of the socket at its correct angle of inclination. But the same requirement also demands an absolute cleanness of the articulating surfaces of the socket and ball; any tiny chip of bone cement in the articulating area will inevitably destroy the adsorption layer and expose parts of the ceramic surfaces to dry friction.

One additional warning may be useful: In repositioning, sometimes, the ceramic ball snaps into the socket. Such a snapping, however, can, under unfortunate conditions, create tiny local damage to the ceramic surfaces, which, if they do not result in an immediate loosening of one or several particles, might remain silent, but can lead to destruction later. Thus, the reposition of ceramic balls into ceramic sockets must be done slowly, and as smoothly as possible.

3.1.2. The Material Aspect

The quality of the surface is primarily determined by the quality of the bulk material. A completely pore-free surface requires a completely dense material as a necessary condition. It also demands fine-grained material, because larger grains of this kind of ceramic carry intragrain pores caused by the sintering process.

Generally, the demand for a pore-free surface, necessitating a density nearly matching the theoretical, single-crystal value, on the one hand, and for a fine-grain structure on the other hand, are contradicting, and could be solved only by the application of a technological trick. To explain this, a brief look into the sintering process is useful: Oxide ceramics are produced from powders. These fine-grained powders are compacted into what the production experts call green bodies. These bodies are particle agglomerates with up to 50% of the final density. They are either already pressed or they are machined as closely as possible to the final shape, but with larger dimensions accounting for the remaining necessary 50% further densification.

In the subsequent firing process, the particle agglomerates are transformed into dense, polycrystalline bodies. This densification process is called sintering, and the associated densification is called shrinkage. In some materials, the sintering is mostly made possible, or at least is facilitated, by the melting of one or more of the components, as is the case, e.g., in the firing of stoneware and porcelains. In sintering alumina ceramics, which is a single-phase material, no liquid phase can assist the sintering process: All the densification must rely on diffusion processes, with the driving force being the reduction of surface energy if the particles grow larger (the surface area is proportional to square of the diameter). Generally, an increase of the average grain size, by a factor of 5–10, is necessary to reach approx 90–95% of the theoretical density. Even with a starting grain size below 1 µ (1 µm, or one-millionth of a meter, or .001 mm), the sintered body must have an average grain size of approx 5 µm, implying the presence of larger particles of up to 10 µm, which usually contain internal holes (*see* Fig. 9 [left]).

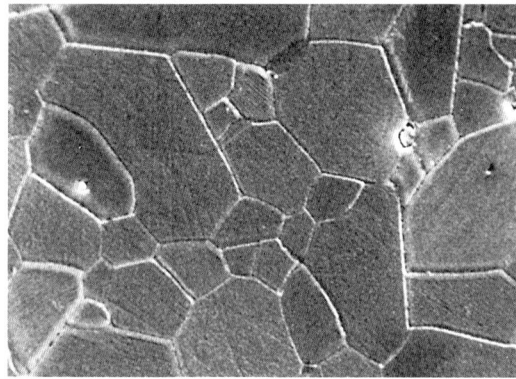 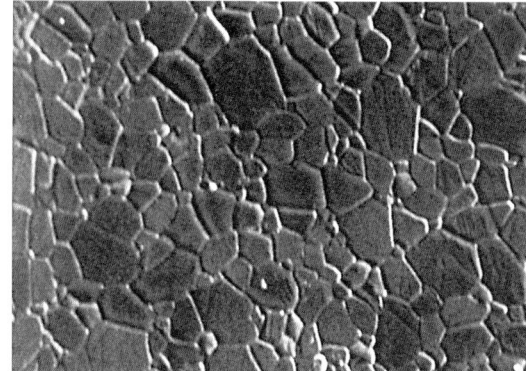

Fig. 9. Surfaces of different alumina ceramic components for articulating surfaces. (Left) Material used in first-generation ceramic medical devices, sintered in air only. (Right) Presently used quality, sintered and HIPed (Biolox forte). The samples were especially etched, in order to improve the visibility of the grain boundaries.

Because the evaluation of the early alumina ceramic components of joint replacements had indicated that this ceramic needs further improvements *(14,86)*, all concerned had to find unconventional ways for reducing the average grain size and the width of the grain size distribution. A drastic, additional reduction of the grain size of the starting powders is not possible, for several reasons. The solution was found in the application of a relatively new technology called hot isostatic pressing (HIPing). In order to employ this process for the purpose concerned, the sintering process is not carried beyond a state of densification at which no open bulk porosity remains, but at which the grains have not yet grown beyond the desired size. If such parts are then taken to temperatures somewhat below the values necessary for grain growth and final densification, and are simultaneously put under pressures on the order of magnitude of 1000 atmospheres, the remaining internal pores can be eliminated without any additional grain growth. Prosthetic components thus treated have average grain sizes of markedly below 2 µm, and hardly any grains in excess of 5 µm, and a density of more than 3.98 g/cm^3, or 99.5% of their theoretical value *(15,87,88)*. The microradiograph in the right part of Fig. 9 gives an example of such a material. The comparison of the two microradiographs indicates the degree of improvement.

3.1.3. Surface Treatment

After sintering and HIPing, the surfaces of the parts are in the so-called "as-fired" state. Because of the special mobility of surface atoms or ions, the surface can reach a high degree of thermodynamic equilibrium, usually resulting in a crystallographically stable and biologically inert state, with well-rounded edges at grain boundaries. But this surface is by no means flat. As the hardness of the corundum ceramic is exceeded by diamond only, this is the most appropriate grinding material. In a first step of surface machining, grinding tools equipped with a relatively coarse diamond powder are used for a first flattening. In further steps, with smaller-grained, diamond-coated tools, the surfaces are more smooth. Microscopically, much of this process consists of scratching and breaking of material and crystals, so the binding forces holding the single corundum particles in position are of high importance. The HIPing of the material contributes considerably to increasing these forces and improving the grinding results. After the last grinding step with the smallest-grained diamond tools, the remaining fine scratches are removed in an extended polishing process, although the brightness of a polished alumina ceramic surface is no indication for its functional quality. Even though the remaining damage of less well-prepared surfaces is of dimensions below detectability with the naked eye, light reflected from the undamaged portions will still be sufficient for a glamorous view.

3.1.4. Dimensions of artificial joint gap

From the viewpoint of friction, a needle bearing, such as used in wristwatches, employing ruby

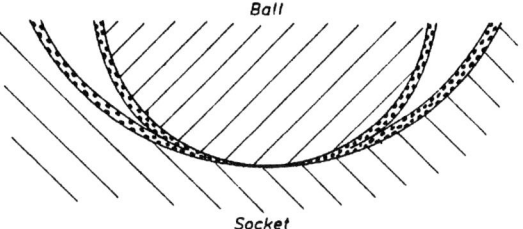

Fig. 10. Schematic and much exaggerated demonstration of squeezing out the adsorbed layer under high pressures.

sockets, would be the maximum solution. With the loads acting on a hip joint, the pressures in the contact areas would completely destroy the adsorbed layers, and the high stresses in the small contact area would even surpass the strength of the ceramic. Such a situation is schematically shown in Fig. 10. A complete match along the total hemispherical interface would minimize the pressures, but would result in high frictional torque, because of the deformation of the ball from spherical to some more flattened shape under the acting forces. In addition, unavoidable production tolerances had to be accounted for, and a compromise had to be found. The artificial joint gap is kept safely outside the ranges of tolerance by all manufacturers, but this also poses a problem: Because neither the dimensions of the artificial joint gaps nor the tolerance fields are generally defined in standards, the combination of balls and sockets from different manufacturers can lead to problems *(89)*. The old general requirement, "Never mix and match," is to be obeyed.

3.1.5. Another Design Consideration

The dangers resulting from an eventual snapping of the ceramic ball into the ceramic socket in repositioning of the joint had been mentioned in subheading 3.1.1. But there is still another danger, possibly causing such a snapping of the ball into the socket: If the neck of the femoral component of the prosthesis meets the rim of the socket, the ball might be lifted out of socket and, in returning to its correct position, damage the articulating surfaces. Such an event must also be avoided for other reasons, because, e.g., any such contact causes a torque on the socket, resulting in a completely unphysiological shear loading along the implant–tissue interface. Such contacts may have been responsible for some socket loosenings.

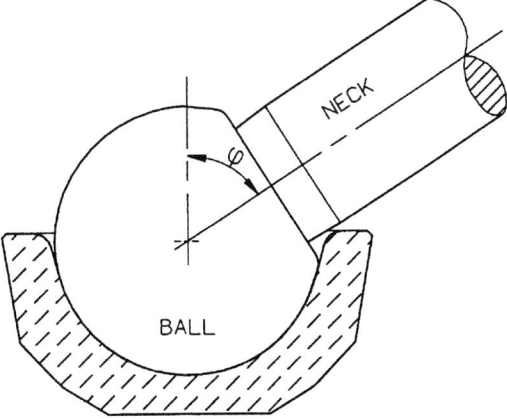

Diameter of		Range of motion (2φ)
Ball	Neck	in degrees
26	12	125
30	12	133
30	15	120
32	15	124
38	27	89

Fig. 11. Range of angular motion of THRs as a function of the ratios of the diameters of balls and necks.

To keep the range of angular motion in an artificial hip joint as large as possible, first, the ratios of the diameters of the balls and the necks must be chosen as large as possible, from the point of view of the safety of the neck material. Figure 11 shows the situation schematically, and gives some values for the ranges of motion for some standard diameters *(15,90)*. But even if the ball–neck ratio is in the favorable range, there are stems that, if used with the smallest neck length, may allow for contacts of the collars to the rims of the sockets. The use of such stems should be carefully avoided. Finally, this is another reason for the surgeon to choose the angle of inclination of the socket within the correct limits.

3.2. Zirconia Ceramics

During the 1970s, the mechanical strength of some zirconia ceramics was increased considerably *(91)*. In a chemically pure version, zirconium oxide undergoes a usually incomplete phase transition in passing from temperatures above 1000°C to room temperature. Because this transition is inherently associated with a change in volume, no dense, solid pieces can be sintered from pure zirconia. If, however, some other oxides, such as calcium oxide, magnesium oxide, and yttrium oxide are added in appropriate amounts, the high-temperature phase of this solid solution can be maintained (stabilized), with a second phase precipitated into this matrix at about 1000°C. These materials are often referred to as partially stabilized zirconia (PSZ) and yttria tetragonal zirconia polycrystalline (Y-TZP) ceramics. Bend strengths of up to twice of those of alumina ceramics could be achieved with such two-phase materials, in which the precipitated phase acts as a toughener. Following the basic principle of surgery, to sacrifice as little as possible of living tissue, the higher strength possibly allowing for smaller components, motivated efforts to evaluate the employment of these materials for joint replacements *(92)*, e.g., in particular, for patients in Japan. This early enthusiasm had soon to be cautioned: The raw materials from which zirconia is derived are always contaminated by at least one-tenth percent urania and thoria, which cannot be completely removed. Thus, zirconia ceramics are usually radioactive to the legal limit for implant purposes *(93)*. This handicap could be compensated for by using very sophisticated and expensive decontamination procedures for the raw materials.

However, it is exactly the two-phase state, which provides for the high mechanical strength of this material, that makes some versions of zirconia ceramics unsuitable for its most important potential application: If a co-precipitated powder (Y-TZP) is used, one of the two phases of the resulting ceramic is not sufficiently stable in aqueous environments *(94)*. These effects, of course, exclude this material completely from any application for ceramic–ceramic articulation, because the chemically controlled surface roughening by the leaching of the soluble phase can result in catastrophic wear, as shown by Toni et al. *(75)* and others *(95,96)*. But this effect also excludes this type of zirconia ceramic from applications in which it must articulate against PE. In 1996, the British Medical Device Agency (MDA) published a warning *(97)* concerning the use of heads made from zirconia ceramics for joint replacements: "The MDA is aware that steam sterilization may lead to surface roughening of zirconia ceramic heads. As a consequence of roughening, increased wear of the ultra-high-mol-wt-polyethylene (UHMWPE) acetabular components has occurred necessitating early revision. In the interest of improved safety, the zirconia ceramic component suppliers have advised that if resterilization is considered necessary, then steam sterilization must not be used."

In contrast to this version, zirconia ceramics manufactured from coated Y-TZP powders are very stable in hydrothermal environments *(98)*. They can, thus, be used safely in combination with PE sockets. Table 6 *(99,100)* contains a comparison of medical-grade alumina ceramic with different zirconia ceramics. The combination of heads with sockets of this zirconia ceramic, made from coated powders, remains controversial. Although Willmann et al. *(101)* found high wear rates, according to which they concluded that medical-grade zirconia ceramic (Y-TZP, according to SO/DIS 13356) should not be used for acetabular cups, Chevalier et al. *(102)* reported more favorable results, and even recommended the bearing combination of alumina ceramic against zirconia ceramic. The higher bend strength of some zirconia ceramics can, therefore, be used for a marked size reduction of ceramic components of hip arthroplasty, but with much caution only. Here again, the old rule, "Never mix and match," should be obeyed.

The difficult relations of allowed, dangerous, and not recommended material combinations are summarized in Table 7 *(97,103)*. These observations strongly suggest an utmost caution in the application of zirconia ceramic components for all articulating applications.

4. PE–Alumina–Ceramic Combination

Observation of a marked reduction of the amount of wear of PE in the articulation with alumina ceramic, compared to all versions of metals used in hip arthroplasty *(104)* constituted a

Table 6
Comparison of Typical Properties of Biomedical-grade Alumina Ceramic and Some Zirconia Ceramics

Property	Alumina ceramic	Y-TZP ceramic	Mg-PSZ ceramic
Composition	Al_2O_3 (+ MgO)	$ZrO_2 + Y_2O_3$	ZrO_2 + MgO
Structure	Polycrystalline corundum	Polycrystalline tetragonal zirconia	Partially stabilized zirconia
Standards	ISO 6474[a]	ISO 13356	None
Elastic modulus	380 GPa	210 GPa	210 GPa
Hardness	2000 HV 0.1	1250 HV 0.1	1250 HV 0.1
Bend strength	>500 MPa	>900 MPa	>500 MPa
Fracture toughness	4 MPa/m$^{1/2}$	8 MPa/m$^{1/2}$	10 MPa/m$^{1/2}$
Average grain size	<2 μm	<0.5 μm	30 μm

[a]Specifications for alumina ceramic mentioned here differ from those given in the 1994 edition of this standard, in order to allow for a direct comparison with the values for the zirconia ceramics.

Table 7
Material Combinations for Articulation in Hip Replacements

Pairs of materials	Characteristic wear properties	Kind of evidence	Comments
Metal–metal (present generation)	1–6 μm/yr, depending on kind of Co-Cr-Mo alloy	in vivo	Metal wear particles might cause systemic problems (50–52)
PE[a]–metal	Wearing of cup about 0.2 mm/yr and more	In vivo long-term	Standard
PE[a]–alumina ceramic[b]	Wearing of cup about 0.1 mm/yr and less	In vivo long-term	Standard
PE[a]–zirconia ceramic[c]	Wearing of cup about 0.1 mm/yr	In vivo midterm	Warning: one of these ceramics only
Alumina ceramic[b]–alumina ceramic	Hardly detectable, order of 0.005 mm/yr	In vivo long-term	By far most wear-resistant pairing
Alumina ceramic–zirconia ceramic[d]	Controversial; see text	in vitro	**Caution:** at present not recommended
Zirconia ceramic[d]–zirconia ceramic	Controversial; see text	In vitro	**Caution:** can be dangerous

[a]UHMWPE.
[b]Medical grade alumina ceramic with specifications shown in the right column of Table 3.
[c]Zirconia ceramic manufactured from Y-TZP powders (e.g., Ziolox).
[d]All zirconia ceramics.

major breakthrough in this field of reconstructive surgery, as well as in the application of this ceramic. After some initial, partially exaggerated expectations, further experimental studies and early, as well as midterm, clinical results have firmly established that it is possible to reduce the wear of the PE by at least a factor of two (105). In more recent studies 3× less PE particles released from the ceramic on PE prostheses were found in autopsy specimens, as well as in biopsies from revision arthroplasties of prostheses that had been implanted for 4–8 yr. The newly established synovium surrounding prostheses with ceramic heads appeared 20% reduced in thickness, with mino villous transformations, compared to implants with metal heads (106). A study of 369 prostheses, using carefully evaluated X-ray images, found average protrusions of the 32-mm heads of the femoral components into the sockets of more than 0.2 mm/yr for Co-alloy heads and 0.1 mm or less/yr for alumina ceramic ones, after an initial 5-yr period with higher rates for both materials *(107)*.

In this application, the quality of the surface finish of the ceramic ball is of utmost importance. Because the two principal material characteristics mentioned and discussed in subheading 3.1.2., a fine-grain structure and a high density, are inevitable prerequisites for a sufficiently high-finish, top-quality ceramic heads must be used only.

4.1. Metal-backed PE Sockets

Mechanically, the combination of PMMA bone cement with the PE socket can be regarded approximately as a composite unit. The stiffness of a PE socket, with its relatively higher wall thickness, but lower modulus of elasticity, is similar to that of the PMMA cement backing, with its higher modulus but usually lower average thickness. Previous estimates have shown that the stiffness of this composite unit matches relatively well with the stiffness of the pelvis. Thus, under load changes, they can be expected to deform similarly.

However, toward the end of the 1970s, finite element calculations of the stresses and strains in the pelvis adjacent to the acetabular socket, as a function of their stiffness, seemed to indicate a more favorable stress distribution for stiffer sockets. This led to the introduction of metal-backed acetabular components of THRs, in which the side of the socket facing the bony tissue consisted of a metal shell containing a liner of PE.

Subsequently, similar combinations of alumina ceramic shells with PE liners were suggested, but were never used in Europe, because of the expected high stress concentration within the PE part. The much stiffer ceramic was expected to result in considerably higher stress concentrations within the relative thin PE, with much faster work-hardening, and, thus, an increased wear rate. The metal-backed sockets, however, soon found large-scale application in both cemented and noncemented systems.

Toward the end of the 1980s, follow-up studies *(108–111)* with large numbers of patients, and extending up to 10 yr, revealed significantly higher wear rates with such modular, metal-backed sockets than with either directly anchored or cemented PE-only sockets. A simultaneously presented finite element analysis of the stress and strain field inside the PE inlay confirmed the higher stress concentrations as the cause of increased wear *(112)*. Comparisons of such metal-backed sockets with PE liners from different suppliers even revealed that, in at least one case, gaps had deliberately been provided between the metal backing and the PE liner, thus further increasing the work-hardening effect *(113–114)*.

Sometimes, a marked contribution of a PE liner to the damping and shock-absorbing capacity of the lower extremities has been suggested. Earlier estimates on the strong limitations of such a favorable influence have recently been confirmed by detailed calculations *(115)*.

Thus, from all of the aspects discussed above, the application of these metal–PE modular devices must be reconsidered critically *(116)*.

5. Sockets with Alumina Ceramic Inserts

All previous experiences have shown that the material combination of alumina ceramic against itself, for the articulating surfaces in total hip endoprostheses, allows for the lowest wear rates. This present state of the art is clearly summarized in Table 7. In order to utilize this knowledge for further increases of the survival rates of hip replacements, metal-backed ceramic sockets have been suggested, evaluated experimentally and clinically, and have stood the test of short- and midterm carefully followed applications *(21–23,117,118)*. They can be regarded as a promising further step ahead in this field of reconstructive surgery.

But, as usual, any new device has some aspects demanding particular attention, of which those producing and handling them must be aware. The metal-backed ceramic sockets are no exception. The additional interface that this device necessitates, between the metal backing and the alumina ceramic insert, must be regarded critically. Three issues demand particular attention: The design of the metal backing, involving the choice of the anchoring mode of the socket in its bony environment; the shape and reliable fixation of the alumina ceramic insert; and the interaction of the modular socket with the femoral component.

5.1. Metal Backings

The outside contour of any socket is primarily determined by the intended mode of fixation, either via PMMA bone cement or directly. If new cements with features of bioactivity are possible, then demand for specially contoured sockets cannot yet be decided.

There is no reason why metal backings of ceramic inserts for cement fixation should have another outside contour than those consisting completely of PE or ceramic, offering relatively wide spaces for cement penetration and rotational stabilization. However, the additional cement layer actually makes such an acetabular component to a three-layered device.

An example of a metal-backed socket with a ceramic insert used for cement fixation, is the Vario 1 socket *(119)*, which is a hemispherical titanium shell with circular grooves.

For the direct, cement-free anchorage, several differently designed metal backings have been suggested and tested. Hemispherical sockets can be inserted without sacrificing much bony tissue; some have been supplied with additional means such as screws, pegs, or fins, for initial and rotational stabilization, and some are differently coated, for better osseointegration. Metal backings of conical shape are mostly equipped with self-cutting threads; some also carry coatings. Most of these components are made of commercially pure Ti or Ti alloys, but some are made of the Co-Cr-Mo alloys.

One of the hemispherical backings is another version of the Vario socket: This Vario II socket carries four parallel, pointed pegs asymmetrically arranged to additionally provide initial and long-lasting rotational stability, and, if correctly oriented, shift the main load direction more laterally. Short-term results are promising. The Duofit, Samo (Cadriano Emilia, Italy) hemispherical metal cups are provided with four peripherally arranged fins. They consist of Ti and are HA-coated *(21)*. Another hemispherical metal backing is made of commercially pure Ti, and is also coated with HA. This SPH PEG socket is to be press-fitted, and carries small pegs only. Its relatively wide openings are intended to allow the surgeon to verify achievement of the correct position *(23)*. The Eska spherical cup is made of the Co-Cr-Mo alloy Endocast (Krupp, Germany), and is coated with a particular, open-spaced, cast mesh resembling the structure of cancellous bone (Tripo-metal). Early clinical results are promising *(120)*. A variation of the Ti, HA-coated Furlong H.A.C. prosthesis, with holes for screw fixation, has been in clinical use since 1991. The 228 cases consecutively inserted between 1991 and 1994 were reviewed in 1996 *(22)*. 95% of the patients obtained excellent-to-good results, reaching values of over 80 points on the Harris score.

The hemispherical metal shell of the Link FGK socket (Waldeman Link, Hamburg, Germany) is made of the Tilistan Ti-6A1-4V alloy, and carries a four-turn self-cutting thread. In contrast to all others, it is provided with a PE liner into which the ceramic insert is placed. This additional PE liner is claimed to facilitate the intraoperational insertion of the ceramic insert. An additional PE ring, placed in front of the ceramic insert, is to protect the ceramic from any contact with parts of the femoral components. Early results with 79 patients are encouraging *(121)*.

Most of these hemispherical metal backings are similar to, or variations of, previously used sockets, and have stood the test of early and mid-term follow-up observations. Figure 12 gives examples of hemispherical and conical devices and the many possible combinations and alternatives available, even intraoperationally, if so desired.

Metal backings carrying threads are mostly conically shaped. These metal threads can be kept much thinner than those of the previous solid ceramic sockets, so they are self-cutting and, thus, make their insertion much less demanding in effort and time. The metal component of the Kaiserswerther socket resembles the shape of a conical ring with three turns of outside threads. Of 269 sockets implanted between September 1990 and December 1996, eight, or 3%, caused problems *(118)*. The similarly shaped metal backing of the Axis socket is made of Ti and is HA-coated. The results of 248 sockets inserted between 1994 and June 1995 are promising *(117)*. The SI-Screw Ring (Implant Science GmBH, Hamburg, Germany) metal backing is made from a Co-Cr alloy, with an additional plasma-sprayed Ti powder coating. It is also conically shaped, and supplied with threads. In a total of 85 implanted sockets, with an average follow-up period of 4.75 yr (aver-

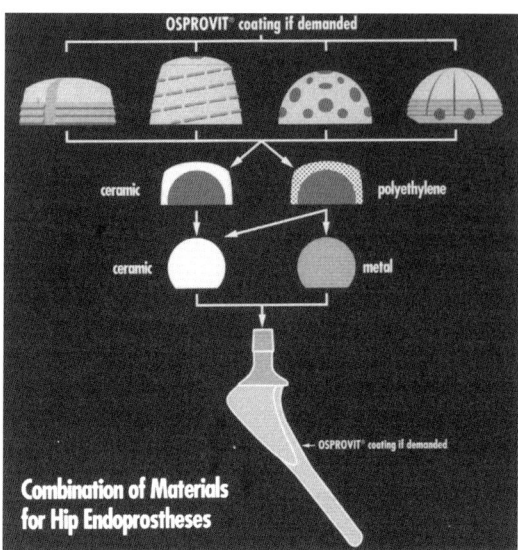

Fig. 12. Schematic examples of metal-backed sockets (top row) with alternative ceramic inserts or PE liners (second row) and ceramic and metal heads, which can be fixed to the same type of stem, if desired. (Osprovit is the trade name for HA coatings from CeramTec AG.)

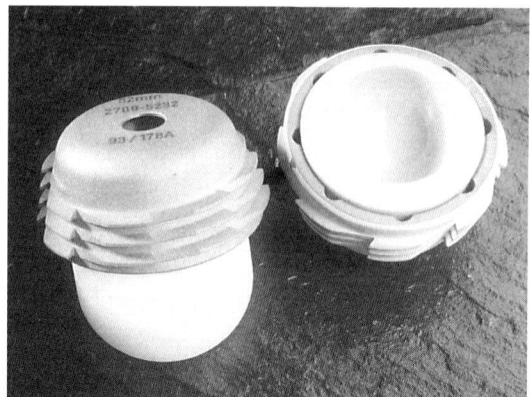

Fig. 13. Example of threaded conical metal-backed socket with an alumina ceramic insert and femoral head (Biolox forte). The metal shell is coated with HA (plasma-sprayed). Axis-system according to D. Stock, Braunschweig, Germany.

age age of patients at the time of operation was 60.6 yr), two had to be revised (2.3%) because of aseptic loosenings not associated with the acetabular components of the prosthetic devices *(122)*. Most of these metal backings are also modifications of previous designs. Figure 13 gives an example.

5.2. Joining Ceramic Insert to Metal Backing

In the wide range of engineering applications of oxide ceramics, several joining techniques for combinations with other materials are well established, such as gluing, cementing, soldering, screwing, or clamping. The first three involve the introduction of at least one additional material, the biocompatibility of which may be critical. The necessity of not only an initial sterilization, but also for further autoclaving, must also be considered. This excludes all presently known gluing and cementing techniques. Remember Boutin's problems with his first generation of ceramic balls containing a glued-in bushing, mentioned in subheading 3. Whether a diffusion-soldering process, recently developed for the fixation of an alumina ceramic ring onto the pergingival portion of Ti dental implants *(123,124)*, employing as intermediate metals niobium (Nb) and tantalum (Ta), can be extended to so much larger parts, remains to be seen. Direct screwing of ceramics onto metals is also not feasible, because of the stiffness mismatch and normal clamping cannot be used, because of the dangers of local stress concentrations inside the ceramic.

Thus, the joining technique that has already stood the test of millions of implantations for more than two decades offers a well-established solution to this joining problem: the Morse taper fixation of alumina ceramic balls on the metal stems. This kind of fixation is even more appropriate for the acetabular insert than for the femoral head: In the latter case, the ceramic surrounds the metal component, resulting in tensional stresses inside the ceramic; the ceramic insert is comprised by the metal backing, and, thus, is compressionally loaded only. This kind of fixation has the further advantage that it can be handled routinely intraoperationally, if the cone angle is chosen correctly, as is discussed in the following paragraph. Many details on the design of ceramic inserts have recently been discussed by Blömer *(115)*.

As with the femoral component, the Morse cone fixation of the ceramic insert in the metal backing of the socket must be self-locking. This can be achieved with a relatively wide range of cone angles between 1:2 and 1:20. The most-used cone for the alumina ceramic femoral heads, such as the Biolox forte heads (Ceram Tec AG, Plochingen, Germany) is 1:10. Since 1986, this same cone geometry has also been used successfully for ceramic metal-backed sockets. However, with this cone angle, a ball, once fixed, cannot be removed from its metal counterpart, at any rate, not intraoperatively. Following this requirement, 1:3 cones (taper angle of 18 degrees) were introduced for the sockets in 1994. They provide for a reliable torsional fixation, but also allow for an exchange of the ceramic component intraoperationally, as well as at later intervention, if necessary. Experience shows that the cone angle, α_c of the ceramic insert must always be some angle minutes larger than the cone angle of the metal backing, α_b, thus $\alpha_a > \alpha_b$, depending on the kind of metal. If the dimensions are chosen correctly, the ceramic insert will always remain under compressional stresses applied along sufficiently large interfacial areas (to avoid stress concentrations).

The probability of occasional subluxations of ceramic heads can be much reduced by special design features: One is the shift of the center of rotation of the ball into the socket by some millimeters, as shown schematically in Fig. 14. Another is the rounding of the edges at the opening of the ceramic insert, as indicated in the lower part of Fig. 14. Because this area is intended to temporarily contribute to articulation, it must also be highly polished. The PE ring placed in front of the opening of the ceramic insert of the Link FGK socket mentioned above *(121)* can also be regarded as an attempt at reducing the dangers of subluxation.

The dimensions and other design details of the ceramic inserts must precisely match the requirements of the individual type of metal backing. This demands close cooperation between manufacturers of the metal components and the ceramic experts. Such metal backings from unauthorized suppliers should neither be used nor prepared by a shop in the clinic or around the corner. For the safety of the patient, and for his own welfare, the clinician should again remember the slogan, "Never mix and match."

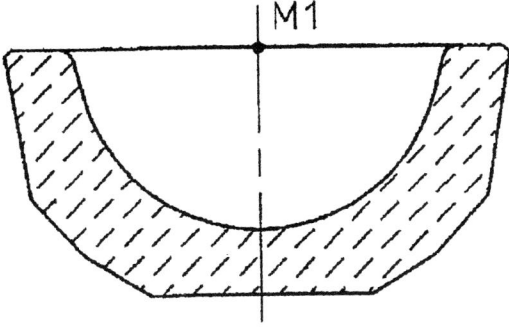

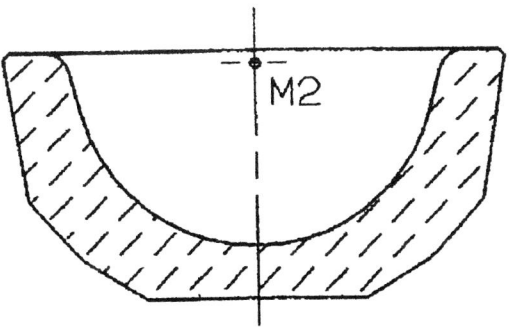

Fig. 14. Cross-section through alumina ceramic insert, with the indication of the positions of the center of rotation of the ceramic balls (not shown). (Top) M 1, the center of rotation identical with center of hole of the socket. (Bottom) M 2, center of rotation of ball shifted inward and edges of inlay opening rounded.

5.3. Interaction Between Socket and Femoral Component

Contacts between the rims of the sockets and the femoral components must be avoided in any THR system. This is the more true for systems containing modular components, because the different materials, as well as the interfaces joining them, demand additional attention. Thus, if, e.g., the neck or the collar of a femoral shaft touches the insert of a socket only, the interface between the insert and its shell will experience shear forces, which had not been designed to withstand this interface. Therefore, all concerned must exclude such contacts as far as possible. Short-necked combinations of stems and balls, together with

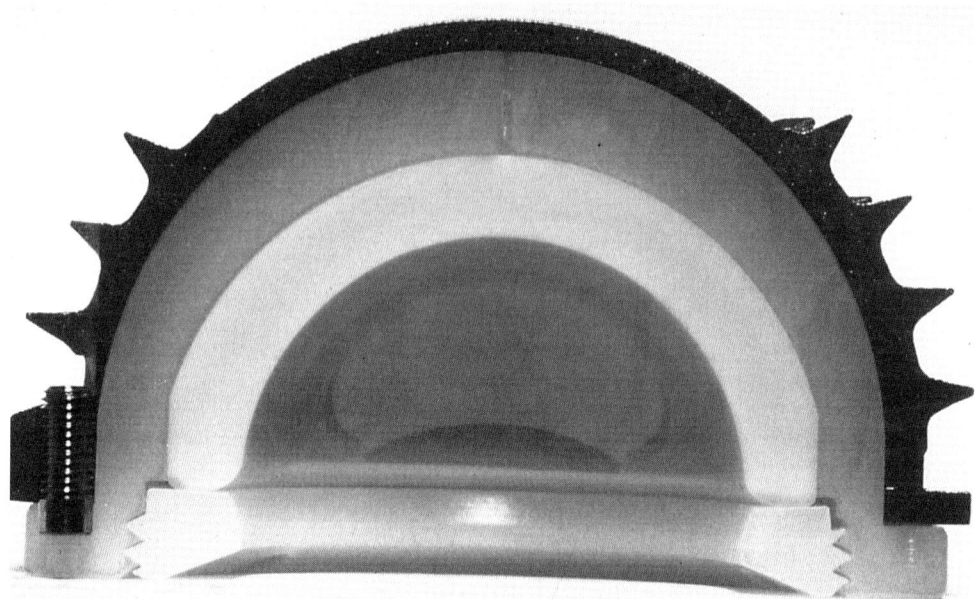

Fig. 15. Cross-sectional view of the Link FGK socket, with PE ring protecting the rim of the alumina ceramic inlay. If its inside diameter is chosen slightly smaller than the diameter of the ball, this PE ring can contribute to preventing luxations. Source: Waldemar Link.

large collars, should be used with utmost care. Also, metal backings of modular sockets must not protrude much above the level of the opening plane of their inserts, because this may additionally confine the angular range of motion (15,125).

The problem of luxations and several of their causes has already been mentioned. Nevertheless, the majority of the 1–3% early complications of the clinical follow-ups, mentioned in the foregoing paragraph, are subluxations. Even if this percentage is in agreement with the overall probability of these early problems in THRs generally, it needs further attention, because, in the case of ceramic articulating against ceramic, the aforementioned snapping in a closed reposition demands particular attention (126). Therefore, any attempt to further decrease the danger of subluxations should be carefully followed. One worthwhile suggestion may be an extension of Lubinus' introduction of an additional PE ring covering the rim of the ceramic insert, and intended to prevent contacts between this rim and the neck of the femoral shaft (121). If the inside diameter of this ring is made slightly smaller than the diameter of the ball, it can contribute to preventing subluxa-

tions (Fig. 15). Because it is not loaded in normal walking, the production of PE wear particles, resulting from this ring, should be negligible.

Critical evaluation of the metal-backed sockets with alumina ceramic inserts presented in this chapter has shown that this concept has already passed the preliminary design and development phases, and that it has stood the test of limited size, and early and mid-term clinical follow-up studies. Any prognosis on the 10-, 15-, and 20-yr success rates rests with the long-term safety of these systems.

6. Safety Aspects

The responsibility for the safety of any implant system rests with whoever must handle it, either directly or indirectly. Many such aspects were discussed earlier in this chapter in subheading 3, on the prerequisites for low wear and their realization, and will not be repeated here, but were also considered, at several other occasions. The importance of these safety concerns were apparent throughout discussions. This will be accounted for by the following evaluations of the more material and engineering-oriented safety issues.

One of the chief concerns in the application of ceramics in medicine is the inherent difference of the stress and strain behavior between metals and ceramics. If a piece of metal is put under a not-too-high tensional stress, it will first become longer, and, if the load is taken away, will return to its original length. Such a deformation is called elastic. If the tensional stress is increased more and more, a threshold value will be reached, beyond which the piece of metal will not return completely to its original shape, but will retain some of the deformation. The piece has, thus, changed its shape: It has been deformed plastically. Under further raised stresses, the metal piece will, in most cases, after more deformations, finally break. A piece of ceramic behaves similarly within the region of stresses causing elastic deformations.

However, most ceramics deform much less under the same stress than metals: Ceramics are much stiffer and retain their shape nearly without any lasting deformation, until they break. This behavior is called brittleness. The details of the stress and strain behavior of the metals was scientifically well understood in the 1920s and the next decade. For ceramics, the detailed description of their mechanics followed, 2–3 decades later. Now, their fatigue processes can also be described in all necessary details, allowing for well-based material evaluations and lifetime predictions.

This increasing knowledge was continuously applied to the components of ceramics in medical applications, in particular to the ceramic balls and their conical fixation onto the femoral shafts *(127–130)*. It was used for further refinements of the conical fixation system, such as the inclusion of the neck length variations into the ceramic heads *(131)*. This detailed understanding of the mechanics of brittle materials even allows for a testing procedure by which all pieces that will not survive a preselected period of time under predetermined stress levels can be eliminated *(132)*. This proof testing has routinely been applied to ceramic femoral heads, since the late 1970s *(133)*.

All these efforts have led to a safety level hardly surpassed by other devices. One of the main supplier of these balls, CeramTec AG, has gathered all ceramic head damages ever reported in the literature *(75)*: 82 heads from a total of 10,313 had fractured or 0.8%, since 1970. If the heads supplied before the introduction of proof testing, about 1980, are excluded, the figures are: From a total of 5,225 heads, 11, or 0.2%, suffered a fracture. A detailed analysis indicated that, in a large number of these cases, the safety rules regarding the machining and handling of the metal cone had been violated severely *(134–136)*. And still, all newly available technical possibilities have been, and are, employed further, such as the replacement of the mechanical engraving of serial number and size by a laser inscription, causing much less damage to the surface of the alumina ceramic *(137)*. Table 8 contains an attempt to demonstrate the safety level of ceramic femoral heads by comparing the revision rates in total hip arthroplasty, from different points of view. Thus, a revision rate of less than .01%, because of problems of ceramic heads of the present generation, must be seen in the light of a total of more than 10% revisions from other causes within 10 yr po.

All these experiences, and the knowledge derived from handling of the balls, have been applied to the ceramic inserts of the modular sockets *(138,139)*. As for this relatively new component, no standards are available, but existing rules from neighboring fields can be used as guidelines. The requirements can be deduced from the data given in Table 9; essential features of a testing device are shown schematically in Fig. 16. In order to reduce the time required for these tests, the number of cycles is reduced to 10 million, but the peak loads are doubled. A detailed evaluation *(138)* has shown that this even increases the safety margin. The torsional stability of the ceramic insert within the metal backing is tested in an arrangement schematically shown in Fig. 17, and, for the push-out resistance, in Fig. 18. Because proof testing of alumina ceramic heads must be regarded as standard today, all inserts of this material should also be proof-tested and inspected piece by piece, as, e.g., is done for all Biolox forte ceramic components. Results from some tests are summarized in Table 10 (according to ref. *138*).

As a result of all these precautions, no material-related failure of these alumina ceramic inserts has been reported. In order to maintain this high safety margin, close cooperation between clinicians, material scientists, and engineers must be

Table 8
General Revision Rates of Total Hip Replacements in Different Time Periods and with Different Material Combinations

Cause of revision	Percentage of revisions	Comments
Aseptic loosening	About 10% within 10 yr po	All systems with PE sockets
Stem fractures	About 2%	Some stem systems have much lower rates
Septic loosenings	About 0.3–1%	
Compiled fractures of first-generation ceramic heads (all systems)	Up to 10% for some systems	(75)
Compiled fractures of first-generation ceramic heads (one system: Biolox)	0.026	(136)
Fractures of second-generation ceramic heads (same system)	0.014	(136)
Compiled fractures in the first development clinics (first- and second-generation Biolox heads)	0.06	Homburg (Saar) (144)
Compiled fractures of one system (Biolox) for all generations	0.015	Study involving 500,000 cases (145)
Compiled fractures of third-generation ceramic heads of one system (now called Biolox forte)	0.004	(136)

One or the other single system may deviate considerably from these average values.

Table 9
Essential Loading Values to be Accounted for in Design of Components of Total Hip Replacements

Kind of influence	Resulting requirement
Weight of patient	Up to 100 kg, resulting in a force at rest of approx 1 kN
Load including accelerations	Up to 10 times body wt, thus up to 10 kN
Average walking frequency	About 1 Hz
Steps/yr	On average, roughly 1 million
Total number of load changes for a survival time of 30 yr	30 million
Requirement for reliable functioning for 30 yr	10–20 million load changes with peak loads of 10 kN (about 2200 lb) will be realistic, because most of the loadings will remain much below 10 kN.
Possible applicable standards	FDA, EN 14630, ISO 7206-05, ISO 7206-6, ISO 6474

maintained, and even intensified (140). Products not meeting the required level must be identified in order to protect patients from avoidable suffering.

Conclusion

The results of early experimental studies on the compatibility of the bulk alumina ceramic and its wear particles had been confirmed by the follow-up evaluations of first-generation total hip prostheses. The conclusions drawn from the animal experiments, regarding the possibilities of cement-free fixations of acetabular components, have not stood the test of 5- and 10-yr clinical observations. Obviously, the stress and strain fields around acetabular sockets are more complicated, and possibly too much changing under load and in time than could be deduced from the relatively short animal experiments, in contrast to the area of dental implantology, in which the histologically documented load-controlled adaptation of

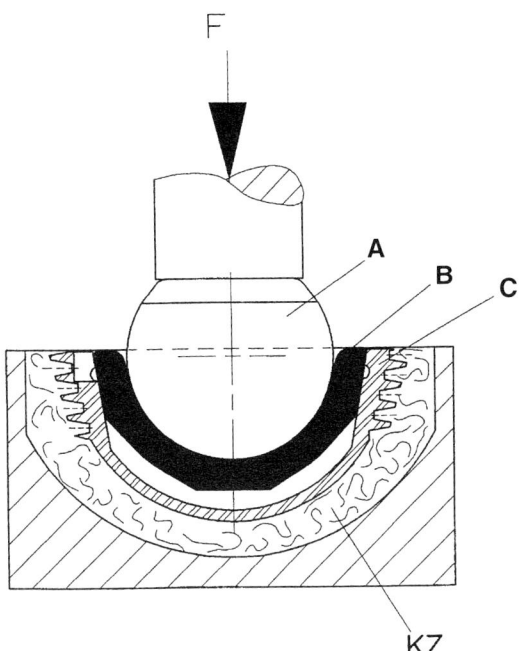

Fig. 16. Cross-sectional view of the arrangement for testing the resistance of alumina ceramic heads and inserts to load changes, with peak loads of 20 kN for 10 million cycles under Ringer solution. F, direction of alternating load; a, ceramic head; b, ceramic insert; c, metal backing; KZ, bone cement.

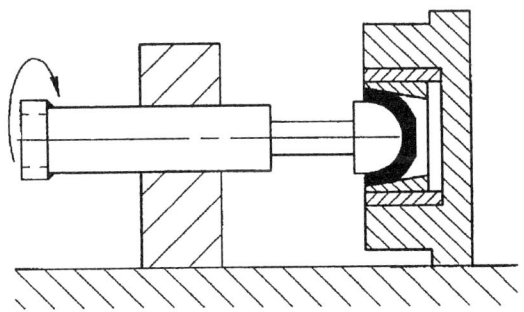

Fig. 17. Cross-sectional view of the testing equipment to determine the torsional stability of alumina ceramic inserts in their metal backings.

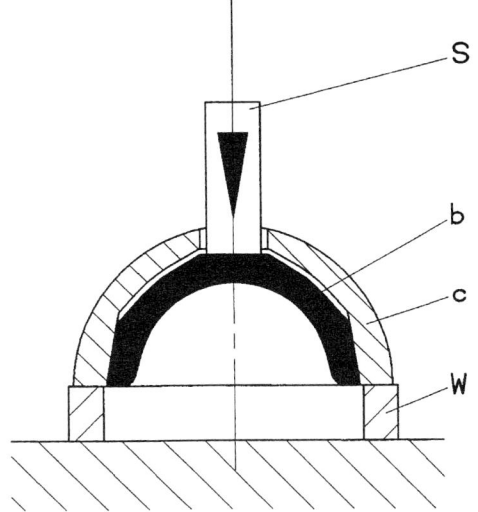

Fig. 18. Cross-sectional view of the testing device to measure the push-out resistance of an alumina ceramic insert in a metal backing. S, piston for load application to the insert; b, ceramic insert; c, metal backing; W, support.

Table 10
Results of Mechanical Strength Tests of Typical Ceramic Components for THRs

Critical component	Typical strength data
28-mm ball with Euro-cone 12/14	Average load at fracture 60 kN
	No single value below 20 kN
XLW 18 Biolox forte inlay[a] for heads of 28 mm diameter, type 28/37 and 28/39[b]	Average load at fracture 50 kN[c]
	No single value below 20 kN

[a]XLW 18 is a standard and typical Biolox forte insert of CeramTec. XLW stands for extremely low wear; 18 gives the taper angle.

[b]The numbers 37 and 39 refer to the outside diameters of the inlays.

[c]Inlays with openings for bone screws for the fixation of the metal cage, or with grooves for rotational stabilization inside PE intermediate inlays have somewhat lower values.

the bony tissue and its stability in time was well confirmed in follow-up studies of more than 20 yr.

The most important result of the early implant systems, with articulating surfaces consisting completely of alumina ceramic, is the confirmation of the high wear resistance of this material combination. In addition, careful observations of these prostheses over time, and evaluations of retrieved implants, opened the possibility to identify some problem areas and, consequently, initiated modifications to reduce risks to levels equal to, or even much lower than, those of the most successful other implant systems, as can clearly be seen in Table 8. There are well-based expectations of even further improvements of long-term survival rates. The marked reduction in the number of wear particles, their size in and below the 1 µm region, and their bioinertness indicate a high probability for a considerable reduction, if not complete avoidance, of the most important remaining cause of the late aseptic loosenings. A near-complete review of all previous experiences with ceramic components in hip arthroplasty, and of the steps that have led to the new metal-backed ceramic sockets, was given in a set of symposia, the content of which is available in three booklets *(141–143)*.

Consequently, the implant systems with metal-backed sockets and alumina ceramic inserts, in combination with femoral heads of the same material, offer the most promising treatment for the great majority of patients concerned. Which of the different metal backings and femoral stems presently clinically employed, and additionally suggested, will be best suited for which indication, remains to be seen from future follow-up studies. Accounting for observations with previously introduced new material combinations and design features, far-reaching deviations from well-established experiences should be avoided.

References

1 Harris WH, Barrack RL, and Mulroy RD Jr. Effect of improved cementing techniques on femoral component loosening in total hip replacements in patients 50 years of age or less. *59th Ann. Mtg Am. Acad. Orthop Surg,* Feb. 1992; Washington, DC, American Academy of Orthopedic Surgeons, Park Ridge, IL, no. 88.
2 Kavanagh BF, Coventry MB, DeWitz M, and Wallrichs S. 1992. Twenty-year follow-up of Charnley low friction arthrosplasty of the hip. *59th Ann. Mtg Am. Acad. Orthop Surg.*, Feb. 1992; Washington, DC, American Academy of Orthopedic Surgeons, Park Ridge, IL, no. 90.
3 Galante JO, Lemons J, Spector M, Wilson PD Jr, and Wright TM. Biological effects of implant materials. *J Orthop Res,* 1991; 9: 760–775.
4 Willert HG and Puls G. Reaction of bone bone cement in hip replacements. *Arch Orthop Unfall Chir,* 1972; 72: 33–71.
5 Heimke G. Aspects and modes of fixation of bone replacements, in *Osseo-Integrated Implants*, vol. I, *Basics, Materials, and Joint Replacements* 1990; (Heimke G, ed.) CRC, Boca Raton, pp. 1–29.
6 Weber BG. Total hip replacement with rotations-endoprosthesis. *Clin Orthop* 1970; 72: 79–84.
7 Willert HG, Semlitsch M, Kriete U, and Zichner L. Clinical experience with Mueller total hip endoprostheses of different designs and materials, in *Mechanical Properties of Biomaterials* 1980; Hastings GW and Williams DF (eds), Biomaterials, Wiley, Chichester, pp. 85–101.
8 Charnley J. Arthroplasty of the hip, a new operation. Lancet, 1961; 1129–1132.
9 Hulbert SF, Young FA, Mathews RS, Klawitter JJ, Talbert CD, and Stelling FH. Potential of ceramic materials as permanent sceletal prostheses. *J Biomed Mater Res* 1970; 4: 433–456.
10 Hentrich RL, Graves GA, Stein HG, Bajpai PK. Evaluation of inert and resorbable ceramics for future clinical applications. *J Biomed Mater Res* 1971; 5: 25–51.
11 Griss P, v Andrian-Werburg H, Krempien H, and Heimke G. Biological activity and histocompatibility of dense Al_2O_3/MgO ceramic implants in rats. *J Biomed Mater Res Symp* 1973; 4: 453–462.
12 Dörre E, Beutler H, and Geduldig D. Anforderungen an oxidkeramische Werkstoffe als Biomaterial für künstliche Gelenke. *Arch Orthop Unfall-Chir* 1975; 83: 269–278.
13 Griss P, Krempien H, v Andrian-Werburg H, Heimke G, and Fleiner R. Experimentelle Untersuchung zur Gewebsverträglichkeit oxidkeramischer (Al_2O_3) Abriebteilchen. *Arch Orthop Unfall Chir* 1973; 76: 270–279.
14 Griss P and Heimke G. Five years experience with ceramic-metal-composite hip endoprostheses. I. Clinical evaluations. *Arch Orthop Traumat Surg* 1981; 98: 157–164.
15 Heimke G and Griss P. Five years experience with ceramic-medal-composite hip endoprostheses. II. Mechanical evaluations and improvements. *Arch Orthop Traumat Surg* 1981; 98: 165–171.
16 Griss P, Heimke G, Werner E, Bleicher J, and Jentschura G. Was bedeutet die Resorption des Calcar femoris nach der Totalendoprothesenoperation der Hüfte? Eine vergleichende Studie an Charnley-Müller- und Oxidkeramikendoprothesen (Typ Lindenhof). *Arch Orthop Traumat Surg* 1978; 92: 225–232.
17 Chillag KJ, Berg E, Heimke G, and Lunceford E

Jr. Lindenhof acetabular component: an eleven year follow-up study, *Bioceramics* 1990; (Heimke G, ed.), vol. 2, German Ceramic Society, Cologne, pp. 429–435.

18 Fritsch E, Remberger H, and Mittelmeier H. Biocompatibility of alumina-ceramic in total hip replacement. Macroscopic and microscopic findings on capsular tissues after long-term implantation. *Die Keramikpaarung BIOLOX in der Hüftendoprothetik*, 1996; (Puhl W, ed.), Ferdinand Enke Verlag, Stuttgart, pp. 12–17.

19 Lintner F, Böhn G, Huber M, Willmann G, and Wais R. Morphologisch-morphometrische Untersuchungen zum Einbauverhalten keramischer Pfannen und deren Partikelfreisetzung, 1996; Ferdinand Enke Verlag, Stuttgart, pp. 18–23.

20 Bos I, Henβge EJ, and Willmann G. Morphologic characteristics of joint capsules around hip prostheses with alumina on alumina combinations. Histologic investigations of revision and autopsy cases, 1996; Ferdinand Enke Verlag, Stuttgart, pp. 24–30.

21 Bonicoli F, Rughini L, Lunati PP, Di Puccio G, Secone St, and Bonicoli E. Ceramic insert in uncemented press-fit titanium total hip prostheses. Our clinical experience in fifty-nine cases, in *Performance of the Wear Couple BIOLOX forte in Hip Arthroplasty*, 1997; (Puhl W, ed.), Ferdinand Enke Verlag, Stuttgart, pp. 38–42.

22 Rueda D, Álvarez M, Barahona F, and Gómez Canedo J. Ceramic inserts in metal cups. A five-year experience, 1997; (Puhl W, ed.), Ferdinand Enke Verlag, Stuttgart, pp. 43–49.

23 Fenollosa J, Aparasi JM, and Seminario P. Ceramic-ceramic in THR: Fifteen years of experience with 262 cases, 1997; (Puhl W, ed.), Ferdinand Enke Verlag, Stuttgart, pp. 51–57.

24 Hench LL, Splinter RJ, Allen WC, and Greenlee K. Bonding mechanisms at the interface of ceramic prosthetic materials. *J Biomed Mater Res Symp* 1971; 2: 117–141.

25 Hench LL and Ethridge EC. *Biomaterials, an Interfacial Approach*, 1981; Academic, New York.

26 Heimke G. Structural characteristics of metals and ceramics, in *Metal and Ceramic Biomaterials*, vol. I, 1984; (Ducheyne P and Hastings GW, eds), CRC, Boca Raton, FL, pp. 7–61.

27 Clark IC and Willmann G. Structural ceramics in orthopaedics, in Bone Implant Interface, 1994; (Cameron HU, ed.), Mosby, St. Louis, pp. 203–252.

28 Willmann G. Production of medical grade alumina. Br Ceramic Trans 1995; 94: 38–41.

29 Willmann G. Ceramic components for total hip arthroplasty. *Orthop Int Ed* 1997; 5: 269–277.

30 Heimke G, Beisler W, von Andrian-Werburg H, Griss P, and Krempien B. Untersuchungen an Implantaten aus Al_2O_3-Keramik. Ber Dt Keram Ges 1973; 50: 4–8.

31 Boutin P. Arthroplastie totale de la hanche par prothèse en alumine frittée. Etude expérimentale et premières applications cliniques. *Rev Chir Orthop* 1972; 58: 229–246.

32 Griss P, Krempien B, von Andrian-Werburg H, Heimke G, Fleier R, and Diehm T. Experimental analysis of ceramic-tissue interactions. A morphologic, fluorescenseoptic, and radiographic study of dense alumina oxide ceramic in various animals. *J Biomed Mater Res Symp 5* 1974; I: 39–48.

33 Griss P, Heimke G, Krempien B, Silber R, Haehner K, and Merkle B. Erste Erfahrungen mit der Keramik-Metallverbundprothese. *Medizin Orthop Tech*, 1975; 6: 159–162.

34 Osborn JF. In *Fortschritte der Kiefer- und Gesichtschirurgie XXVIII* 1983; (Pfeifer G und Schenzer N eds), Georg Thieme Verlag, Stuttgart.

35 d'Hoedt B. Influence of implant materials and material surfaces on blood clotting: a scanning electron microscopic study, in *Tissue Integration in Oral and Maxillofacial Reconstruction*, 1986; (Steenberge D, ed.), Excerpta Medica, Amsterdam, pp. 46–50.

36 Dörre E, Beutler H, and Geduldig D. Anforderungen an oxidkeramische Werkstoffe als Biomaterial für künstliche Gelenke. *Arch Orthop Unfall-Chir* 1975; 83: 269–276.

37 Dörre E and Dawihl W. Mechanische und tribulogische Eigenschaften keramischer Endoprothesen. *Biomed Tech* 1978; 23: 305–310.

38 Griss P, Heimke G, von Andrian-Werburg H, Krempien B, Reipa S, Lauterbach HJ, and Hartung HJ. Morphological and biomechanical aspects of Al_2O_3 ceramic joint replacement. Experimental results and design considerations for human endoprostheses. *J Biomed Mater Symp* 1975; 6: 177–188.

39 Heimke G, Schulte W, Griss P, Jentschura G, and Schulz P. Generalization of biomechanical rules for the fixation of bone, joint, and tooth replacements. *J Biomed Mater Res* 1980; 14: 537–543.

40 Heimke G. Disuse atrophy and adaptive remodeling in the implant carrying femur. *Semin Arthroplasty* 1993; 4: 261–276.

41 Schulte W. FRIALIT Tübingen implant system in *Osseo-Integrated Implants*, vol. II, *Implants in Oral and ENT Surgery*, 1990; (Heimke G, ed.), CRC, Boca Raton, pp. 2–33.

42 Heimke G, Griss P, Jentschura G, and Werner E. Die Aussagefähigkeit histologischer Befunde zur Beurteilung von Knochenersatzwerkstoffen. *Arch Orthop Traumat Surg* 1978; 91: 267–276.

43 Heimke G, Griss P, Werner E, and Jentschura G. Effects of mechanical factors on biocompatibility tests. *J Biomed Eng* 1981; 3: 209–213.

44 Soltesz U, Siegele D, and Baudendiestel E. Might biomechanical effects influence biocompatibility tests in bone? in *Clinical Implant Materials, Advances in Biomaterials,* vol. 9, 1990; (Heimke G, Soltesz U, and Lee AJC, eds), in Biomaterials, vol. 9. Elsevier, Amsterdam, pp. 657–662.

45 Harms J and Mäusle E. Tissue reaction to ceramic implant material. *J Biomed Res* 1979; 13: 67–87.

46 Griss P, Werner E, Buchinger R, Büsing CM, and Heimke G. Zur Frage der unspezifischen Sarkomentstehung um Al_2O_3-keramische Implantate. *Arch Orthop Unfall Chi* 1977; 90: 29–40.

47 Nothdurft H. Experimentelle Sarkomauslösung durch eingeheilte Fremdkörper. Strahlentherapie, 1956; 100: 192–210.

48 Nothdurft H. Tumorerzeugung durch Fremkörperimplantation. Abhandl. Dtsch. Akad. Wissenschaft, Klasse für Medizin, 1960; 80–89.

49 Ott G. Fremdkörpersarkome, in *Experimentelle Medizin, Pathologie und Klinik,* vol. 32, 1970; Springer, Berlin, pp.

50 Gillepsie WJ, Framton CMA, Henderson RJ, and Ryan PM. Incidence of cancer following total hip replacements. *J Bone Joint Surg* 1988; 70-B: 539–542.

51 Black J. Does corrosion matter? *J Bone Joint Surg* 1988; 70-B: 517–520.

52 Heimke G. Biomaterial highlights. II. Materials for biomedical applications: high long-term success rates might pose new problems. *Adv Mater* 1989; 7: 234–236.

53 Bouchard PR, Black J, Albrecht BA, Kaderly RE, Galante O, and Pauli BU. Carcinogenicity of CoCrMo (F-75) implants in the rat. *J Biomed Mater Res* 1996; 32: 37–44.

54 Streicher RM, Schön R, and Semlitsch MF. Investigation of the tribological behaviour of metal-on-metal combinations for artificial hip joints. *Biomed Technik* 1990; 35: 101–111.

55 Heimke G. Role of alumina ceramics in surgical implants, in (Vincenzini P, ed.), *Ceramics in Substitutive and Reconstructive Surgery,* 1991; Elsevier, Amsterdam, pp. 567–581.

56 Ehrl PA and Frenkel G. Experimental and clinical experiences with a blade vent-abutment of Al_2O_3-ceramic in the shortened dental row-situation of the mandible. In (Heimke G, ed.), *Dental Implants, Materials and Systems* 1980; Carl Hanser Verlag, München, pp. 63–67.

57 Schulte W. Das enossale Tübinger Implantat aus Al_2O_3 (Frialit™). Der Entwicklungsstand nach 6 Jahren. Zahnärztl. Mitt. 1981; 71: 2–20.

58 Büsing CM, d'Hoedt B, Schulte W, and Heimke G. Morphological demonstration of direct deposition of bone on human aluminium oxide ceramic dental implants. *Biomaterials* 1983; 4: 125–127.

59 Heimke G, d'Hoedt B, and Schulte W. Ceramics in dental implantology, in *Biomaterials and Clinical Applications,* 1987; (Pizzoferrato A, Marchetti PG, Ravaglioli A, and Lee AJC, eds.), Elsevier, Amsterdam, pp. 93–104.

60 d'Hoedt B and Lucas D. Statistische Ergebnisse des Tübinger Implantates. *Dtsch zahnärztl Z,* 1981; 36: 551–562.

61 Heimke G, Schulte W, and d'Hoedt B. Influence of material and dimension on the gingival attachment to implants. *Clin Mater* 1986; 1: 147–150.

62 Heimke G. *Werkstoffprobleme im pergingivalen Bereich von Implantaten. Jahrbuch für orale Implantologie* 1993; Quintessenz Verlags, Berlin, pp. 13–17.

63 Plester D and Jahnke K. Ceramic implants in otologic surgery. *Am J Otol* 1981; 3: 104–108.

64 Weerda H, Zöllner C, and Ritter KH. Die Tracheopexi mit Stützgerüsten. Eine experimentelle und klinische Studie. *Laryngol Rhinol Otol* 1984; 64: 556–561.

65 Godbersen GS. Septumstütze aus Aluminiumoxydkeramik. *Laryn Rhinol Otol* 1985; 64: 290–291.

66 Polack FM and Heimke G. Ceramic keratoprostheses. *Ophthalmology* 1980; 87: 693–698.

67 Polack FM. Clinical results with a ceramic keratoprosthesis. *Cornea* 1983; 2: 185–196.

68 Boutin P. THA using alumina-alumina sliding and metallic stem: 1330 cases and an 11 years follow-up, in *Orthopedic Ceramic Implants,* 1981; (Oonishi H and Ooi Y, eds), Proc Jap Soc Orthop Ceram Implants, pp. 11–19.

69 Boutin P Personal communication, 1976.

70 Boutin P. Les protheses totale de la hanch en alumine. L'ancrage direct sans ciment dans 50 cas. *Rev Clin Orthop* 1974; 60: 233–245.

71 Boutin P. L'arthroplastie totale de la hanche par prothèse en alumine. Résultats de 150 cas d'ancrage direct de la pièce acétabulaire. *Int Orthop* (SICOT) 1977; 1: 87–94.

72 Boutin P, Christel P, Dorlot JM, Meunier A, De Roquancourt A, Blanquaert et al. Use of dense alumina-alumina ceramic combination in total hip replacement. *J Biomed Mater Res* 1988; 22: 1203–1232.

73. Mittelmeier H. Selbsthaftende Keramik-Metall-Verbundprothesen. *Med Orthop Tech* 1975; 97: 152–159.
74. Salzer M, Zweymüller K, Locke H, Zeibig A, Stark N, Plenk H, and Punzel G. Further experimental and clinical experience with aluminum oxide endoprostheses. *J Biomed Mater Res* 1976; 10: 847–856.
75. Toni A, Sudanese A, Terzi S, Tabaaroni M, Calista F, and Giunti A. Ceramics in total hip arthroplasty, in *Encyclopedic Handbook of Biomaterials and Bioengineering*, Part B: *Applications*, vol. 2, 1995; (Wise DL et al., eds.), M. Dekker, New York, pp. 1501–1544.
76. Mittelmeier H. 4 Jahre Erfahrung mit dem Autophor-Keramik-Hüftsystem. *Med Orthop Techn (MOT)* 1980; 100: 19–30.
77. Griss P, Hackenbroch MH, Jäger M, Preussner B, Schäfer Th, Seebauer R, Eimeren W van, and Winkler W. Ten year results of total hip replacement. A retrospective multicenter study based on a 10% random sample of 39,000 total hip replacements, in *Aktuelle Probleme in Chirurgie und Orthopädie*, 1981; (Buri C, Herfarth D, and Jäger M, eds.) H. Huber, Bern.
78. Mulroy RD Jr and Harris WH. Effect of improved cementing techniques on component loosening in total hip replacement. *J Bone Joint Surg* 1990; 72-B: 757–760.
79. Willert H-G, Semlitsch M, Buchhorn G, and Kriete U. Materialverschleiss mit Gewebereaktion bei künstlichen Gelenken (Histopathologie, Biokompatibilität, biologische und klinische Probleme). *Orthopäde* 1978; 7: 62–83.
80. Henssge EJ, Bos I, and Willmann G. Al_2O_3 against Al_2O_3 combination in hip endoprostheses. Histologic investigations with semiquantitative grading of revision and autopsy cases and abrasion measures. *J Mater Sci, Mater Med* 1994; 5: 657–661.
81. Sedel L, Kerboull L, Christel P, Meunier A, and Witvoet J. Alumina on alumina hip replacement. Results and survivorship in young patients. *J Bone Joint Surg* 1990; 72-B: 658–663.
82. Willmann G, Kemmer U, and Zweymüller K. Investigation of retrieved femoral Biolox heads. In *Bioceramics*, (Andersson OH and Yil-Urpo A, eds.), vol. 7, 1999; Butterworth-Heinemann, Oxford, pp. 377–381.
83. Mahoney OM and Dimon JH. Unsatisfactory results with a ceramic total hip prosthesis. *J Bone Joint Surg* 1990; 72-A: 663–671.
84. Heimke G, Berg E, and Chillag K. Correspondance to the editor. *J Bone Joint Surg* 1991; 73-A: 1112–1113.
85. Walter A. Wear screening of ceramic-to-ceramic components for total hip replacements by ring-on-disc device joint simulator test, in *Ceramics in Clinical Applications*, 1987; (Vincenzini P, ed.), pp. 159–168.
86. Walter A and Plitz W. Wear mechanism of alumina-ceramic bearing surfaces of hip joint prostheses, in *Biomaterials and Biomechanics* (Ducheyne P, van der Perre G, and Aubert AE, eds.), Elsevier, Amsterdam, 1983; pp. 55–60.
87. Willmann G, Pfaff HG, and Richter HG. Steigerung der Sicherheit von keramischen Kugelköpfen für Hüftendoprothesen. *Biomed Tech* 1995; 40: 342–346.
88. Walter A. On the material and the tribology of alumina-alumina couplings for hip joint prostheses. *Clin Orthop* 1992; 282: 31–36.
89. Blencke B-A. Zur Austauschbarkeit von Keramik-Kugelköpfen verschiedener Endoprothesen-Systeme. *Z Orthop*, 1987; 125: 188–189.
90. McTighe T, Trick LW, and Koeneman JB. Design considerations for cementless total hip arthroplasty, *Encyclopedic Handbook of Biomaterials and Bioengineering*, Part B: *Applications*, vol. 1, 1995; (Wise DL, et al., eds.), M. Dekker, New York, pp. 573–612.
91. Claussen N. Umwandlungsverstärkte keramische Werkstoffe. *Z Werkstofftech* 1982; 13: 138–145.
92. Garvie RC, Urbani C, Kennedy DR, and McNeuer JC. Biocompatibility of magnesia partially stabilized (Mg-PSZ) ceramics. *J Mater Sci* 1984; 19: 3224–3229.
93. Cieur S, Heindl R, and Robert A. Radioactivity of a femoral head of zirconia ceramics, in *Bioceramics*, vol. 3, 1992; (Hulbert SF, ed), Rose Hulman Institute of Technology, Terre Haut, IN, pp. 367–371.
94. Nakajima K, Kobayashi K, and Murata Y. Phase stability of Y-PSZ in aqueous solutions, in *Advances of Ceramics*, (Claussen N, Rühle M, and Heier HA, eds.), vol. 12, *Science and Technology of Zirconia II*, 1984; American Ceramic Society, Columbus, OH, pp. 339–345.
95. Willmann G. Oxide ceramics for articulating components of total hip replacements, in *Bioceramics*, vol. 10, (Sedel L and Rev C, eds), Elsevier, Amsterdam, pp. 123–126.
96. Früh HJ, Willmann G, and Pfaff HG. Wear characteristics of ceramic-on-ceramic for hip endoprostheses. *Biomaterials*, 1997; 18: 873–876.
97. Medical Device Agency Adverse Incidence Center. Zirconia ceramic heads for modular total hip femoral components: advice to users on resterilization, 1996; Notice Medical Device Agency SN 97617, London, June 1997.

98. Richter HG, Burger W, and Osthues F. Zirconia for medical implants: the role of strength properties, in *Bioceramics* 1994; (Andersson OH and Ylil-Urpo A, eds), Butterworth-Heinemann, Oxford, pp. 104–106.
99. Willmann G. Ceramics for total hip replacement. *Orthopedics* 1998; 21: 173–177.
100. Calès B and Stéfani Y. Yttria-stabilized zirconia for improved orthopedic prostheses, in *Encyclopedic Handbook of Biomaterials and Bioengineering,* Part B: *Applications,* vol. 1, 1995; (Wise DC, et al., eds), M. Dekker, New York, pp. 415–452.
101. Willmann G, Früh HJ, and Pfaff HG. Wear characteristics of sliding pairs of zirconia (Y-TZP) for hip endoprostheses. *Biomaterials,* 1996; 17: 2157–2162.
102. Chevalier J, Cales B, Drouin JM, and Stefani Y. Ceramic-ceramic bearing systems compared on different testing configurations, in *Bioceramics,* vol. 10, 1997; (Sedel L and Rey C, eds), Elsevier, Amsterdam, pp. 271–274.
103. Bosdorf K, Mollenhauer I, Willmann G, and Boenick U. Werkstoffe für Hüffendoprothesen: Alternativen zu den Standardmaterialien. *Biomed Tech* 1995; 40: 356–362.
104. Semlitsch M, Lehmann M, Weber H, Dörre E, and Willert HG. New prospects for a prolonged functional lifespan of artificial hip joints using the material combination polyethylene/aluminum oxide ceramic/metal. *J Biomed Mater Res* 1977; 11: 537–542.
105. Streicher RM, Semlitsch M, and Schön R. Ceramic surfaces as wear partners for polyethylene, in *Bioceramics,* vol. 4, 1991; (Bonfield W, Hastings GW, and Tanner KE, eds), Butterwortth-Heinemann, Oxford, pp. 9–16.
106. Bos I, Meeuwssen E, Henβge, EJ, and Löhrs U. Unterschiede des Polyäthylenabriebs bei Hüftgelenkprothesen mit Keramik- und Metall-Polyäthylenpaarung der Gleitfächen. EineUntersuchung an Operations- und Autopsiematerial. *Z Orthop* 1991; 129: 507–515.
107. Zichner L and Lindenfeld T. In-vivo Verschleiß der Gleitpaarungen Keramik-Polyethylen gegen Metall-Polyethylen. *Orthopäde* 1997; 26: 129–134.
108. Jensen RE, Collier JP, Mayor MB, McNamara JL, and Surprenant VA. Potential mechanisms for acetabular component failure: a retrieval analysis. *Proc 59th Ann Mtg Am Acad Orthop Surg* Feb 1992; Washington, DC, American Academy Orthopedic Surgeons, Park Ridge, IL, no. 66.
109. Parsley BS. Current concerns with modular metal-backed acetabular components, 1992; no. 95.
110. Cates HE, Faris PM, Keating EM, and Ritter MA. Polyethylene wear with cemented metal-backed acetabular cups in total hip arthroplasty, 1992; no. 96.
111. Ritter MA, Keating EM, Faris PM, and Brugo G. Metal-backed acetabular cups in total hip arthroplasty. *J Bone Joint Surg* 1990; 72-A: 672–675.
112. Gabriel SM and Bartel DL. Metal backing and wear in acetabular components for total hip arthroplasty. *Proc 38th Ann Mtg Orthop Res Soc,* February 1992; Washington, DC, Orthopedic Research Society, Park Ridge, IL, pp. 47.
113. Fehring TK, Hurley PT, Braun E, Mobley Jr C, Wang P-L, and Griffin WL. Modular acetabular components: Are they really metal backed? *Proc: 59th Ann Mtg Am Acad Orthop Surg,* Feb. 1992; Washington, DC, American Academy Orthopedic Surgeons, Park Ridge, IL, 92.
114. Hurley PT, Fehring TK, Braun E, Mobley Jr C, Wang P-L, and Griffin WL. Polyethylene liners in modular porous acetabular components: a comparative analysis. 1992; American Academy Orthopedic Surgeons, Park Ridge, IL, 94.
115. Blömer W. Design aspects of modular inlay fixation, in *Performance of the Wear Couple BIOLOX forte in Hip Arthroplasty,* 1997; (Puhl W, ed), Ferdinand Enke Verlag, Stuttgart, pp 95–104.
116. Heimke G. Orthopedic reconstruction: taking the right approach. *Adv Mater* 1992; 4: 476–679.
117. Franke C and Stock D. Monolithische versus modular aufgebaute, zementfreie Keramik-Hüft-Endoprothesen, in *Performance of the Wear Couple BIOLOX forte in Hip Arthroplasty,* 1997; (Puhl W, ed), Ferdinand Enke Verlag, Stuttgart, pp. 62–64.
118. Maaz B and Schlegel TJ. Erfahrungen mit dem Kaiserswerther Pfannensystem (Metallschraubring mit Keramikinlay), 1997; Ferdinand Enke Verlag, Stuttgart, pp. 61.
119. Widhalm R, Karner A, and Gebhart Ch. Die Variopfanne mit Pressfitverankerung und Keramik-Gleitpaarung. Konzepte und erste Ergebnisse, 1997; Ferdinand Enke Verlag, Stuttgart, pp 77–80.
120. Quack G, Willmann G, Krahl H, and Grundei H. Weiterentwicklung des ESKA-Spongiosametall-Pfannensystems durch die BIOLOX*forte Gleitpaarung, 1997; Ferdinand Enke Verlag, Stuttgart, pp. 65–76.
121. Lubinus P. Das Konzept des funktionsgeschützen Keramiklagers (FGK), 1997; Ferdinand Enke Verlag, Stuttgart, pp. 85–89.
122. Menge M and Hesse J. Mittelfristige Ergebnisse

mit dem SI-Schraubring mit Keramik-Inserts. 1997; Ferdinand Enke Verlag, Stuttgart, pp. 81–84.
123. Gibbesch B, Elssner G, and Petzow G. Microstructure and mechanical properties of Ti-Ta/alumina and Ti-Nb/alumina joints for dental implants. *Int J Oral Maxilofac Implants* 1989; 4: 131–137.
124. Gibbesch B, Elssner G, and Petzow G. Investigation of titanium-alumina joints with intermediate tantalum and niobium layers. *Biomaterials,* 1992; 13: 455–461.
125. Oonishi H, Clark IC, and Amino H. New design features of high-quality alumina-alumina ceramic combination in total hip replacement, in *Bioceramics 5,* 1992; (Yamamuro T, Kokubo T, and Nakamura T, eds), Kobunshi Kankokai, Kyoto, pp. 403–408.
126. Kaddick C, Steinhauser E, Köhler D, and Gradinger R. Determination of resistance to luxations/repositions of total hip joint prostheses, *Bioceramics in Orthopaedics: New Applications,* 1998; (Puhl IW, ed), Ferdinand Enke Verlag, Stuttgart, pp. 25–28.
127. Richter H, Seidelmann U, and Soltész U. Slow crack growth and failure prediction for alumina in simulated physiological media, in *Evaluation of Biomaterials,* 1980; (Winter GD, Leray JL, and de Groot K, eds), Wiley, Chichester, UK, pp. 227–232.
128. Seidelmann U, Richter H, and Soltész U. On the structural safety of ceramic hip-joint heads, in *Biomaterials,* 1980, 1982; (Winter GD, Gibbons DE, and Plenck H Jr, eds), Wiley, Chichester, UK, pp. 213–218.
129. Soltész U and Heimke G. Stress analysis in ceramic hip-joint heads of various shapes and fittings, in *Biomechanics: Principles and Applications,* 1982; (Huiskes R, van Campen D, and de Wijn J, eds), Martinus Nijhoff, The Hague, pp. 283–290.
130. Seidelmann U, Richter H, and Soltész U. Failure of ceramic hip endoprostheses by slow crack growth: lifetime prediction. *J Biomed Mater Res* 1982; 16: 705–713.
131. Kleer G, Soltész U, Benzing U, and Siegele D. Structural safety and stress distribution in ceramic hip-joint-heads for different neck lengths, in *Biomechanics: Basic and Applied Research, Selected Proceedings of the Fifth Meeting of the European Society of Biomechanics,* (Bergmann G, Kölbel R, and Rohlmann A, eds), September 1986; Berlin, pp. 773–378.
132. Schäfer R, Soltész U, and Siegele D. Proof testing of ceramic hip joint heads, in *Bioceramics,* vol. 2, 1990; (Heimke G, ed), German Ceramic Society, Cologne, pp 172–179.
133. Richter HG and Willmann G. Reliability of ceramic components for total hip endoprostheses, in *Die Keramikpaarung BIOLOX in der Hüftendoprothetik,* 1996; (Puhl W, ed), Ferdinand Enke Verlag, Stuttgart, pp 77–83.
134. Heimke G. Safety aspects of the fixation of ceramic balls on metal stems, in *Bioceramics,* vol. 6, 1993; (Ducheyne P and Christiansen D, eds), Butterworth-Henemann, Oxford, pp 283–288.
135. Heimke G. Safety of ceramic balls on metal stems of hip arthroplasty. *Adv Mater* 1994; 6: 165–170.
136. Willmann G. Wie sicher sind keramische Kugelköpfe für Hüftendoprothesen? *Mat-wiss Werkstofftech* 1996; 27: 280–286.
137. Willmann G. Steigerung der Sicherheit von keramischen Kugelköpfen für Hüftendoprethesen. *Biomed Tech* 1995; 40: 342–346.
138. Willmann G, Kälberer H, and Pfaff H-G. Ceramic cup inserts for hip endoprostheses. *Biomed Tech* 1996; 41: 98–105.
139. Willmann G, Kälberer H, and Pfaff H-G. Ceramic acetabular cups for total hip replacements. Part 2: Component testing and reliability. *Biomed Tech* 1996; 41: 284–290.
140. Willmann G. BIOLOX® forte heads and cup inserts for THR: What the surgeon should know, in *Performance of the Wear Couple BIOLOX forte in Hip Arthroplasty* 1997; (Puhl W, ed), Ferdinand Enke Verlag, Stuttgart, pp 105–116.
141. W. Puhl, ed. *Die Keramikpaarung BIOLOX in der Hüftendoprothetik,* 1996; Ferdinand Enke Verlag, Stuttgart.
142. W. Puhl, ed. *Performance of the Wear Couple BIOLOX forte in Hip Arthroplasty,* 1997; Ferdinand Enke Verlag, Stuttgart.
143. W. Puhl, ed. *Bioceramics in Orthopaedics: New Applications,* 1998; Ferdinand Enke Verlag, Stuttgart.
144. Fritsch EW and Gleitz M. Ceramic femoral head fractures in total hip arthroplasty. *Clin Orthop Rel Res* 1996; 328: 129–136.
145. Semlitsch M, Weber H, and Steger R. 15 Jahre Erfahrungen mit Ti-6A1-7 Nb-Legierung für Gelenkprothesen. *Biomed Tech* 1995; 40: 347–355.

15

Applied Aspects of Calcium Phosphate Bone Cement Application

F. C. M. Driessens, M. G. Boltong, I. Khaïroun, E. A. P. De Maeyer, M. P. Ginebra, R. Wenz, J. A. Planell, and R. M. H. Verbeeck

1. Nature of Calcium Phosphate Bone Cements

Calcium phosphate bone cements (CPBCs) consist of a powder and an aqueous liquid, which are mixed to form a paste that sets at room or body temperature under the formation of a precipitate that contains at least one calcium phosphate (CaP) *(1–4)*. In the system, $Ca(OH)_2$-H_3PO_4-H_2O, a limited number of CaPs can precipitate *(5,6;* Table 1). Among these CaPs, monocalcium phosphate monohydrate precipitates only from very acidic aqueous solutions, which are for that reason cytotoxic. Moreover, octacalcium phosphate precipitates only after very long induction times, which are impractical to form CPBCs. The composition of the apatite can vary continuously from CDHA to hydroxyapatite (HA), so that no definite border between the pH ranges exists at which a Ca-deficient or stoichiometric apatite precipitates. If the system contains also Na^+ and/or CO_3^{2-} ions, these ions will be incorporated at least partially into the apatite precipitate. Finally, there is no easy way to distinguish between amorphous calcium phosphate (ACP) I and ACP II. For these reasons, the CPBCs known are of the brushite type, the apatite type, or the ACP type.

Apart from the compounds that can precipitate in CPBC, other Ca-containing compounds can be used as constituents of the CPBC powders (Table 2).

Because the ions Na^+, K^+, Mg^{2+}, Ca^{2+}, Zn^{2+}, Cl^-, SO_4^{2-}, carbonate, and phosphate are regular constituents of the body fluids *(5)*, it is obvious that solid compounds containing these ions can be used safely in the powder of the CPBCs, because of the absence of cytotoxicity. Sulfates and phosphates of Na^+ and/or K^+ can effectively be used in the liquid of CPBCs to accelerate or retard their setting, as will be shown in subheading 3. From the phosphates, only orthophosphates are suitable as components of biomaterials, because pyrophosphates, metaphosphates, and polyphosphates hydrolyze to orthophosphates in contact with body fluids. Some compounds, not containing Ca, are not yet used as constituents in the liquid or the powder of CPBCs, but may be attractive for that purpose (Table 3; *3*).

CaP bone cements gain their strength by two different mechanisms. In the case of dicalcium phosphate dihydrate (DCPD) or apatite cements, when the precipitate is crystalline, strength is gained by entanglement of the precipitating crystals *(7)*. This mechanism is comparable to the setting of gypsum products. However, in the case of ACP cements, strength is gained by a sol–gel transition *(8)*. In both cases, the rate of setting and the increase in strength with time are increased

From: *Biomaterials Engineering and Devices: Human Applications,* Volume 2
Edited by D. L. Wise, et al. © Humana Press, Inc., Totowa, NJ

Table 1
CaPs that Can Precipitate at Room or Body Temperature in the system $Ca(OH)_2$-H_3PO_4-H_2O

Ca/P	Calcium phosphate	Formula	pH
1.35	Amorphous calcium phosphate I (ACP I)	–	4–9
1.35	Amorphous calcium phosphate II (ACP II)	–	4–9
0.5	Monocalcium phosphate monohydrate (MCPM)	$Ca(H_2PO_4)_2 \cdot H_2O$	0–2
1.0	Dicalcium phosphate dihydrate (DCPD) (brushite)	$CaHPO_4 \cdot 2H_2O$	2–6
1.33	Octocalcium phosphate (OCP)	$Ca_8(HPO_4)_2(PO_4)_4 \cdot 5H_2O$	5.5–7.0
1.5	Calcium deficient hydroxyapatite (CDHA)	$Ca_9(HPO_4)(PO_4)_5(OH)$	6.5–8.0
1.67	Hydroxyapatite (HA)	$Ca_{10}(PO_4)_6(OH)_2$	9.5–12

Table 2
Ca-containing Reagents Other than Those of Table 1, Which Are also Suitable as Constituents of CPBC Powders

Ca/P	Reagents	Formula
1.0	Dicalcium phosphate (DCP)	$CaHPO_4$
1.5	β-tricalcium phosphate (β-TCP)	$\beta\text{-}Ca_3(PO_4)_2$
1.5	α-tricalcium phosphate (α-TCP)	$\alpha\text{-}Ca_3(PO_4)_2$
2.0	Tetracalcium phosphate (TTCP)	$Ca_4(PO_4)_2O$
1.42	Sodium whitlockite (SWH)	$Ca_{10}Na(PO_4)_7$
1.0	Rhenanite (RH)	$CaNaPO_4$
1.0	Calcium potassium phosphate (CPP)	$CaKPO_4$
1.0	Calcium sodium potassium phosphate (CSPP)	$Ca_2NaK(PO_4)_2$
1.33	Magnesium tricalcium phosphate (MTCP)	$MgCa_8(PO_4)_6$
1.28	Magnesium whitlockite (MWH)	$Ca_9Mg(HPO_4)(PO_4)_6$
0.84	Magnesium calcium phosphate	$Ca_5Mg_4(PO_4)_6$
0.5	Calcium zinc phosphate (CZP)	$CaZn_2(PO_4)_2$
2.0	Spodiosite (SP)	Ca_2PO_4Cl
1.67	Chloroapatite (CLA)	$Ca_{10}(PO_4)_6Cl_2$
∞	Calcium carbonate (either calcite or aragonite)	$CaCO_3$
∞	Dolomite (DOL)	$CaMg(CO_3)_2$
∞	Calcium sulfate anhydrous	$CaSO_4$
∞	Calcium sulfate hemihydrate	$2CaSO_4 \cdot H_2O$
∞	Calcium sulfate dihydrate	$CaSO_4 \cdot 2H_2O$
1.67	Calcium phosphate sulfate	$Ca_{10}(SO_4)(PO_4)_6$
∞	Calcium fluoride	CaF_2

considerably by decreasing particle size of the cement powder ingredients, and by increasing temperature (9,10). Even a temperature rise from room temperature to body temperature has a considerable effect on the rate of setting.

2. Biocompatibility and Bone Histology of CPBCs

The first CPBC was of the apatite type, based on a mixture of tetracalcium phosphate and dicalcium phosphate (11). It was not mutagenic nor toxic (12). Quantitative testing confirmed the absence of cytotoxicity (13). Testing cytotoxicity of five other CPBCs, and one magnesium phosphate cement in a static human fibroblast culture (14), revealed that contact cytotoxicity is mostly caused by pH values deviating more than 2 units from 7.0. It is expected that none of the known CPBCs will show any cytotoxicity in a dynamic, buffered system resembling more the tissue conditions in the living body. Therefore, the chance for

Table 3
Other Compounds Suitable as Additives for Improving Properties of CaP Cements

Component	Compounds
Sodium	NaF, Na_2CO_3, $NaHCO_3$, Na_2SO_4, orthophosphates of Na, Na_2SiO_3
Potassium	KF, K_2CO_3, K_2SO_4, orthophosphates of K, K_2SiO_3
Magnesium	$MgHPO_4$, $Mg_3(PO_4)_2 \cdot xH_2O$, MgF_2, $MgCO_3$, MgO, $Mg(OH)_2$, $MgSO_4$
Zinc	$Zn_3(PO_4)_2 \cdot 4H_2O$, ZnF_2, $ZnCO_3$, $ZnSO_4$, ZnO, $Zn(OH)_2$
Biopolymers	Proteins, peptides, proteoglycans, glycosaminoglycans, carbohydrates
Organic acids	Citric acid, malonic acid, pyruvic acid, tartaric acid
Inorganic acids	Phosphoric acid
Synthetic polymers	Polylactic acid, polyglycolic acid
Growth factors	TGF-β, osteocalcine, GLA proteins

contact toxicity upon implantation of CPBCs is very small, and adverse cellular reactions are probably caused by implantation damage.

As for CaP ceramics, systemic toxicity is completely absent (15), because excess Ca and phosphate ions are excreted by the kidneys, but there is a fine-tuned mechanism to keep enough Ca and phosphate in the bone (16).

Very interesting is the interaction of CPBCs with cells occurring in and near bone. Osteoclasts in culture resorb CPBCs of the apatite type (17). Osteoblasts and osteoprogenitor cells grow and differentiate on apatite-type CPBC surfaces, and excrete collagen (18–21). So apatite-type CPBCs are open for the processes occurring during bone remodeling. It is expected that, upon implantation in bone, the apatite-type CPBCs will be taken up in the local remodeling of bone. There is abundant evidence now for the fact that apatite-type CPBCs are replaced gradually by new bone tissue, and that cellular activity is responsible for this transformation (22–28). This could be derived from experiments in which apatite-type CPBC cylinders were implanted subcutaneously in rats, so that no cellular contact occurred, but there was continuous contact with extracellular fluid (30). Because there was no change in weight, composition, and strength in these cylinders, it was inferred that cellular activity is indispensable for the CPBC transformation into new bone, i.e., osteotransduction (29). As the result of cellular activity, the apatite-type CPBCs are even osteoinductive. This was shown by implantation in dorsal muscles of dogs, in which the cement degraded at its interface with the soft tissue, while new bone was simultaneously formed (31).

The behavior of DCPD-type CPBCs upon implantation is quite different, as would be expected from the higher solubility of DCPD, compared to that of apatite, and from the fact that body fluids are undersaturated with respect to DCPD. Consequently, DCPD dissolves spontaneously into body fluids, without any cellular activity. In fact, passive resorption is found upon implantation of DCPD-type cements into the bone of rabbits and dogs (32–37). The same allegedly holds for some ACP-type CPBCs (32), which may be in line with expectations, because, in the physiological range of pH, the solubility of ACP II is comparable to that of DCPD (5,6), so that body fluids are also undersaturated with ACP II, which thus will dissolve spontaneously upon implantation. Whether the body is able to form new bone at the same rate, with which these DCPD-type or ACP-type cements dissolve, mostly depends on local recovery and healing potential. Therefore, when CPBCs of the DCPD type, of some ACP types, or of the mixed DCPD-ACP-type, are implanted in bone, their transformation into new bone may seem faster than that of apatite-type cements. Consequently, complete loss of structural coherence between the implant and the surrounding bone may occur. This certainly does not happen with implantation of apatite-type cements. The most rapid resorption possible of a bone-substituting material, such as a CPBC, is therefore not advantageous.

3. Initial and Final Setting Times

These are measured mostly with Gilmore needles. The light-and-wide needle is used to determine the initial setting time, t_1. At that moment, the cement paste has already reached some stiffness. In fact, it has by then passed the stage for moldability, without serious damage to the cement structure for quite some time (*see* subheading 6). But the method is quick and easy. With the heavy-and-fine Gilmore needle, one can measure the final setting time, t_F, beyond which it is possible to touch the cement without causing any damage (39).

The setting times decrease with decreasing liquids:powder ratio (40,41), with smaller particle size of the active powder ingredient (41), and with higher seed contents (42). Mostly, the setting of apatitic CPBCs must be accelerated for practical use. This can be done effectively by using solutions of Na_2HPO_4 or $NaH_2PO_4 \cdot 2H_2O$ as cement liquid (43). On the other hand, the setting of DCPD-type CPBCs must be retarded, and this can be done by addition of Ca pyrophosphate, Ca sulfate dihydrate, or Ca sulfate hemihydrate to the powder (44). In general, for dental applications, t_I should be about 2–4 min; for orthopedic applications, it may be as long as 15 min, depending on the wishes of the surgeon (45,46).

4. Cohesion Time

Animal experiments (28), using an α-tricalcium phosphate (α-TCP)-based apatite cement, revealed that this cement disintegrated upon early contact with blood or other body fluids. Other investigators (47) had the same problem with a tetracalcium phosphate (TTCP)–dicalcium phosphate-based apatite cement. Indications were found that the early cohesion of cement pastes could be improved by dissolving compounds, such as Na alginate, in the cement liquid (48–51). The problem was systematically tackled by the development of a method to determine the cohesion time (t_C), the time necessary to develop enough resistance to disintegration by early contact with fluids (52). It is clear that implantation of a cement paste can not be done before this t_C is reached. On the other hand, implantation should be done long before the initial setting time t_I, i.e., in the dough state of the paste. Recently (53), it was shown that t_c can be reduced considerably by dissolving amounts of the following cohesion promoters into the cement liquid: hydroxyethyl starch, Na dextran sulfate, starch, α-, β- or γ-cyclodextrine, hyaluronic acid potassium salt, Na alginate, and Na chondroitine sulfate. The disadvantage of addition of such biochemical ingredients is that extensive animal testing is then unavoidable before admission to the market is allowed. Therefore, it is better to reduce the cohesion time of CPBCs by adding inorganic constituents, and by proper milling of the cement powders (54,55).

5. Strength

Among mechanical properties, chiefly the compressive strength (C) of CPBCs is measured (56). For that purpose, cylindrical specimens are prepared, with a height of 12 mm and a diameter of 6 mm. An appropriate cross-head speed is 1 mm/min. A comparative study of the strength and some other characteristics of some experimental and commercial CPBCs retrieved on the market was done (57; Table 4).

It may be argued that, for load-bearing applications, a CPBC must at least have the compressive strength of trabecular bone. The highest value for human trabecular bone is about 30 MPa (58). In this respect, it can be seen from Table 4 that only three cements, i.e., Norian SRS, Experimental 3, and Biocement D, are adequate. The values for t_I and t_F for the latter are also clinically attractive.

However, the elasticity coefficient for CPBCs may be quite different from that of trabecular bone, so that also the tensile strength and the toughness of CPBCs may become important for certain applications. This can only be tested by clinical and animal trials, in combination with mechanical testing.

6. Injectability and Dough Time

Most researchers in the field of CPBCs feel that the ideal CPBC should have the highest possible injectability (I%). For this reason, some authors (59,60) even made qualitative measurements. In order to make considerations about I% really operational, a test was designed (61) to measure it quantitatively with a commercial syringe, which was accepted as standard for that test. In this way, I% is obtained (57) by extrusion, immediately after mixing the cement in a mortar, filling the syringe with the paste, and extruding the paste from the syringe 2 min after the start of mixing

Table 4
Injectability (I%), Initial Setting Time (t_I) (min), Final Setting Time (t_F) (min) and Compressive Strength at 24 h (C) (MPa) of some Commercial and Experimental CPBCs

Product	C	t_I(20°C)	t_I(37°C)	t_F(20°C)	t_F(37°C)	I%
Norian SRS	33 (5)	22 (1)	6½ (½)	37 (1)	8½ (½)	83 (1)[a]
Cementek	8 (2)	36 (1)	9½ (½)	64 (2)	17 (1)	81 (1)
Biocement D	83 (4)	6½ (½)	2¾ (¼)	11 (1)	6½ (½)	94 (1)
Experimental 1	4 (1)	70 (5)	11 (1)	>200	19 (1)	96 (1)
Experimental 2	15 (5)	90 (15)	9 (1)	180 (30)	24 (1)	92 (1)
Experimental 3	44 (14)	5 (½)	n.d.[b]	7 (½)	n.d.[b]	n.d.[b]

[a] Standard deviations in parentheses.
[b] n.d. = not determined.

liquid and powder. In this respect, Biocement D is among the best products (Table 4).

The dough time of a CPBC can be described as the time up to which the cement paste can be deformed without doing any harm to the final structure of the hardened cement, and is situated somewhere between the t_C and the t_I. Therefore, a method to determine the dough time experimentally consisted of determining the time after which deformation results in decreased strength after complete hardening (62), but this method is very crude. However, the test on the I% can be used to approach the dough time. The I% of a CPBC paste decreases rapidly with increasing viscosity of the paste, and is very sensitive to the moment of entanglement of the precipitating crystals. When the opening of the syringe is small (e.g., 2 mm) and the force of extrusion is limited to the average hand force, I% drops to zero at this moment. In this way, the dough time of a CPBC can be determined, with an accuracy of approx .25 min, by plotting the I% as a function of time after the start of mixing and extrapolation of the curve to zero. From the above considerations, it is clear that a CPBC should be applied after the cohesion time, but before the dough time.

7. Mixing Powder and Liquid

The first method used to mix the powder and the liquid of a CPBC into a paste was by hand in a mortar. Although this method was indispensable for the chemical development of these materials, it is not suitable in the hands of clinicians and their assistants, because the properties of the resulting cement depend on the intensity and duration of mixing by hand. Therefore, in order to make a CPBC product ready for the market, the dispensing and dosage of powder and liquid, their sterilization, and their mixing should be made independent of any operator, and should be completely automatized.

8. Admixtures

It seems to be an illusion to think that CPBCs can be made tough and fatigue-resistant by incorporation of biopolymers, such as collagen, cellulose, or chitosan, into their structure (63,64). It is the authors' experience that, with such additives, the strength of CPBCs decreases dramatically, probably because these additives hinder the entanglement of the growing crystals of the precipitating CaP (65).

But there may be other reasons for trying to incorporate additives. Several authors have incorporated antibiotics or drugs, such as cephalexin, norfloxacin, gentamicin, tobramycin, and vancomycin, and, consequently, have determined their release in vitro (66–70) and in vivo (70). It has been claimed that, in this way, osteomyelitis can be treated effectively. In any way, during about 2 wk, effective doses of antibiotics are realized around the implant.

Other authors (71–73) have incorporated bone morphogenetic proteins (BMPs) into CPBCs. It was claimed that this combination was a favorable augmentation material (71). However, there is considerable doubt whether addition of BMPs leads to advantages in the stimulation of bone repair or augmentation that the CPBCs do not already have on their own account (72,73).

9. Clinical Applications and Animal Experimentation

The following dental and orthopedic applications are claimed for CPBCs (74).

1. Cavity bases and liners to protect the pulp
2. Materials for capping exposed pulps
3. Materials to replace or promote regeneration of bone mineral lost because of periodontal disease
4. Direct filling materials
5. Buildup of alveolar ridges in edentulous patients
6. Endodontic filling materials for root canals
7. Material to cement retention pins
8. Material to fill alveolar sockets to prevent resorption of alveolar ridges
9. Replacement of bone that is surgically removed or lost because of trauma
10. Cement for implanting or replanting teeth
11. Luting cement in dentistry and orthopedic surgery
12. Investment mold material
13. Material that will promote bone growth in its vicinity
14. Mineralizing polish in dentistry in place of pumice
15. Root cement for remineralizing and desensitizing of exposed root surfaces

As far as published data reveal, the chief application realized up to now is the filling of surgical bone defects caused by cysts or bone cancer. However, an increasing number of animal experiments are being published, for example:

1. Obliteration and reconstruction of the cat frontal sinus (75), which was successful.
2. Repair of bone defects in the long bones of dogs (76). Successful.
3. Repair of bone defects in the mandibles of rabbits (77). Four/16 implants were lost before setting, because of intense bleeding. The rest were successful.
4. Repair of cranial defects in the rabbit (78). Problem similar to item 3.
5. Augmentation onto cranial bone under the periosteum of rabbits (78). Complete success.

Probably, many studies will follow in the near future, as manufacturers proceed rapidly in making their systems suitable for clinical use.

10. Final Remarks

CPBCs are promising in dentistry, orthopedics, and plastic surgery, for regeneration and augmentation of bone in many applications. It is expected that clinical research will increase rapidly, because many manufacturers have made their systems suitable for the clinical situation. The most rapid resorption upon implantation is found with DCPD-type CPBCs, which resorb passively, and thus with possible loss of coherence of the bone–implant construction. The desired rate of resorption is found with nano-apatite-type CPBCs, which comprise all present-day commercial materials. These materials are taken up in the local remodeling of the bone, which depends, according to Woolf's law, primarily on the stress distribution within the skeleton. ACP-type cements, such as α-BSM (Etex α), transforms, within about 3 d, spontaneously into a nano-apatite, so that it is invalid to claim a better and faster resorption for this material (38) than that found for competing nano-apatite materials, such as Bone Source, Norian SRS, or Biocement D.

The nano-apatitic CPBCs form a case of good biomimetics, perhaps the best there is among biomaterials. In fact, the apatitic part of bone mineral is also a nano-apatite. Probably for that reason, the nano-apatitic CPBCs are taken up in the natural bone remodeling process, rather than being phagocytized like polymethylmethacrylate debris. The nano-apatites are recognized as belonging to the body.

Acknowledgments

F. C. M. D. gratefully acknowledges a grant from the Bijzonder Onderzoeksfonds of the University of Ghent. E. A. P. D. M. is senior research assistant of the Fund for Scientific Research (Flanders) Belgium.

References

1 Driessens FCM, Boltong MG, Bermudez O, Planell JA, Ginebra MP, and Fernandez E. *J Mater Sci Mater Med* 1994; 5: 164–170.

2. Drissens FCM. *Fourth Euro Ceramics* 1995; 8: 77–83.
3. Driessens FCM, Planell JA, and Gil FJ. Calcium phosphate bone cements, in *Encyclopedic Handbook of Biomaterials and Bioengineering. Part B. Applications*, Vol. 2, 1995; (Wise DJ et al., eds), M. Dekker, New York, 1995, pp. 855–877.
4. Driessens FCM, Fernandez E, Ginebra MP, Boltong MG, and Planell JA. *An Quim Int Ed* 1997; 93: S38–S43.
5. Drissens FCM and Verbeeck RMH. *Biominerals* 1990; CRC, Boca Raton.
6. Christoffersen MR, Christoffersen J, and Kibalczyc W. *J Crystal Growth* 1990; 106: 349–354.
7. Fernandez E, Gil FJ, Best SM, Ginebra MP, Driessens FCM, and Planell JA. *J Biomed Mater Res* 1998; 41: 560–567.
8. Driessens FCM, De Maeyer EAP, Fernandez E, Boltong MG, Berger G, Verbeeck RMH, Ginebra MP, and Planell JA. *Bioceramics* 1996; 9: 231–234.
9. Ginebra MP, Fernandez E, Driessens FCM, Boltong MG, Muntasell J, Font J, and Planell JA. *J Mater Sci Mat Med* 1995; 6: 857–860.
10. Ginebra MP, Fernandez E, Driessens FCM, Boltong MG, and Planell JA. *Bioceramics* 1997; 10: 481–484.
11. Brown WE and Chow LC. *J Dent Res* 1983; 62: 672.
12. Gruninger SE, Sien C, Chow L, O'Young A, Tsao NK, and Brown W. *J Dent Res* 1984; 63: 200.
13. Yoshikawa M, Toda T, Oonishi H, Kushitani S, Yasukawa E, Hayami S, Mandai Y, and Sugihara F. *Bioceramics* 1994; 7: 187–192.
14. Driessens FCM, van Loon JA, van Sliedregt A, and Planell JA. *11th Eur Conf Biomater* 1994; Pisa, pp. 344–346.
15. Fischer-Brandies E, Dielert E, Bauner G, Feder FH, Reidel G, and Möllenstedt S. *Dtsch Zahnärztl. Z.* 1989; 44: 436–437.
16. Driessens FCM, Verbeeck RMH, and van Dijk JWE. *Acta Stomatolog Belg* 1990; 87: 107–124.
17. De Bruijn JD, Bovell YP, Planell JA, and Driessens FCM. *5th World Biomater Congress,* 1996; Toronto, p. 121.
18. Yoshimine Y, Sumi M, Isobe R, Anan H, and Maeda K. *Biomaterials* 1996; 17: 2241–2245.
19. Knabe C, Driessens FCM, Planell JA, Gildenhaar R, Berger G, Reif D, et al. *23rd Ann Meeting Soc Biomater* 1997; New Orleans, p. 340.
20. Oreffo ROC, Driessens FCM, Planell JA, and Triffitt JT. *13th Eur Conf Biomater* 1997; Göteborg, p. 86.
21. Oreffo ROC, Driessens FCM, Planell JA, and Triffitt JT. *Advances in Tissue Engineering and Biomaterials* 1997; University of York, UK.
22. Hong YC, Wang JT, Hong CY, Brown WE, and Chow LC. *J Biomed Mater Res* 1991; 25: 485–498.
23. Constantino PD, Friedman CD, Jones K, Chow LC, Pelzer HJ, and Sisson GA. *Arch Otolaryngol Head Neck Surg* 1991; 117: 379–384.
24. Sugaware A, Nishiyama M, Kusama K, Moro I, Nishimura S, Kudo I, Chow LC, and Takagi S. *Dent Mater J* 1992; 11: 11–16.
25. Kurashina K, Kurita H, Hirano M, De Blieck JMA, Klein CPAT, and De Groot K. *Mater Sci Mat Med* 1995; 6: 340–347.
26. Kurashina K, Kurita H, Kotani A, Takenchi H, and Hirano M. *Biomaterials* 1997; 18: 147–151.
27. Vasconsalos M, Afonso A, Branco R, Planell J, Driessens F, and Cavalheiro J. *Fifth World Biomater Congress* 1996; Toronto, p. 61.
28. Jansen JA, De Ruijter JE, Schaeken HG, Van Der Waerden JPCM, Planell JA, and Driessens FCM. *J Mater Sci Mat Med* 1995; 6: 653–657.
29. Foster MM, Shige AG, and Davies JE. *24th Ann Meeting Soc Biomater* 1998; San Diego, p. 188.
30. Driessens FCM, Boltong MG, Zapatero MI, Verbeeck RMH, Bonfield W, Bermudez O, et al. *J Mater Sci Mat Med* 1995; 6: 272–278.
31. Li Y, Yuan H, and Zhang X. *24th Ann Meeting Soc Biomater* 1998; San Diego, p. 428.
32. Constantz BR, Barr BM, Qniaoit J, Ison IC, Baker JT, McKinney L, et al. *Fourth World Biomater Congress,* 1992; Berlin, p. 56.
33. Lemaitre J, Munting E, and Mirtchi AA. *Rev Stomatol Chir Maxillofac.* 1992; 93: 163–165.
34. Bohner M, Lemaitre J, Ohura K, and Hardouin P. *Ceramic Trans* 1995; 48: 245–259.
35. Munting E, Mirtchi AA, and Lemaitre J. *J Mater Sci Mat Med* 1993; 4: 337–344.
36. Ohura K, Bohner M, Hardouin P, Lemaitre J, Pasquier G, and Flantre B. *J Biomed Mater Res* 1996; 30: 193–200.
37. Frayssinet P, Gineste L, Conte P, Fages J, Rouquet N, and Lerch A. *Bioceramics* 1997; 10: 493–496. (*See also* Frayssinet P, Gineste L, Conte P, Fages J, and Rouquet N. *Biomaterials* 1998; 19: 971–977).
38. Ailova M, Tofighi A, Knaack D, and Lee DD. *24th Ann Meeting Soc Biomater* 1998; San Diego, p. 275.
39. Driessens FCM, Boltong MG, Bermudez O, and Planell JA. *J Mater Sci Mat Med* 1993; 4: 503–508.
40. Bermudez O, Boltong MG, Driessens FCM, and Planell JA. *J Mater Sci Mat Med* 1994; 5: 67–71.
41. Ginebra MP, Boltong MG, Driessens FCM, Bermudez O, Fernandez E, and Planell JA. *J Mater Sci Mat Med* 1994; 5: 103–107.

42. Chow LC, Takagi S, Constantino PD, and Friedman CD. *Mat Res Soc Symp Proc* 1991; 179: 3–24.
43. Driessens FCM, Boltong MG, Planell JA, Bermudez O, Ginebra MP, and Fernandez E. *Bioceramics* 1993; 6: 469–473.
44. Mirtchi AA, Lemaitre J, and Munting E. *Biomaterials* 1989; 10: 634–638.
45. Ginebra MP, Fernandez E, Boltong MG, Bermudez O, Planell JA, and Driessens FCM. *Clin Mater* 1995; 17: 99–104.
46. Driessens FCM, Khaïroun I, Boltong MG, and Planell JA. *Bioceramics* 1997; 10: 279–282.
47. Miyamoto Y, Ishikawa K, Fukao H, Sawada M, Nagayama M, Kon M, and Asaoka K. *Biomaterials* 1995; 16: 855–860.
48. Ishikawa K, Miyamoto Y, Kon M, Nagayama M, and Asaoka K. *Biomaterials* 1995; 16: 527–532.
49. Miyamoto I, Ishikawa K, Takuchi M, Yuasa M, Kon M, Nagayama M, and Asaoka K. *Biomaterials* 1996; 17: 1429–1435.
50. Ishikawa K, Miyamoto Y, Takuchi M, Toh T, Kon M, Nagayama M, and Asaoka K. *J Biomed Mater Res* 1997; 36: 393–399.
51. Kurashina K, Kurita H, Hirano M, De Blieck JMA, Klein CPAT, and De Groot, K. *J Mater Sci Mat Med* 1995; 6: 340–347.
52. Fernandez E, Boltong MG, Ginebra MP, Driessens FCM, Bermudez O, and Planell JA. *J Mater Sci Lett* 1996; 15: 1004–1005.
53. Khaïroun I, Driessens FCM, Boltong MG, and Planell JA. *J Mater Sci Mat Med* 1998; 9: pp. 667–671.
54. Khaïroun I, Boltong MG, Driessens FCM, and Planell JA. *Biomaterials* 1997; 18: 1535–1539.
55. Khaïroun I, Boltong MG, Driessens FCM, and Planell JA. *J Biomed Mater Res (Appl Biomater)* 1997; 38: 356–360.
56. Bermudez O, Boltong MG, Driessens FCM, and Planell JA. *J Mater Sci Mat Med* 1993; 4: 389–393.
57. Driessens FCM, Boltong MG, De Maeyer EAP, Vercruysse CWJ, Wenz R, and Verbeeck RMH. *Bioceramics* 1998; 11: 231–233.
58. Yaszemski MJ, Payne RG, Hayes WC, Langer R, and Mikos AG. *Biomaterials* 1996; 17: 175–185.
59. Lemaitre J, Andrianjatovo H, Biourge C, Ohura K, and Harodouin P. *Oberflächen Werkstoffe* 1994; 9: 13–18.
60. Chow LC, Markovic M, Takagi S, and Cherng M. *Innov Technol Bio Med* 1997; 18: 11–14.
61. Khaïroun I, Boltong MG, Driessens FCM, and Planell JA. *J Mater Sci Mat Med* 1998; 9: 425–428.
62. Ginebra MP, Fernandez E, Boltong MG, Bermudez O, Planell JA, and Driessens FCM. *Clin Mater* 1995; 17: 99–102.
63. Sugihara F, Minamikawa K, Oonishi H, Mandai Y, Nagatoni K, Yasukawa E, Kushitani S, and Tshuji E. *Bioceramics* 1994; 7: 193–198.
64. Yoshikawa M, Toda T, Oonishi H, Kushitani S, Yasukawa E, Hayami S, Mandai Y, and Sugihara F. *Bioceramics* 1994; 7: 187–192.
65. Boltong MG, Driessens FCM, and Planell JA. Unpublished results.
66. Otsuka M, Matsuda Y, Yu D, Wong J, Fox JL, and Higuchi WI. *Chem Pharm Bull* 1990; 38: 3500–3502.
67. Nachiondo JM, Poser RD, Goodman SB, and Constantz BR. *20th Ann Meeting Soc Biomaterials* 1994; Boston, p. 146.
68. Anderson JR and Berrey BH. *42nd Ann Meeting Orthopaedic Research Society,* 1996, Atlanta, p. 440.
69. Takano I, Ishi Y, Shimoda M, Takashima Y, and Sazaki S. *Bioceramics* 1996; 9: 267–270.
70. Hamanishi C, Kitamoto K, Tanaka S, Otsuka M, Doi Y, and Kitahashi T. *J Biomed Mater Res (Appl Biomat)* 1996; 33: 139–307.
71. Kamegai A, Shimamura N, Naitou K, Nagahara K, Kanematsu N, and Mori M. *Biomedical Mater Eng* 1994; 4: 291–307.
72. Ohura K, Hamanishi C, Tanaka S, and Matsuda N. *Bioceramics* 1996; 9: 247–250.
73. Ongpipattanakul B, Nguyen T, Zioncheck TF, Wong R, Osaka G, De Guzman L, Lee WP, and Beck LS. *J Biomed Mater Res* 1997; 36: 295–305.
74. Brown WE and Chow LC. 1985; US Patent 4518430.
75. Friedman CD, Constantino PD, Jones K, Chow LC, Pelzer HJ, and Sisson GA. *Arch Otolaryngol Head Neck Surg* 1991; 117: 385–389.
76. Munting E, Mirtchi AA, and Lemaitre J. *J Mater Sci Mat Med* 1993; 4: 337–344.
77. Kurashina K, Kurita H, Kotani A, Takenchi H, and Hirano M. *Bioceramics* 1996; 9: 259–261.
78. Kurashina K, Kurita H, Kotani A, Kobayashi S, Kyoshima K, and Hirano M. *Biomaterials* 1998; 19: 701–706.
79. Lee DD, Rey C, and Aiolova M. 1996; International Patent WO 96/36562.

16

Osteointegration and Dimensional Stability of Poly(D,L–Lactide-Co-Glycolide) Implants Reinforced with Poly(Propylene Glycol-Co-Fumaric Acid)

Histomorphometric Evaluation of Metaphyseal Bone Remodeling in Rats

Joseph D. Gresser, Kai-Uwe Lewandrowski, Debra J. Trantolo, and Donald L. Wise

I. Introduction

Internal fixation devices (IFDs), fabricated from biodegradable (resorbable) polymers, have several advantages, compared to metallic devices: They do not corrode; they may be constructed with moduli closer to that of normal bone than metal devices, and, thus, as a corollary, avoid stress shielding; and finally, resorbability obviates the need of a second surgical procedure for removal. However, to ensure dimensional stability during degradation, and to match modulus and strength to that of bone, it is necessary to introduce a reinforcing structure for those applications to plate fixation. One approach is to use as the major structural element a poly(D,L-lactide-co-glycolide) (PLGA), which is dispersed within a three-dimensional (3-D) network, or scaffold, of poly(propylene fumarate) (PPF) crosslinked with a vinyl monomer, such as vinyl pyrrolidone (VP).

This crosslinked network locks the PLGA chains in place. Because the crosslinks of the network terminate at hydrolytically labile fumarate ester bonds, the crosslinked network remains hydrolytically degradable.

This scaffolding concept is best termed "molecular reinforcement." PLGA and PPF, an unsaturated polyester, form a compatible blend. PPF and the vinyl monomer are crosslinked as a deformable blend, using benzoyl peroxide (BP) as a crosslinking initiator. This plasticized composite is then pressurized and heated to induce crosslinking in compression molding. The authors hypothesize that this molecularly reinforced composite will have improved mechanical properties (strength and modulus in compression, tension, and bending), in comparison with unreinforced PLGA, when used for plating of bone fractures. The support to the main structural element, PLGA, should protect the device against dimensional instability, such as warping or bowing, arising from unequal rates of degradation on the surfaces exposed to tissue fluid, and on the surface adjacent to bone.

The chief goal of the experiments described herein was to develop a temporal history of the healing of critical-size defects made in the rat tibia in relation to the degradation and dimensional stability of the molecularly reinforced device.

2. Background and Significance

2.1. Historical Use and Developmental Problems of Plate Fixation

Metal plates are commonly used in the operative treatment of bone fractures. Rigid metal plates stabilize the fracture site, maintain good contact between bone fragments, and allow early weight-bearing and patient mobility. However, it was recognized that treatment with rigid metal plates may cause localized bone atrophy because of stress shielding and interference with blood circulation, and the weakened bone may refracture after plate removal (1). Therefore, attempts were directed toward development of plates that would exert less stress protection on bone. Limited-contact dynamic compression plate systems (LC-DCP) were introduced. These plates consist of cold-worked pure titanium (Ti), and represent implants with a track record of outstanding biocompatibility. In fact, the first prospectively controlled clinical series on the use of Ti dates back to 1966, and was reported to be most successful (2). Pure Ti also became the material of choice for implants to be used in patients suffering from metal allergy.

Today, a long-term and well-documented experience with these implants exists. Although results are favorable, and confirm the outstanding biocompatibility of pure Ti (3), long-term problems with these plates persist, because stress protection cannot be fully eliminated. Therefore, it is generally admitted that plate fixation of fractures results in reduced stress and subsequent structural adaptation of bone, with bone loss (2). In fact, many investigators view the lack of callus healing and the long-term overprotection of the underlying bone in the application of rigid plates for diaphyseal fractures as undesirable consequences.

Thus, an ideal bone plate would provide rigid fixation to ensure stabilization of bone fragments at the early stage after fracture, but at the late stage, osteoporosis induced by stress-shielding effect of the plate should be prevented.

Potential solutions offered to overcome this dilemma include use of less-rigid plate-fixation systems, modification of the timing of plate removal, and use of biologically degradable materials for plates, so that stress shielding can be minimized.

The use of less-rigid plate-fixation systems has been demonstrated, and flexible fixation of fractures, with minimally invasive surgical techniques, has become increasingly popular. However, it has been recognized that such techniques can lead to relatively large fracture gaps and considerable interfragmentary movements. Claes et al. (4) investigated the influence of the size of the fracture gap, interfragmentary movement, and interfragmentary strain on the quality of fracture healing. A simple diaphyseal long bone fracture was modeled by means of a transverse osteotomy of the right metatarsus in sheep. Although this study involved the use of an external ring fixator, and not a plate, it demonstrated that the treatment of simple diaphyseal fractures with a more flexible fixation can only be improved if sufficient reduction of the fracture is achieved. Because the healing process was inferior when the gap was larger than 2 mm, this study demonstrated that better control over flexible fixation methods is needed to prevent large interfragmentary gaps. Therefore, the basic principle of adequate fracture reduction remains, and must be taken into account when designing any new type of plate with reduced stress protection.

Modification of time of removal of plate implants has been considered, and there are clinical situations with the symptomatic patient when removal of plates is part of standard management. At some centers, it is common practice to remove forearm plates after fracture healing is completed, because it is felt that stress shielding under the metal plate may be associated with late clinical problems caused by insufficiency fractures around the implants. However, increasing concern has been expressed about the complications and morbidity associated with implant removal (5).

The use of biologically degradable materials

for plates, so that stress shielding can be minimized, has been investigated since the late 1980s. The development of composites of metal plates and polymeric interest (hybrid plates), and purely polymeric plate implants, has primarily stemmed from the need for better plating techniques in the growing skeleton in oral-maxillofacial and craniofacial applications. Other investigators have focused on the development of axially flexible internal fixation plates for use in long bone fracture reconstruction.

Ferguson et al. *(6)* have designed a hybrid bone plate system that combines the torsional and bending rigidity of a metal plate with the axial compliance of a polymer insert. A finite element model was used to study the performance of biodegradable polymer inserts in the plate system. The flexible plate reduced stress-shielding effects at the fracture site, when subjected to an axial load. The bending strength of the plate was not compromised by the addition of the polymer inserts. Biodegradable inserts further enhanced the performance of the new plate design, transferring less of the axial load to the plate as the inserts broke down.

Similar observations were confirmed by others *(7)*, using in vitro and in vivo models with axially flexible plates. These studies have shown that plate implants that have moderate bending and torsional stiffnesses, and low axial stiffness, will provide adequate fixation to achieve callus union, and they also permit the underlying bone to share the physiological stresses needed for bone remodeling. These drastic changes in mechanical demands on an internal fixation plate during the early healing phase and the postunion remodeling phase are critical considerations in the design of a new type of internal bone fixation plate.

Thus, there is a strong case for bioresorbable plate implants, not only on the basis of clinical considerations (because such implants do not need to be removed, and perioperative and operative risks are eliminated), but also on the basis of considerations of the physiology of a fractured bone undergoing healing. Ideally, bioresorbable plate implants should provide sufficient initial internal fixation during the early healing phase, while allowing normal remodeling to occur secondary to their progressive degradation, in the later *postunion phase*.

2.2. Resorbable Plating Devices and Their Complications

The concept of rigid initial internal fixation during the early healing phase and the more flexible internal fixation during the later postunion remodeling phase has been demonstrated in purely bioresorbable implant plates. These were originally developed for oral-maxillofacial and craniofacial applications. For example, Peltoniemi et al. *(8)* used Ti miniplates and biodegradable self-reinforced poly-L-lactide (SR-PLLA) plates, and assessed the consolidation of experimental craniotomy. Two sagittal (2.3–2.5 mm wide and 22 mm long) symmetrical craniotomy lines were made in the skulls of eight young sheep. One craniotomy line was covered with a biodegradable SR-PLLA plate, and the other with a Ti miniplate. The SR-PLLA plates promoted better osteotomy healing in the dynamically growing skull of young sheep than did the Ti plates.

In analogous study, Peltoniemi et al. *(9)* later demonstrated the biocompatibility and the degradation process of the SR-PLLA plate, with cross-sectional histology, histomorphometry, and oxytetracycline chloride fluorescence studies after 6, 12, 20, 52, and 104 wk postoperatively. The consolidation pattern supported the principle of guided tissue regeneration; through the wide, resorbable plate, osseous bridging proceeded evenly throughout the line; Ti plating led to bulky, uneven growth in the bone margins. All SR-PLLA-plated osteotomy lines had healed completely by 20 wk, but none of the Ti-plated lines had consolidated during a follow-up of 1 yr.

In comparison, Suuronen et al. *(10)* used totally biodegradable fixation devices in the fixation of mandibular osteotomy in sheep. Mandibular unilateral body osteotomies were fixed with biodegradable SR-PLLA multilayer plates and screws in nine sheep. The unoperated sides acted as control. The follow-up times were 6, 12 and 24 wk, after which radiological, mechanical, and histological studies were carried out. The results showed that the SR-PLLA plates and screws were strong enough to fix the osteotomy, and that the osteotomies healed mostly with callus formation.

Getter et al. *(11)* created fractures in the mandibles of six dogs, which, after reduction, were fixed with biodegradable plates and screws fabricated from polylactic acids (PLA). Those authors reported that, at 24 wk, the devices could not be palpated, suggesting a high degree of resorption. Hollinger and Battistone *(12),* reported on unpublished work of A. F. Tortorelli, stated that the latter worker, performing a similar experiment with PLA plates, observed that the plates warped as they biodegraded, causing the retaining screws, also fabricated from PLA, to pull loose from the bone.

The problem of warping may be caused by the accumulation of acidic degradation products (glycolic acid, lactic acid) between the plate and the underlying bone. The accumulation of degradation products appears to be the cause of sterile sinus formation, which occurs in approx 8% of patients *(13).* This is a delayed acute inflammatory response that is nonbacterial, and may, in the case of slowly degrading PLLA, occur as late as 3 yr postoperatively. Another possible consequence of the acidic accumulation between plate and bone is autocatalyzed hydrolysis on the protected surface, which may occur more rapidly than on the outer surface. This is not a proven point: Bos et al. *(14)* used slowly degrading PLLA plates and screws to repair mandibular fractures in six dogs. The devices were removed at 3–9 wk after fixation. Ten samples taken from different sites on each plate showed no difference in decrease of mol wt. However, the relatively short period over which these observations were made may have not been adequate to reveal differential hydrolysis. The reference by Hollinger and Ballistone *(12)* to Tortorelli's work *(15)* suggests that warping occurred over longer time periods.

To prevent warping, plates have been reinforced by incorporation of fibers. Parsons et al. *(16)* incorporated high modulus carbon fibers into PLA: This approach compromised the biodegradability of the device. Skirving et al. *(17)* explored a completely nondegradable, carbon-fiber-reinforced plate prepared from an epoxy cement. However, this did not solve the problem of warping. Some plates displayed permanent shape distortion acquired in vivo. Reinforced and completely biodegradable plates were prepared by Christel et al. *(18),* who embedded fibers of poly(glycolide) in PLA plates. Since then, considerable interest has focused on the concept of SR IFDs. These are materials in which the reinforcing element has the same chemical composition as the surrounding polymeric medium. Tormala et al. *(19)* have described methods of preparation. Bundles of poly(glycolide) sutures were sintered into rods in cylindrical molds by compression at 205–232°C under pressure. Tormala *(20,21)* also investigated SR-PLLA that were prepared by mechanical deformation of nonreinforced material, i.e., by free (hot) drawing or die drawing in the range between the glass transition and crystalline melting temperature. Weiler and Gogolewski *(22)* demonstrated an enhancement of mechanical properties (flexural and yield strength) on solid-state extrusion of rods prepared by melt extrusion of poly(D-lactide).

In addition to warping and deformation, implants have been noted to demonstrate focal areas of progressive degradation. This was observed particularly at screw holes and at osteotomy sites, suggesting that the bone not only responds to the implant, but also vice versa; a similar response would occur in the implant while it is undergoing hydrolytic degradation. Conceivably, the strain field within bones fixed with bioresorbable implants promotes this focal progression of degradation, possibly because of implant fatigue and microfractures which in turn will accelerate the implant degradation. In addition, it appears totally reasonable to assume that bioresorbable implants, used in the fixation of long bones that are under eccentric axial load, are more susceptible to such a phenomenon.

To date, the use of bioresorbable plate implants in the fixation of long bone fractures is unprecedented. The authors have set out to develop a bioresorbable SR plate for such application. Such implants must be materially improved toward their potential clinical application, before they may be applied in humans. As a suitable clinical application for resorbable plate fixation, the internal fixation of forearm fractures, specifically fractures of the radius and the ulna, appear as areas where such a fixation device would be needed.

3. Rationales for Molecular Reinforcement of PLGA

PLGAs undergo bulk degradation rather than surface degradation, which implies that the rate of water penetration is greater than the rate of polymer hydrolysis. In certain situations, this might result in homogeneous hydrolytic degradation throughout the body of the material, but this is not the case with the PLGAs. It is known, in fact, that hydrolytic degradation of PLGAs does not occur homogeneously throughout the material, nor even homogeneously over the surface and inward. The rate of degradation at various loci on or within the implant depends on the pH of the microenvironment, the availability of water at various points, and the crystallinity of the polymer.

PLGAs are semicrystalline, the extent of crystallinity depending on the lactide:glycolide ratio, the extent to which the lactide moiety is optically active or racemic, and the fabrication procedures. Water penetration, or absorption, and therefore hydrolysis, is more rapid through the amorphous regions than through the crystallites; thus, the crystalline content tends to increase during the early stages of hydrodegradation.

As the device absorbs water, the more hydrophilic and amorphous regions will swell. The swelling is nonisotropic, not only because of the existence of amorphous and crystalline regions, but because the concentration of water at any point in the polymer will depend on time and the accessability of water to the front and back surfaces of the device. The nonisotropic swelling can cause deformations (including bowing), and can exert pressure against the screws that anchor the device against the bone. Thus, deformation and swelling tend to pull the screws out of the bone.

Heterogeneous hydrolysis is also a function of the accessibility of water to the surfaces of the plate. The surface in contact with bone is obviously less accessible to water than is the surface in contact with soft tissue. This promotes differential rates of hydrolysis.

Accompanying these processes is the effect of pH in the microenvironment of the plate. Degradation products formed within the interior do not diffuse away as rapidly as those formed on the surface. The internal lowering of the pH results in autocatalysis, and the interior will degrade more rapidly than the exterior.

To minimize deformations, the authors include the linear PLGA chains within a crosslinked network of PPF. This should control the deformation by anchoring the chains within this relatively stable structure, which is slowly degradable by virtue of its ester bonds, but lends stability by virtue of its vinyl linkages.

3.1. Biomechanical Considerations

Ideally, a molecularly reinforced IFD should degrade at rates commensurate with the course of bone healing. The stages of healing have been described by Heppenstall *(23):* stage of induction (up to approx 4 d); stage of inflammation (approx 3–4 d); stage of soft callus (3–4 wk); stage of hard callus (begins at 3–4 wk to 3–4 mo); and stage of remodeling (several months to several years).

When hard callus formation is complete (in an average of about 2 mo), the fracture is considered to be clinically and radiographically healed. Thus, ideally, the molecularly reinforced IFD could be substantially resorbed in 3–4 mo (13–17 wk). Actually, after 25–50 d, the fracture is sealed with hard immature bone, which responds to stresses by remodeling like uninjured bone, and thus significant degradation can be accepted by about 2 mo. Adams *(24)* has pointed out that healing of most human bones is virtually complete in about 8 wk, with about 50% recovery of mechanical properties of intact bone in about 3 wk.

The reported mechanical properties of human bone are summarized in Table 1. Mechanical properties of the molecularly reinforced material should be similar to those of human bone. The values shown in Table 1, reported in the literature for wet compact bone, represent targets for this program.

4. PPF-Based Biomaterials

4.1. Analytical Characterization of Crosslinked PPF Biomaterials

Studies conducted to characterize the chemistry of the PPF crosslinking determined the average length and density of the VP crosslinks between PPF units, using a PPF-based bone cement. The formulation consisted of PPF (38% w/w), a soluble calcium salt (27%), VP (10%), BP (1.25%), and unreactive viscosity control agents (31%). After completion of the crosslinking, the material was extracted sequentially with water, ethanol, and methylene chloride, to isolate the insoluble

Table 1
Mechanical Properties of Wet Compact Bone[a]

Stiffness		GPa	1–30	Tormala et al. (19)
Bending	Modulus,	GPa	6–30[b]	Fung (25)
	Strength,	MPa	160	Fung (25)
Torsion	Modulus,	GPa	3.2 (femur)	Fung (25)
	Strength,	MPa	54.1 (femur)	Fung (25)
Tension	Modulus,	GPa	14.9–18.9	Fung (25)
	Strength,	MPa	124–174	Fung (25)
Compression	Modulus,	GPa	8–9[c]	Fung (25)
	Strength,	MPa	170 (femur)	Fung (25)

[a] Except as otherwise noted.
[b] Poly(L-lactide) and Poly(D,L-lactide)-reinforced with calcium phosphate fibers.
[c] Equine long bones.

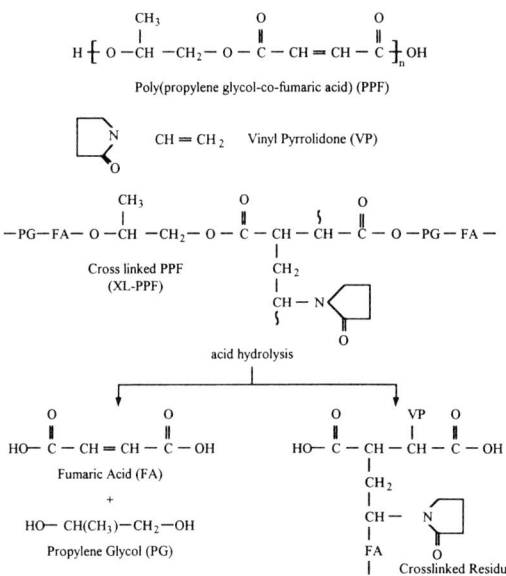

Fig. 1. Structural formulas.

crosslinked poly(propylene fumarate) (XL-PPF). This insoluble residue was hydrolyzed in two steps: first, in 6 N hydrocloric acid (HCl) at room temperature for 48 h, and then in 6 N HCl at 60°C for 6 h. Samples from each hydrolysis were sent for elemental analysis, and indicated that hydrolysis was complete after the first step (C, H, N: 53.85 ± 0.03, 6.56 ± 0.06, 3.83 ± 0.07).

Based on the structures shown in Fig. 1, the weight fraction of each element in the hydrolyzed residue is related to the ratio VP:fumaric acid (FA) moieties by the following equations:

$f_N = 14.007x[116.072y + 111.139x]^{-1}$
$f_C = [48.04y + 72.06x][116.072y + 111.139x]^{-1}$
$f_H = [4.032y + 9.072x][116.072y + 111.139x]^{-1}$
$f_O = [64.00y + 16.00x][116.072y + 111.139x]^{-1}$

where $x{:}y$ is the mol ratio of VP:FA moieties. The $x{:}y$ ratios calculated from these equations are given below give mean value of 1.16 ± 0.65.

These measurements suggest about one VP/FA in the crosslinked residue. The mol ratio of VP monomer:FA units in the starting PPF in the formulation is 5.24. Thus, if one VP unit is linked to one FA unit, there are approx four free fumarate double bonds per crosslink, and it can be tentatively assumed that the structure of the crosslinked PPF is as shown in Fig. 1. This type of analytical protocol will be repeated with formulations of molecularly reinforced IFDs. The accuracy of this information will be improved by including elemental analysis of the crosslinked PPF, both prior to hydrolysis and after, and is supported by analysis of free fumaric acid in the soluble products of hydrolysis.

In a study of similar PPF-based bone cements crosslinked with VP, Gresser et al. (26) have shown that >90% of the PPF is crosslinked over a wide range of PPF:VP weight ratios, varying from 0.33 to 2.0, but that the fraction of VP used in forming crosslinks depended on the PPF:VP ratio. At the highest PPF:VP ratio explored (1.7), approx 67% of the VP was incorporated, the remainder being polymerized to poly(vinyl pyrrolidone) (PVP). In the present study, the PPF:VP ratio is 1.4. Extrapolation of their results leads to an estimate of about 60% of the VP incorporated into the crosslinks.

4.2. Biocompatibility of Crosslinked PPF Biomaterials

These PPF-based bone cements have been evaluated with respect to osteoconductive and biocompatibility properties. The authors employed the cement in an injectable format for fixation in the rat femoral osteotomy model, and examined degradation of the cement in relation to metaphyseal bone remodeling in vivo. Negative and positive controls, with loose and rigid internal fixation, were included for comparison. Results of this study showed that foreign body reactions were absent at the sites where the cement was injected. Osteoclastic activity and new trabecular bone formation was noted at the interface between the metaphyseal bone and the cement. Degradation of the cement resulted in cavitation. These cavitations were sites of invasion by vascular and bony tissues. Intimate contact between the bone cement and the endosteal surface of the cortex was found. Quantitative histomorphometric analysis corroborated these observations. Findings of this study showed in vivo compatibility of the bone cement in this model, and support the concept of osteoconductivity.

5. Design Considerations of Molecularly Reinforced PLGA Implants

PLGAs undergo hydrolytic degradation in aqueous environments, with the generation, and eventual metabolic elimination, of glycolic and lactic acids as carbon dioxide and water. The specific polymer chosen for use as a resorbable plate for bone fracture repair has a lactide:glycolide ratio of 85:15, and is identified as PLGA-85:15 (or simply as PLGA, unless otherwise specified). Although initial mechanical properties may be sufficient, the progressive hydrolytic degradation of PLGA results in decreased strength and modulus with time, and thus may not give adequate fixation to healing fractures. To maintain adequate strength over time, the authors have investigated reinforcing the PLGA with PPF, also a polyester subject to hydrolytic degradation. PPF, however, also contains an unsaturated C=C double bond, which can be crosslinked in the presence of a suitable vinyl monomer. The authors have chosen N-VP as the crosslinking agent, arguing that, by analogy with PVP, the linear fragments produced by hydrolysis of the crosslinked PPF (XL-PPF) should also be water-soluble, and thus capable of elimination from the body.

6. Molecular Reinforcement of PLGA

Molecular reinforcement of PLGA with XL-PPF, was approached with two objectives: first, development of a protocol for effecting the crosslinking of the PPF in the presence of PLGA, to form an interpenetrating network; and second, a method for fabricating the final device shape. Thus, the authors investigated preparing a homogeneous blend (an IPN of PLGA and PPF crosslinked in solution), and compared this to a system comprising micronized PLGA blended with previously crosslinked and micronized PPF. Because extrusion can be a continuous process, and is therefore well-suited to production of devices with constant cross-sections, and because the high content of PLGA, a thermoplastic polymer, which, the authors argued, would allow the composite to be extruded, this method was the first choice for fabrication techniques. Further, extrusion would permit preparation of a large number of samples for three-point bending from a single extruded rod. However, in spite of the high PLGA content, extrusions were difficult.

The authors therefore investigated compression-molding rods from a blend of PLGA and PPF plasticized with the requisite quantity of VP, the monomer chosen as the liquid crosslinking agent, and an initiator, BP. This plasticized and easily deformable blend was loaded into a mold, which was first pressurized at room temperature, and then heated, still under pressure, to induce crosslinking. Following crosslinking in the mold, the samples were removed from the mold and subjected to 2.5 Mrad of γ-irradiation, first to cure, i.e., to induce further crosslinking, and, second, to sterilize, the samples, the sterilization method of choice for these types of materials. Because the length:diameter ratio of these preliminary compression-molded samples was too low for evaluation of flexural modulus and strength in three-point bending, samples were tested for hardness at each stage, i.e., after compression, but before crosslinking, and again after irradiation.

All materials were compared against extruded or compression-molded PLGA as a standard. On the basis of these comparisons, the authors have identified compression molding (or transfer molding) at room temperature of PLGA/PPF/VP/BP, followed by crosslinking under pressure at elevated temperature, and again by γ-irradiation, as the method of choice. The composition of the charge to the mold, PLGA(3):PPF(1):VP(0.7):BP (0.1), appeared to work well, and formed the start of investigations.

6.1. Materials

PLGA-85:15 was purchased from Boehringer-Ingelheim (Resomer 858, article no. 640671, lot 261703), and purified before use, by precipitation from an acetone solution (50 mg/mL) into 2-propanol (Isopropyl alcohol [IPA]). (Note: the designation, −85:15 following PLGA refers to the lactide:glycolide mol ratio in the copolymer. The lactide moiety in Resomer 858 is the racemic D,L-lactide.)

PPF (batches 86-1–2 and 91-2–3) were synthesized by direct esterification of fumaric acid with propylene glycol, using p-toluene sulfonic acid as a catalyst. The weight average mol wt were 4470 and 3620, with polydispersities of 2.10 and 1.74, respectively, as measured by gel permeation chromatography (Jordi, Bellingham, MA).

PPF was crosslinked with VP (Aldrich, cat. no. V340-9, lot 09231MY), using BP (Aldrich, no. 17,998-1, lot MZ06613KY) as the initiator. VP was vacuum-distilled and stored at −4°C.

Glacial acetic acid (glHAc) (Fisher, cat. no. A38C-212, lot FL 030,589) was used as received.

6.2. Reinforcement Protocols

Several techniques were explored for reinforcing the PLGA with XL-PPF. The efficacy of these techniques in creating an IPN of XL-PPF was judged by comparison of bending strength and modulus of extruded rods to PLGA-only controls. For simplicity, these various sample protocols will be designated by Roman numerals, as indicated below.

6.2.1. Extrusion Techniques

1. PLGA control
2. *In situ* PPF–PLGA crosslinking: PPF, PLGA, VP, and BP were co-dissolved in glHAc, and the PPF was crosslinked *in situ*, followed by lyophilization of the glHAc before extrusion.
3. Dry-mixed PLGA + X-PPF: PPF was first crosslinked *ex situ*, then micronized and dry-mixed with micronized PLGA prior to extrusion. (This sample was an additional control formulated to reflect basic material properties in lieu of IPN.)

6.2.2. Compression-molding Techniques

1. *In situ* crosslinking with simultaneous molding: PPF, PLGA, VP, and BP were co-dissolved in acetone, and, following evaporation of the acetone, the plasticized blend was molded to a desired shape under pressure at room temperature, followed by heating under pressure in the mold (10,000 psi, 70°C, 30–60 min) to crosslink the PPF *in situ*. Samples were then subjected to 2.5 Mrad of γ-irradiation for simultaneous completion of crosslinking and sterilization.

Typical formulations are given in Table 2.

Of the various methods explored, protocol IV proved superior. Crosslinking under pressure yielded smooth cylindrical specimens. Crosslinking was demonstrated by an increase of hardness, as measured by a Shore Type D durometer. Hardness was first measured after compression, but before heating.

To do this, the face plate of the mold was removed, and the exposed cross-section was tested. After replacing the plate and repressurizing, the mold was heated to 70°C with heating tapes for 30 min–1 h. After cooling, the plug was removed and hardness tested. Samples were then γ-irradiated (Isomedix, Northborough, MA), after which a final hardness measurement was made. Results are given in Table 3.

The constancy of weight following molding, until after irradiation, suggests that any residual

Table 2
Formulations for Reinforcement Protocols

	I PLGA control	II In situ XL-PPF in PLGA/glHAc	III XL-PPF + PLGA dry-mixed	IV Crosslink PPF after molding
PLGA-85:15 g	As needed	3.00	6.60[a]	3.00
PPF, g		1.00	2.20	1.00
VP, g		0.70	0.66	0.70
BP, g		0.10	0.22	0.10
glHAc, mL		14	None	–
Acetone, mL		–	None	15

[a]PLGA was added after the PPF had been separately crosslinked. The glHAc used in the crosslinking was removed by lyophilization prior to combining with the PLGA.

Table 3
Hardness Testing of Crosslinked Molded Specimens (Protocol IV)

Sample ID[a]	Weight after molding (mg)	Wt after irradiation (mg)	Wt %	Hardness before heating	Hardness after heating	Hardness after irradiation
–1	214.2	215.5	+0.14	5–7	20–25	50
–3	277.7	278.2	+0.18	5–7	37	50
–4	204.5	204.4	–90.05	5–7	20	60
–5	246.2	246.6	+0.16	5–7	17–20	55

[a]Sample reference prefix 101-21.

Table 4
Experimental Formulations: Protocol II

Formulation	97-27-A	97-27-B	97-27-C	97-27-D
PLGA–85:15, g	3.0010	3.0015	3.0009	3.0016
PPF, g	1.0014	1.0015	1.0012	1.0007
VP, g	0.7057	1.7006	0.7020	0.7036
BP, g	0.1019	0.1007	0.1018	0.1016
HAc, mL	16	14	14	14
Total wt., g	4.8100	5.8043	4.8059	4.8076
ΣWt% PPF + VP + BP	37.63	48.29	37.56	37.56

solvent (acetone) left after evaporation may have been further reduced during molding.

6.3. Characterization of Experimental Formulations

Formulations used for *in situ* crosslinking (protocol II) are given in Table 4. Formulations A, C, and D are similar in composition, but, in each, variations in the addition of VP to the reaction mixture, as well as length of heating time, were explored. Formulation C is best with respect to its mechanical properties. All components of formulation C were mixed prior to reaction at 100°C, at which temperature crosslinking occurred rapidly. Following reaction, the glHAc was removed by lyophilization. Prior to extrusion, half of each

Table 5
Weight Loss on Extraction with IPA

Sample ID	97-27-A	97-27-B	97-27-C	97-27-D
Initial wt	2.2591	2.4311	2.1332	1.7455
After washing	1.9741	2.2529	2.0170	1.5971
Δ%	−12.62	−7.33	−5.45	−8.50

batch was extracted with IPA, and mechanical testing was conducted for comparison with the unextracted samples. The rationale for the IPA extraction step was to remove soluble components, including unreacted monomer (if any) and PVP.

One purpose of this experiment was to determine optimum conditions for performing the crosslinking, with respect to the protocol for adding the VP to the glHAc–PLGA–PPF solution. Thus, formulations A, C, and D have the same overall compositions. The optimum addition was eventually the simplest: All components were present when the crosslinking was initiated. The second purpose of this experiment was to determine the extent of crosslinking, given a standard composition. This was anticipated to be the sum of the weights of VP, PPF, and BP, or perhaps less, if some VP homopolymerized to PVP. After removal of the HAc by lyophilization, half of the matrix was extracted with IPA, to remove PVP. After drying and weighing, the material was extracted with methylene chloride (MC), to determine the quantity of XL-PPF, based on its insolubility in this solvent. PLGA dissolves readily in MC.

Results of IPA extractions are summarized in Table 5. Samples lost an average of 8.5 ± 3.0%, by weight, on extraction with IPA. This is probably PVP, generated by homopolymerization of VP. Gresser et al. *(26)* have shown that the quantity of PVP formed is inversely proportional to the weight ratio of PPF:VP. Solubility tests were run on samples that had not been extracted with IPA. Samples underwent rapid dissolution. A test run on pure PPF (not crosslinked, no PLGA) showed negligible insolubles.

The results of the MC extractions are shown in Table 6. The percent of MC insolubles ranged from 46 to 62% (mean = 54.3 ± 7.2). The authors speculate that the XL polymer network involves only the VP, PPF, and BP. If so, the percent of insolubles would correspond to the percent of these components, which, in samples A, C, and D, accounts for 37.6% of the total, and, in B, for 48.3%, as shown in Table 6. The Δ% is the percent weight increase over the expected weight. The last row gives the % increase in weight relative to the PLGA content of the formulation, and thus expresses the percent of PLGA that may have been incorporated into the crosslinked network.

This unexpected increase may result from the incorporation of PLGA into the XL (crosslinked) network. This could happen by either or both of two mechanisms. First, chain transfer processes could generate radicals on the PLGA chains by abstraction of a hydrogen atom, possibly the tertiary hydrogen of the lactide moiety. These radicals could then react with PPF unsaturation, covalently linking PLGA with PPF. HAc is known as a good chain transfer agent. The second mechanism for incorporating PLGA is by transesterification reactions in which propylene glycol-fumaric acid ester bonds are broken with formation of propylene glycol-lactic acid or propylene glycol-glycolic acid ester bonds. In addition, fumarate may participate in transesterification by reaction with the hydroxy moiety of the lactate or glycolate residues, forming fumaric acid-lactic acid or fumaric acid-glycolic acid linkages. The quantity of PLGA incorporated can be calculated. The Δ% listed in the next to last row of Table 6 represents the incorporated PLGA. Thus, the percent of the PLGA that is incorporated into the network is the Δ% divided by the % of PLGA in the formulation, which is noted in the last row. This calculation does not take into account the quantity of PVP that may have been lost. Samples used in this test had not been previously extracted with IPA. The percent of insolubles would probably have been higher, if the samples had been first extracted with IPA.

Table 6
MC Insoluble Fraction

Sample ID	97-27-A	97-27-B	97-27-C	97-27-D
Initial wt	0.2323, 0.2160	0.2073	0.2208	0.2144 (0.2203)[a]
Wt insol.	0.1267, 0.1050	0.1251	0.1374	0.0981 (0.0164)
% Insoluble	54.54, 48.61	60.35	62.23	45.76 (7.44)
Wt% VP–PPF–BP	37.6	48.3	37.6	37.6
Wt% MC insol	54.5, 48.6	60.4	62.2	45.8
$\Delta\%$	+14.0 (mean)	+12.1	+24.6	+8.2
$\Delta\%/\%$ PLGA	22.4	23.3	39.5	13.1

[a]Numbers in ( ) in last column are for PPF alone, not XL, no PLGA.

6.4. Flexural Modulus, Strength, Stiffness, and Swelling

Flexural strength, modulus, stiffness, and swelling were measured on samples incubated in phosphatesterified at 37°C for 21 d. Measurements of rod diameter, before immersion and on removal from the bath, were made to judge swelling deformation. Formulations included unmodified PLGA-85:15 as a control (I), PPF crosslinked with VP in the presence of PLGA in gl HAc (II), and micronized PLGA-85:15 dry-mixed with micronized XL-PPF prior to extrusion (III).

Mechanical testing was performed at the Orthopedic Biomechanics Laboratory of the Beth Israel Deaconess Medical Center, Boston, MA, under the direction of Wilson C. Hayes, Ph.D. Three-point bending tests were conducted on the specimens obtained from the extrusion-based protocols (i.e., specimen types I, II, and III). Testing was performed on a TA-XT2 Texture Analyzer (StableMicro Systems, Surrey UK; Texture Technologies, Scarsdale, NY), equipped with a 5 kg–0.1 g load cell, and had a sample support diameter of 1.57 mm. The top loading point was displaced at a rate of 0.1 mm/s until failure. Load and displacement data were recorded using Stable Micro-Systems XTRA-Dimensions software, version 3.7J, and a PC. The real-time-generated graph immediately identifies the maximum load and slope of the curve (stiffness). From these data, the flexural modulus and strength were calculated from the following:

$$\text{Flexural strength} = \frac{8Wl}{\pi d^3}$$

$$\text{Flexural modulus} = \frac{32}{\pi^2} \frac{Pl^4}{d^4 v}$$

where W = load at fracture (Newtons [N]); l = span between supports, (m); d = rod diameter, (m); P = load at midpoint (N); v = vertical displacement (m).

The results are presented in Figs. 2–5. Although, in all cases, unreinforced PLGA performed better (higher modulus and strength at all time-points, higher stiffness from d 4, and least swelling), several other points should be mentioned: Results suggest incorporation of PLGA into the network. This should dramatically improve performance if devices were fabricated using compression molding. The *in situ* cross-linked PPF–PLGA (protocol II) showed approximately the same degree of swelling as did the PLGA control, up to d 11. Again, the compression molding should reduce swelling by minimizing micropores produced by the stresses of extrusion. Although values are lower than desired, materials produced under protocol II showed good constancy in strength and stiffness over the 21-d incubation.

7. Preliminary In Vivo Biocompatibility Evaluations

7.1. Animal Model and Operative Procedure

An in vivo biocompatibility study in rats was conducted, using the tibia defect model of Gerhart et al. *(27)*. Adult male Sprague-Dawley rats, weighing approx 400 g, were used as the animal model (Charles River Laboratories, Wilmington, MA). A total of 60 animals, divided into five sets of 12 animals, were operated. Each set consisted of four groups of three animals each. This allowed

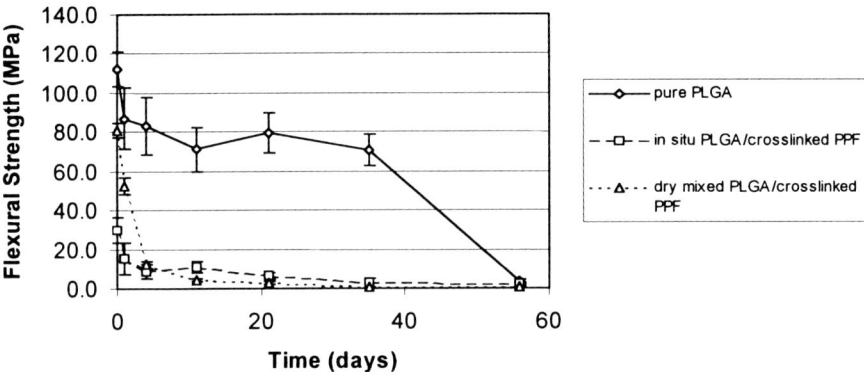

Fig. 2. Flexural strength of PPF-reinforced systems.

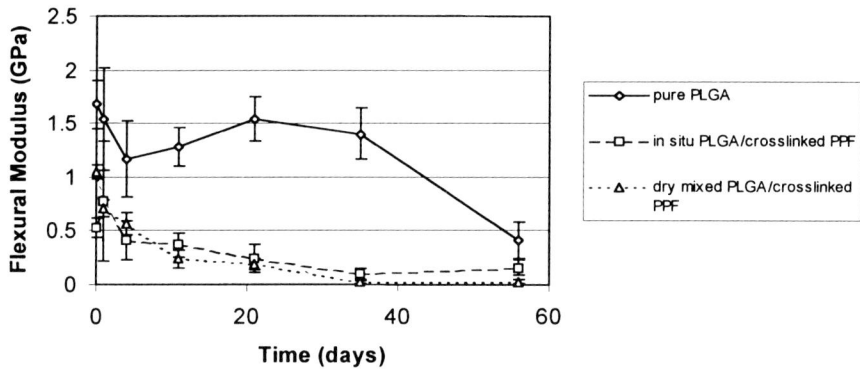

Fig. 3. Flexural modulus of PPF-reinforced systems.

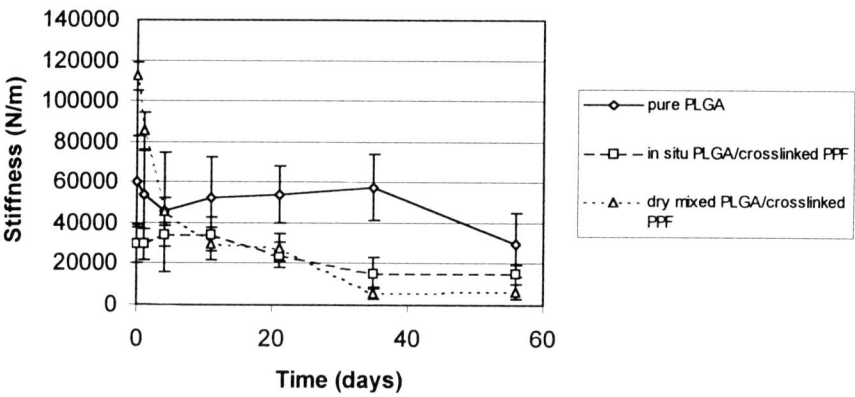

Fig. 4. Stiffness of PPF-reinforced systems.

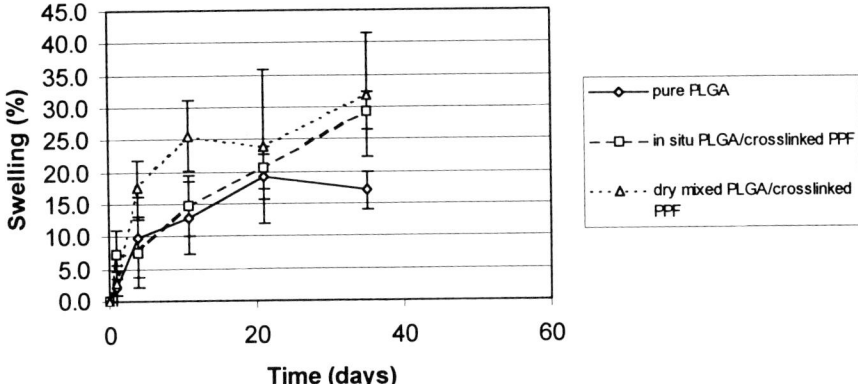

Fig. 5. Swelling of PPF-reinforced systems.

development of a temporal sequence for sacrificing animals at 4 and 10 d, and 3, 5, and 8 wk.

The rats were anesthetized with an intramuscular injection of ketamine HCl (100 mg/kg) and xylazine (5 mg/kg). They were given an intramuscular prophylactic dose of penicillin G (25,000 U/kg), and the surgical site was shaved and prepared with a solution of betadine (povidone-iodine) and alcohol (Dura-Prep; 3M Health Care, St. Paul, MN). The tibia defect model of Gerhart et al. *(27)* was employed by creating a 1-mm drill hole in the medial aspect of the proximal tibia with use of Dremel Flex Shaft drill equipped with a sterile drill bit. Polymer implants that were not treated with γ-irradiation were sterilized in ethylene dioxid. Implants of types I–IV were then inserted, and the wounds were closed in layers, in standard surgical fashion.

7.2. Evaluation of Animal Studies

Following sacrifice, bone specimens were retrieved. After stripping of soft tissues, bone specimens were then fixed in 10% buffered formalin. Thereafter, specimens were decalcified in ethylenediamine tetraacetic acid and paraffin-embedded. Longitudinal 5-μm-thick sections of the bone specimens were cut and stained with hematoxylin and eosin (H&E). Slides were examined for bone resorption and new bone formation at the proximal tibial metaphysis. Newly formed bone was readily identified by the presence of osteoid and woven bone.

Prior to histologic analysis of specimens retrieved from animals at 8 wk, Micro-computed tomography (CT) scans were obtained, which allowed direct visualization of the new trabecular bone surrounding the implant, by generating 3-D reconstructions. These reconstructions allowed measurements of the thickness of the new bone cuff surrounding the implant.

Differences in the remodeling index at sacrifice were analyzed for statistical significance by employing an analysis of variance test, allowing repeated measures and testing for covariates. Homogeneity of variances and covariances was tested with the use of post hoc Leven's test. A p-level of 0.05 was considered significant.

7.3. Histologic Findings

Good biocompatibility in type I implants, which were the unmodified PLGA-85:15 controls, was seen. There was increasing coverage of the implant with newly formed trabecular bone over time. At 8 wk postoperatively, there was a uniform layer of new bone in intimate contact with the implant, and there was no fibrous tissue between the implant and the newly formed trabecular bone cuff. With use of histomorphometric methods, this layer was noted to be on the order of 200–300 μm. The integrity of the implant was preserved throughout the time period studied (8 wk), and only initially an inflammatory response, as evidenced by the presence of polymorphonuclear cells, macrophages, and lymphocytes, was seen (Fig. 6A–D).

In type II implants, which were the *in situ* cured 85:15-5PLGA/XPPF (crosslinked with VP in the presence of PLGA in glHAc), similar find-

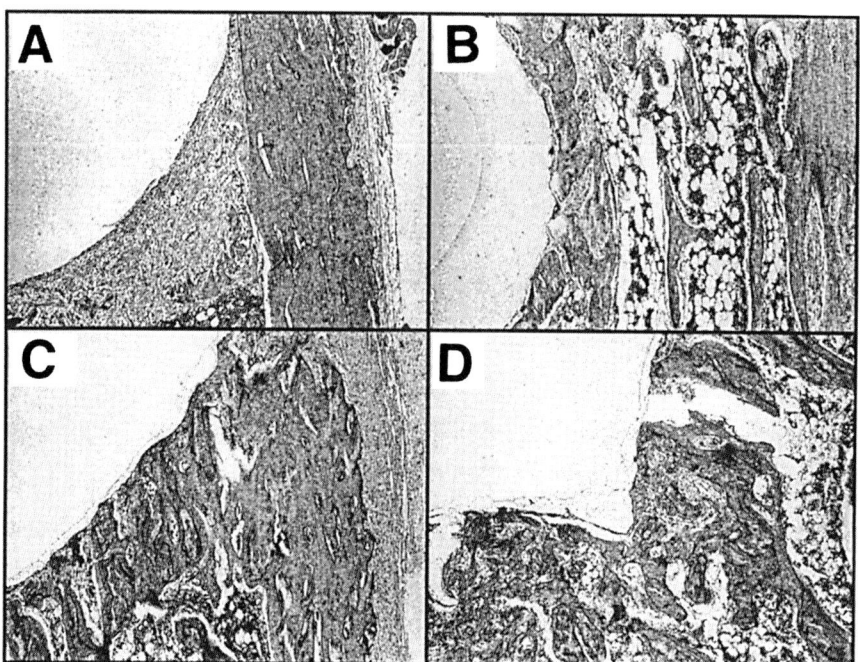

Fig. 6. Photomicrograph of a longitudinal sections (H&E) of rat tibias, in which a pure PLGA-85:15-based bioresorbable bone implant (control) was placed. Plates A–D represent the following different postoperative time intervals: **(A)** 1 wk postoperatively; (× 10). The implant surface is intact. There is little accompanying infiltration with PMNs, consistent with early postoperative changes. Additionally, there is newly formed woven bone in close proximity to the implant. **(B)** 3 wk postoperatively; (× 10). There is increasing contact between the implant and a surrounding, more tightly packed woven-form bone cuff without any interposition of fibrous tissues. **(C)** 5 wk postoperatively; (× 10). The surrounding woven bone cuff is denser than at 3 wk postoperatively. The implant remains intact. **(D)** 8 wk postoperatively; (× 10). There is intimate contact between the entirely intact implant and the new woven bone cuff that has formed tightly around it. Occasionally, there is bone marrow between the newly formed bone traculae.

ings were noted. However, surface erosion of the implant by microfragmentation, with an accompanying inflammatory response, as evidenced by the appearance of multinucleated osteoclasts and macrophages, was seen as early as 1 wk. This was also noted on sections of specimens evaluated at later time-points, with the residual implant remaining structurally stable. At 5 wk, a newly formed woven bone cuff had formed around the implant. This bone cuff was surrounding the entirety of the implant at 8 wk postoperatively. At that time, a moderate inflammatory response was still noted. With use of histomorphometric methods, this layer was noted to be on the order of 100–200 μm (Fig. 7A–D).

In type III implants, which were the micronized 85:15-PLGA/XPPF dry-mixed implants (prior to extrusion), rapid disintegration was noted as early as day po wk 1. The implant was found to break down from its periphery to its center, and was completely disintegrated at 8 wk postoperatively, at which time there was no implant identifiable.

Multiple fragments were noted. Occasionally, these fragments were surrounded by fibrous tissue, and some new trabecular bone formation in the proximity of the implant was noted. At 8 wk postoperatively, a thin new bone cuff formed around the implant. With use of histomorphometric methods, this layer was found to be on the order of 50 μm (Fig. 8A–D).

In type IV implants, which were crosslinked *in situ* and simultaneously molded and γ-irradiated, there was increasing coverage of the implant with newly formed trabecular bone over time. At 8 wk

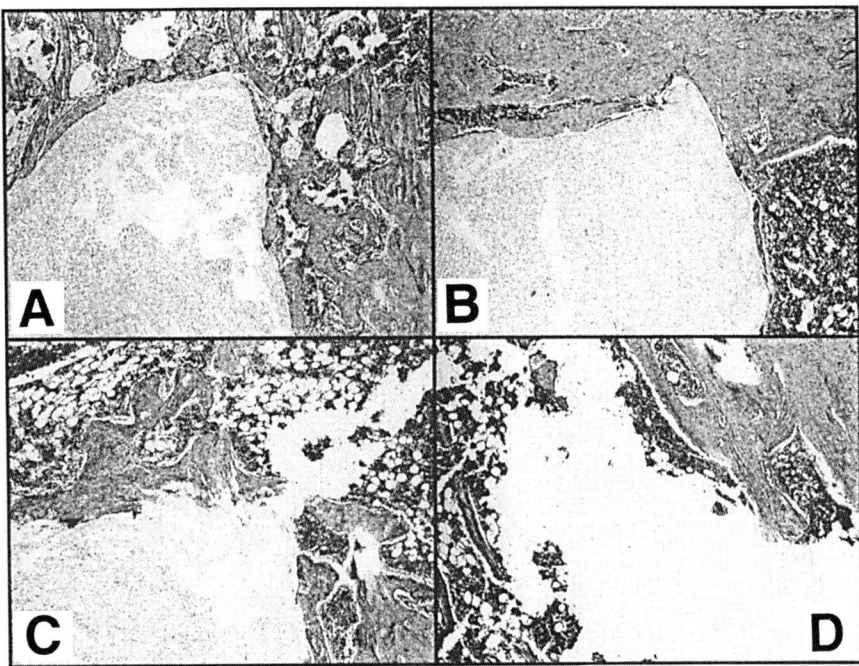

Fig. 7. Photomicrograph of a longitudinal sections (H&E) of rat tibias, in which an *in situ* cured 85:15 PLGA/XPPF molecular reinforced implant was inserted. Plates A–D represent the following different postoperative (po) time intervals: **(A)** 1 wk postoperatively, (× 10). The implant is relatively intact, and there is some reactive bone formation around it. **(B)** 3 wk postoperatively, (× 10). There is moderate implant surface erosion. However, the implant remained grossly intact. There is increasing bone formation around it, which is accompanied by a moderate inflammatory reaction. **(C)** 5 wk postoperatively, (× 10). The implant is unchanged to previous time-points. There is a clearly defined, newly formed woven bone cuff round it, with a decreased inflammatory reaction. **(D)** 8 wk postoperatively, (× 10). The implant is not present in this plate. Gross histologic findings are similar to the 5-wk time-point.

postoperatively, the surrounding new bone cuff was noted to be on the order of 100–150 µm. Although some surface erosion was present initially (1 wk postoperatively), the implant showed little surface erosion, and remained structurally intact throughout the po course. A moderate inflammatory response was seen initially, but this response appeared to have decreased at later po time-point (Fig. 9A–D).

7.4. Micro-CT Scanning

As shown in Fig. 10A, 3-D reconstruction of the newly formed bone cuff surrounding a type I implant revealed that the unmodified PLGA-85:15 control served as a good osteoconductor. A uniform layer of trabecular bone had formed on top of the implant, and volumetric measurements corresponded with histomorphometric analysis, showing that the thickness of this newly formed trabecular bone cuff was approx 100 µm. Only few apparent defects in this surrounding trabecular bone cuff were seen. In addition, these 3-D reconstructions clearly demonstrated a moderate extent of remodeling in the adjacent trabecular bone of the rat tibia metaphysics.

As shown in Fig. 10B, 3-D reconstruction of the newly formed trabecular bone cuff surrounding a type II implant demonstrated this cuff to be slightly thicker, and volumetric measurements corresponded with histomorphometric measurements, indicating a thickness of the trabecular bone cuff of approx 200–300 µm. In contrast to type I implants, 3-D reconstruction of the trabecular bone of the rat tibial metaphysis surrounding the implant demonstrated more vigorous remodeling of the adjacent trabecular bone of the rat tibia

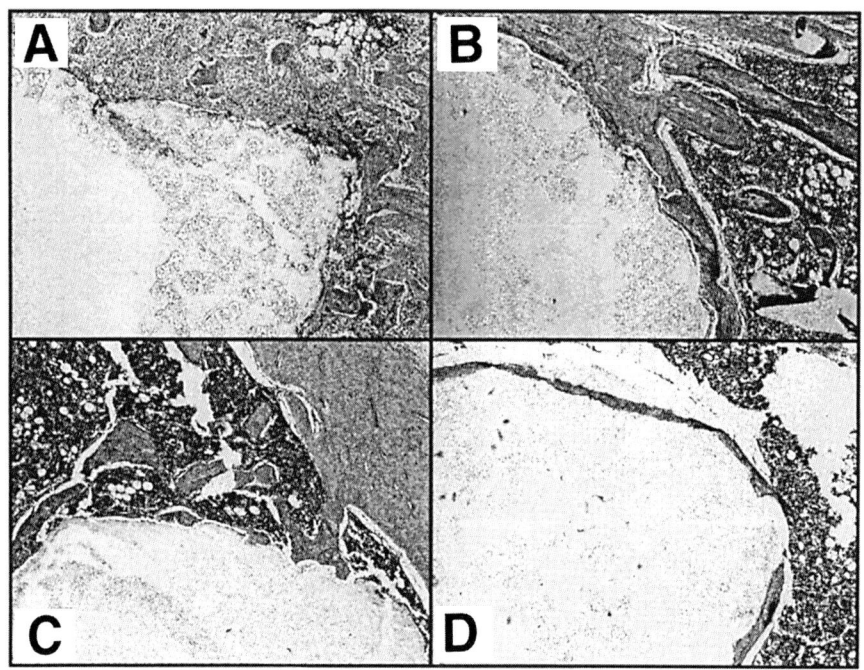

Fig. 8. Photomicrograph of a longitudinal sections (H&E) of rat tibias, in which a dry-mixed 85:15-PLGA/XPPF implant was inserted. Plates A–D represent the following different po time intervals: **(A)** 1 wk postoperatively (× 10). The implant is undergoing disintegration. There is moderate infiltration with PMNs and macrophages. **(B)** 3 wk postoperatively (× 10). Surface erosion and disintegration of the implant continued, and has involved a larger section of the implant. There is a thin surrounding newly formed bone cuff that is accompanied by inflammation, as evidenced by the bone marrow infiltration with inflammatory cells. **(C)** 5 wk postoperatively (× 10). There is increasing inflammation in the surrounding new bone cuff. **(D)** 8 wk postoperatively (× 10). Total disintegration of the implant is noted. A thin bone cuff with a moderate accompanying inflammatory response remains around the implant.

metaphysis. In fact, volumetric measurements confirmed that the trabecular bone volume in the proximal metaphysis was higher than in type I implants, where unmodified PLGA-85:15 was used. This indicated a greater tissue response to the *in situ* PPF-crosslinked implants, and corresponds with histologic findings presented above.

8. Summary and Conclusions

All materials were compared against extruded or compression-molded PLGA as a standard. On the basis of these comparisons, the authors have identified compression molding (or transfer molding) at room temperature of PLGA/PPF/VP/BP, followed by crosslinking under pressure at elevated temperature, and again by γ-irradiation, as the method of choice. The composition of the charge to the mold, PLGA(3):PPF(1):VP(0.7):BP (0.1), appears to work well, and will form the compositional and procedural basis for investigations.

Preliminary in vivo biocompatibility evaluations in rats showed that both the unmodified PLGA-85:15 control implants and the implants comprised of PPF crosslinked with VP in the presence of PLGA in glHac had acceptable osteoconductive properties. No foreign body or inflammatory response was observed. Histologic evaluation and analysis by micro-CT scanning demonstrated that the implants comprised of PPF crosslinked with VP in the presence of PLGA in glHac (type II) seemed to provoke a more vigorous response of the surrounding trabecular bone in the rat tibia

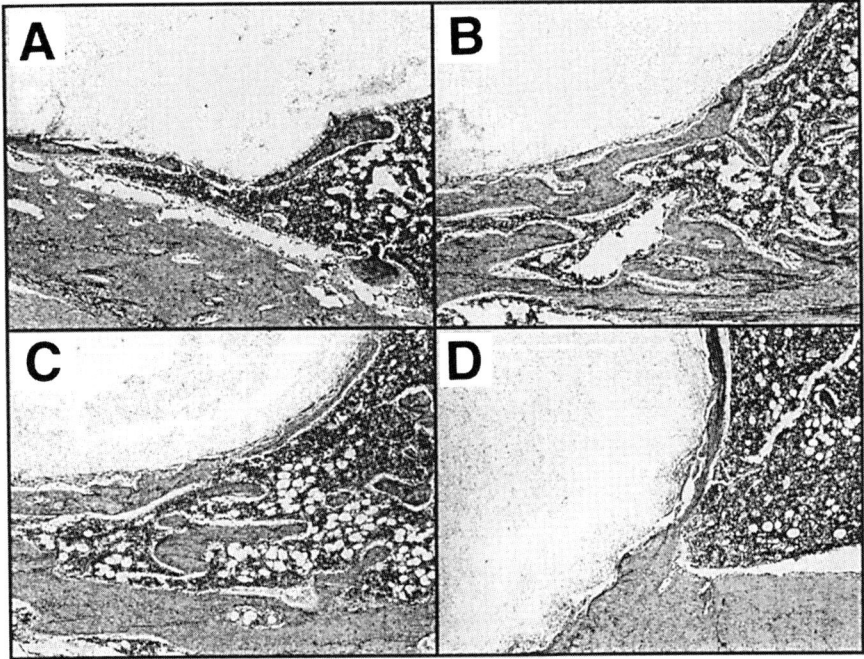

Fig. 9. Photomicrograph of a longitudinal sections (H&E) of rat tibias, in which a 85:15-PLGA/XPPF implant crosslinked *in situ* simultaneously molded and γ-irradiated was inserted. Plates A–D represent the following different po time intervals: **(A)** 1 wk postoperatively (× 10). The implant is intact but shows some surface erosion. There is an accompanying inflammatory response and a bone cuff started to form around the implant. **(B)** 3 wk postoperatively(× 10). There is increasing bone formation around the implant, and a thin newly formed bone cuff developed around the entirety of the implant. **(C and D)** 5 and 8 wk postoperatively (× 10). No change from previous time-point.

metaphysis. As evidenced by histologic analysis, this also involved the production of a thicker, newly formed trabecular bone cuff and ingrowth of bone into the surface of the implant.

Support for the reinforcement potential of XL-PPF is suggested in a recent study by Yaszemski et al. *(28)*, who measured the compressive strength and modulus over a 12-wk period of a composite of PPF crosslinked with VP, and containing β-tricalcium phosphate and sodium chloride. The value of both parameters increased with degradation time, and remained above the minimum values acceptable for trabecular bone substitutes. A compressive strength of 21.3 ± 0.4 MPa and modulus of 696 ± 53 MPa were measured after 12 wk for a composite material with an initial strength of 18.0 ± 4.6 MPa and modulus of 113 ± 0 MPa.

9. Future Developmental Goals

In situ crosslinking of PPF with VP in the presence of PLGA, and in glHAc solution, is a facile reaction. However, the drawback is that the low density of the lyophilized product requires that the material be severely deformed in molding or extrusion. This deformation results in disruption of the XL-PPF–PLGA network, and subsequent reformation of a continuous material, but with boundaries across which PPF networks do not penetrate. The same applies to the dry-mixed extrudates. Thus, these approaches did not result in improvements in mechanical properties (swelling on exposure to water, stiffness, nor either flexural modulus or strength).

The authors have shown how this can be resolved. It is important to start with a homoge-

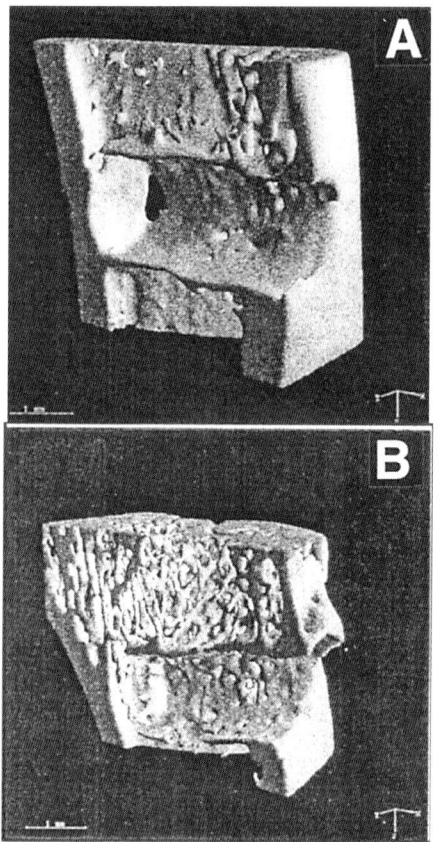

Fig. 10. **(A)** 3-D reconstruction of micro-CT scans of the proximal rat tibial metaphysis. A type I implant (unmodified PLGA-85:15 control) was used. There is a newly formed bone cuff surrounding the implant undergoing moderate remodeling. Cone-shaped empty space in the center indicates implantation site of the implant. Note thin new bone cuff (approximate thickness, 100 µm). Bar in the left lower corner of the image indicates a length of 1 mm. **(B)** 3-D reconstruction of micro-CT scans of the proximal rat tibial metaphysis. A type II implant (PPF crosslinked with VP in the presence of PLGA in glHac) was used. There is a newly formed bone cuff surrounding the implant undergoing substantial remodeling. Cone-shaped empty space in the center indicates implantation site of the implant. Note thick new bone cuff (approximate thickness 200–300 µm). Bar in the left lower corner of the image indicates a length of 1 mm.

neous nonporous blend of all components, without the void volume left by solvents removed by lyophilization (the purpose of crosslinking in glHAc was to ensure homogeneity of the PPF and PLGA blend). When the components are dissolved in a low-boiling solvent, such as acetone, followed by evaporation of the acetone, a plasticized homogeneous blend forms (because of the presence of VP), which can be loaded into a mold, subjected to pressure at room temperature (transfer or compression molding) to form the desired shape, followed by heating, while still under pressure in the mold to effect *in situ* crosslinking. Further crosslinking occurs on sterilization by γ-irradiation, leading to a product with a hardness equivalent to that of compression-molded PLGA. Such a process leads to continuity of both the PLGA and XL-PPF components, and a strong nonporous device of the desired shape.

Therefore, initial work should include a more focused analytical and mechanical characterization of the compression-molded plates produced by the protocol summarized above. Based on these analyses, blends will be compositionally optimized by varying the crosslink density in the molecular network, for development of in vitro and in vivo corollaries to mechanical strength and dimensional stability, using PLGA-only plates as a control. Given this in vitro/in vivo optimization of a molecularly reinforced plate, the structural performance of a selected formulation should then be more thoroughly characterize in a small (rat) animal model system.

Acknowledgments

The authors wish to thank Dr. Joseph Alroy, DVM, Associate Professor in Pathology, Tufts University Schools of Medicine and Veterinary Medicine for his assistance in the histologic analysis of this study. Furthermore, the authors are indebted to Shrikar Bondre and Eric Gusek for their assistance with animal care. This work was supported in part by National Institutes of Health/National Institute of Arthritis, Musculoskeletal and Skin Diseases (NIH/NIAMS) Grant No. 1 R43 AR 44450-01A1 (J.D.G.), and NIH/NIAMS Grant AR 45062 (to K.-U.L.).

References

1 Cheal EJ, Mansmann KA, DiGioia AM 3rd, Hayes WC, and Perren SM. Role of interfragmentary

1. strain in fracture healing: bovine model of a healing osteotomy. *J Orthop Res* 1991; 9: 131–142.
2. Cordey J, Perren SM, and Steinmann S. Stress protection in plate osteosynthesis: myth or reality? *Helv Chir Acta* 1989; 56: 235–259.
3. Matter P and Burch HB. Clinical experience with titanium implants, especially with the limited contact dynamic compression plate system. *Arch Orthop Trauma Surg* 1990; 109: 311–313.
4. Claes L, Augat P, Sugar G, and Wilke HJ. "Influence of size and stability of the osteotomy gap on the success of fracture healing", *J Orthop Res* 1997; 15: 577–584.
5. Bednar DA, Grandwilewski W. "Complications of forearm-plate removal", *Can J Surg* 1992; 34: 428–431.
6. Ferguson SJ, Wyss UP, Pichora DR. "Finite element stress analysis of a hybrid fracture fixation plate", *Med Eng Phys* 1996; 18: 241–250.
7. Woo SL, Lothringer LS, Akeson WH, Coutts RC, Woo YK, Simon BR, and Gomez MA. "Less rigid internal fixation plates: historical perspectives and new concepts", *J Orthop Res* 1984; 1: 431–449.
8. Peltoniemi HH, Ahovuo J, Tulamo RM, Tormala P, and Waris T. "Biodegradable and titanium plating in experimental craniotomies: a radiographic follow-up", *J Craniofac Surg* 1997; 8: 446–451.
9. Peltoniemi HH, Tulamo RM, Pihlajamaki HK, Kallionen M, Pohjonen T, Tormala P, Rokkanen PU, and Warris T. "Consolidation of craniotomy lines after resorbable polylactide and titanium plating: a comparative experimental study in sheep", *Plast Reconstr Surg* 1998; 101: 123–133.
10. Suuronen R, Manninen MJ, Pohjonen T, Laitinen O, and Lindqvist C. "Mandibular osteotomy fixed with biodegradable plates and screws: an animal study", *Br J Oral Maxillofac Surg* 1997; 35: 341–348.
11. Getter L, Cutright DE, Bhaskar SN, and Augsburg JK. Biodegradable intraosseous appliance in the treatment of mandibular fractures", *J Oral Surg* 1972; 30: 344.
12. Hollinger JO and Battistone GC. "Biodegradable bone repair materials: synthetic polymers and ceramics", *Clin Orthop Related Res* 1986; 207: 290–305.
13. Bostman OM. "Current concepts review: absorbable implants for the fixation of fractures", *J Joint Bone Surg* 1991; 73: 148–153.
14. Bos RRM, Rozema FR, Boering G, Nijenhuis AJ, Pennings AJ, and Verwey AB. "Bioabsorbable plates and screws for internal fixation of mandibular fractures: a study in six dogs", *Int J Oral Maxillofac Surg* 1989; 18: 365–369.
15. Tortorelli, unpublished work.
16. Parsons JR, Alexander H, Corcoran SF, Karoluk JM, and Weiss AB. "Development of a variable stiffness absorbable bone plate", *Proceedings of the 7th Northeast Bioengineering Conference* 1979; Pergamon, New York, p. 162.
17. Skirving AP, Day R, MacDonald W, and McLaren R. "Carbon fiber reinforced plastic (CFRP) plates versus stainless steel dynamic compression plates in the treatment of fractures of the Tibiae in dogs", *Clin Orthop Related Res* 1987; 224: 117–124.
18. Christel P, Chabot F, Leary JL, Morin C, and Vert M. Biodegradable composites for internal fixation, in *Biomaterials* 1982; (Winter GD, Gibbon DF, and Plenk H, eds), Wiley, New York, pp 271–280.
19. Tormala P, Vasenius J, Vainionpaa S, Laiho J, Pohjonen T, and Rokkanen P. "Ultra-high-strength absorbable self-reinforced polyglycolide (SR-PGA) composite rods for internal fixation of bone fractures: *in vitro* and *in vivo* study", *J Biomed Mater Res* 1991; 25: 1–22.
20. Tormala P. "Biodegradable self-reinforced composite materials: manufacturing structure and mechanical properties", *Clin Mater* 1992; 10: 29–34.
21. Tormala P. "Biodegradable self-reinforced absorbable polymeric composites for applications in different disciplines of surgery", *Clin Mater* 1993; 13: 35–40.
22. Weiler W and Gogolewski S. "Enhancement of the mechanical properties of polylactides by solid-state extrusion", *Biomaterials* 1996; 17: 529–535.
23. Heppenstal RB. Fracture healing, in *Basic Orthopaedic Biomechanics* 1991; (Mow VC and Hayes WC, eds), Raven, New York, pp. 35–64.
24. Adams JC. *Outline of Fractures: Including Joint Injuries* 1978; Churchill Livingston, New York.
25. Fung YC. *Biomechanics: Mechanical Properties of Living Tissues* 1981; Springer-Verlag, New York, pp. 383–389.
26. Gresser JD, Hsu SH, Nagaoka H, Lyons CM, Nieratko DP, Wise DL, Barabino GA, and Trantolo DJ. "Analysis of a vinyl pyrrolidone/poly(propylene fumarate) resorbable bone cement", *J Biomed Mater Res* 1995; 29: 1241–1247.
27. Gerhart TN, Renshaw AA, Miller RL, Noecker RJ, and Hayes WC. "*In vivo* histologic and biomechanical characterization of a biodegradable particulate composite bone cement", *J Biomed Mater Res* 1989; 23: 1–16.
28. Yaszemski MJ, Payne RG, Hayes WC, Langer R, and Mikos AG. "*In vitro* degradation of a poly(propylene fumarate) based composite material", *Biomaterials*, 1996; 17: 2127–2130.

17

Particulate Metal in Late Aseptic Loosening of Cemented Total Hip Arthroplasties

Jochanan H. Boss, David G. Mendes, and Ines Misselevich

1. Introduction

Success of total joint replacements, whether cemented or otherwise, depends on attainment of stable fixation of the alloplastic components to bone. The morphological scene at the implant–bone interfaces provides a crucial clue in understanding aseptic loosening of prosthetic components, which is the leading failure mode of artificial joints. The granulomatous interfacial membrane (GIM), separating the alloplastic component from bone, constitutes the hallmark of aseptically loosened arthroplasties. The GIM unbinds a formerly stable component: bony anchorage. Prosthetic failures are also caused by physical mishaps, such as femoral stem–cement debonding, cup-head impingement, stem-related cement splitting, cement defects, dissociation of a metallic–polyethylene (PE) backing, and fractures of a femoral stem or an acetabular cup. However, these accidents are exceptions, and the biologically driven formation of the GIMs accounts for most prosthetic failures.

Without the capacity for self repair, any substance, no matter how strong initially, will ultimately fail, given sufficient repetitive loading *(1)*. Prosthetic breakdown products accumulate in the effective joint space *(2)*. Submicron- to micron-sized, ingestible, but undigestible, polymeric and metallic particles recruit and activate leukocytes, primarily cells of the mononuclear phagocytic system. The leukocytes, primarily macrophages ingesting wear debris, profusely secrete proinflammatory and osteoclast-activating factors. Acting in concert, the enhanced bone resorption, amplified recruitment of further leukocytes, and boosted proliferation of fibroblasts sustain the expansive growth of the GIMs. Likewise, the ensuing implant instability, which intensifies the breakdown of the alloplastic components, and the negative bone balance cooperate in propagating the growth of the GIMs. This cycle finalizes the failure of intraosseous devices, in general, and of arthroplasties, in particular *(3)*.

Polymethylmethacrylate (PMMA) is successfully employed in fixation of alloplastic components to their bony beds. Indeed, the survival rates of cemented arthroplasties have become the gold standard against which success of cementless joint replacements is measured. Two theories vie with each other to explain aseptic loosening of cemented components. First, initially achieved mechanical anchorage is lost as a result of stress-induced microfractures of the buttressing, interlocking osseous and acrylic projections. Second, all cemented components are condemned to loosen, because the formation of ever-expanding GIMs is inherent in the cementation procedure. Mallory *(4)* has forewarned that the interfacial events kick off "a race between the life of the patient and the life of the prosthesis" *(4)*.

Prosthetic debris is derived from PMMA, PE,

and metallic parts of the artificial joints. Nevertheless, the cement has been made a scapegoat for prosthetic failure, so much so that the term "cement disease" is commonly used interchangeably with aseptic loosening *(5)*. Heat-induced bone necrosis (consequent on the exothermic methylmethacrylate polymerization reaction and bone reaming), as well as tissue-damaging effects of the cement, outlasting methylmethacrylate monomer and additives, are implicated in the formation of the GIMs. It is contended that the cement never becomes osseointegrated, because the acrylic mantle is separated from the bone by a soft tissular membrane at all times. These premises are unsubstantiated. In fact, cementation does not raise the temperature to levels at which osteocytes die. That the osseous and hemopoietic tissues near the cement are viable a few days after implantation attests to the nontoxicity of the PMMA *(6–8)*. Charnley first recorded, and other researchers *(9)* have since confirmed, that cement osseointegrates where a stable interfacial situation prevails. Because osseointegration bears witness to biocompatibility, cement is decidedly not endowed with those innate pernicious properties blamed for prosthetic failure *(10)*. Loosened, uncemented implants are also separated from the underlying bone by a GIM. It is circular to argue that PMMA is inherently harmful to bone because loosened cemented arthroplasties are surrounded by GIMs. In the context of bone balance, acrylic particles inhibit new bone formation to a lesser degree than either interfacial movements or PE particles *(11)*.

2. Materials and Methods

The morphological aspects of the GIMs were reviewed by literature perusal and histological study of the authors' collection of aseptically loosened cemented total hip joint replacements. The microscopic features of GIMs of artificial joints, loosening after a service period of less than 15 yr, i.e., short-term survivorship, were compared to those of arthroplasties serving successfully for more than 15 yr, i.e., long-term survivorship. Special attention was paid to the amounts of the different kinds of prosthetic debris deposited in the GIMs.

3. Results

3.1. Short-Term Surviving Cemented Hip Prostheses

Perceiving similarities to synovitis, Goldring et al. *(12)* have introduced the term of "synovial-like membrane" for the GIMs. In view of the role of the GIMs in osteolysis, Santavirta et al. *(13)* have stressed the aggressive quality of the prosthetic debris-induced granulation tissue. The GIMs display a nearly three-layered texture, namely, the inner synovial-like, the middle inflammatory-granulomatous, and the outer, mostly fibrotically sclerosed, layers *(14)*. Large cement chunks are identified as optically empty, polycyclic spaces containing tiny, black, birefringent barium sulphate ($BaSO_4$) grains; they are surrounded by mono- and polykaryonic macrophages (the so-called giant cells) and concentrically oriented collagenous fibers. Micron-sized acrylic particle-induced fibrosis is accompanied by lymphohistiocytic infiltrates. The bubbly cytoplasm of PMMA particle-ingesting macrophages comprises tiny, grayish, birefringent, $BaSO_4$ grains (the PMMA having been dissolved by solvents used in preparation of the sections; the $BaSO_4$ is preserved). Evaluation of the periprosthetic tissues evidences the minor participation of the cement breakdown products in the formation of the GIMs: When compared to the exuberant reactions induced by PE debris, the PMMA-induced granulomatous response is trivial.

The dominant characteristic is the presence of broad sheets of closely packed, plump, foamy, mono-, bi-, and polykaryonic macrophages. Histochemical, polarization optical, and electron microscopical studies have disclosed that phagocytosis of countless, submicron- to micron-sized PE particles bestows on the macrophages a distinct foamy aspect *(15)*. In agreement with the tribological setting at, and mode of generation of, wear debris from the acetabular insert, release of large shreds is limited, so that PE fragment-provoked giant cell granulomas are scarce in the GIMs of artificial hip joints *(16–19)*. Whatever their size, the PE breakdown products are the prevalent species of prosthetic detritus in the GIMs of short-term surviving hip arthroplasties. Hence, aseptic loosening of cemented artificial hip joints equals Müller's concept of the PE disease *(20)*.

Metallic particles are recognizable as 1–5-µ-sized, nonbirefringent, black specks within the macrophages or between the collagen fibers. Macrophages, which have ingested PE debris as well as metallic particles, exhibit black grains on the foamy cytoplasmic background, unless they are overburdened by the metallic dust to such an extent that all cellular details are obscured. Metallic debris is generally present in only small amounts in the GIMs of the short-term surviving cemented hip joint replacements *(21)*. Metallosis, the grossly appreciable black staining of the periprosthetic tissues, is not infrequently encountered at revision operations of aseptically loosened, uncemented artificial hip joints, especially those with titanium- or titanium alloy-based parts. However, metallosis is rarely seen around cemented components, and then only in cases in which abrasion has occurred as a result of harsh mechanical conditions *(22–24)*.

3.2. Long-Term Surviving Cemented Hip Prostheses

The GIMs obtained at autopsy, or retrieved at revision operations performed for aseptic loosening after more than 15 yr of service, typically display certain distinctive features. Extensive osseointegration of the cement mantle and an inverse ratio of the polymeric to the metallic wear particles are the remarkable findings. Osseointegrated cement segments alternate with cement segments disjoined from the bone by a thin layer of fibrous tissue or a typical GIM. The filmy fibrous layer, not more than a few cells thick, contains some aggregated foamy macrophages filled with submicron- to micron-sized PE particles. Focally, the acrylic mantle closely apposes a dense shell of newly formed bone. Where present, the GIMs consist, for the most part, of a densely textured or hyalinized collagenous tissue, within which sheets of foamy macrophages are scarce and small *(25,26)*. Expansive GIMs, akin to those of the short-term surviving arthroplasties, are present in a minority of the long-term surviving artificial hip joints, in which the acrylic mantles have become entirely separated from the underlying bone by a synovial-like membrane.

Cement chunks are blandly incorporated in hypocellular and hyalinized fibrous tissue. They are encircled by coarse, concentrically arrayed collagen fibers, which abut directly on the PMMA. Conspicuous by its absence is an enclosing macrophagic barrier (Fig. 1), the prototypic reaction pattern of soft and hard tissues to nonresorbable polymers. Elsewhere, many $BaSO_4$-grain-laden macrophages are strewn in the fibrous tissue, close to the cement slabs (Fig. 2), in numbers far greater than usually encountered in the GIMs of the short-term surviving joint replacements.

When compared with GIMs of the short-term surviving arthroplasties, not much PE debris is present in the periprosthetic tissues of most long-term surviving artificial hip joints. Correspondingly, sheets of foamy macrophages are few and small, but many single or grouped, plump macrophages, massively overburdened by micron-sized metallic particles, prevail at sites where, in the absence of osseointegrated cement, a GIM has developed (Fig. 3). In addition, randomly dispersed, large, 10–300 µ-sized, jagged metallic fragments are present extracellularly, among the macrophages or the collagen fibers, as well as within giant-celled granulomas. Much metallic debris occasionally accumulates in sizable foci of coagulation necrosis.

Abundant PE debris, and the granulomatous response thereto, are the rightfully accepted perspectives of the GIMs surrounding loosened alloplastic components of short-term surviving cemented hip arthroplasties. As if vicariously supplanting for these characteristics, metallic particles and the macrophagic response thereto constitute the principal species of prosthetic breakdown products and the overwhelming reaction pattern, respectively, in the GIMs of many long-term surviving cemented hip replacements.

4. Discussion

Biofunctionality defines those mechanical and physical properties that enable an implant to perform in the manner planned at the time of its design. Foreign body-induced reactions, by themselves, do not set limits to an implant's biofunctionality. Biocompatibility expresses the capacity of an implanted device to successfully perform, with

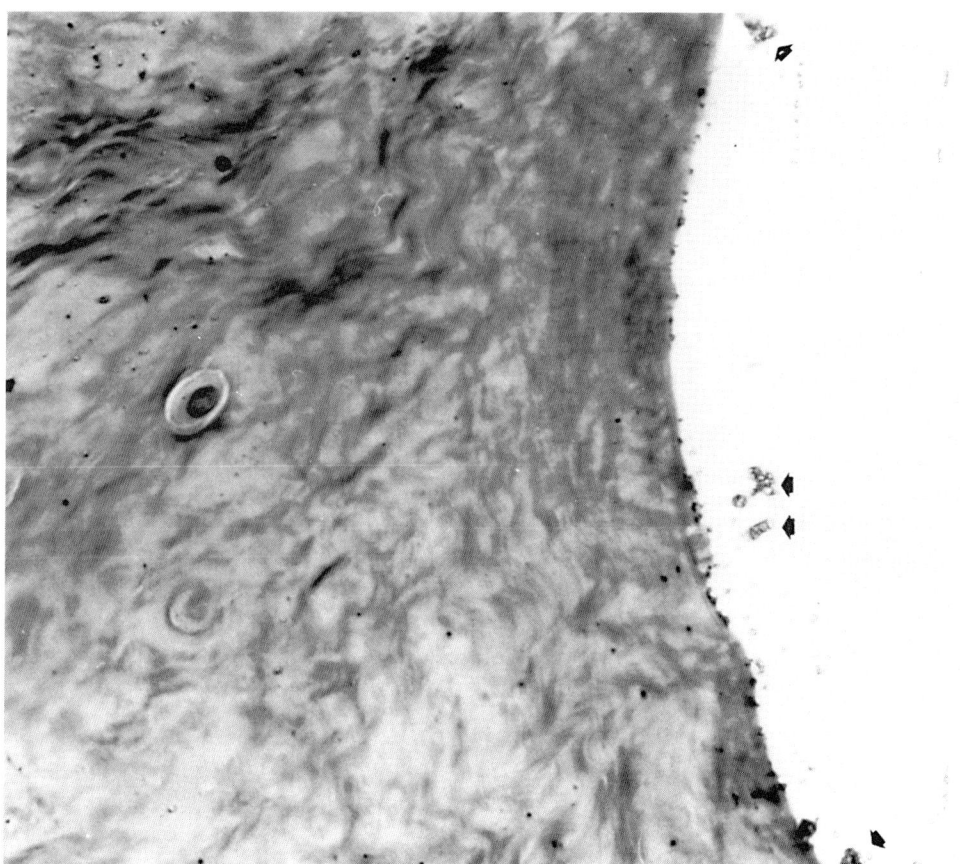

Fig. 1. Cement chunk blandly incorporated in hypocellular fibrous tissue. Optically empty space surrounded by coarse, concentrically arrayed collagen fibers, without an intervening macrophagic barrier. Some $BaSO_4$ grains (arrows) are present in the roundish space (from which the cement was dissolved by the solvents used for the preparation of the section). Section of plastic-embedded sample stained by Goldner's technique. ×320.

appropriate host inflammatory and granulomatous responses, in specific applications. By these formulations, contemporary biomaterials in bulk form are biofunctional and biocompatible (10). In the context of aseptic loosening of cemented hip arthroplasties, formation of a bone-resorbing GIM can be ascribed to neither untoward effects of the cement nor to cementation. The concept of cement disease (5) is misleading because it suggests a linear relationship between a material and the cause of prosthetic failure. In analyzing the behavior of implants, in general, it is fallacious to only exploit insights gained from observations made on what failed, rather than on what succeeded.

Exuberant granulomatous reactions to PE breakdown products are found in the GIMs of cemented artificial hip joints loosening after short periods of service. It may be anticipated *a priori* that wear at the articulating surface of the acetabular insert would produce ever increasing amounts of particles with increasing duration of service, thus progressively amplifying the granulomatous reaction to the PE debris. This is not what is actually observed at the bone–implant interfaces of most long-term surviving cemented hip arthroplasties, in which the macrophagic response to metallic particles prevails over the granulomatous reaction to PE particles. Adverse mechanical settings at the articulating surfaces are probably responsible for excessive generation of PE particles early on. Accumulating in, and disseminating throughout, the effective joint space, the abound-

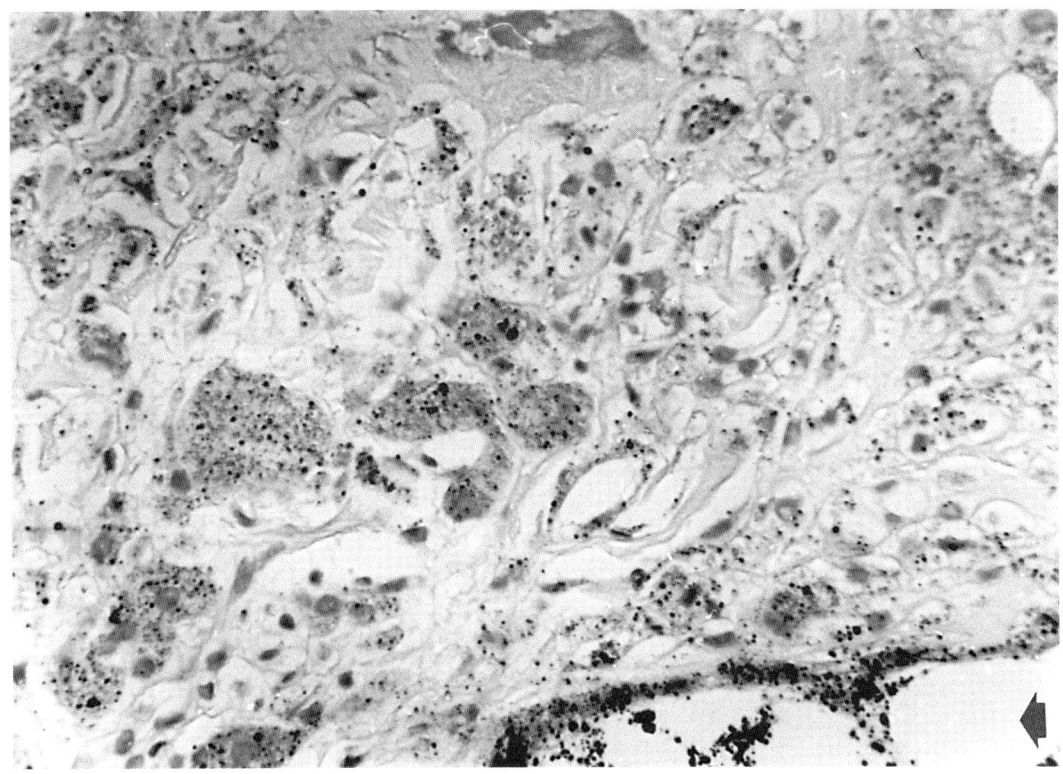

Fig. 2. Many, large BaSO$_4$-grain-laden macrophages scattered close to a cement chunk (arrow). Despite dissolution of the cement, numerous BaSO$_4$ particles remain within the formerly PMMA-containing space. H&E ×500.

ing PE debris stimulates the formation of the bone-resorbing GIM, the mediator of the premature loosening process. If other adverse accidents do not interfere with the effective performance of a cemented artificial hip joint, proper mechanical settings keep the joint contact forces within a sustainable range. Generation of PE wear products being minimized, and absence of a luxuriant GIM facilitating osseointegration of the cement mantle, long-term survivorship is achievable. In fact, this is the morphologic scene at the interfaces of cemented hip arthroplasties that successfully served for more than 15 yr. This view turns attention away from the biomaterials' chemical properties, emphasizes the significant role of the implant's mechanical and tribological history, and directs awareness to the primacy of the physical circumstances operative in the loosening process *(18,27–29)*.

Microscopic assays are customary in semi-quantifying the absolute and relative amounts of the different species of prosthetic breakdown products polluting the periprosthetic tissues. Using this analytical modality, the present survey shows that, at the bone–implant interfaces of most long-term surviving cemented total hip arthroplasties, the metallic particles, and the macrophagic response thereto, typically prevail over the PE particles and the granulomatous reaction thereto. It is a demanding task to confidently appraise the contribution of individual species of prosthetic breakdown products to GIM formation. With this reservation in mind, two generalizations are proposed. First, under optimal mechanical circumstances, wear of the articulating surface of the metallic femoral head proceeds unabated, in the face of limited generation of polymeric wear from the PE acetabular socket. Second, the metallic particles provide a crucial force in the recruitment and activation of the mononuclear phago-

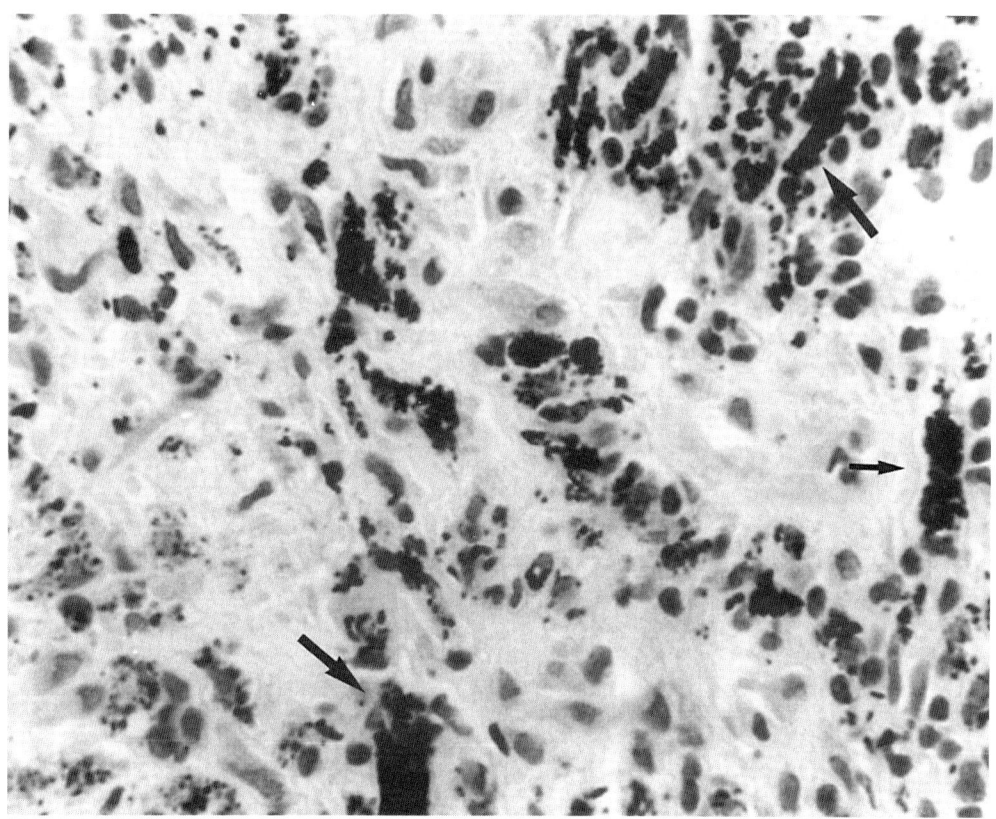

Fig. 3. Single and grouped, plump, metallic-particle-laden, macrophages. Some large, jagged metallic fragments (arrows), measuring ~ 100μ or more, are strewn between the phagocytes, which have ingested the micron-sized metallic debris. Section of plastic-embedded sample stained by von Kossa's technique with McNeal's counterstain. ×320.

cytes, lymphocytes, and fibroblasts, which lead to enlargement of the GIMs. Thus, the metallic breakdown products appear to participate significantly in triggering the processes involved in late aseptic loosening of artificial hip joints (30).

Many failed hip arthroplasties are believed to have been loose from the time of their implantation, as a result of insufficient initial fixation or early loss of fixation (31). In contrast, Mjöberg (32) contends that instability and migration of prosthetic components are drawn-out, ongoing processes, activated upon cyclic loading of the artificial joints. There is little to hinder osseointegration of the cement mantle in the absence of a GIM. Indeed, lengthy cement segments directly contact mineralized bone or osteoid seams in most cases of long-term surviving hip arthroplasties. Osseointegration being a biomaterial's affirmation of biocompatibility (4), the cement is not endowed with those innate toxic properties to which some authors have attributed prosthetic failure (5). The bland incorporation of cement chunks in the fibrous tissue, without an intervening macrophagic barrier, further reaffirms the biocompatibility of PMMA in bulk form. To the authors' knowledge, this inoffensive in vivo behavior of the cement has not been stressed by other investigators. The authors can offer no ready explanation for the absence of a segregating macrophagic barrier, except to point out the analogy with cement osseointegration, in which bone, a mineralized collagenous and noncollagenous connective tissue, abuts on PMMA, without the mediation of an enclosing reactive-type tissue. These large cement slabs appear to disintegrate with time, as evinced by the clustered $BaSO_4$-grain-laden macrophages in their environs. This macrophagic response to released and interstitially deposited $BaSO_4$ grains is of phenomenological interest, but, being quantitatively trivial, hardly contributes to the formation of the GIMs.

Al-Saffar et al. *(33)* have recently described the potential of macrophages ingesting metallic particles to produce cytokines involved in the build-up of GIMs, as well as in the mobilization and activation of osteoclasts. Particulate metals may be causally linked to loosening processes directly, via GIM formation, or indirectly, via cellular hypersensitivity reactions. The metallic and polymeric breakdown products are evidently equally effective in their capacity to produce bone-resorbing GIMs. Dorr et al.'s *(34)* perception of a "small particles disease," as the quintessence of the aseptic loosening process, conveys the common final pathway leading to prosthetic failure.

The activated macrophages synthesize both bone-resorbing and osteogenic factors *(29)*. Macrophage activation at the bone–implant interface may provide the osteogenic cytokines essential for bone growth onto, and into, the recesses of the cement mantle. In the absence of a GIM, the enhanced bony anchorage achieved by the segmentally osseointegrated components explains the long-term survival of the cemented hip arthroplasties. Long-lasting stability of an intraosseous implant is a prerequisite for successful long-term performance. Success or failure of intraosseous devices depends, in part, on a positive bone balance, which, in its turn, depends on the effects of interfacially osteogenic factors overruling the effects of bone-resorbing mediators *(35,36)*. On searching the literature, the authors have found no quantitative data relating interfacially released cytokines to the duration of survivorship of artificial joints. The notion that the equilibrium between factors, negatively and positively affecting bone balance, is shifted in the direction of the former in short-term, and in the direction of the latter in long-term, surviving joint replacements, is conjectural.

Macrophages and lymphocytes are attracted to sites where prosthetic detritus accumulates. Particulate PE copiously accumulates in the effective joint space of patients whose cemented total hip arthroplasties loosen within a decade or so of implantation, and the luxurious granulomatous response to this wear species dominates the scene in the interfacial membranes. In most patients whose cemented artificial hip joints loosen 15 or more yr postoperatively, the macrophagic reaction to metallic particles is the most prominent feature of the interfacial membranes. The different amounts of polymeric vs metallic debris, in patients with short-term vs long-term surviving cemented hip arthroplasties, are indicative of unequal wear rates of the acetabular socket and femoral head, and probably also of different loading modes of the alloplastic components. Excessive wear of the acetabular insert is incompatible with long-lasting success of a hip joint replacement. Likewise, wear of the femoral head may generate a glut of metallic particles, frustrating long-term survival of a hip arthroplasty.

References

1 Dye SF. Future of anterior cruciate ligament restoration. *Clin Orthop* 1996; 325: 130–139.

2 Schmalzried TP, Jasty M, and Harris WH. Periprosthetic bone loss in total his arthroplasty. Polyethylene wear debris and the concept of the effective joint space. *J Bone Joint Surg* 1992; 74A: 849–863.

3 Shanbag AS, Jacobs JJ, Black J, Galante JO, and Glatt TT. Cellular mediators secreted by interfacial membranes obtained at revision total hip arthroplasty. *J Arthroplasty* 1995; 10: 498–506.

4 Mallory TH. *Current Concepts in Joint Replacement.* 1988; tape no. 6 (Greenwald S, ed), Mt. Sinai Medical Center, Cleveland, OH.

5. Jones LC and Hungerford DS. Cement disease. *Clin Orthop* 1987; 225: 192–206.

6 Boss JH, Shajrawi I, Dekel S, and Mendes DG. Bone–cement interface: Histological observations of the interface of cemented arthroplasties within the immediate and late phases. *J Biomater Sci Polymer Edn* 1993; 3: 221–230.

7 Boss JH, Shajrawi I, and Mendes DG. Nature of bone-implant interface: The lessons learned from implant retrieval and analysis in man and experimental animal. *Med Progr Technol* 1994; 20: 119–142.

8 Garino JP, Lotke PA, Sapega AA, Reilly PJ, and Esterhai JL. Osteonecrosis of the knee following laser-assisted arthroscopic surgery. A report of six cases. *J Arthroscop Related Surg* 1995; 11: 467–474.

9 Kwong LM, Jasty M, Mulroy RD, Maloney WJ,

Bragdon C, and Harris WH. Histology of the radiolucent line. *J Bone Joint Surg* 1992; 74B: 67–73.

10. Boss JH, Shajrawi I, Aunullah J, and Mendes DG. Relativity of biocompatibility. A critique of the concept of biocompatibility. *Isr J Med Sci* 1995; 31: 203–209.

11. Goodman S, Aspenberg P, Song Y, Regula D Jr, Doshi A, and Lidgren L. Effects of intermittent micromotion versus polymer particles on tissue ingrowth: Experiment using a micromotion chamber implanted in rabbits. *J Appl Biomater* 1994; 5: 117–123.

12. Goldring SR, Schiller AL, Roelke M, Rourke CM, O'Neill DA, and Harris WH. Synovial-like membrane at the bone-cement interface in loose total hip replacements and its proposed role in bone lysis. *J Bone Joint Surg* 1983; 65A: 575–584.

13. Santavirta S, Konttinen VT, Bergroth V, Eskola A, Tallroth K, and Lindholm S. Aggressive granulomatous lesions associated with hip arthroplasty. Immunopathological studies. *J Bone Joint Surg* 1990; 72A: 252–258.

14. Johansson NA, Bullough PG, Wilson PD Jr, Salvati EA, and Ranawat CS. Microscopic anatomy of the bone-cement interface in failed total hip arthroplasties. *Clin Orthop* 1987; 218: 123–135.

15. Schmalzried TP, Jasty M, Rosenberg A, and Harris WH. Histologic identification of polyethylene debris using oil red O stain. *J Appl Biomater* 1993; 4: 119–125.

16. Campbell P, Ma S, Yeom B, McKellop H, Schmalzried TP, and Amstutz HC. Isolation of predominantly submicron-sized UHMWPE wear particles from periprosthetic tissues. *J Biomed Mater Res* 1995; 29: 127–131.

17. McKellop HA, Campbell P, Park S-H, Schmalzried TP, Grigoris P, Amstutz HC, and Sarmiento A. Origin of submicron polyethylene wear debris in total hip arthroplasty. *Clin Orthop* 1995; 311: 3–20.

18. Schmalzried TP, Jasty M, Rosenberg A, and Harris WH. Polyethylene wear debris and tissue reactions in knee as compared to hip replacement prostheses. *J Appl Biomater* 1994; 5: 1185–190.

19. Isaac GH, Wroblewski BM, Atkinson JR, and Dowson D. Tribological study of retrieved hip prostheses. *Clin Orthop* 1992; 276: 115–125.

20. Müller ME. Lessons of 30 years of total hip arthroplasty. *Clin Orthop* 1992; 274: 12–23.

21. Betts F, Wright T, Salvati EA, Boskey A, and Bansal M. Cobalt-alloy debris in periarticular tissues from total hip revision arthroplasties. Metal contents and associated histologic findings. *Clin Orthop* 1992; 276: 75–82.

22. Buchert PK, Vaughin BK, Mallory TH, Engh CA, and Bobyn D. Excessive metal release due to loosening and fretting of sintered particles of porous-coated hip prostheses. *J Bone Joint Surg* 1986; 68A: 606–609.

23. Scales JT. Black staining around titanium alloy prostheses an orthopaedic enigma. *J Bone Joint Surg* 1991; 73B: 534–536.

24. Boss JH, Shajrawi I, Luria M, and Mendes DG. Necrotizing granulomas within the periprosthetic tissues of cemented and cemented total arthroplasties. *Vet Comp Orthop Traumatol* 1995; 8: 107–113.

25. Collier JP, Bauer TW, Bloebaum RD, Bobyn JD, Cook SD, Galante JO, et al. Results of implant retrieval from postmortem specimens in patients with well-functioning long-term total hip replacement. *Clin Orthop* 1992; 274: 97–12.

26. Boss JH, Misselevich I, Behar J, and Mendes DG. Histologic analysis of the periprosthetic tissues of long-term surviving cemented total hip arthroplasties. *J Long-Term Eff Med Implants* 1996; 6: 73–90.

27. Jacobs JJ, Shanberg A, Glatt TT, Black J, and Galante JO. Wear debris in total joint replacement. *J Am Acad Orthop Surg* 1994; 2: 212–220.

28. Manley MT and Serekian P. Wear debris. An environmental issue in total joint replacement. *Clin Orthop* 1994; 298: 137–146

29. Boss JH, Shajrawi I, and Mendes DG. Significance of mechanical factors in the evolution of the aggressive interfacial membrane of orthopaedic intraosseous implants, in *Biomedical Engineering: Recent Developments* 1994; (Vossoughi J, ed), University of the District of Columbia, Washington, DC, pp 1121–1124.

30. Salvati E, Betts F, and Doty SB. Particulate metallic debris in cemented total hip arthroplasty. *Clin Orthop* 1993; 293: 160–173.

31. Krismer M, Stöckl B, Fischer M, Bauer R, Mayrhofer P, and Ogon M. Early migration predicts late aseptic failure of hip sockets. *J Bone Joint Surg* 1996; 78B: 422–426.

32. Mjöberg B. Fixation and loosening of hip prostheses: a review. *Acta Orthop Scand* 1991; 62: 500–508.

33. Al-Saffar N, Khwaja HA, Kadoya Y, and Revell PA. Assessment of the role of GM-CSF in the cellular transformation and the development of erosive lesions around orthopaedic implants. *Am J Clin Pathol* 1996; 105: 628–639.

34. Dorr LD, Bloebaum R, Emmanuel J, and Meldrum J. Histologic, biochemical and ion analysis of tissue and fluids retrieved during total hip arthroplasty. *Clin Orthop* 1990; 261: 82–95.

35. Boss JH, Shajrawi I, Alperson M, and Mendes

DG. Inhibition of osteogeneseis by foreign body granulomatous response to bony debris. *Orthop Int Edn* 1994; 2: 447–453.

36 Boss JH, Shajrawi I, Soudry M, Anullah J, Solomon H, and Mendes DG. Studies on a novel anterior cruciate ligament polyethylene fiber prosthesis: the histomorphological pattern of organization and bony anchorage of a polyethylene fiber prosthesis in the stifle of the goat. *Clin Mater* 1994; 15: 61–67.

18

Injectable and Bioresorbable Poly(Propylene Glycol-Co-Fumaric Acid) Bone Cement

Debra J. Trantolo, Kai-Uwe Lewandrowski, Joseph D. Gresser, and Donald L. Wise

1. Introduction

Acrylic-based bone cements are currently used in many orthopedic procedures, including prosthesis fixation or filling of bony defects. They provide immediate structural support, but they are biologically inert *(1–4)*, and act not only as barriers to fracture healing, but also undergo degradation because of fatigue resulting in implant loosening and bone loss *(3,5–11)*.

A biodegradable bone cement that would provide immediate structural support, and subsequently allow normal bone healing and remodeling, would have immediate orthopedic and maxillofacial applications. The utility of biodegradable, or resorbable, cements for temporary support during bone healing has been recognized *(12–18)*. An injectable format would assure that the cement could also be used in minimally invasive procedures, allowing the costs of treatment to remain low. Resorbability eliminates the need for implant removal and therefore reduces the potential for long-term implant complications associated with foreign materials *(19)*.

The authors have demonstrated the feasibility of a resorbable and injectable bone cement. Part A of the two-part formulation includes an unsaturated polyester, poly(propylene glycol-co-fumaric acid) (PPF), a vinyl monomer, a combination of hydroxyapatite (HA) and calcium carbonate as a buffering filler that improves the osteoconductive properties of the cement by increasing porosity during its rapid dissolution, and an accelerator. Part B contains an initiator suspended in a nonreacting fluid vehicle and an inhibitor to control mixing and working time. Upon mixing, the two parts cure via crosslinking of the PPF by the monomer, and this crosslinking results in a hard cement degradable by hydrolysis. The use of HA as part of the filler supports osteoconductivity *(20)*, thus promoting bony ingrowth, while acting as a buffer in combination with the more soluble buffer, Ca carbonate, thereby preventing the potential formation of sterile abscesses that have been attributed to the acidic degradative products of some resorbable materials *(21–23)*.

In the authors' studies, select formulations demonstrated reasonable injectability and cure times in vitro, and promising results in vivo, in both the rat tibial defect and the rat femoral osteotomy model. These studies have allowed direct further development, more rapidly, toward preclinical optimization of the formulation. The authors developed a versatile resorbable bone cement, using in vitro and in vivo models for materials characterization that involve radiographic, biomechanical, histological, and histomorphometric evaluation of bone healing.

2. Background

An injectable, resorbable cement is potentially capable of induction of bony ingrowth as resorption of the cement progresses. In addition, it will undergo a buffered hydrolytic degradation that may eliminate sterile abscess formation, which is a well-recognized complication of other bioresorbable bone fixtures. As an adjunct to healing, a bone cement with such properties could provide structural support to stabilize and support a fracture, a bony defect, or an implant, over the extended period of time required for natural healing to occur. This cement appears particularly applicable in select clinical situations.

The major first-generation clinical applications for a resorbable bone cement include its use as an adjunct to healing of simple fractures with little or no displacement, which are generally treated conservatively, including those of the ankle, foot, and lateral tibial plateau. Later-stage development could be potential use of the cement in the fixation of surface-textured orthopedic implants (total joint replacements, e.g., artificial hip joints). Other potential applications of this new type of cement may include its use as a void filler in spinal fusions *(24)*, in which autologous bone grafting is often necessary, and crushed lyophilized and demineralized allogeneic bone is used when autologous bone stocks are insufficient. In these cases, an injectable, resorbable bone cement, with both osteoconductive and osteoinductive properties, could provide new minimally invasive treatment modalities, or could even serve as a bone substitute.

2.1. Cements for Fracture Fixation

Each year in the United States there are over 1.1 million bone fractures. Although some of these are severe enough to require surgical procedures to implant internal fixation devices, over 580,000 are fresh fractures that are managed conservatively. Nonoperative treatment is preferred in simple fractures, when minimal or no displacement is present, and soft tissues are well intact. These types of fractures are frequently encountered in the ankle *(25–30)* and foot *(31)*. As such, transverse fibular fractures at, or distal to, the ankle joint (Danis-Weber type A), low spiral fractures of the lateral malleolus and avulsion of the medial malleolus (Dyputren; Danis-Weber type B), avulsion fractures of the posterior malleolus (Volkmann's triangle), and nondisplaced vertical fractures of the neck of the talus (Hawkins type I) *(32)* may be treated with anatomical (less than 2 mm displacement, or posterior malleolar fragment <25% of joint surface) *(27,33)* reconstruction by closed reduction and splinting or short leg casting, with molding to prevent secondary displacement.

With the use of minimally invasive techniques, a resorbable bone cement having both osteoconductive and osteoinductive properties could be used by injecting it into the fracture site, under fluoroscopic control. This may help to prevent complications, such as repeated displacement, instability, and malunion *(27,34)*. The use of the cement may also warrant conservative treatment in patients with relative indications for operative management, including older patients, for whom long leg casting would make mobility difficult; irreducible fractures, or ones that have slipped in the cast; obese legs, which limit the capability of casts to maintain reduction; and noncompliant patients, such as chronic alcohol abusers *(35)*. In addition, patients with relative contraindications to operative treatment, such as vascular insufficiency, diabetes mellitus, soft tissue blisters, abrasions, contusions, or burns, could be successfully managed in a minimally invasive fashion, thus eliminating peri- and postoperative risk factors. Finally, patients with severe osteoporosis may benefit from the use of this osteoconductive and osteoinductive bone cement as an adjunct to conservative treatment of their fractures *(27)*. Aside from its use in the treatment of ankle and foot fractures, a resorbable and osteoconductive cement may be applicable for the treatment of undisplaced or minimally displaced lateral tibial plateau fractures that would normally warrant conservative treatment (depression <1 cm and valgus instability <10 degrees), but that bear the potential for worsening of displacement and thus joint surface incongruency *(36)*.

2.2. Comparisons to Cements for Fixation of Fractures and Orthopedic Implants

Polymethylmethacrylate (PMMA)-based cements have been used, with well-recognized complications *(2,20,37–41)*, for many years. A resorbable, osteoconductive bone cement may prove superior to PMMA-based cements, for a variety of reasons. First, it cures at body temperatures, thus preventing osteonecrosis, which is known to occur in PMMA-based cements (20,41). Second, osteoconductivity and increasing porosity, while undergoing dissolution, may maintain intimate bone–cement contact, stimulating bony ingrowth, which may provide continuous structural support; resorbability may eliminate long-term complications secondary to cement failure caused by fatigue or fragmentation (2,20). Resorbability would also eliminate the problem of cement removal, which can be technically very difficult (37–40). Third, hypersensitivity reactions (7,23,42), leading to bone loss because of osteolysis (2,8,43–45), and other complications, such as urological complications (46–49), are not to be expected, because of the resorbable format of the cement. Because of a growing aging patient population with an ever increasing frequency of muskuloskeletal injuries, these anticipated material properties are of clinical significance.

2.3. Comparisons to Other Injectable Bone Cements

Although there are several HA-based bone materials, the cement by Norian is the only cement that is injectable. It consists of a unique formulation of Ca carbonate and Ca triphosphate salts that undergoes continuous mineralization, once mixed in a solution. The injectable cement cures within 10 min, to form a carbonated apatite, and reaches its full mechanical strength within 12 h. This material resembles the structure of HA found in bone, and, in fact, was found to stimulate bone ingrowth. In comparison, the authors' injectable bone cement relies on a different developmental concept, by providing initial mechanical support while undergoing dissolution. In contrast, the Norian cement relies on the body's ability to incorporate it by ongoing resorption and concomitant new bone formation.

The authors' injectable bone cement dissolves by hydrolytic degradation and dissolution of the Ca salts. Therefore, the rate of degradation is determined by its composition, and, thus, is independent of the recipient bed. In fact, faster resorption times are anticipated for the PPF-based bone cement than those reportedly seen with the Norian cement. In short, the injectable cement may find its place in fixation of simple fractures, resulting in expediting of the healing process. The Norian cement on the other hand seems to function as a void filler that thereby provides fracture fixation, as indicated by initial clinical trials conducted at Massachusetts General Hospital, where the Norian cement is currently being tested in comminuted distal radial fractures and fractures of the wrist and hand. In addition to resorbability, a PPF-based bone cement may also serve as a slow-release carrier of growth factors: a unique material property that is unparalleled by the Norian cement.

3. Cement Design and Composition

A low-viscosity biodegradable cement has been formulated, which can be delivered to a bone repair site via a syringe, and which cures *in situ*. The cure reaction is based on the crosslinking of the unsaturated polyester, PPF, with the vinyl monomer, vinyl pyrrolidone (VP). Fillers include both soluble and insoluble components, which control the rate of degradation, as well as the development of porosity and osteoconductivity, to facilitate bony ingrowth. Further degradation depends on hydrolysis of the ester bonds. The authors summarize studies with three formulations.

These three types of cement formulations all varied with respect to the filler composition. The fillers were calcium gluconate (CG), a very soluble filler, designed to facilitate bony ingrowth, with developing porosity; CG–HA, a filler combination designed to support bony ingrowth, using concepts of both developing porosity and osteoconduction; and CG–HA–poly(lactic acid) (PLA), a filler designed to facilitate not only bony ingrowth, as above, but also potentially protection and controlled release of therapeutic adjuncts to bone healing. All of the final embodiments of these three formulations displayed reasonable viscosities for injectability (~50 centipoise [CP]), and working (6–7 min) and hardening (10–12 min) times. Of these, the one containing the CG–HA filler combination will serve as the basis for further development, based on its favorable in vitro physiochemical and mechanical properties, and encouraging early-stage in vivo compatibility, reported herein.

Table 1
Cement Formulations

Formulation	CG	CG–HA	CG–HA–PLA	PART
PPF[a]	38.03	38.03	38.03	A
Calcium gluconate	27.06	6.76	6.76	A
Hydroxyapatite	–	20.29	13.53	A
Poly(D,L-lactide)[b]	–	–	6.76	A
1-Vinyl 2-pyrollidinone[c]	10.37	10.37	10.37	B
Ethanol[d]	8.21	8.21	8.21	B
Peanut oil	15.09	15.09	15.09	B
Benzoyl peroxide	1.25	1.25	1.25	C
Sample ID	79–70	79–34	79–57	

[a]Wt avg. mol wt = 7280; dispersity = 3.4.
[b]Particle size = 45–90 µ.
[c]This is referred to as vinyl pyrollidone (VP) in the text. The VP is used as a carrier for the accelerator, N,N-dimethyl-p-toluidine (DMPT). The DMPT was dissolved in the VP to form a solution containing 0.685% (w/w) of DMPT.
[d]Hydroquinone (HQ), serving as an inhibitor, was dissolved in the ethanol to form a solution containing 0.455% (w/w) HQ.

4. Formulations and Elemental Analysis

PPF was synthesized by direct esterification of fumaric acid (FA) with propylene glycol (PG), as described by Gresser et al. *(16)*. The weight average mol wt and dispersity of this polymer, as determined by gel permeation chromatography, were 7280 and 3.4, respectively.

A cement of composition given in Table 1 (CG filler only) was prepared and cured for the purpose of analyzing the ratio of FA:VP units that participate in the crosslinks.

The cured pellets were crushed and sequentially extracted with water, ethanol, and methylene chloride to isolate the insoluble crosslinked PPF (XL-PPF). This insoluble crosslinked residue was hydrolyzed in 6 M HCl at 37°C for 48 h, and a portion of this was hydrolyzed again under more rigorous conditions (6 M HCl, 60°C, 6 h), to ensure complete hydrolysis. The remaining insoluble materials from the first and second hydrolyses were isolated, dried over phosphorus pentoxide (P_2O_5), and sent for elemental analysis of carbon, hydrogen, and nitrogen (C, H, N) in duplicate (Galbraith Laboratories, Knoxville, TN). Results are given in Table 2.

The elemental analyses of the two samples are virtually identical, indicating that hydrolysis was

Table 2
Analysis of Residue Remaining After Extraction and Hydrolysis of Cured Cement

	Element	Results
First hydrolysis	C	53.83 + 0.03%
	H	6.54 + 0.09
	N	3.81 + 0.11
Second hydrolysis	C	53.87 + 0.00
	H	6.59 + 0.01
	N	3.85 + 0.04

complete in the first step. Thus, the N content is taken as the mean of the four results: 3.83 + 0.07% (standard deviation [SD]). Based on the structures shown in Fig. 1, the weight fraction of each element in the hydrolyzed residue is related to the ratio of VP to FA moieties by the following equations:

$$f_N = 14.01x[116.07y + 111.14x]^{-1}$$
$$f_C = [48.04y + 72.06x][116.07y + 111.14x]^{-1}$$
$$f_H = [4.03y + 9.07x][116.07y + 111.14x]^{-1}$$
$$f_O = [64.00y + 16.00x][116.07y + 111.14x]^{-1}$$

where f_o is the fraction of oxygen and $x{:}y$ is the mol ratio of VP:FA moieties. The $x{:}y$ ratios calculated from these equations are given below.

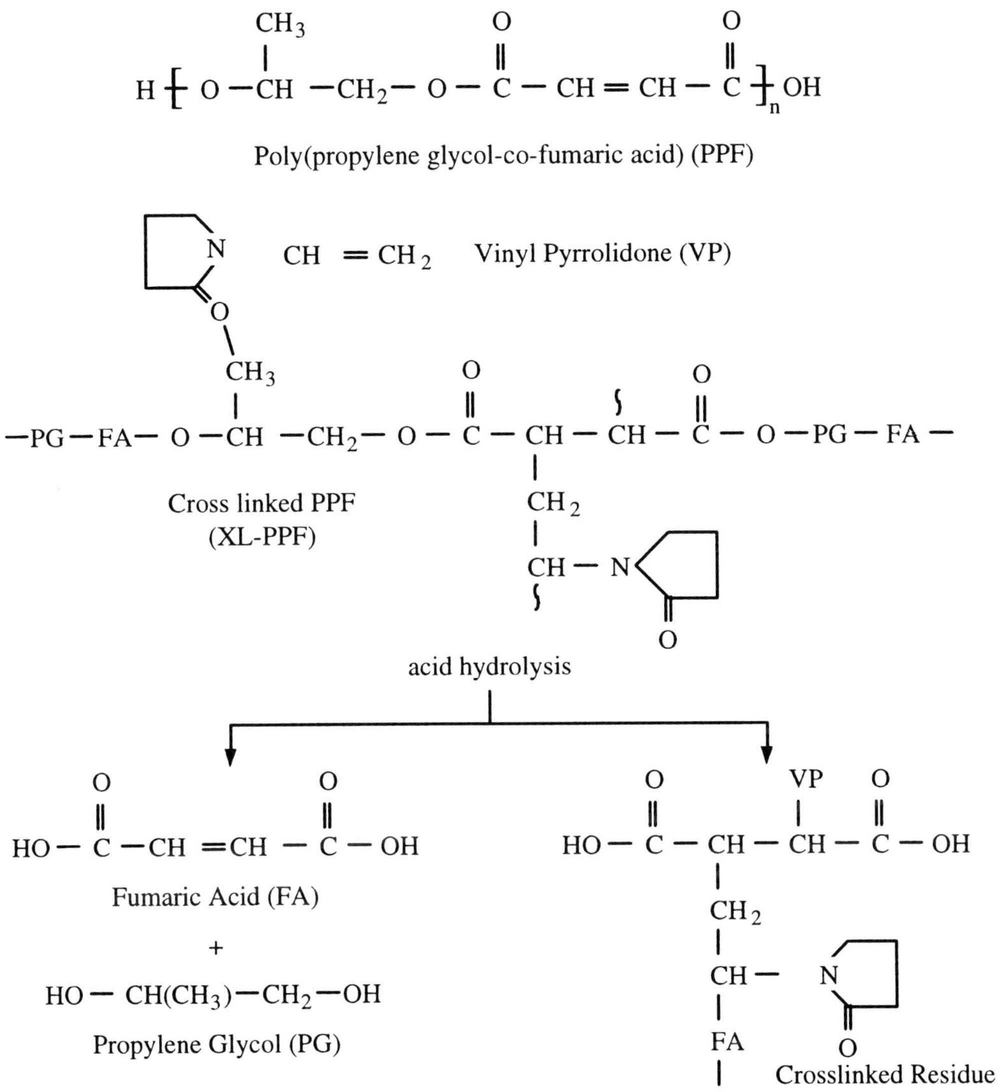

Fig. 1. Schematic of cement chemistry.

Poly(propylene glycol-co-fumaric acid) (PPF)

Vinyl Pyrrolidone (VP)

Cross linked PPF (XL-PPF)

acid hydrolysis

Fumaric Acid (FA)

+

Propylene Glycol (PG)

Crosslinked Residue

$x:y$ = 1.18 (based on C)
= 0.97 (based on O)
= 2.01 (based on H)
= 0.46 (based on N)

Although the precision of these calculated ratios varies, the mean value (1.16 ± 0.65) suggests about one VP/FA in the residue. The mol ratio of VP monomer to FA units in the starting PPF in the formulation is 5.24. Thus, if one VP unit is linked to one FA unit, there are approximately four free fumarate double bonds per crosslink.

Thus, one can tentatively assume the structure of the crosslinked PPF to be as shown in Fig. 1.

Additional evidence must still be obtained by elemental analysis of the crosslinked PPF, prior to hydrolysis, supported by analysis of FA in the soluble products of hydrolysis.

In a study of similar PPF cements crosslinked with VP, Gresser et al. *(16)* have shown that over 90% of the PPF is crosslinked over a wide range of PPF:VP weight ratios, varying from 0.33 to 2.0, but that the fraction of VP used in forming crosslinks depended on the PPF:VP ratio. At the

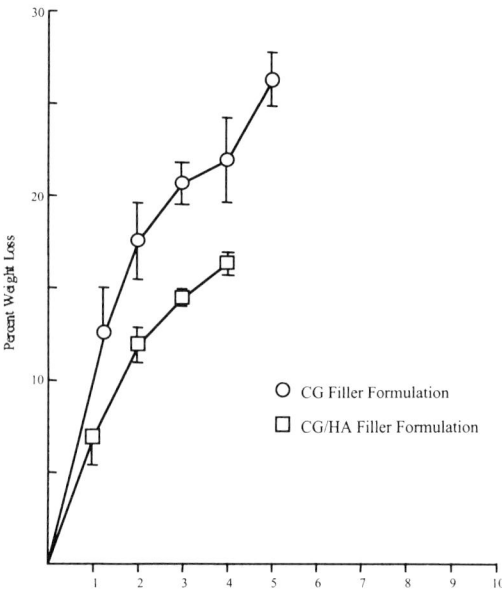

Fig. 2. *In vitro* degradation of cured injectable cement % weight loss as a function of time.

highest PPF:VP ratio explored (1.7), approx 67% of the VP was incorporated, the remainder being polymerized to poly(vinyl pyrrolidone). In the present study, the PPF:VP ratio is 3.7. Extrapolation of these results leads to an estimate of over 90% of the VP incorporated into the crosslinks.

5. In Vitro Evaluation

5.1. Degradation of Cured Cement: Weight Loss as a Function of Time

Two formulations of varying filler solubility (CG filler and CG–HA filler) were tested for weight loss over a 5-wk interval (formulations are given in Table 1). Eight cured pellets, weighing approx 450 mg each, were incubated in 50 mL phosphate-buffered saline. Sample vials were contained in a constant temperature shaker bath set at 37°C and 80 cpm. At each time-point, five samples were removed and dried to constant weight over P_2O_5. The remaining pellets were reserved for mechanical testing. The record of weight loss is presented in Fig. 2. The slower rate of weight loss for the CG–HA formulation results from the lower content of the soluble filler, CG. The data to 5 wk, at which time the experiment was terminated, shows continuing weight loss, but at declining rates. The rate is expected to continue to decline, until only hydrolytic degradation of the XL-PPF and slow dissolution of less-soluble fillers contribute to weight loss.

5.2. Compressive Strength and Modulus of Cured Cement

Compressive strength and modulus of the CG and the CG–HA filler formulations were measured after cure on an Instron 8511 equipped with a 500-lb load cell, and operating at a strain rate of 1 cm/min (0.423 mm/s). Testing followed American Society for Testing and Materials (ASTM) recommendations for acrylic bone cements (ASTM F451). Cured pellets, measuring 6 mm diameter by 12 mm length, were incubated as described in subheading 5.1. Three pellets were removed for testing on a weekly schedule. Results are presented in Table 3 and Fig. 3.

Using midrange values for trabecular bone as a guide, as determined by Carter and Hayes *(50)*, Gerhart et al. *(14)* estimated that compressive strengths greater than 5 MPa and compressive moduli between 45 and 100 MPa (0.045–0.10 GPa) are necessary to permit functional loading of trabecular bone.

The authors' values are consistently higher than those in Table 3, and, furthermore, strength and moduli do not diminish during the period of exposure to the aqueous medium.

5.3. Scanning Electron Microscopy

Scanning electron micrographs (SEM) of the CG filler formulation were taken of pellets used for measurement of degradative weight loss, after removal from the water bath and drying. SEMs were taken after 0, 1, 2, 4, and 5 wk incubation, using an Amray AMR-1000 SEM. During the first 2 wk, the surface shows progressive pitting and development of holes measuring about 3–6 μ. Larger holes of 10–15 μ were also seen. At 3, 4 and 5 wk, surface erosion and pitting are more pronounced. Figure 4 shows SEMs taken of the pellet surface after 1 and two wk incubation. The development of pores is apparent; such pitting was not observed prior to incubation.

Microscopic examination of the as-received CG, using calibrated optics, shows that the particles range in size from approx 1.5 to 10 μ, in the

Table 3
Compressive Strength and Modulus

	CG filler		CG–HA filler	
Time (wk)	Strength (MPa)	Modulus (GPa)	Strength (MPa)	Modulus (GPA)
0	19.67 4.40	0.59 0.17	44.22	0.68
1	26.85 1.40	0.61 0.16	31.51 3.40	0.78 0.16
2	22.81 4.14	0.56 0.12	44.88 6.31	1.55 0.19
3	23.72 1.71	0.52 0.09	35.65 3.41	1.07 0.17
4	22.98 1.39	0.62 0.06	34.29 3.67	1.44 0.08
5	35.20 3.90	0.86 0.07		

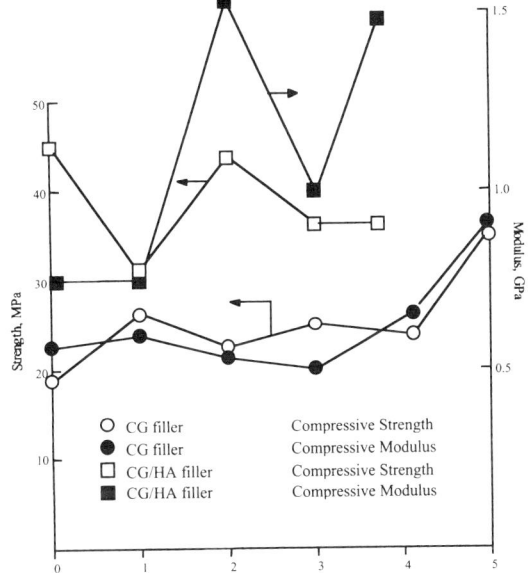

Fig. 3. Compressive strength and modulus of cured injectable cement as a function of incubation time in PBS at 37°C.

range of the observed holes. The authors conclude that holes arise mostly from the early dissolution and leaching of the CG from the pellet.

5.4. Estimated Precure Viscosity

All formulations discussed in this report contain 27.1% filler, although the composition of the filler has been varied. Formulation 79-70 contains only soluble filler, CG; in 79-74, HA replaces much of the CG. Formulation 79-57 contains also PLA as part of the filler. The rationale for inclusion of PLA is that, in certain applications, it may be desirable to include a therapeutic agent

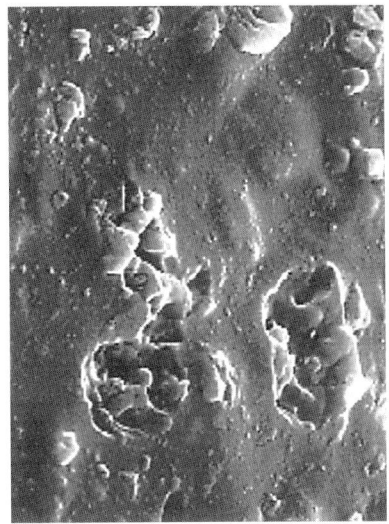

(1 wk) (× 6250)

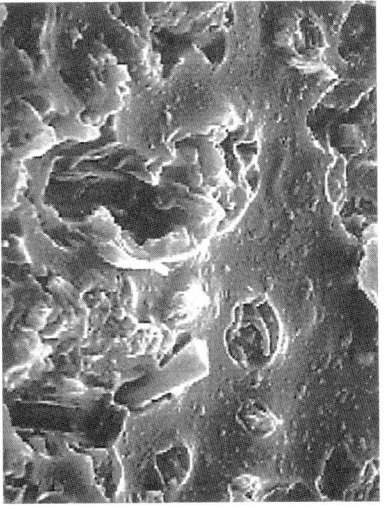

(2 wk) (× 6250)

Fig. 4. SEMs of the CG filler formulation at 1 and 2 wk. Scanned photos have been reduced ~50%.

incorporated into a controlled-release vehicle. In such applications, the PLA also serves to protect the active agents from reaction with the components of the cement during the cure stage, when the PPF is being crosslinked. This formulation was chosen for estimation of precure viscosity.

A plastic syringe (15.7 mm interior diameter) was used to measure flow rates of both PG as a standard and the cement formulation from which the initiator, benzoyl peroxide, had been omitted. This omission allowed repeated measurements to be made, without an increase of viscosity caused by the crosslinking reaction. Flow, induced by a constant force of 2 kg on the plunger (1.03 kg/cm^2), was measured at 21°C. Flow rates of PG and the cement under these conditions are given in Table 5. Viscosity of PG at 21°C was calculated from reported viscosity–temperature data, using the equation

$$\eta^{-1} = A\exp(-E/RT)$$

where η = viscosity at $T°$K; E, the activation energy of the fluidity (reciprocal of viscosity); and A, the pre-exponential factor. The values of A and E, calculated from viscosity–temperature data, are, respectively, 1.08 ± 108 and 38,318 J. Thus, at 21°C, the viscosity of propylene glycol is 58.86 cp, and the cement viscosity was calculated from the relationship

$$\eta_C/\eta_P = F_P/F_C$$

where subscripts C and P refer to the cement and PG, respectively, and F is the measured flow rate. The cement viscosity is therefore approx 50.9 cp. Results are shown for three replicates (Fig. 5).

5.5. Thermochemical Measurements, Working Time, and Shelf Life

The temperature rise during cure was measured by embedding a thermocouple into approx 1 mL of the CG cement formulation, which was held in a 1.5-mL polypropylene snap-cap microcentrifuge tube. The tube was fitted into a block of polystyrene foam for insulation. The temperature, displayed on an Omega digital thermometer, was recorded every 10 seconds for 30 min. This record is presented in Fig. 5. The formulation was mixed at room temperature (22°C) for 1 min before recording began. From the temperature–time recording, it is possible to estimate dough time

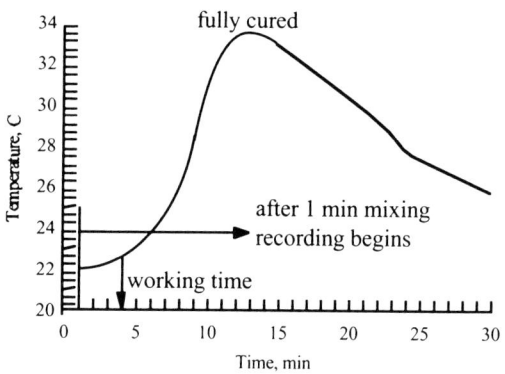

	Flow rate (cm^3/min) at 21°C	Viscosity, cp
Propylene glycol	3.792 ± 0.198	58.86
Precured cement	4.398 ± 0.216	50.92 ± 5.01

Fig. 5. Temperature profile during cure.

(time to development of stickiness), as well as working time to hardness. Following the 1-min mixing period, the temperature rose only about 1°C in approx 4 min, which is consistent with development of stickiness as observed. From about 5 to 9 min, the temperature rose linearly, at a rate of 1.66°C/min. The maximum temperature of 33.6°C (92.5°F) was reached in 12 min, by which time the formulation is hard. The working time is thus about 6–7 min, with hardening of the cement at 10–12 min.

Technical data from Richards Technical (52) allows comparison of results with several commercial bone cements. The times presented in Table 4 are cumulative, and thus represent total time from the start of mixing. From these data, the test formulation compares favorably with commercially available bone cements.

Heat of reaction (enthalpy) caused by polymerization of formulation, was measured by differential scanning calorimetry on a Mettler TA 4000 system. The value of ΔH, measured for three samples of a freshly prepared cement, was 64.5 ± 4.4 J/g, and is consistent with the expected value for vinyl polymerization, corrected for the weight fraction of inert components. The three-part (see Table 1) formulation was stored in a refrigerator for 2 mo, and tested again in triplicate. ΔH was 64.3 ± 4.2 J/g. The constancy of ΔH indicates the

Table 4
Comparison of PPF Injectable Cement with Commercial Bone Cements

Time (min)	Palacos R	Surgical Simplex P	Zimmer	CMW	PPF
Mixing	0.5	0.8	0.8	1.0	1.0
Dough	0.9	7.1	5.0	3.3	4.0
Working	4.4	10.2	7.0	5.0	6.0–7.0
Hardening	6.5	11.5	9.7	6.5	10–12

satisfactory stability of the formulation in this period, and further suggests that the shelf life is expected to be significantly longer than this.

6. In Vivo Evaluation: Biocompatibility in Rats

The biocompatibility of the CG–HA–PPF bone cement was evaluated in male Sprague-Dawley rats (Charles River Breeding Laboratories) weighing approx 200 g. The formulation was tested using both *ex vivo* and *in situ* cures. Precured samples were prepared in a Teflon-coated steel mold, to produce cylindrical rods of approx 1.7 mm in diameter.

Rats were anesthetized with 0.3 mL 10 mg/mL ketamine (Fort Dodge NDA Laboratory) and 0.15 mL 20 mg/mL xylazine (Gemeni). The left rear leg was shaved with an electric clipper, and swabbed with betadine. An incision (approx 1.5 cm in length) was made in the lower ventral portion of the leg, parallel to and exposing the tibia. A hole was drilled into the ventral cortex of the tibia with a Dreml Flex Shaft drill equipped with a sterile drill bit.

Cured cement pellets, sterilized by 2.75 Mrad γ-irradiation, were inserted into the tibial defect, after which the muscle was sutured with prolene 5.0 sutures, and the incision was similarly sutured or closed with wound clips. Twenty-one rats were included in this study, and, in groups of three rats, were sacrificed weekly to 7 wk.

Another 21 rats were used for the evaluation of biocompatibility with *in situ* cure. The cement was injected into the tibial defects and allowed to cure *in situ*. Three rats were sacrificed periodically, at 3 d and at 1, 2, 3, 4, 6, and 7 wk postcementing.

Animals were given food and water ad libitum until sacrifice. The implanted (precured) or injected (*in situ* cured) leg was stripped from soft tissues, and tibia was excised. Specimens were fixed in 10% neutral buffered formalin for 3–5 d, followed by decalcification in 0.5–0.75% nitric acid. The cement was gently removed. The bone was dehydrated in graded alcohols, embedded in paraffin, cut into cross-sections 5-µm-thick sections, stained with hematoxylin and eosin (HOE), and examined microscopically. Specimens were evaluated for bone resorption, new bone formation, and inflammatory or foreign body (FB) responses, such as granuloma for fibrous tissue formation.

Results of the implantation studies, using precured and *in situ* cured cement, have failed to show any adverse FB reaction to the cement. No fluid collections or late inflammatory responses, as indicated by increased fibrous tissue formation or multinucleated FB cells for cellular infiltration, were seen. The bone–cement interface was assessed for new bone formation and bone resorption. In both, *in situ*-cured and precured cement pellets increased remodeling on the bone–cement interface with time, so that, at 7 wk, newly formed woven bone, mirroring the shape of the surface of the removed cement pellet, was seen. In addition, only ingrowth into the cement pellet was observed with this indirect method of evaluation. Fragmentation of the *in situ*-cured cement was occasionally noted. However, this was not accompanied by hypersensitivity reactions. Fragmentation of the cement was felt to be a result of incomplete *in situ* curing, rather than a result of cement failure, because this was not seen in precured cement pellets.

This study using the rat tibial defect model indicated that the injectable bone cement underwent hydrolytic degradation, and was thus resorbable. It also indicated that this cement stimulated bony ingrowth.

7. In Vivo Evaluation in Rat Fracture Model

To further substantiate these observations, and to begin to investigate the fixation of an actual fracture, the authors performed studies in rodents, which were intended to demonstrate feasibility of the use of resorbable bone cement in an injectable format, to fix a fracture and to maintain this fixation over time, while healing of this fracture occurs and the bone cement is undergoing degradation.

7.1. Animal Model

For this purpose, the authors used male Sprague-Dawley rats (Charles River Laboratories) weighing approx 200 g. As listed below, 36 animals were divided into three groups of 12 rats each. Rats were anesthetized with 0.3 mL 10 mg/mL ketamine (Fort Dodge) and 0.15 mL 20 mg/mL xylazine (Gemeni SA). The left rear leg was shaved with an electric clipper, and swabbed with betadine. A midshaft femoral defect was created through the lateral approach to the femur with use of Dreml Flex Shaft drill equipped with a sterile drill bit. Fixation was then achieved with one of the following three methods: an undersized smooth 0.062 in. K-wire; a 0.1 in. threaded K-wire; and a smooth 0.062 in. K-wire, with additional use of injectable cement. Thus, cement-fixed osteotomies were compared to osteotomies with loose (negative control) and rigid fixation (positive control). In the cemented group, the cement was first injected into the proximal and distal portion of the intradmedullary canal, after meticulous homeostasis was achieved. The wounds were then closed in layers in standard surgical fashion.

Per definition, loose fixation was expected to consistently result in nonunion; rigid fixation was expected to result in complete and normal healing of the osteotomy. The augmentation of the loose fixation with cement would therefore indicate the ability of the cement to support a healing fracture, while bone healing and progressive dissolution of the cement are occurring. The midshaft femoral osteotomy model, with use of an undersized intramedullary K-wire, is well recognized in the literature for the study on nonunion. Any alteration to this model that will increase the rigidity of the fixation by presenting rotational instability, will therefore improve the biological outcome, as evidenced by a healing fracture.

7.2. Methods of Evaluation

Animals were evaluated with weekly radiographs taken in antero posterior and lateral views. For this purpose, animals were briefly anesthetized with Enfluran. These radiographs were assessed for position of the intramedullary K-wire and the occurrence of impact fracture or pathological fractures. In addition, healing at the osteotomy site was evaluated by radiographic criteria, such as periosteal bone formation and increasing density of the calcifying callus. Animals were given food and water ad libitum, until sacrifice at 4 wk postoperatively.

After sacrifice, test bones were carefully stripped of soft tissues. Specimens were fixed in 10% neutral buffered formalin for 3–5 d, followed by decalcification of 0.50–0.75% nitric acid. The bone was dehydrated in graded alcohol. While specimens were embedded in paraffin, the intramedullary K-wire was gently removed, which could be done without difficulty in all specimens. Then, center sections, including the osteotomy site, were taken from the test bones, cut into 5-μm-thick sections, stained with H&E, and examined microscopically. Specimens were evaluated for bone resorption, new bone formation, and inflammatory or FB responses, such as granuloma or fibrous tissue formation.

Histomorphometry was done by acquiring images of serial longitudinal H&E-stained sections of the specimen, using a CCD video camera system (TM-745; PULNiX, Sunnyvale, CA) that was mounted on a Zeiss microscope. Images were digitized and analyzed, using Bioscan image software (München, Germany). For each bone specimen, the total cross-sectional area of trabecular bone in the distal and proximal metaphysis was determined on sequential longitudinal sections. Then the intertrabecular space was approximated by measuring the area occupied between the bone trabeculae. A minimum of 10 sections, obtained from different levels of the specimen, was included for this analysis. The spacing between sections of adjacent levels was typically 300 μm. This allowed an approximated total metaphyseal trabecular bone volume, which is actually given

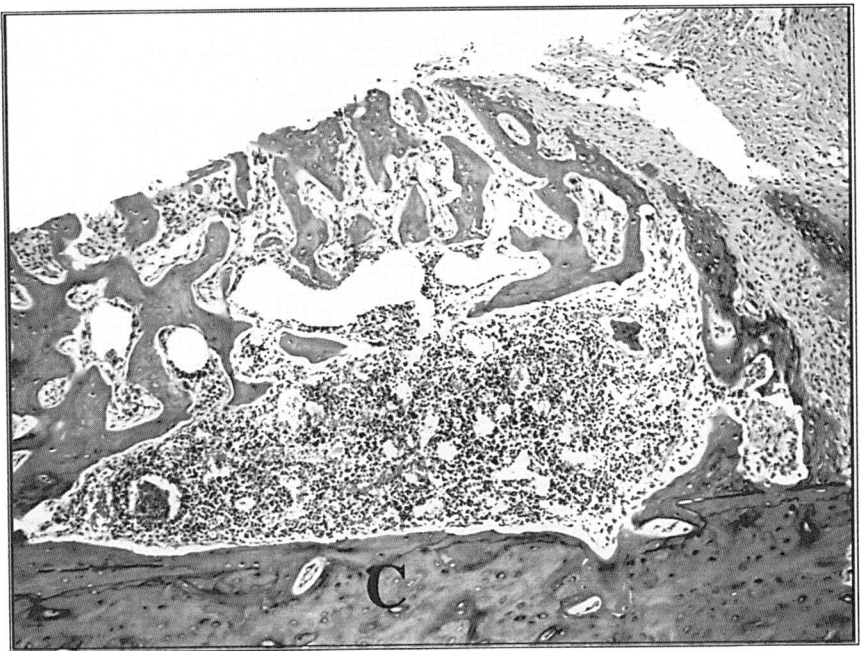

Fig. 6. Longitudinal section through the distal metaphysis of a group A specimen (loose fixation) at 4 wk postoperatively, (H&E, ×2.5). Note a fibrous tissue envelope (white-striped arrowhead) extending over the whole length of the K-wire, and separating it from the adjacent endosteal surface of the inner femoral cortex. There is extensive metaphyseal bone resorption, with widening of the intertrabecular spaces (black dotted line at the two remaining bone trabeculae of this specimen).

in mm^3 (mean ± SD), and an average percentage rate (mean ± SD) of the volume occupied by the trabecular bone within the distal and proximal metaphysis for each bone specimen. To express the extent of metaphyseal bone remodeling in response to the type of internal fixation used in the three different study groups, the remodeling index was defined as the average percentage rate of trabecular bone volume of both the distal and proximal femoral metaphysis, based on 12 animals per study group.

7.3. Results of Repair Process in Rats

As expected, analysis of radiographic studies consistently showed nonhealing osteotomy sites in the group A animals, which were operated with loose internal fixation. Radiographic evidence of bridging callus formation was absent. However, widening of the cortex, consisetnt with pseudoarthrosis formation, was seen (elephant-feet pseudoarthrosis). Animals that received rigid fixation of their femoral osteotomy (group B) showed radiographic evidence of fracture healing. However, complete bony union was not seen, at least not in the time period studied.

With the animals of group C, in which the osteotomy was fixed with an undersized K-wire and the resorbable cement, findings were observed similar to those in group B animals, in which rigid fixation with a threaded K-wire was employed.

Histologic evaluation of H&E-stained sections showed evidence of absence of healing at the osteotomy site in animals of group A. At the osteotomy site, occasional periosteal reaction, with minimal bone formation, was found. However, fibrous tissue was present between the proximal and the distal end of the femoral bone. Sporadically, chondrocytes were seen. In addition, cortical thickening was present at the osteotomy site (Fig. 6).

At the metaphyseal distal and proximal end, fibrous tissue was seen between the implant (K-wire) and the metaphyseal bone. This fibrous tissue envelope extended over the whole length

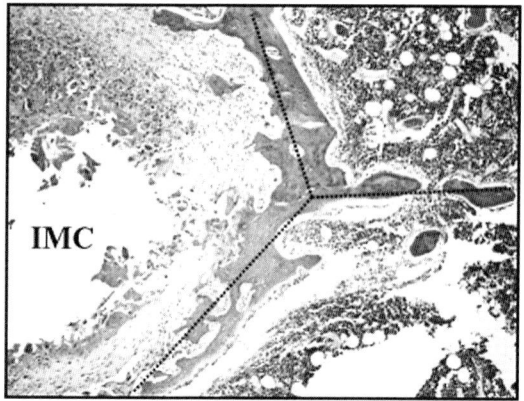

Fig. 7. Longitudinal section through the osteotomy site of a group A specimen (loose fixation) at 4 wk postoperatively (H&E, × 5). Pseudoarthrosis, with periosteal (black open arrowhead) and enchondral bone formation at the osteotomy site, are present. Woven bone formation at the endosteal surface facing the K-wire was noted.

of the K-wire, and separated it from the adjacent endosteal surface of the inner femoral cortex. In the distal and proximal metaphysis, extensive remodeling of the trabecular bone, with widening of the intertrabecular spaces, was noted (Fig. 7).

In group B animals, in which rigid fixation was employed, enchondral and periosteal bone formation was found at the osteotomy site. However, complete bony union was not detected. Moderate cortical remodeling was noted over the entire length of the specimen, but cortical thickening, as observed in group A animals, was absent. Moderate remodeling of the diaphyseal and metaphyseal section of the femoral bone was seen, and widening of the intertrabecular spaces, as in group A animals, was not found (Fig. 8).

In animals in whom the osteotomy was fixed with use of an undersized K-wire and additional injection of the bioresorbable CG–HA–PPF bone cement (group C), findings similar to those in group B animals were noted. Enchondral and periosteal new bone formation was noted at the osteotomy sites. Cortical remodeling was confined to the area directly adjacent to the osteotomy. No cellular infiltrates or extensive fibrous tissue formation, indicative of FB reactions or inflammation, were seen. Active new bone remodeling, with deposition of osteoid, was noted at the interface between the metaphyseal bone and the cement in the distal and proximal diaphyseal and metaphyseal portion of the rat femur (Fig. 9).

At 4 wk postoperatively, the formation of cavitations within the cement was noted. These cavitations were invaded by capillaries with ingrowing endothelial cells (Fig. 10). In addition, osteoclastic and osteoblastic activity was observed in these degradation lacunae. Similar histologic findings were also directly observed at the endosteal cortical surface facing the cement (Fig. 11). Furthermore, osteoid was noted at these sites, indicating intimate contact between the bone cement and the endosteal surface (Fig. 12).

Histomorphometric analysis of diaphyseal and metaphyseal bone remodeling, averaged for the 12 animals for each group and performed at 4 wk postoperatively, corroborated histologic data. The respective data are shown in Table 5.

Differences found in the remodeling index were statistically significant ($p < 0.009$), indicating that there was significantly more cortical bone remodeling, with the approximated trabecular bone volume being the highest in group B, in which rigid fixation was used. In animals in which loose internal fixation was employed (group A), extensive metaphyseal bone resorption, with widening of the intertrabecular spaces, had occurred, and bone trabeculae were rarefied as evidenced by the lowest total trabecular bone volume and remodeling index of all three experimental groups. In the specimens from animals in whom the bioresorbable CG–HA–PPF bone cement was used as an adjunct to the internal fixation device (group C), a significantly lower remodeling index was obtained than in group B animals. The total trabecular bone volume was less than in group B specimens.

8. Summary and Conclusion

Results of this study demonstrated similar biologic outcomes, with comparable histologic findings, in the animals in which rigid fixation with a threaded K-wire (group B) was employed, and in animals in which both a smooth undersized K-wire and the injectable cement (group C) was used. In comparison to group A animals, in which pseudoarthrosis were consistently found, normal fracture healing was noted in group B and C ani-

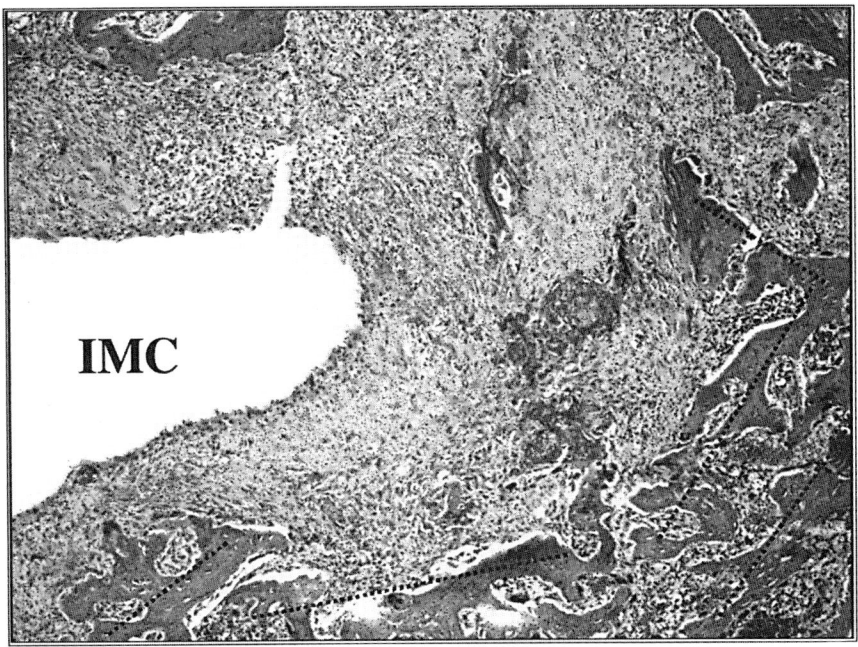

Fig. 8. Longitudinal section through the distal metaphysis of a group B specimen (rigid fixation) at 4 wk postoperatively (H&E, × 2.5). Note moderate remodeling of the metaphyseal trabecular bone, without significant widening of the intertrabecular spaces (black dotted lines indicate newly formed metaphyseal bone trabeculae). As in group A specimens (loose fixation), a fibrous tissue envelope surrounding the K-wire was observed.

mals. Thus, biocompatibility of the cement was demonstrated in a functional setting. In addition, an active intimate bond–cement interface was noted, suggesting that injectable and resorbable bone cement has, as predicted, additional osteoinductive and osteoconductive properties.

Because complete healing of the osteotomies was not seen in any of the three experimental groups, quantitative biomechanical testing could not be performed. However, no pathological fractures were noted in any animal throughout the entire period of the study. This pilot study indicated that the use of injectable resorbable bone cement provided and maintained adequate fixation of a bony defect in this rat midshaft femoral osteotomy model.

Furthermore, the authors demonstrated the following:

1. PPF:VP ratio (3.67) used in the formulations investigated in this study led to an estimated >90% incorporation of the VP into the crosslinked network. Based on elemental analysis, the authors further estimate that the crosslinks are, on average, about one VP unit in length, and that the frequency of crosslinks is about 1/5 fumarate double bonds.
2. In vitro degradative weight loss is initially rapid, because of dissolution of soluble components, and is more rapid for formulations, with a higher proportion of soluble components in the filler. Further weight loss will be slower, depending more on hydrolysis of the fumarate double bonds.
3. SEMs show a developing porosity with time in vitro, with pore size being approximately the diameter of the incorporated soluble components. Thus, by controlling the particle size distribution of the soluble components, a controlled porosity can be established that can facilitate the bony ingrowth.
4. Cure reaction proceeds with a temperature rise to only about 34°C, which, being slightly below body temperature, will not cause thermal damage to adjacent tissues. Further, the kinetics of cure lead to mixing time, dough,

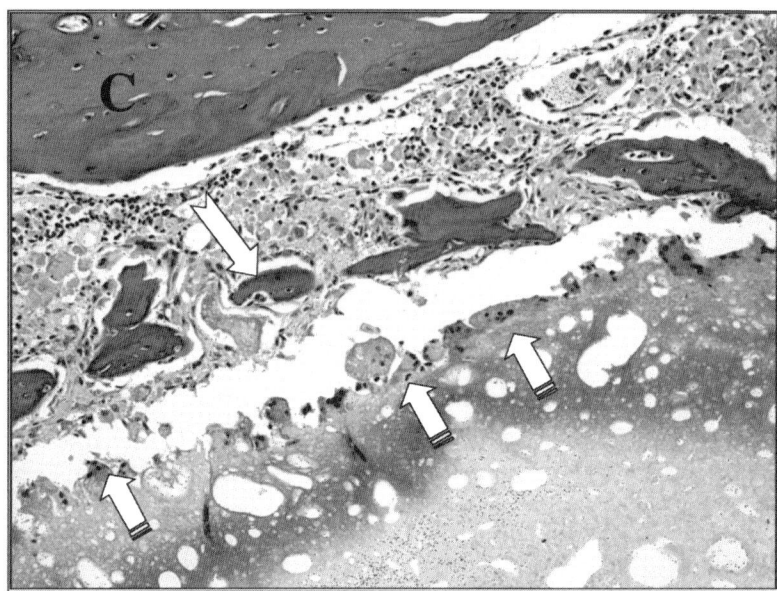

Fig. 9. Longitudinal section through the distal metaphysis of a group C specimen (cement fixation) at 4 wk postoperatively (H&E, × 10), showing intimate contact between the CG–HA–PPF bone cement and the metaphyseal bone. There is osteoblastic activity with osteoid formation at the interface between the cement and the adjacent mesenchymal tissue. Osteoblasts are facing the outer cement surface (white-striped arrowheads). In addition, there is neovascularization and active metaphyseal bone remodeling, as evidenced by the presence of capillaries filled with erythrocytes and multinucleated osteoclasts (black arrowhead).

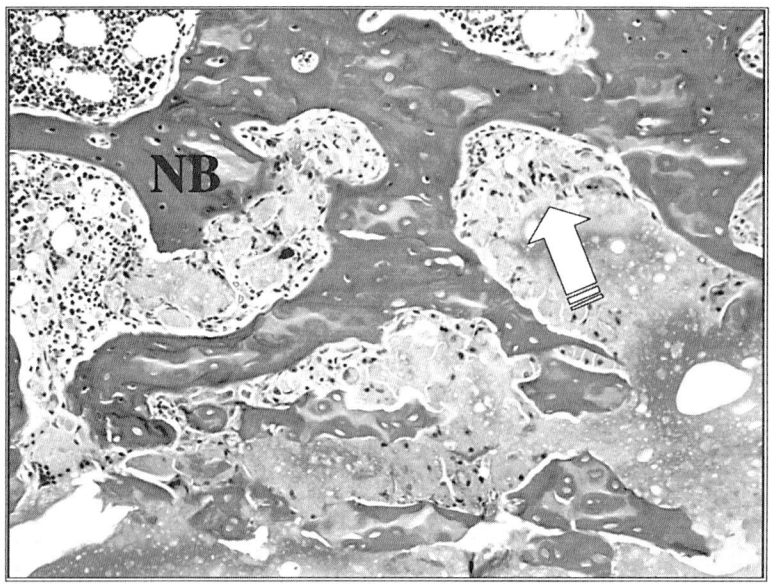

Fig. 10. Longitudinal section through the proximal metaphysis of a group C specimen (cement fixation) at 4 wk postoperatively (H&E, × 10), demonstrating degradation of the cement with formation of cavitations that were invaded by capillaries and ingrowing, newly formed bone. In these cavitations and at the interface between the cement and the invading fibrous tissue, osteoblasts were noted to be lined up against the cement surface, directly depositing new bone onto it (white-striped arrowhead and black open arrowhead).

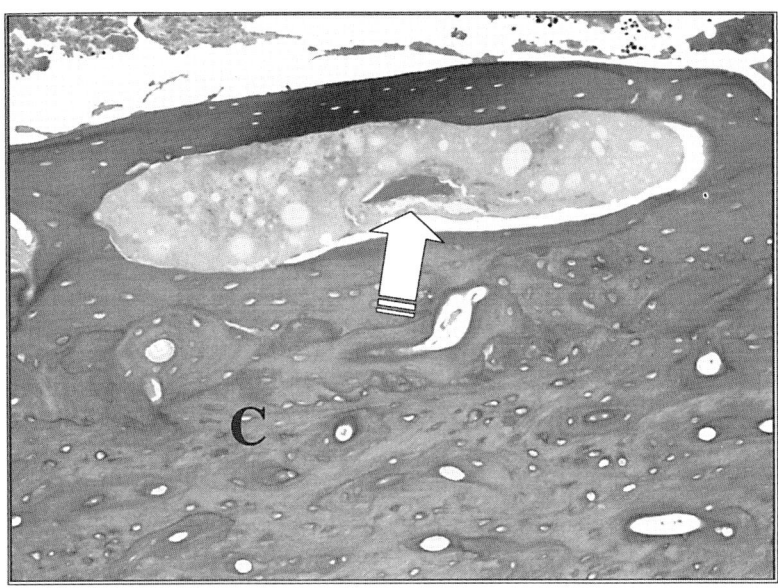

Fig. 11. Longitudinal section through the distal metaphysis of a group C specimen (cement fixation) at 4 wk postoperatively (H&E, × 10), showing the interface between the cement and the endosteal surface of the femoral cortex (notched white arrows) at the metaphyseal–diaphyseal transition zone. Degradation of the cement, with formation of cavitations at 4 wk postoperatively, is present. There is mesenchymal tissue at the interface. In addition, there is osteoid formation at the interface (open black arrowheads) and extensive osteoblastic activity at the cement surface facing the interface (white-striped arrowheads).

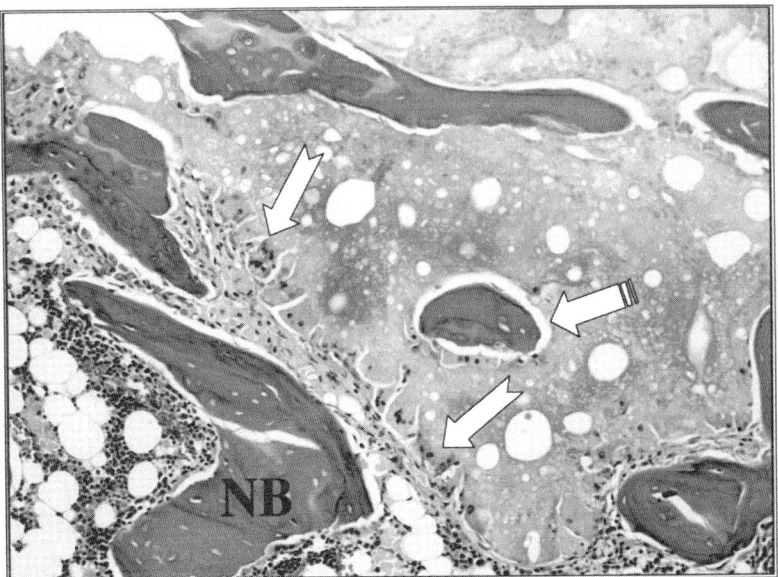

Fig. 12. Longitudinal section through the distal metaphysis of a group C specimen (cement fixation) at 4 wk postoperatively (H&E, × 20). Note intimate contact between the cement and the remodeling endosteal surface of the femoral cortex (white notched arrowhead), with new bone growing within (white-striped arrowhead) and around the cement.

Table 5
Histomorphometric Analysis of Metaphyseal Bone Remodeling Averaged for 12 Animals for Each Group and Performed at 4 Wk Postoperatively

Group	Remodeling index (%) (mean ± SD)	ANOVA p-level	Approximated trabecular bone volume (mm^2) (mean ± SD)	Analysis of variance p-level
A, Loose K-wire	18.2 ± 6.3		6.2 ± 2.1	
B, Rigid K-wire	64.5 ± 9.7	<0.002	15.8 ± 5.3	<0.009
C, Loose K-wire + cement	48.8 ± 8.3		11.4 ± 3.6	

working, and hardening times comparable to commercially available bone cements. The enthalpy of reaction of freshly prepared cement is 64.5 ± 4.4 J/g, a value consistent with that expected for vinyl polymerization, corrected for the weight fraction of polymerizable components in the cement. After refrigerated storage for 2 mo, the enthalpy was 64.3 ± 34.2 J/g, indicating a shelf life significantly greater than 2 mo.

5. The estimated precure viscosity is 50.9 cp, which allows facile delivery of the cement to the surgical site via a syringe.
6. Compressive strengths and moduli exceed the limits for use with trabecular bone, as suggested by Carter and Hayes *(50)* and by Gerhart et al. *(14)*. Compressive strength and moduli remain fairly constant for 3–4 wk in vitro. The strength and moduli were greater for formulations including a higher proportion of HA in the filler.
7. Histology, performed on rat tibial defects filled with precured and *in situ*-cured cement, indicated a high degree of biocompatibility. The *in situ*-cured cement showed some fragmentation, without inflammatory reactions, in the course of observation. This may result from incomplete cure. This observation will be addressed by increasing the cure rate and viscosity of the cements, thereby approximating state-of-the-art cementing techniques.
8. Histologic analysis of midshaft femoral osteotomies in rats, with use of injectable and resorbable bone cement, indicated normal fracture healing in cement-fixed osteotomies, similar to osteotomies in which rigid fixation was performed. From a practical standpoint, the cement was found to be easy to handle and in a suitable injectable format. The cement achieved and maintained sufficient fixation during the concurrent processes of healing at the osteotomy site and degradation of the cement.

On the basis of its favorable in vivo osteoconductive properties reported herein, the authors suggest further development of the PPF bone cement containing the CG–HA filler combination (CG–HA–PPF). It has reasonable viscosity for injectability, and working (6–7 min) and hardening (10–12 min) times, and cures at body temperature *(51)*. It may prove to be of clinical significance once similar in vivo osteoconductive properties an be demonstrated when supporting healing fractures of weight-bearing bones in larger animals and humans.

Acknowledgments

The authors wish to thank Joseph Alroy, DVM, Associate Professor in Pathology, Tufts University Schools of Medicine and Veterinary Medicine for his assistance in the histologic analysis of this study. Furthermore, the authors are indebted to Shrikar Bondre and Eric Gusek for their assistance with animal care. This work was supported in part by National Institutes of Health/National Institute of Arthritis, Musculoskeletal and Skin Diseases (NIH/NIAMS) Grant No. 1 R43 AR44317-01 (J.D.G.), and NIH/NIAMS Grant AR 45062 (K.-U.L.).

References

1 Gerhart TN, Renshaw AA, Miller RL, Noeckler RJ, and Hayes WC. *In vivo* histologic and biomechanical characterization of a biodegradable partic-

ulate composite bone cement. *J Biomed Mater Res* 1989; 23: 1–16.
2. Jasty M, Jiranek W, and Harris WH. Acrylic fragmentation in total hip replacements and its biological consequences. *Clin Orthop Related Res* 1992; 116–128.
3. Nordstrom D, Santavita S, Gristina A, and Konttinen Y. Immune-inflammatory response in the totally replaced hip: a review of biocompatibility aspects. *Eur J Med* 1993; 2: 296–300.
4. Topoleski LD, Ducheyne P, and Cuckler JM. Microstructural pathway of fracture in poly(methyl methacrylate) bone cement, *Biomaterials* 1993; 14: 1165–1172.
5. Anonymous. Case records of the Massachusetts General Hospital. Weekly clinicopathological exercises. Case 34-1990. A 74-year-old man with a failed right-hip replacement, constant pain centered in the right hip, and an osteolytic lesion in the right acetabulum. *N Engl J Med* 1990; 323: 534–539.
6. Bos I, Lindner B, Seydel U, Johannisson R, Dorre E, Henssge J, and Lohrs U. [The cause of loosening in cemented hip joint prostheses. Light and electron microscopy study and laser microprobe mass analysis], [German]. *Z Orthop Grenzgeb* 1990; 128: 73–82.
7. Gil-Albarova J, Lacleriga A, Barrios C, and Canadell J. Lymphocyte response to polymethylmethacrylate in loose total hip prostheses, *J Bone Joint Surg Br* 1992; 74: 825–830.
8. Horowitz SM, Doty SB, Lane JM, and Burstein AH. Studies of the mechanism by which the mechanical failure of polymethylmethacrylate leads to bone resorption, *J Bone Joint Surg Am* 1993; 75: 802–813.
9. Horowitz SM and Purdon MA. Mechanisms of cellular recruitment in aseptic loosening of prosthetic joint implants, *Calcif Tissue Int* 1995; 57: 301–305.
10. Koller W, Muller U, and Henssge EJ. [Reactions of the osseous site following imiplantation of cemented endoprostheses in the femur], [German] *Z Orthopadie Grenzgeb* 1990; 128: 67–72.
11. Willert HG, Bertram H, and Buchhorn GH. Osteolysis in alloarthroplasty of the hip. The role of bone cement fragmentation, *Clin Orthop Related Res* 1990; 108–121.
12. Domb AJ, Manor N, and Elmalak O. Biodegradable bone cement compositions based on acrylate and epoxide terminated poly(propylene fumarate) oligomers and calcium salt compositions, *Biomaterials* 1996; 17: 411–417.
13. Gerhart TN, Hayes WC, and Stern SH. Biomechanical optimizaiton of a model particulate composite for orthopedic applications, *J Orthop Res* 1986; 4: 76–85.
14. Gerhart TN, Miller RL, Kleshinski SJ, and Hayes WC. *In vitro* characterization and biomechanical optimization of a biodegradable particulate composite bone cement, *J Biomed Mater Res* 1988; 22: 1071–1082.
15. Gerhart TN, Roux RD, Hanff PA, Horowitz GL, Renshaw AA, and Hayes WC. Antibiotic-loaded biodegradable bone cement for prophylaxis and treatment of experimental osteomyelitis in rats, *J Orthop Res* 1993; 11: 250–255.
16. Gresser JD, Hsu SH, Nagaoka H, Lyons CM, Nieratko DP, Wise DL, Barabino GA, and Trantolo DJ. Analysis of a vinyl pyrrolidone/poly(propylene fumarate) resorbable bone cement, *J Biomed Mater Res* 1995; 29: 1241–1247.
17. Witschger PM, Gerhart TN, Goldman JB, Edsberg LE, and Hayes WC. Biomechanical evaluation of a biodegradable composite as an adjunct to internal fixation of proximal femur fractures, *J Orthop Res* 1991; 9: 48–53.
18. Yaszemski MJ, Payne RG, Hayes WC, Langer R, and Mikos AG. *In vitro* degradation of a poly(propylene fumarate)-based composite material, *Biomaterials,* 1996; 17: 2127–2130.
19. Jacobsen S, Honnens De Lichtenberg M, Jensen CM, and Torholm C. Removal of internal fixation—the effect on patients' complaints: a study of 66 cases of removal of internal fixation after malleolar fractures, *Foot Ankle Int* 1994; 15: 170–171.
20. Saito M, Maruoka A, Mori T, Sugano N, and Hino K. Experimental studies on a new bioactive bone cement: hydroxyapatite composite resin, *Biomaterials,* 1994; 15: 156–160.
21. Bostman OM. Distal tibiofibular synostosis after malleolar fractures treated using absorbable implants, *Foot Ankle* 1993; 14: 38–43.
22. Liu Y and Rong G. [Absorbable SR-PGA implant in orthopedics: preliminary results of treatment of fractures] [Chinese]. *Chung-Hua Kai Ko Tsa Chih* [*Chin J Surg*] 1995; 33: 51–53.
23. Strycker ML. Biodegradable internal fixation, *J Foot Ankle Surg* 1995; 34: 82–88.
24. Sandhu HS, Kanim LE, Kabo JM, Toth JM, Zeegan EN, Liu D, Seeger LL, Dawson EG. Evaluation of rhBMP-2 with an OPLA carrier in a canine posterolateral (transverse process) spinal fusion model, *Spine* 1995; 20: 2669–2682.
25. Ahl T, Dalen N, Holmberg S, and Selvik G. Early weight bearing of malleolar fractures, *Acta Orthop Scand* 1986; 57: 526–529.
26. Ahl T, Dalen N, and Selvik G. Mobilization after

operation of ankle fractures. Good results of early motion and weight bearing, *Acta Orthop Scand* 1988; 59: 302–306.
27. Anand N and Klenerman L. Ankle fractures in the elderly: MUA versus ORIF *Injury* 1993; 24: 116–120.
28. Bauer M, Bergstrom B, Hemborg A, and Sandegard J. Malleolar fractures: nonoperative versus operative treatment. A controlled study, *Clin Orthop & Related Res* 1985; 199: 17–27.
29. Broos PL and Bisschop AP. Operative treatment of ankle fractures in adults: correlation between types of fracture and final results, *Injury* 1991; 22: 403–406.
30. Broos PL and Bisschop AP. New and easy classification system for ankle fractures, *Int Surg* 1992; 77: 309–312.
31. Karasick D. Fractures and disslocations of the foot, *Semin Roentgenology* 1994; 29: 152–175.
32. Wilson FC. Fractures and dislocations of the ankle, in *Fractures* 1984; (Anonymous) Lippincott, Philadelphia.
33. Harper MC and Hardin G. Posterior malleolar fractures of the ankle associated with external rotation-abduction injuries. Results with and without internal fixation, *J Bone Joint Surg Am* 1988; 70: 1348–1356.
34. Wyss C and Zollinger H. Causes of subsequent arthrodesis of the ankle joint, *Acta Orthop Belg* 1991; 57(Suppl 1): 22–27.
35. Gumann G and Engle A. Emergency treatment of an acute ankle fracture in a chronic alcohol abuser, *J Am Podiatry Assoc* 1984; 74: 453–457.
36. Holm M and Delamarter R. Cast brace and tibial plateau, *Clin Orthop Related Res* 1989; 242: 26.
37. Gray FB. Total hip revision arthroplasty. Prosthesis and cement removal techniques, *Orthop Clin North Am* 1992; 23: 313–319.
38. Mulroy WF and Harris WH. Revision total hip arthroplasty with use of so-called second-generation cementing techniques for aseptic loosening of the femoral component. A fifteen-year-average follow-up study, *J Bone Joint Surg Am* 1996; 78: 325–330.
39. Scholz C, Matthes M, Kar H, and Boenick U. [Removal of bone cement with laser] [German]. *Biomed Technik* 1991; 36: 120–128.
40. Sherk HH, Lane G, Rhodes A, and Black J. Carbon dioxide laser removal of polymethylmethacrylate, *Clin Orthop Related Res* 1995; 310: 67–71.
41. Wykman AG. Acetabular cement temperature in arthoplasty. Effect of water cooling in 19 cases, *Acta Orthop Scand* 1992; 63: 543–544.
42. Wooley PH, Nasser S, and Fitzgerald RH Jr. Immune response to implant materials in humans, *Clin Orthop Related Res* 1996; 326: 63–70.
43. Buchholz HW and Heinert K. Long-term results of cemented arthroplasty. Analysis of complications fifteen years after operation, *Orthop Clin North Am* 1988; 19: 531–540.
44. Murray DW and Rushton N. Macrophages stimulate bone resorption when they phagocytose particles, *J Bone Joint Surg Br* 1990; 72: 988–992.
45. Williams RP and McQueen DA. Histopathologic study of late aseptic loosening of cemented total hip prostheses, *Clin Orthop Related Res* 1992; 275: 174–179.
46. Brandser E, El-Khoury G, Riley M, and Callaghan J. Intravenous methylmethacrylate following cemented total hip arthroplasty, *Skeletal Radiol* 1995; 24: 493–494.
47. Hersh J, Bono JV, Padgett DE, and Mancuso C. Methyl methacrylate levels in the breast milk of a patient after total hip arthroplasty, *J Arthroplasty* 1995; 10: 91–92.
48. McCallum TJ, O'Connor GJ, and Allard MJ. Intravesical methylmethacrylate after revision hip arthroplasty, *J Urol* 1996; 156: 17–77.
49. Tremps Velazquez E, Ramon Dalmau M, Garcia Rojo D, and Cardona Carbonell S. [Ureteral stenosis secondary to methacrylate used in total hip arthroplasty], [Spanish] *Arch Espanoles Urol* 1995; 48: 741–743.
50. Carter DR and Hayes WC. Bone compressive strength: The influence of density and strain rate, *Science* 1976; 194: 1174–1176.
51. David A, Lewandrowski KU, Pommer A, Ostermann PAW, Bähr H, and Muhr G. Interlocking strength of hydroxapatite and titanium coated implants. A biomechanical and histological study, *Orthop Int* 1996; 4: 209–218.
52. Palacos®-R Technical Paper. Richards Technical Publication No. 7395, Smith and Nephew.

19

Development of a Modular Ceramic Knee Prosthesis

W. M. Payten and B. Ben-Nissan

1. Introduction

Degenerative joint disease, recognized as an increasing problem for society, is a direct result of an aging population *(1)*. When patients present with joint pain, their primary concern is the relief of pain and return to a mobile life style. This often requires replacement of skeletal parts, such as hips, knees, elbows, finger joints, shoulder, and teeth, or fusion of vertebrae, and repair or augmentation of the jaw and bones of the skull. The result is a current worldwide orthopedic market valued at over $5 billion; joint replacement represents 68% of this market. The demand for knee replacements is increasing at approx 17%/yr, with some 300,000 knee joints replaced each year in the United States alone *(2)*. This increase results in part from increased confidence in using such prostheses. Unfortunately, results do not reinforce this confidence: Long-term clinical results are scattered *(3)*, and, although the overall rate of failure is reasonably low, it remains unacceptable. A further complication arises because the increase in younger patients undergoing total knee arthroplasty (TKA) may well lead to a higher incidence of eventual failure.

The current orthopedic range of knee prostheses is extensive, and a variety of models are available, but the basic design philosophy is similar for all knee prostheses. TKA involves the replacement or resurfacing of the distal femur, proximal tibia, and patella. The primary aims of such operations are to relieve the patient of pain, correct joint deformity, provide a good range of movement, and improve joint stability. A TKA procedure is generally recommended for patients who present with the following indications *(4)*: a painful joint, with or without any apparent deformity; rheumatoid arthritis; osteoarthritis; traumatic arthritis; or tumor resection.

The typical design of a TKA consists of tibial and femoral components forming the condylar replacements; the femoral component consists of two joined metal runners shaped in a form similar to the natural bone surface. The prosthesis may or may not have a central stem. The tibial component is generally a combination of a metal tray and a plastic running surface that is fixed to the superior side of the metal tray. Both the femoral and tibial prosthetic components come in either cemented (bonded with polymethylmetacrylate) or cementless (bonding through bioactive coating or surface micro- or macrotexturing) types.

From a biomechanics point of view, the human knee has two primary functions: to provide mobility and stability to the lower extremity. The knee joint must allow both flexion and axial rotation to occur, while still maintaining stability. The knee is actually composed of two articulating joints: the patellofemoral and the tibiofemoral joints. The tibiofemoral joint defines the kinematics of flexion, axial rotation, and extension; the patellofemoral joint increases the efficiency of the extensor mechanism. Some compromises must be allowed in the structure of the knee, in order to optimize both mobility and stability. The knee is therefore susceptible to sprains, tears, dislocations, and general wear, which may eventually lead to degenerative joint disease *(5)*.

Research by Collier et al. *(6)*, Moran et al. *(7)*, Windsor et al. *(8)*, and Moreland *(9)* showed that the majority of current total or revision knee replacement failures result from either component loosening or failure of the tibial polyethylene component, caused through wear and cold-flow. High-contact stresses and a high coefficient of friction between the tibial and femoral component are the chief causes *(10,11)*. The use of ceramics, together with an appropriate design, could significantly reduce these problems, offering considerable improvement, compared to that currently obtained by metal designs. However, early ceramic TKA designs achieved only limited success *(12–14)*. This is in contrast to total hip arthroplasties, in which commercially based designs using either alumina or partially stabilized zirconia (PSZ) femoral heads have achieved significant success *(15,16)*. This may be a result of stress profiles occurring in the hip ceramic femoral heads because geometry and loading conditions are simpler to predict.

The efficient and reliable utilization of structural ceramics, despite the prediction of a "new stone-age" since the early 1980s, is still in infancy. In the biomedical field, this is particularly prevalent, with market penetration much lower than expected. The reasons for this are further complicated by economic considerations. However, one of the major factors has been the inability of material scientists and engineers to overcome some of the shortcomings of ceramics, because of inherent brittleness and the scatter of strength data. In order to utilize these materials in biomedical applications, stress and strain distribution must be much better understood than for similar applications of metals.

A major problem with ceramics is that catastrophic failure will occur if loaded in tension to near their maximum strength. In contrast, a metal component, when temporarily overloaded, will often survive because of its ductility. Although ceramic brittleness is not an inherent barrier to mechanical reliability, it complicates the design issue, because of the resultant sensitivity to stress concentrators. Internal flaws lead to a statistical variation in strength that may cause failure at loads that are often well below the desired design stresses *(17–19)*. The distribution of these stresses, their magnitudes, and orientations throughout the structure depends not only on the loading configuration, but also on the geometry of the structure and the properties of its material. This makes the design of a ceramic knee joint prosthesis a complex problem.

The stress distributions within the ceramic and bone can only be solved using numerical methods, such as finite element analysis (FEA) or boundary element analysis. In order to obtain the necessary design information, the geometry, physiology, forces, and boundary conditions must be understood *(20)*. Any design must be able to withstand repeated loads of up to 6.5 × body wt for normal activities, such as walking, as well as transient loads that can be much higher. The majority of FE research on knee anatomical and implant analysis has focused on tibial stresses and fixation, primarily because a high percentage of failures have occurred in this area *(21,22)*. Design and analysis of ceramic femoral components is relatively new, and, as a result of the inherent lack of ductility of these materials, the development of a distal femoral finite element model (FEM) is required.

FEA enables a snapshot of the stresses imposed on the knee during loading to be estimated. However, it provides very limited information on long-term effects of bone adaptation/resorption that occurs around prostheses. Such processes are particularly important in understanding and avoiding prosthesis failure mechanisms. Relatively recent research *(23–28)* enables the use of algorithms that give the analyst the ability to allow the FE mesh to evolve and adapt similarly to real bone, and thereby gain an insight into long-term behavior.

2. Designing with Ceramic Components

The use of ceramics in prostheses is attractive, because their coefficient of friction is close to that of a natural human joint, they are mostly hydrophilic, have excellent resistance to wear, and have biocompatibility. Therefore, ceramics can offer considerable improvements in terms of compatibility, wear rates, and general life extension, beyond those currently obtained by metal replacement parts (29). An example of this is the PSZ or alumina femoral hip components. The use of ceramics and an appropriate design may reduce wear and the amount of contact stress commonly seen with the current knee implant designs.

Unfortunately, attempts at designing a ceramic knee have met with only limited success, by attempting to manufacture the entire femoral component from ceramic material (12). That design used an alumina femoral component bearing onto an ultra-high-molecular-weight-polyethylene (UHMWPE) tibial tray. Initial follow-up clinical results were promising (13), showing no metallosis and UHMWPE debris or wear to either component; however, a high incidence of tibial and femoral compartment subsidence, with loosening of the ceramic from the bone, did occur. Oonishi et al. (13) felt that this was caused by the waffling pattern used on the ceramic to obtain fixation, rather than by the use of bone cement. Alumina ceramics are stiff in comparison to bone, and this tended to allow a layer of membranous fibrous tissue to form, rather than bone ingrowth, because of unacceptable micromotion. Clinical results of other ceramic knees have also been reported: A brief review of these prosthesis was reported by Koshino (14). Although these prostheses were made from alumina ceramics, their design incorporated an intermedullary stem to stabilize the femoral component, and bone cement was used to achieve fixation. No long-term follow-up results were reported. Recently, Atsui et al. (30) reported that unicompartmental replacement with ceramic knee prosthesis using a Kyocera knee was performed in 10 patients. The follow-up period of 24–68 months showed no deterioration, and all of the patients showed marked improvement of pain relief, although there were few complications.

2.1. Porous Biomaterials and Interfaces

Current metallic knee designs increasingly use porous coatings at the bone interface surface to provide fixation (31,32). In the case of the tibial component, this is usually augmented with screws

**Table 1
Different Types of Microfixation Methods for Implants**

Micro- and macrotextured coating (sintered bead, wires)
Plasma-sprayed metallic and ceramic materials
Thin-film bioactive coatings

that enter from the tray, either vertically downwards into the cancellous bone, or at an angle into the stronger cortical bone. This system provides initial support while bone ingrowth into the porous coating occurs. A number of coatings are currently in use that generate mechanical interlocking and surface reactive bonding (Table 1).

The attraction of the first two fixation methods is that, if solid bone ingrowth occurs, then a significantly larger interface surface area is available to distribute and transfer loads between the components and the bone. Currently, the most popular method is the sintered bead coating or the sintered mesh system, plasma-sprayed with a mixed calcium phosphate (CaP) coating.

2.2. Porous-coated Implant with Cortical Bone Screws

CaP ceramics were first proposed by Albee and Morrison in 1920s, for biomedical applications. They observed that tricalcium phosphate, injected into defects, demonstrated more rapid bone growth and union than the untreated defects. Hydroxyapatite (HA) was first identified as being the mineral component of bone by De Jong (33). However, it was not until about 25 yr ago that synthetic HA, $(Ca_{10}[PO_4]_6(OH)_2)$, was accepted as a potential biomaterial for use in orthopedics, bone grafts, and dentistry. It is one of a limited number of materials that will form strong chemical bonds with bone in vivo, while remaining stable under the harsh conditions encountered in the human body. These properties place HA and other CaPs into the class of biomaterials known as surface-active or bioactive materials. The only other inorganic materials that fall into this highly specialized classification are the biocompatible glasses and glass ceramics (34).

Most metallic orthopedic and dental implants are bioinert, do not bond chemically to bone, as does HA, and, consequently, they can become encapsulated by fibrous tissue. Thus, the only means of biofixation is mechanical interlock, in which the implant must be manufactured in such a way that it possesses surface porosity with interconnections of 100 µm and pore sizes of 150 µm or larger in diameter *(35)*, or be suitably surface-macrotextured, so that hard bony tissues can grow into the implant and anchor it in place *(36)*. Other methods available at present, to fix implants firmly in place, are the use of screws or bone cements. If the implant does not integrate well with the surrounding bone, or is not held rigidly with a fastening device, the implant will be subjected to micromovement, and surrounding bone will remodel. This may lead to implant loosening over a period of time.

Brittleness, poor fatigue resistance, and reduced strength, because of porosity, preclude monolithic HA from use in load-bearing situations. It is presently restricted to applications that involve non-weight-bearing conditions in service, such as bone fillers and bone graft substitutes in orthopedics, as well as ossicular bone replacements and materials for maxillofacial reconstruction *(37)*. Coating a load-bearing substrate, such as titanium (Ti) metal, with HA overcomes the physical inadequacy of HA. At the same time, it combines the beneficial properties of both materials.

During the past two decades, various coating methods were proposed to increase bioactivity, and hence accelerate and improve early bone–implant bonding *(38)*. Methods for applying a ceramic coating include dip-coating into a powder suspension, pulsed-laser deposition, electron beam evaporation combined with ion beam mixing, electrophoretic deposition, sputter coating, and plasma spraying. Of these processes, only plasma spraying is used commercially.

One of the most recent coating methods is the thin bioactive layers produced by the sol-gel deposition techniques. The term "sol-gel" is currently used to describe any chemical procedure or process capable of producing ceramic oxides from solutions (aqueous or alkoxide). The overall process has been explained in various comprehensive review papers and books *(39,40)*. Although commonly used for producing glasses and oxides, it has more recently been utilized to produce other more complex materials, as well as nonoxide ceramics.

A porous coating used alone results in poor short-term fixation, because bony ingrowth into the prosthesis takes several weeks. In thick porous coatings, gaps of up to 1 mm between HA coating and bone has been shown to be bridged by the healing process, leading to an early fixation. The attachment to bone in HA-coated implants in 3 wk was reported, which is half the time required for the uncoated implants *(41)*. This increased bond strength, associated with accelerated osteoconductivity, is very important in clinical applications in which initial bone attachment determines the success rate of an implant.

Studies performed by Hirschhorn, cited by Lutton *(42)*, and Bobyn *(43)*, showed 7 and 8 wk are required before sufficient strength and bonding occurs. Any micromovement occurring during the bone ingrowth period will result in the formation of a fibrous tissue at the interface, which has inferior load-sharing characteristics, and subsequent loosening of the prosthesis becomes more likely. A combination of porous coating and macrotexturing or cortical bone screws has been shown to offer the best long-term solution. The use of the cortical screws provides immediate short-term fixation, and therefore weight-bearing, for 6–8 wk, during which time sufficient bone ingrowth occurs. The load is progressively transferred from the screws and onto the interface. Extensive use of this approach has been utilized in the Huckstep Hip, and the follow-up studies *(15,16,42,44)* showed excellent clinical results. In the Huckstep Hip, a flame-sprayed porous alumina coating was used with transcortical screws.

2.3. Ceramic Knee Femoral Component

The ceramic knee prosthesis developed in this work by the authors incorporates a modular approach in which a number of prosthesis sizes and components are available to cover most surgical contingencies. To ensure that the benefit of using ceramics is obtained without compromising the reliability, the design must minimize tensile stress while still enabling the options of intramedullary stems and reliable bone fixation. This is achieved by shielding of the ceramic component via a base plate incorporated between the ceramic femoral component and the femoral resected bone. The Ti alloy (or a cobalt-chromium alloy) base plate is attached to the ceramic, using clips

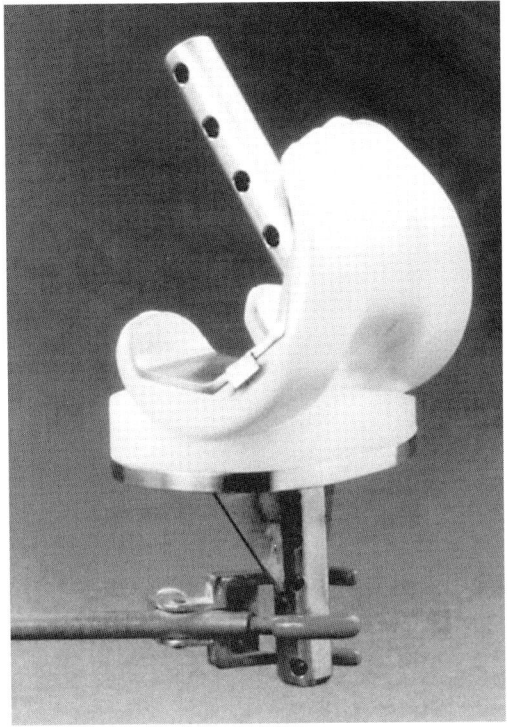

Fig. 1. Prototype of the ceramic knee.

Table 2
Design Objectives

1. Avoid the use of bone cement.
2. Incorporate screws for short-term stable fixation or for revision, if necessary.
3. Include the option of a Morse taper fixed central stem.
4. Bone bonding by the use of a thin bioactive coating or bone ingrowth into a porous coating for long-term fixation.
5. Anatomical surfaces on both femoral and tibial implants.
6. Utilize both single tibial tray and two half-tibial trays.

Table 3
Surgical Cases

1. Primary knee replacement, eg. osteoarthritis, fractures, and so on.
2. Previously failed knee replacement (revision).
3. Severely comminuted distal femoral fractures or proximal tibial fractures.
4. Partial destruction of the knee (lateral or medial proximal tibia, distal femur).

located on the medial and lateral sides (Fig. 1). Because of its shape, the base plate has a high stiffness in the medial-lateral (M-L) direction, which is necessary to withstand transient varus–valgus loading. A Ti alloy stem having the same dimensions and design as the Huckstep nail *(15,45)* can be fitted to the base plate via a Morse taper. This stabilizing intramedullary femoral stem with cross nailing may be required for revision or difficult cases. The base plate functions as the attachment point for the stem, thus minimizing any stress concentrations in the ceramic. This has been a problem in the only ceramic-stemmed single-piece designs. Results from clinical trials of Oonishi et al. *(13)* showed the difficulties in attaching ceramic directly to bone. The use of a metal backing plate, as utilized in this current design, with an appropriate biocoating, overcomes these problems without resorting to the use of bone cement. Fixation is provided by the cross-nailing, and bioceramic coating provides bone ingrowth into the metal plate. The use of a clipped base plate, not intimately bonded to the PSZ ceramic condyle component, enables the reduction of stresses on the inside corners of the ceramic.

The ceramic design developed in the current work uses a system of nine curves to describe the medial, lateral, and patellar track. Each one of these curves is placed to conform to the anatomical curves of the femur. Each track uses three curves, and each curve is tangent to the next. The tibial- and femoral-conforming surfaces, when coupled, will allow a −10- to +12-degree M-L rotation and an anteroposterior (AP) displacement of at least 13 mm. The posterior-distal transition angle equals 20.

2.4. Modular Ceramic Knee Configurations

The ceramic knee has been designed to achieve a number of objectives (Table 2), for specific surgical cases (Table 3), and has a number of available options (Table 4).

2.5. Biocompatibility

The Ti alloy used for both the base plates and screws, the polyethylene tibial inserts, and the

Table 4
Surgical Options

1. Primary total knee incorporating a PSZ femoral component and Ti base plate, articulating on a UHMWPE insert attached to a tibial Ti base plate. Transcortical screws are optional.
2. Revision replacement for severe fractures is possible by using modified ceramic condyles and Ti base plate, incorporating a groove or slot, to guide an extended finger of the UHMWPE insert. The femoral and tibial component will include long stems and 4.5-mm locking transcortical screws located through the Ti stem.

magnesia-stabilized partially stabilized zirconia magnesium ([Mg]-PSZ) all have current U.S. Food and Drug Administration approval as materials for implantation purposes. Both active and silent-type tests have been undertaken with PSZ material *(42,46,47)*. There was no adverse reaction to the implants, and the tissue response to Mg-PSZ was considered to be biocompatible and bioinert.

2.6. Manufacture

Aluminum femoral test pieces were manufactured on University of Technology, Sydney, Aus, and commercial numerical control (NC) mills to check the AUTOCAD (*Autodesk*) drawings. After revisions to the drawings, the prototypes were green-machined at ANSTO Engineering development section from PSZ blocks, which had been cold-isostatically pressed at ICI Advanced Ceramics, Melbourne (currently Carpenter). Tool paths developed by SURFCAM were used to direct a four-axis mill fitted with a special mandrel mounted in a rotary table. The green-machined ceramic was then fired at ICI to produce the finished product.

2.7. Surgical Implantation

Preliminary surgical implantation of the prosthesis in a cadaver was performed at the University of New South Wales, Sydney, Aus under the direction of Huckstep, Etherington, and Pollack. A comlete set of cutting guides and jigs were designed and manufactured to locate the cutting blades, and align the prostheses and transcortical nails. These trials proved that the design could be successfully used in the surgical environment.

3. FE Analysis

FEA was an essential part of the development and validation process for the PSZ modular ceramic knee prosthesis. Although three-dimensional (3-D) models of the tibia were developed, analysis focused on simplified two-dimensional (2-D) models, because of the number of arrangements and the associated difficulties of modeling the interface conditions. On the femoral side, determination of ceramic prosthesis stresses was the dominating factor, so models focused on this aspect. On the tibial side, which is historically more prone to problems of bone collapse and bone resorption, the models focused on bone stresses and adaptation.

3.1. Femur

2-D models of the femur were analyzed in both the sagittal and transverse (frontal) planes. In the sagittal plane, the major loads were the ground reaction force and patella-femoral contact force. In the transverse plane, a range of varus–valgus loads were modeled. The open-beam-type arrangement of the prosthesis in the transverse plan was simulated by determining the moment of inertia in the plane, and including the stiffness by adjusting the material and thickness properties in the M-L plane. Both 2-D and 3-D analyses of the ceramic component were undertaken and compared with experimental strain gaging for comparison. Because of the complexity of interface conditions between the ceramic, the base plate, and the bone, a series of studies were carried out modeling different conditions. The design was modeled with and without coupling between the ceramic condyles and Ti base plate, and including or omitting the central stem.

Incorporating the effects of the nonmodeled third dimension is necessary for 2-D cases. For the 2-D models considered here, a mixture of the plane-stress method, utilizing the composite material approach of McNiece et al., *(48)*, and standard-thickness approach is used.

3.2. Interface Modeling

It has long been recognized that bone–prosthesis interface stresses play a crucial role in the long-term stability of implants. In recent years, interface problems have been solved using specialized elements *(49,50)*. When analyzing multi-component systems with interfaces merged, the side nodes of different elements with varying stiffness are coincident on the interface side, and must be shared. The FEM solution will enforce the displacement compatibility, and therefore stresses across the interface nodes, producing a smoothly contoured distribution. In reality, however, stresses at the interface would normally be discontinuous *(51)*. The effect on bone and prosthesis can be significant.

In this work, models were analyzed assuming both full and zero bonding, incorporating intermediate interface properties between the PSZ ceramic, Ti alloy base plate, and bone. Frictional gap elements were used to model the interface between the plate and bone. Justification for the use of these is based, first, on the principle that intimate and fully bonded interfaces would not occur, and, second, if element interfaces were not included, frictional movements would not be possible between the components. Finally, because this porous interface region is only several microns thick, a large number of conventional elements would be needed through the interface, to ensure that the aspect ratio of the elements at the interface is appropriate.

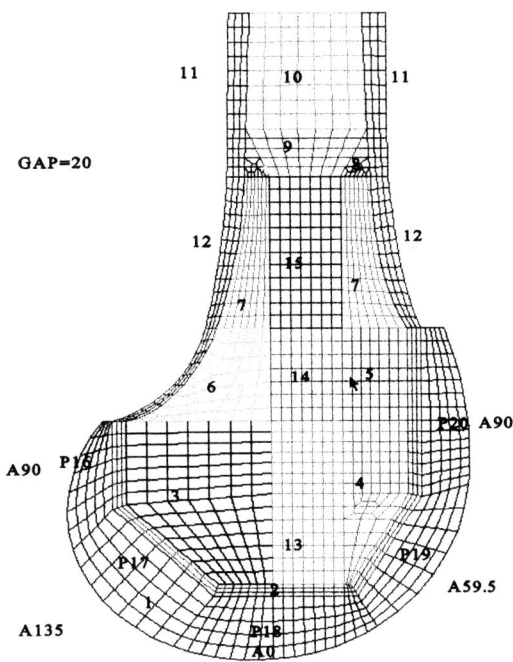

Fig. 2. Material positions: femoral model sagittal plane.

3.3. Element Type

All 2-D models were meshed using 2-D plain strain, four-node linear quadratic elements. 3-D verification models used 3-D eight-node elements, and the bone adaptation work used 2-D plain stress eight-node parabolic elements.

3.4. Material Properties

Material properties were taken from a number of sources *(21,22,49,50,52–54)*. Depending on the model, up to 17 material and 21 real constants were used (Figs. 2–4). All bone properties for this study were assumed to be linear elastic and isotropic. Range of bone mechanical properties utilized are given in Tables 5A–C and 6A,B. Delineation of zones is complex, and data on the distal femoral bone is limited (primarily cortical properties), so the zones are somewhat arbitrarily modeled. The various major areas shown in Table 7 were included. Mechanical properties of Mg-PSZ is given in Table 8.

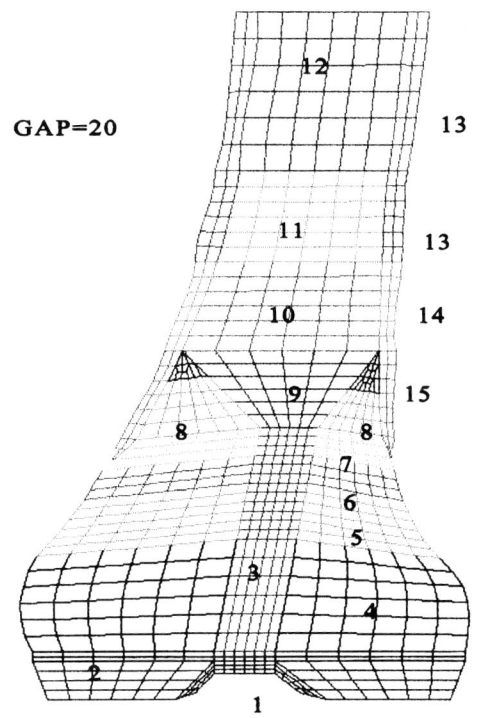

Fig. 3. Material map: femoral model frontal plane.

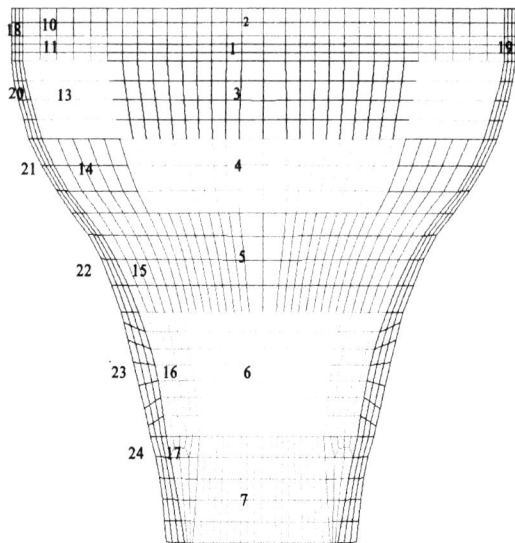

Fig. 4. Material map: tibial model frontal plane.

3.5. Geometrical Properties

The prosthesis was modeled to be medium–large size M-L = 73 mm and A-P = 61 mm. The femoral component thickness was 400 mm, and the base plate thickness 2.53 × 4.00 mm. Moment of inertia of the various knee components were taken from the 3-D CAD drawings, which were obtained from computed tomography scans. The appropriate pseudomoment of inertia was then calculated and a thickness derived for this moment, to ensure correct stiffness in the 2-D plane.

3.6. Loading Conditions

Frontal or sagittal plane models preclude the use of many of the ligaments and muscles as their force direction acts out of the plane of modeling. In the sagittal plane, joint reaction and patella forces were taken for a walking gait of 1.4/ms, starting with zero degrees flexion at heel-strike to toe-off (55,56). The applied and reactive forces must be balanced by the use of a force-couple between the ground and patella reaction force. This couple balances the patella load with the contact point load on the distal femur, to offset the lack of restraining geometry and soft tissues usually supplied by the cruciate ligaments and posterior portions of the joint capsule, which are not included. In the frontal or transverse plane, the ground reaction force plus a varus or valgus moment was analyzed. The forces used in the design and modeling process are adapted from Rohrle et al. (56). Figures 5–7 indicate that the maximum force on the knee is reached during the terminal phase of the gait, just prior to toe lift-off, occurring 1.09 s after initial heel-strike.

Table 5A
Tibial Bone Mechanical Properties*

Bone type	Symbol	Young's modulus (MPa)	Poisson's ratio
Cortical Bone	A	15,000	0.28
Cancellous Bone	B	600	0.32
	C	360	0.32
	D	180	0.32
	E	60	0.32

*See Lewis et al., 1982 (52).

Table 5B
Tibial Bone Mechanical Properties

Bone type	Young's modulus elastic (MPa)	Poisson's ratio
Compact bone	14,000	0.3
Trabecular bone		
Subchondral	700	0.2
Intramedullary	350	0.2

Adapted with permission from ref. 53.

Table 5C
Tibial Bone Mechanical Properties

Material	Young's elastic modulus (MPa)	Poisson's ratio	Yield strength (MPa)
Proximal cortical	1000	0.24	24.4
Distal cortical	5000	0.31	71.3
Cortical articular condylar	800	0.23	21.0
Outer trabecular	320	0.20	11.4
Subchondral trabecular	440	0.21	14.0
Inner cancellous	100	0.18	5.3

*See Beaupre et al., 1986 (21).

Table 6A
Properties of Tibia in Frontal and Sagittal Plane*

Region	Young's elastic modulus (MPa)	Poisson's ratio	Yield strength (MPa)
1	1000	0.24	24.4
2	5000	0.31	71.3
3	320	0.20	11.4
4	440	0.21	14.0
5	100	0.18	5.3
6	800	0.23	21.0

*See Vasu et al., 1986 (22).

Table 6B
Cancellous Material Curves*

Linear relationships
$E_1 = 1.55p - 62.21$ MPa $G_{12} = 0.53p - 13.19$ MPa
$E_2 = 2.01p - 72.80$ MPa $G_{13} = 0.48p - 27.74$ MPa
$E_3 = 4.36p - 41.24$ MPa $G_{23} = 0.66p - 8.93$ MPa

Power law relationships
$E_1 = 0.52p^{1.16}$ MPa $G_{12} = 0.08p^{1.26}$ MPa
$E_2 = 0.79p^{1.14}$ MPa $G_{23} = 0.29p^{1.13}$ MPa
$E_3 = 2.84p^{1.07}$ MPa $G_{13} = 0.22p^{1.15}$ MPa

See Ashman et al., 1989 (54).
where p = density.

Table 7
Material Regions

1. Condylar surface
2. Subcondylar bone
3. Inner cancellous
4. Distal cancellous
5. Hard trabecular
6. Soft trabecular
7. Proximal cortical
8. Distal cortical

Table 8
Material Properties of ICI Mg-PSZ

Properties	Temperature (°C)	Value
Flexural strength four-point bend (MPa)	20	820
	820	430
Tensile strength (MPa)	20	450
Compressive strength (MPa)	20	1990
Fracture toughness K_{ic} (MPa.m$^{-1/2}$)	20	8–12
	800	5
Weibull modulus (m)	20	>30
Modulus of elasticity (GPa)	20	205
Poisson's ratio	20	0.31
Hardness (Hv$_{0.3}$Kg.mm^{-2})	20	1120
Density (g.cm^{-3})	20	5.74
Mean coefficient of thermal expansion $\times 10^{-6}$ °C	25–400	10.2
Thermal shock resistance down-shock DT		375°C
Specific heat (J.g^{-1}.k^{-1})	20	0.47
Thermal conductivity (W.mK^{-1})	20	3.08
	400	2.44
	800	2.26

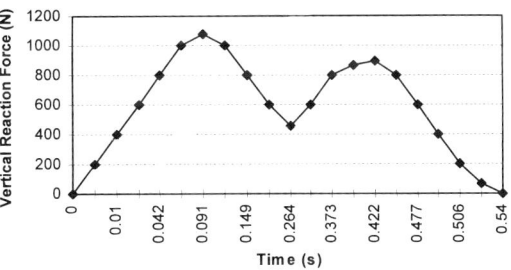

Fig. 5. Foot–ground reaction forces. Adapted with permission from ref. 56.

4. Results

On the femoral side of the design, the emphasis is on the behavior of the coupled modular design; the tibial analysis concentrates on bone and interface stresses. The models include the range of loads encountered during normal activities. 2-D femoral cases were analyzed in the sagittal plane (Table 9) and transverse plane, (Table 10); the special loading conditions for transverse plane analysis are shown in Table 11. In all cases in which a stem is used, the stem is assumed to be bonded, and, in every case study, a body wt of 70 kg, with 6.5× load, was used.

4.1. Sagittal Plane
4.1.1. Gait Stresses at Toe-off

Sagittal plane models were analyzed based on the gait data detailed above. The quasistatic analysis extended over the entire gait range, from heel-strike to toe-off, in case 6. The remaining models were analyzed at the position of maximum stress occurring just prior to toe off (56). Details of the first principal stress (S1P) for the selected

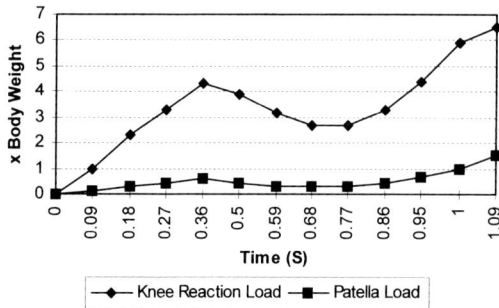

Fig. 6. Calculated patella and knee reaction load as a function of time. Adapted with permission from ref. 56.

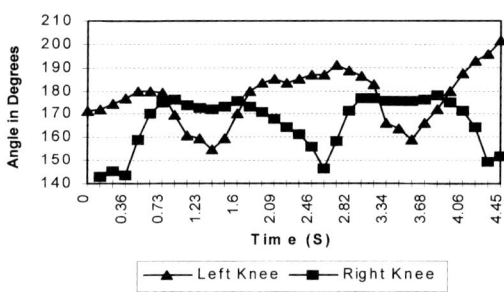

Fig. 7. Angles vs gait diagram. Adapted with permission from ref. 56.

Table 9
Case Studies (Sagittal Plane)

Ceramic only
    Case 1. Ceramic only (no base plate): Bonded
    Case 2. Ceramic only (no base plate): Unbonded
    Case 3. Ceramic + stem (no base plate): Unbonded

Ceramic and base plate
    Case 4. Ceramic + base plate + stem: Fully bonded
    Case 5. Ceramic + base plate: Bonded, base plate + bone: Unbonded
    Case 6. Ceramic + base plate + stem: Unbonded, base plate + bone: Unbonded
    Case 7. Ceramic + base plate: Unbonded, base plate + bone: Unbonded (no stem)

Table 10
Case Studies (Transverse Plane)

Ceramic only
    Case 3. Ceramic + stem (no base plate): Unbonded
Ceramic and base plate
    Case 4. Ceramic + base plate: Fully bonded
    Case 5. Ceramic + base plate: Bonded, base plate + bone: Unbonded
    Case 6. Ceramic + base plate: Unbonded, base plate + bone: Unbonded

Table 11
Transverse Model Loading Conditions

1. Even medial and lateral loading
2. 50 Newton valgus load
3. 150 N valgus load
4. 220 N valgus load

interface and design conditions are shown in Figs. 8–14.

The range of resultant stress for the seven selected cases show the variety of stresses that can be experienced by the femoral component, depending on design attachment configuration. Stresses vary from 17 MPa, in the case of the ceramic-only component perfectly bonded (Fig. 8, case 1), to 69 MPa, when the ceramic is detached from the base plate, which has a frictional interface to the bone, (Fig. 13, case 6). The location of the maximum stress is dependent on the design and interface conditions. In the case of the ceramic-only (cases 1 and 2), this point occurs at the posterior internal distal angle for both the bonded and unbonded cases, rising to a maximum stress of 35 MPa in the latter. If a stem is included, (case 3), and the system is treated as unbonded, then the maximum stress moves from the inside surface to the external anterior flange, resulting in a maximum stress of 58 MPa. The modular design incorporating a base plate changes the stress pattern significantly. If the system is fully bonded (case 3), then a maximum stress of 24 MPa occurs on the anterior flanges (Fig. 10). This contrasts to cases 1 and 2, in which the maximum stress occurs on the inside corner, as described above, this paragraph. If the ceramic component and the tray are unbonded, and the tray is bonded or unbonded to the underlying bone (cases 5 and 6), then the maximum stress occurs on the inside surface of the Ti tray, increasing from 56 to 69 MPa, respectively (Figs. 12 and 13). The maximum stress, which occurs on the

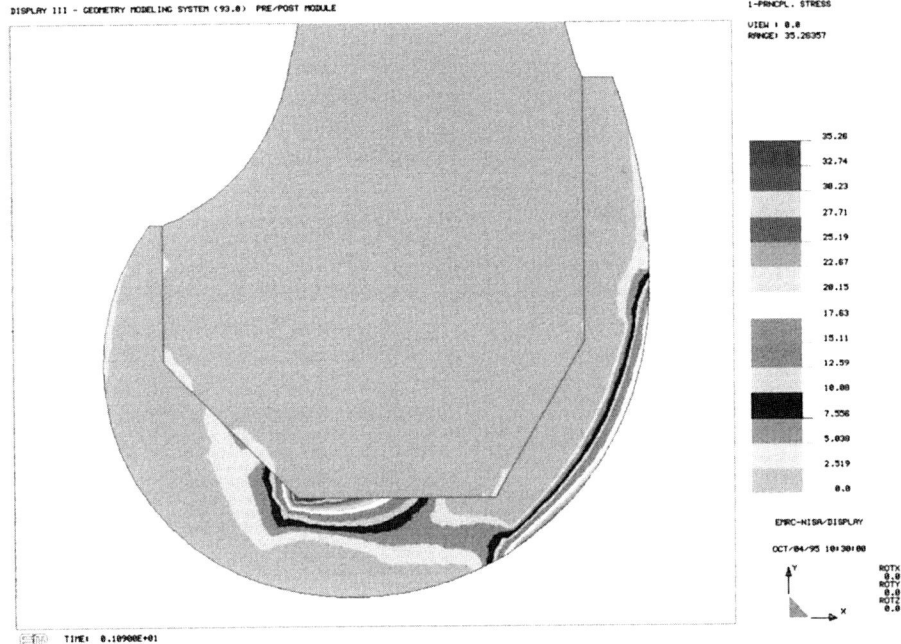

Fig. 8. First principal stress (S1P), case 1.

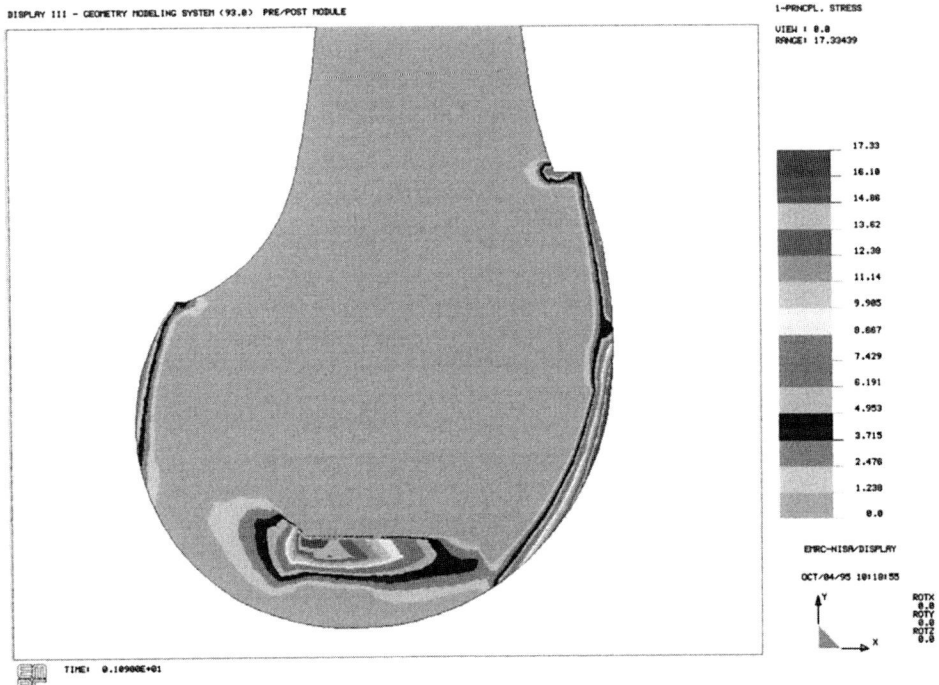

Fig. 9. First principal stress (S1P), case 2.

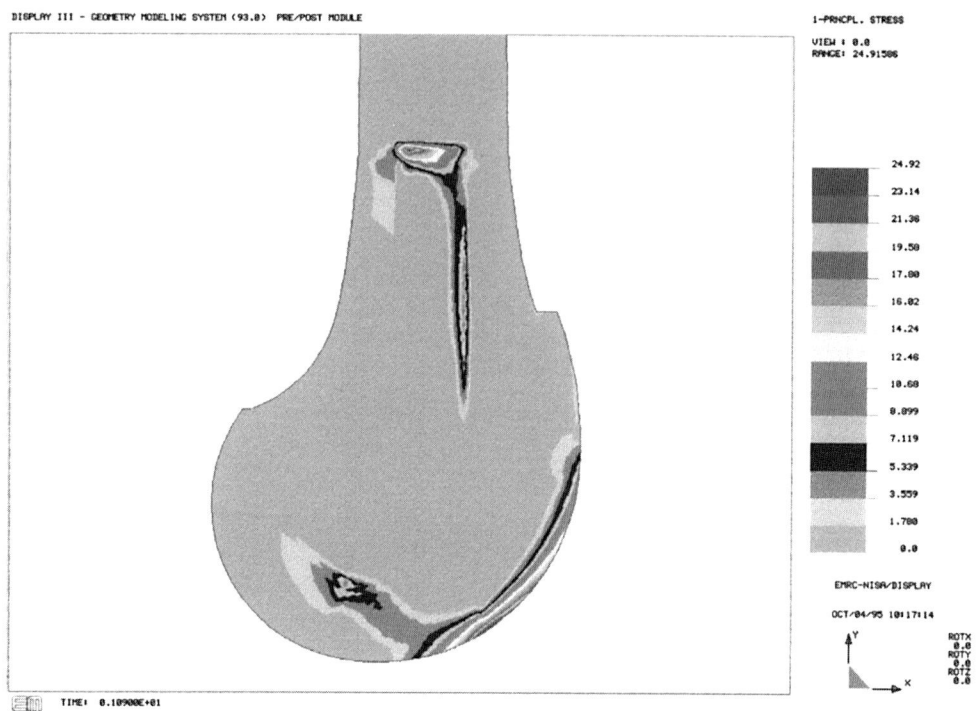

Fig. 10. First principal stress (S1P), case 3.

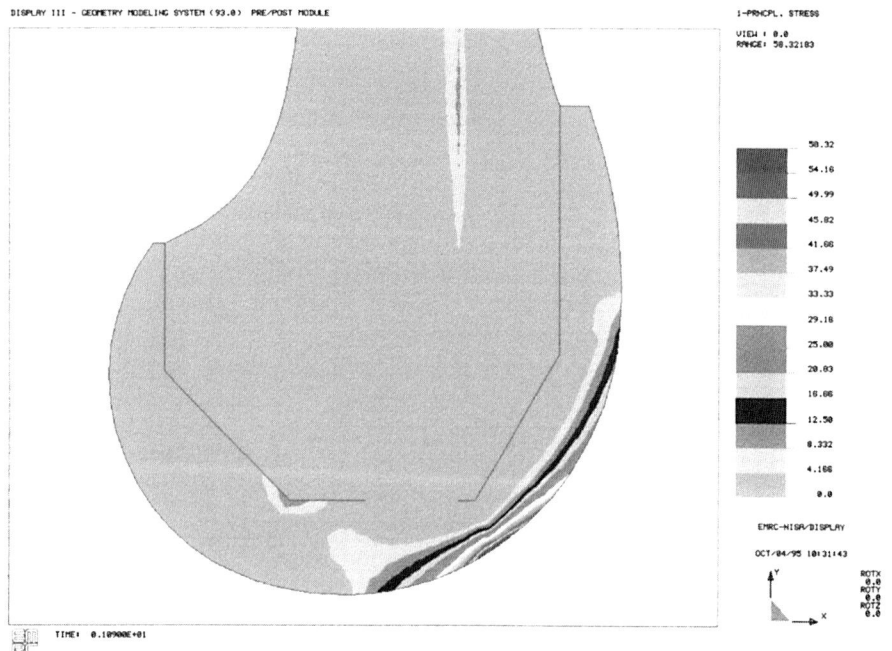

Fig. 11. First principal stress (S1P), case 4.

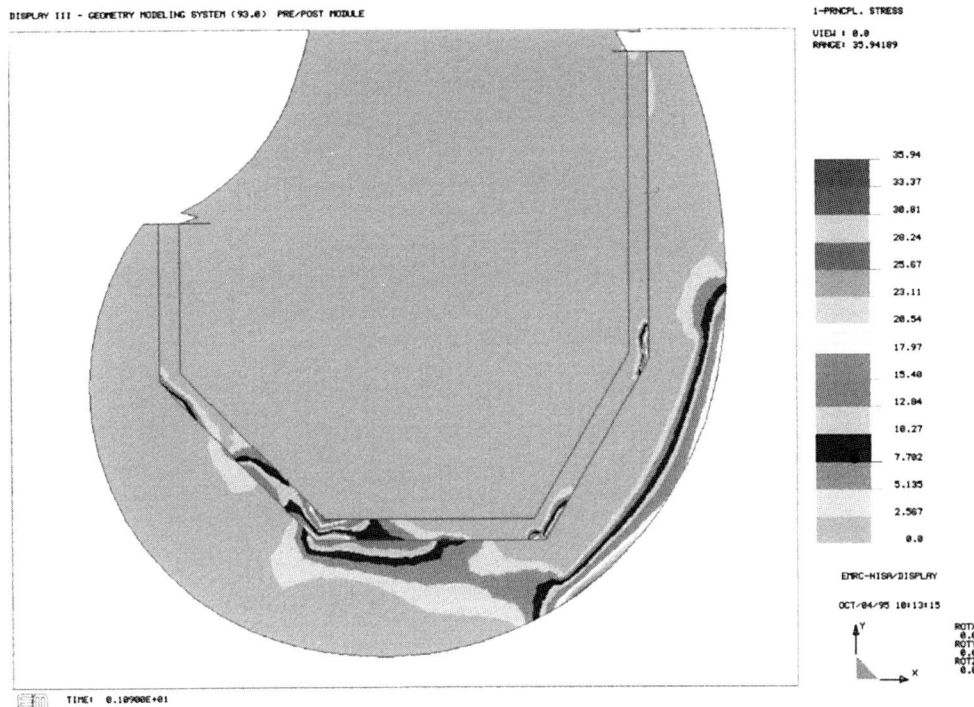

Fig. 12. First principal stress (S1P), case 5.

anterior flange of the ceramic, is approx 10 MPa below that occurring in the Ti, in both cases. If the stem is removed (case 7), the stresses decrease to 36 MPa in the Ti base plate and 28 MPa on the anterior flanges of the ceramic component (Fig. 14). This is similar to the situation seen in the ceramic component alone, in which the stem also increased the maximum stress. Comparisons of the first principal stress and third principal stresses are shown in Figs. 15 and 16.

Maximum compressive stresses (i.e., the third principal stresses) occur on the inside distal anterior corner of the ceramic, in both the bonded and unbonded cases. Stresses range from −14 MPa in case 1 to −181 MPa in case 7. The comparison of the designs, with and without stems, show significant differences when the ceramic surfaces are unbonded (Figs. 10, 13, and 14). Stresses increase from 35 to 58 MPa in the ceramic with no base plate, and from 24 to 69 MPa with a stem incorporated. Thus, if limited bonding occurs between the bone and the ceramic, then the most suitable design is that with a tray but no stem. This conclusion must be tempered, however, by the possibility of only minimal bone ingrowth occurring. The component will then be free to move, resulting in possible tipping of the component.

The stress contours for the unbonded cases, incorporating the tray (cases 5 and 6) are complex. This can be visualized by observing the vector magnitudes and directions of the principal stresses (Fig. 17). This vector plot from case 6 shows how the ground reaction force interacts with the patella reaction load. The patella force induces compression at the point of application. A force couple is generated, resulting in compression stress on the inside anterior corner and tension stress on the anterior surface. The larger ground reaction force results in compression at the point of application, as well as in the stem. This induces a tensile stress on the inside posterior corner. The application of the ground reaction force is plainly seen in the bonded cases (cases 1 and 4), but is significantly increased in the unbonded systems, in which base

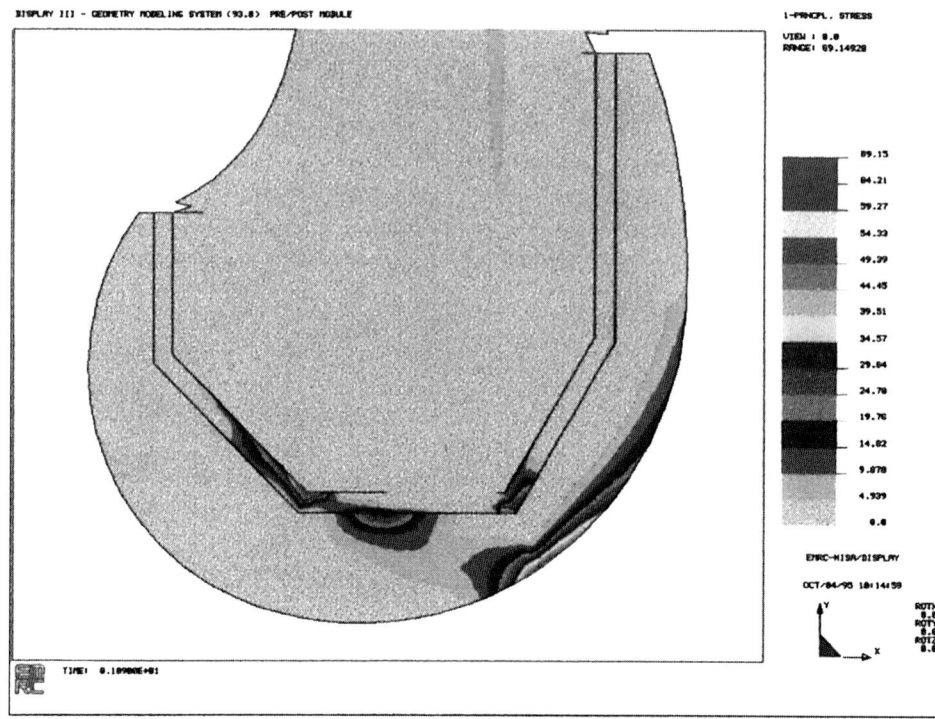

Fig. 13. First principal stress (S1P), case 6.

plates are included (cases 6 and 7). This results from a partial decoupling of the ceramic component from the metal base plate during loading. The interface status showed that the application of the ground reaction force is not through the base plate, but is relocated to a position directly superior to the force application point. The force then becomes distributed and applied to both anterior and posterior positions on the rear internal distal corner.

The above cases show the importance of incorporating the effect of the bone–prosthesis interface. If perfect bonding is assumed between the prosthesis and bone, then the resulting system stress are low, and there is little cause for concern. In this case, a ceramic prosthesis by itself would suffice. However, there are significant problems with this assumption. The first is that, in reality, perfect bonding of the prosthesis to the bone can never be guaranteed. Some micromotion may be experienced: This was the primary cause of failure of the first single-piece ceramic components (14). Micromotion has also been noted in the proximal femoral hip replacement system, as well as the tibial system (49,50,57), loosening and growth of fibrous tissue is common. The first reason can be considered to be of physiological significance. The second reason is based on the correctness of the FEM. The basic problem results from the large differences between the bone and prosthesis material properties, which can vary by three orders of magnitude, from 200 MPa in bone, to 200 GPa in ceramic, giving an ill-posed problem in terms of stiffness. Although the deflections may be equal, the stresses will be smeared across the interface, leading to incorrect stresses on both the hard and soft side of the model: This is seen in case 1 and case 5, (Figs. 8 and 11). The intimate bonding also means that a Poisson's ratio effect results; the applied load causes relative movement between the two vertical faces of the prosthesis, this movement being resisted by the bone. If perfect bonding is assumed between the bone and prosthesis, then reduction in calculated stresses will be observed; hence, this assumption may result in incorrectly determined stresses. Finally,

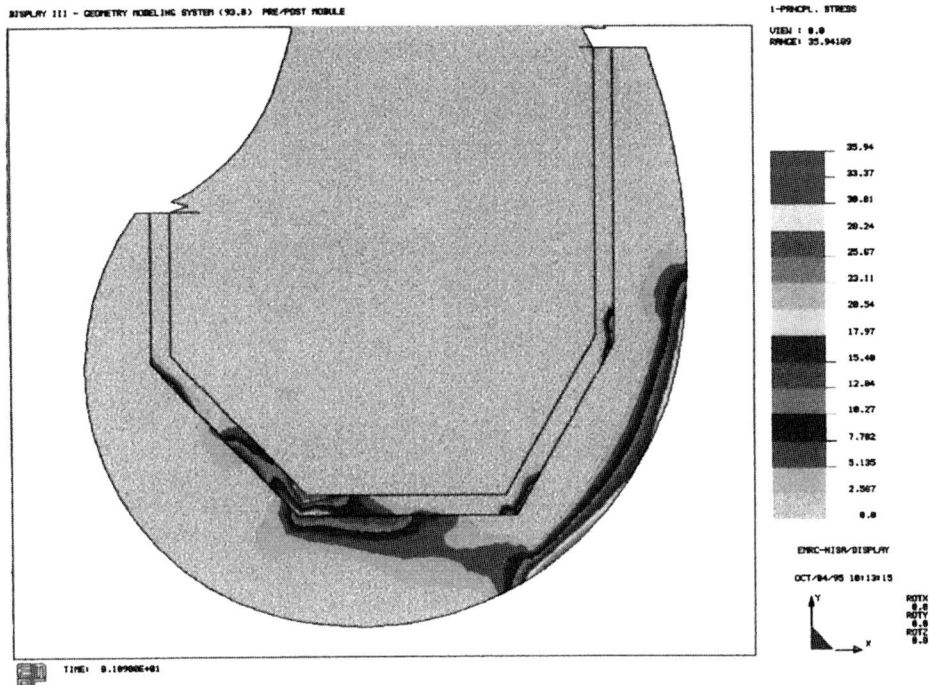

Fig. 14. First principal stress (S1P), case 7.

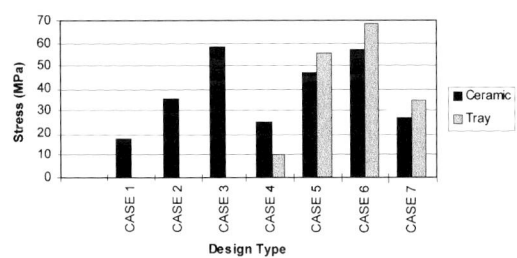

Fig. 15. Comparison of first principal stresses (S1P) for all cases. C, ceramic; T, tray.

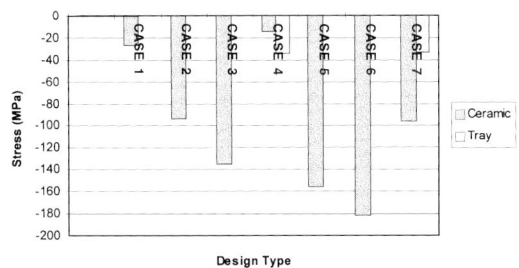

Fig. 16. Comparison of third principal stresses (S3P) for all cases. C, ceramic; T, tray.

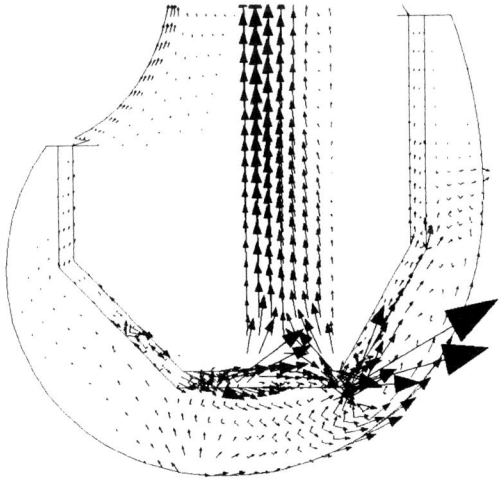

Fig. 17. Vector plot first (light gray) and third (black) principal stresses. Length of arrow indicates magnitude.

the use of a perfectly bonded interface means that the assumption of no interface shearing exists. The importance of recognizing that an interface exists is crucial, with the real situation probably being between the two extremes. Preferably, the

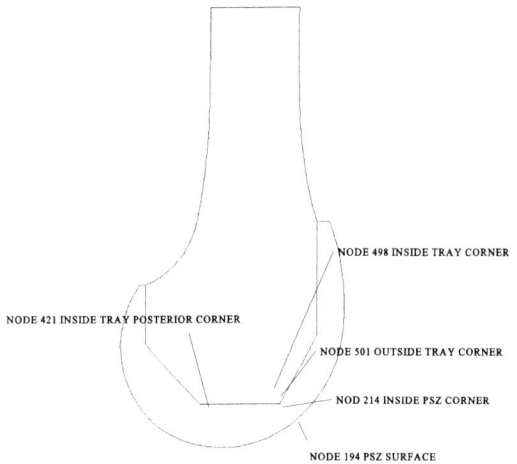

Fig. 18. Node high-stress locations.

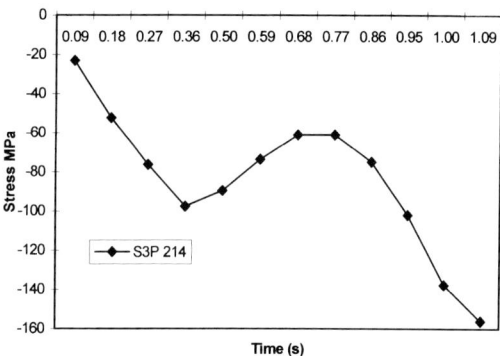

Fig. 20. Third principal stresses (S3P) throughout ground phase of motion case 6 for node 214.

use of a static frictional coefficient would provide a more accurate answer: Values of between 0.2 and 0.65 were used by Rakotomanana et al. *(49)*. This was at best an educated guess, in the absence of reliable data; the assumption of no bonding is a conservative approach.

4.1.2. Quasistatic Analysis of Case 6 from Heal-strike To Toe-off

Case 6 was analyzed from heel-strike to toe-off, incorporating the ground reaction force, the patella reaction load, and the gait angulation during motion. Using the load curves for ambulatory gait, the peak stresses occur at the terminal phase of gait, just prior to toe-off. A lower peak occurs just after heel-strike, which then decreases in accordance with the load curve during midphase, before finally increasing at toe-off, because of the antagonist behavior of the hamstrings and quadriceps. Figs. 19 and 20 detail S1P and S3P stresses at node locations shown in Fig. 18.

Peak stresses occur on the external front surface of the ceramic prosthesis, and at the interior corner of the metal base plate, because of the ground reaction force. The peak value of compression occurs on the front internal surface. During the ground-contact phase, the angulation does not vary more than 12–16 degrees from the anatomical axis, with the result that the component stress closely follows the load curve. The results for the femoral analysis do not provide conclusive

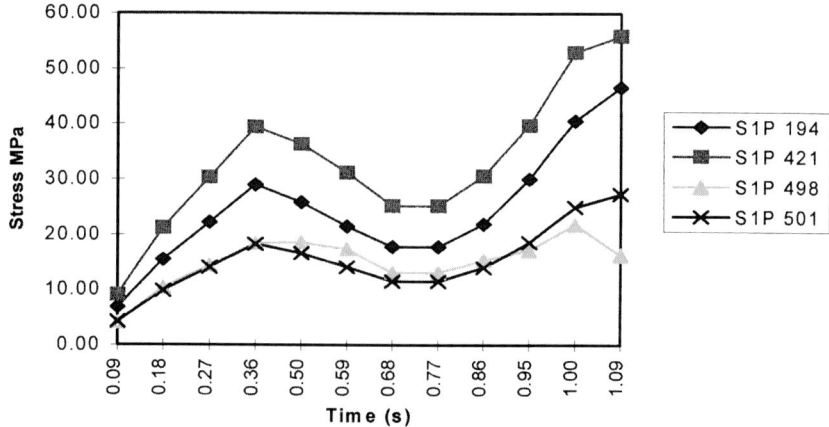

Fig. 19. First principal stresses (S1P) throughout ground phase of motion case 6 for nodes shown in Fig. 18.

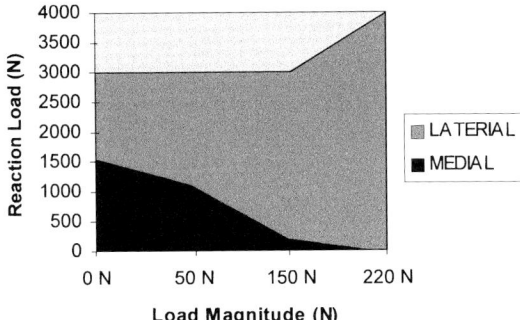

Fig. 21. Transverse plane stresses at ground force of 3× body wt, under incresing lateral (varus) load 0 to 220N.

reasons for using a base plate in this plane. Stresses in the sagittal plane show an increase in the stress when both a base plate and a stem are used; however, ceramic stresses are marginally reduced when a base plate is incorporated and a stem is omitted. Femoral models in the sagittal plane show only part of the resultant stresses; varus–valgus stresses cannot be modeled, because they occur out of the sagittal plane. These stresses can only be resolved in the frontal or transverse plane.

4.2. Transverse Plane Stresses

Frontal plane stresses were based on a varus force increasing from 0 to 220 N and a ground reaction load of 3× body wt. As the varus load increases, the distribution of the combined load on the medial and lateral compartments changes from even at 0 N to 100% lateral at 220 N. Four cases are considered, as shown in Fig. 21. These lateral and medial loads are also present in the tibial compartments. Above 150 N, accessory muscle forces are required to keep the joint in static equilibrium. The total reaction force increases to 4000 N, at which time the force on the medial condyle has reduced to zero. This is seen in the shape rise of the lateral force (Fig. 21). Any further increase in varus force will cause joint lift-off to occur on the medial compartment. Of the four cases analyzed, all included the stem. Figures 22 and 23 show the first principal stresses for cases 3 and 6 at 220 N.

Stress contours (Figs. 22 and 23) illustrate the effect of an unevenly distributed load on the femoral condyles in the transverse plane on the stem and prosthesis. Stresses in case 3 (the ceramic and integral stem design) reach a peak stress of 182 MPa, which occurs at a position slightly proximal of the condylar stem junction point, within the ceramic stem. Stresses at this location could be well over 2.5× greater, if the higher load of 6.5× body wt is assumed. This loading could result in tensile stresses up to 456 MPa, which exceed the tensile stress of 450 MPa of PSZ. For case 6, the modular design, the use of the base plate increases the stress to a maximum of 225 MPa, which is 43 MPa higher than in the ceramic and stem design (case 3). The stresses in case 6 are, however, located in the Ti tray, and not within the ceramic. The tray, because of its inherent stiffness, results in a 90% reduction in the ceramic stresses, to 18 MPa. If 6.5× body wt is assumed, then the resultant stresses in the modular design could exceed 450 MPa in the tray. Although these stresses will cause some local yielding in the Ti stem, the plasticity will be confined to a localized area of the stem thickness. The inherent ductility of the metal will allow this type of short-term transient overload, but the ceramic-only designs may fail catastrophically under the same load conditions. For each of the selected designs, the S1P and S3P, plus the maximum shear stress for the ceramic, base plate, and the stem (if large in magnitude), are plotted for the increasing load from 0 to 220 N, (Figs. 24 to 27).

Stresses increase in all components as the varus load is increased. However, this increase is not linear, with applied load being minimal up to 50 N load, before rising more rapidly as the load is raised to 150 and 220 N. The lowest system stresses are again seen when the prosthesis is intimately bonded to the bone (case 4). In this arrangement, a maximum stress of 18 MPa occurs in the ceramic component and 44 MPa in the base plate, under a 220 N valgus load. If a ceramic with no base plate is modeled, and full bonding is assumed between the ceramic and the bone, then the system stresses are similar, with the ceramic maximum stresses increasing marginally to 46 MPa. When the design arrangements are treated as interface systems, stresses rapidly increase in both the ceramic and stem. A comparison of the S1P, S3P, and the maximum shear stress at 220 N are shown for the four analyzed cases (Fig. 28).

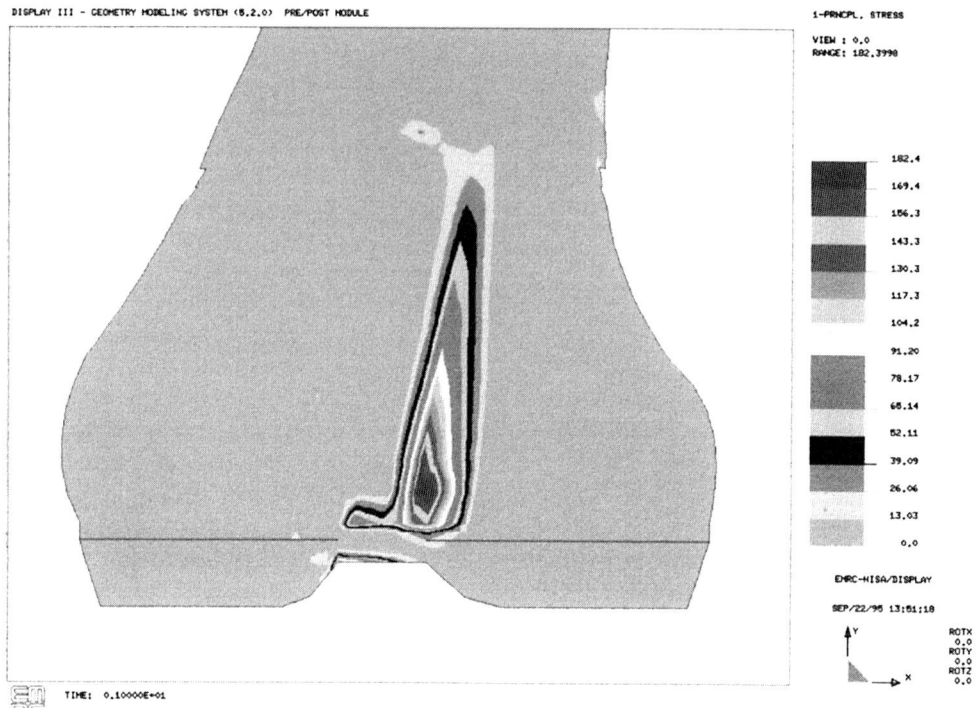

Fig. 22. First principal stresses for case 3 at 220 N varus load.

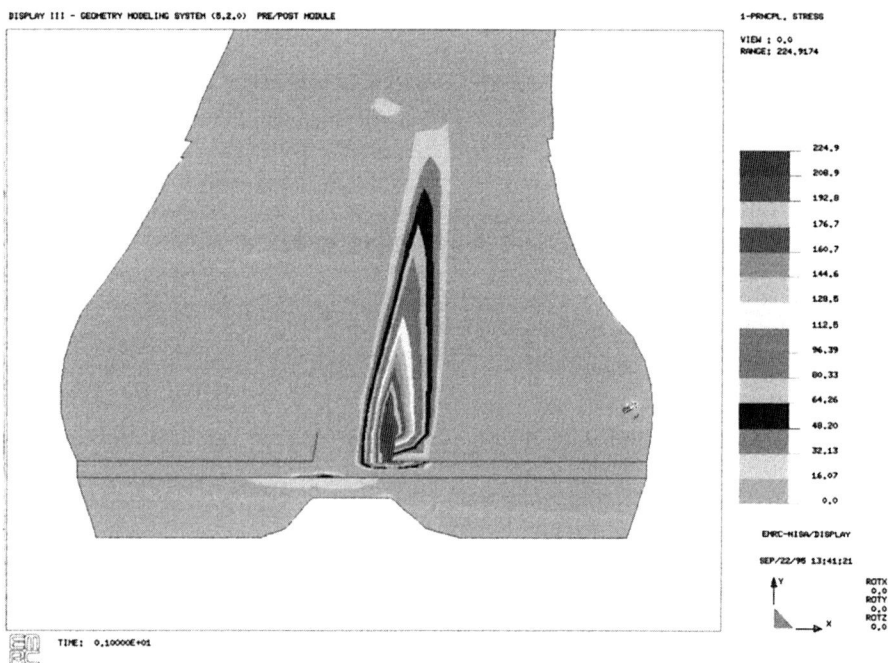

Fig. 23. S1Ps case 6 at 220 N varus load.

Modular Ceramic Knee Prosthesis

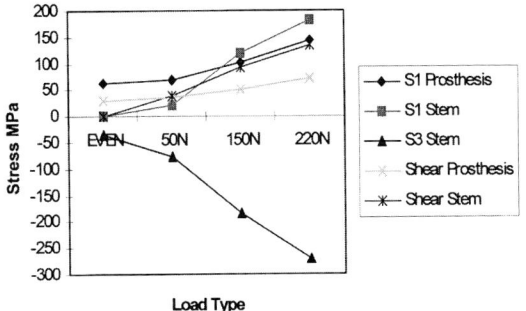

Fig. 24. S1P and S3P and shear stresses for case 3: ceramic with stem: unbonded.

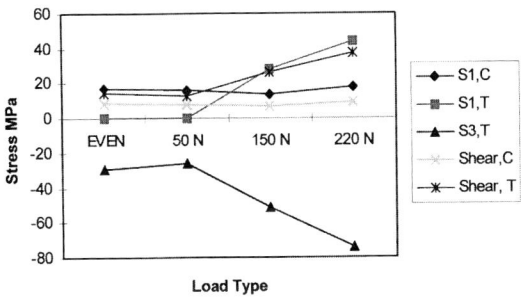

Fig. 25. S1P and S3P and shear stresses for case 4: ceramic and tray design, all bonded. The first points represent an even load on both the medial and lateral condylar surfaces; C denotes ceramic and T the tray.

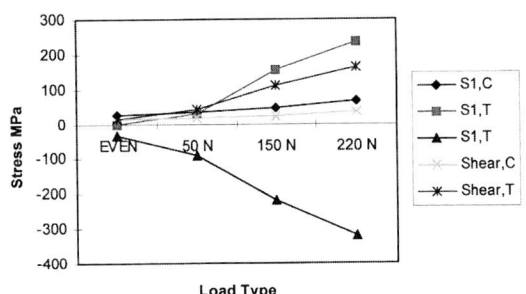

Fig. 26. S1P and S3P and shear stresses for case 5: ceramic and tray: bonded; tray and bone: unbonded. C denotes ceramic and T the tray. The first points represent an even load on both the medial and lateral condylar surfaces.

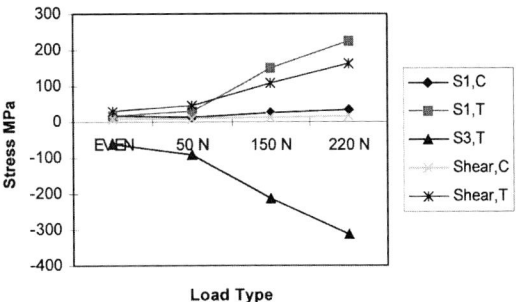

Fig. 27. S1P and S3P and shear stresses for case 6: ceramic and tray: unbonded; tray and bone: unbonded. C denotes ceramic and T the tray. The first points represent an even load on both the medial and lateral condylar surfaces.

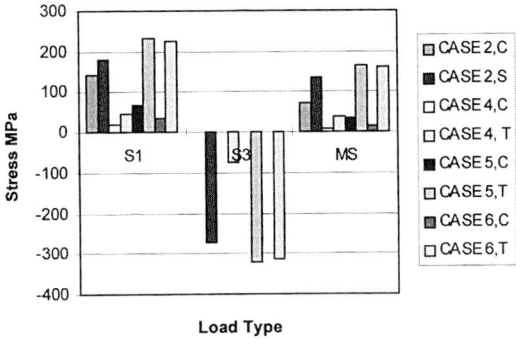

Fig. 28. Comparison of various designs at a load of 220 N medial force.

The change in ceramic stresses for the loads and design arrangements considered are shown in the surface plot (Fig. 29).

The results of Figs. 28 and 29 confirm the stress-shielding effect of the base plate in the transverse direction. Case 6, the modular ceramic Ti design, shows the lowest ceramic stresses, even though the total system stresses are slightly higher than the ceramic-only (case 2) stresses. Figure 29 also shows that the rate of stress increase is minimized in case 6. As the load is increased from 50 to 220 N, the stresses stay almost constant, with an increase of 1 MPa (within the errors of the analysis). In contrast, the unattached ceramic stemmed design (case 3) starts with a stress in the ceramic condyles of 63 MPa, rising to a maximum stress of 142 MPa at a load of 220 N.

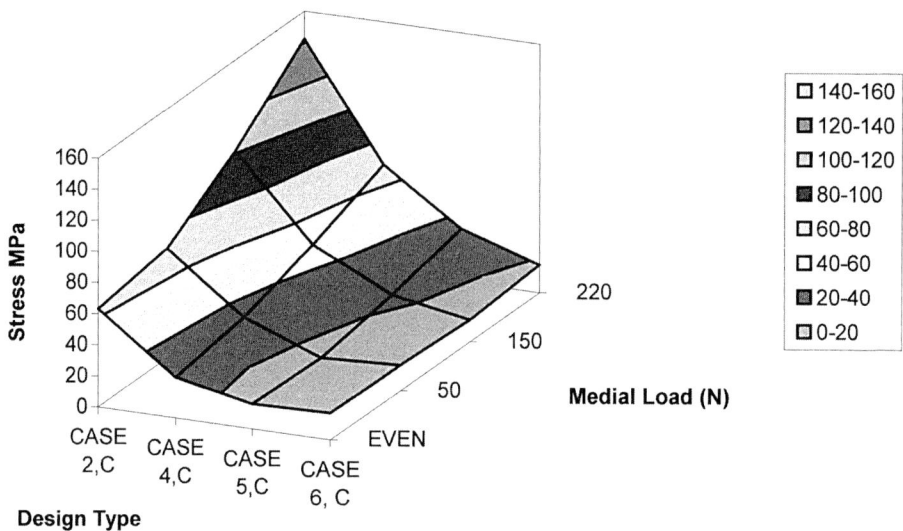

Fig. 29. Ceramic component stresses for the design cases considered under various medial loading conditions.

4.3. Femoral Prosthesis Conclusions

The major stresses occurring in ceramic femoral knee prosthesis have been determined. The results show that, if all loading cases and interface cases are not considered, then the system stresses can be seriously underestimated. In order to incorporate the major loads that the femoral prosthesis will experience, modeling and analysis should be carried out in both the sagittal and transverse planes. In the sagittal plane, the ground reaction force and the patella reaction force are dominant. In the transverse plane, the ground reaction force is again dominant; however, varus–valgus moments should be incorporated. In the transverse plane, the models are more complicated than in the sagittal plane, and the properties and thickness must include the moments of inertia of the various components, to correctly include the out-of-plane effects. Results indicate that, if complete fixation is achieved, then all of the proposed designs, including the ceramic and integral stem, would survive the loads expected in service. If incomplete bonding is assumed, then the stemmed ceramic prosthesis will result in failure of the stem near where it joins the ceramic condyles. Stresses are also high in the base of the patella track: This is undesirable, because wall thickness of the ceramic at this location is only 2.1 mm. Failure of the stem may or may not cause catastrophic failure of the entire prosthesis. However, this is a possibility, because the stresses shown in Fig. 23 are highest where the stem meets the thinnest part of the prosthesis, and this point is also close to the high stresses in the patella track in both the transverse and sagittal planes. The other cause of failure may be as a consequence of a fractured stem. The remaining condylar prosthesis may have limited bonding, causing increased movement with eventual loosening and failure, similar to that experienced by Oonishi et al. *(13)* and Koshino *(14)*.

The uncertainty of intimate bonding occurring between the prosthesis and the bone indicates that the best design solution is the ceramic design incorporating a Ti alloy base plate, either with or without the stem. The base plate can be coated in a number of ways, so that fixation is less of a problem. In this case, if bone stocks are of good quality and the prosthesis is being used as a primary replacement, then a very short stem or a design without a stem would be recommended. However, for revision design, in which bone quality is compromised, a metal stem and base plate design becomes mandatory, to ensure reasonable fixation is obtained.

Results indicate that normal gait stresses will not be of significant magnitude to cause failure through fatigue. However, transient stresses, particularly varus and valgus moments, could exceed the failure stress in the case of the ceramic-only design (case 3).

Based on this analysis, the major design issue is one of protecting the prosthesis from these types of very high loads, which occur infrequently. In these high load cases, the use of a shielding base plate, on which temporary overload stresses may cause small amounts of local yielding to occur in the tray and localized bone collapse in areas adjacent to the stem, could be the best option. This will shield the ceramic from these transient loads that could result in instantaneous failure.

The above conclusions indicate the reasons behind evaluating stresses in both the sagittal and transverse planes. The applied loads on each model are different, because they correspond to forces that operate only within these planes. This is not strictly true in a 3-D sense, because components of the loads are not completely orthonormal, giving vectors in all three axes. When simplifying these forces into the X, Y, and Z planes, certain forces are lost. When analyzing in only one plane, out-of-plane forces cannot be included, because of the nature of the model. Therefore, stress resultants only pertain to the planer loads applied to the model. Thus, depending on the magnitudes of the loads in the different planes, it is unknown prior to the analysis which loads may cause the highest stress on the model. The requirement is then to analyze the femoral model in both the two major planes.

The results showed that stresses, from moments occurring in the abducting–adducting couple, result in an increase in the interpenetrating gait force on a single condyle. These results can only be obtained in either a 3-D model or in models analyzed in the transverse plane. Modeling only in the sagittal plane would have failed to arrive at the maximum system stress.

4.4. Verification of Femoral Prosthesis Models

To verify FEA results, a prototype was machined from aluminum, having a Young's modulus of 70 GPa and a Poisson's ratio of 0.3. This prosthesis was loaded with an equivalent patella reaction force, to give peak tensile stress values on the outer surface. Strain gages were located at various positions. Force was applied on the anterior surfaces, and the posterior condyle fingers were constrained. This was done to crudely simulate a patella load. In order to distribute the load evenly across the prosthesis, negatives of the anterior and posterior load surfaces were machined. Similar loads were applied to the equivalent 2-D and 3-D FEMs and boundary element models (BEM). An evenly increasing load, terminating at 1000 N, was applied using an Instrom 1000 tensile testing machine.

The success or failure of the proposed ceramic design will only be known after lengthy and costly patient implant trials. Prior to this, confidence in the design can be gained by a combination of calculations and experimental verifications under a range of functional loadings. The FEMs and FEA are themselves complicated, because of the wide range of loading conditions and material data used. Although there are standard methods available to check the numerical accuracy of the FEA calculations, and to ensure that the selection of mesh and element type is appropriate, it is very prudent to crosscheck the results, using a second method, in addition to direct comparison with experimental results.

In this work, the FEA results were first compared to those obtained from the BEM, and, second, from a experimentally strain-gaged ceramic component, under an imposed anteroposterior (AP) static load condition of 1300 N. In addition, the use of both 2-D and 3-D models provide a further verification that the results were correct.

From a numerical viewpoint, models were checked for aspect ratio, warpness, and screw. A normal check and boundary line check were also performed. The 2-D models were analyzed using FEA (NISA, EMRC) and BEM (BEASY, Computational Mechanics). Because the initial 3-D results showed consistently higher values than the experimental results, models were reanalyzed using a number of different element types (solid, thick-shell, and hybrid). Models incorporated both a general and a smooth geometry, and were analyzed with three element types, an eight-node isoparametric element (type 4), a general thick-shell element (type 5), and a hybrid element for modeling relative thin-to-thick models (type 9). The final aspect was reliability testing of the unsupported component in the AP aspect over 10 million

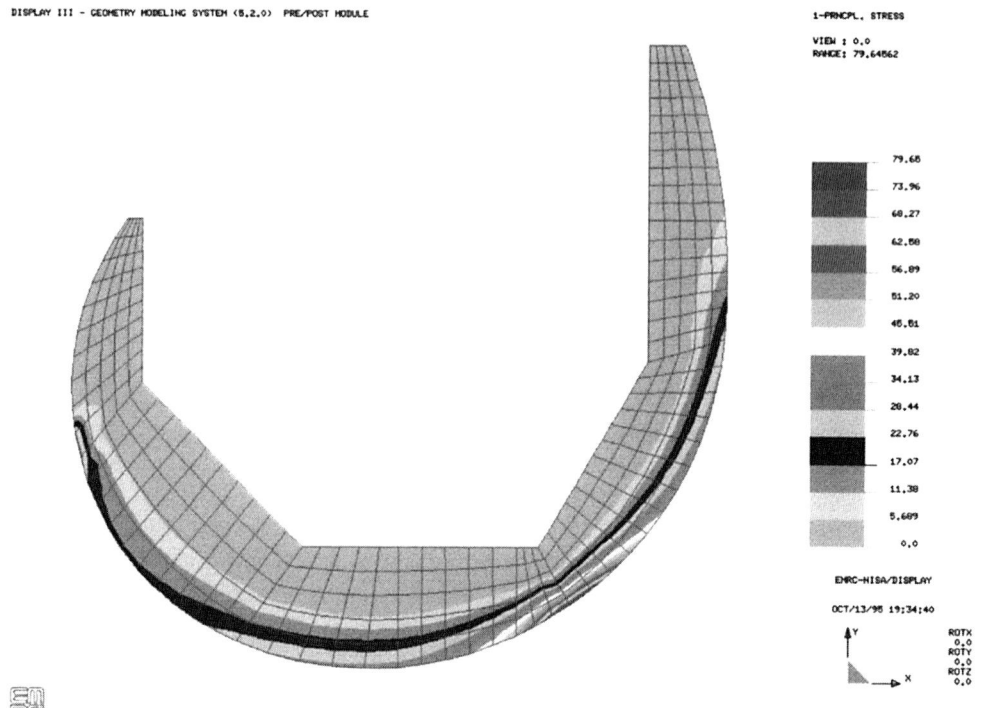

Fig. 30. 2-D FEA, S1P, verification model.

cycles (Mc) using the equivalent load of 6.5× body wt. This was paralleled by computational reliability assessment, using CARES3 on a CRAY-YMP at the NASA-Lewis Research Laboratories, Cleveland, OH.

4.5. FEA/BEM/Strain Gage Results

Figure 30 shows the S1P on the ceramic 2-D FEM under the 1300 N AP load. Figures 31 and 32 show the first principal stress for the 3-D general model and the 3-D smoothed model, using type 9 hybrid elements. As shown, in all cases, the maximum stress is located on the anterior medial and lateral surfaces.

Table 12 and corresponding Figs. 33 and 34 show comparisons between the S1P and S3P for the various models, types of elements used, and position of stresses. The stresses are the maximum stress occurring on the anterior bottom surface of the prosthesis.

For the 3-D models, stresses were also measured at five locations (Table 13). These were the medial, lateral, and patella tracks at the location of highest stress (in the center of each track) and the lateral and medial tracks at the center point (the position located where the medial and lateral tracks are tangent to the horizontal AP direction). The comparison is illustrated in Fig. 35.

Agreement between all models was reasonable. The 2-D models showed very good agreement with stresses of 80 MPa for the FEA model and 81 MPa for the BEM (Table 12). The location of the maximum stress under the patella load was on the anterior outside edge of the flanges for both models (Fig. 30). The S3P also compared well, with a difference of 1 MPa between the two methods. For the 2-D models, predicted stresses were 23% higher than the experimentally determined values. The 3-D models also compared favorably with the 2-D models, giving stresses between 80 and 90 MPa (Table 13). These stresses were also 20–25% higher than the experimentally determined tensile stresses.

The results from the analyses involving different element types showed large variations, ranging from 64 MPa, using thick-shelled elements,

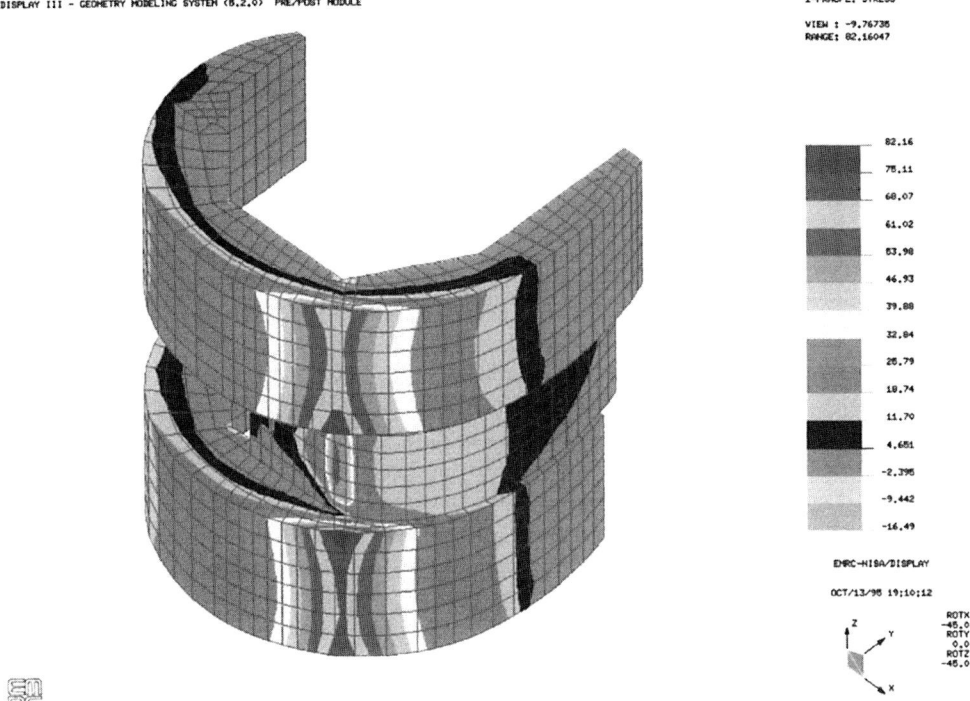

Fig. 31. 3-D general model S1P verification.

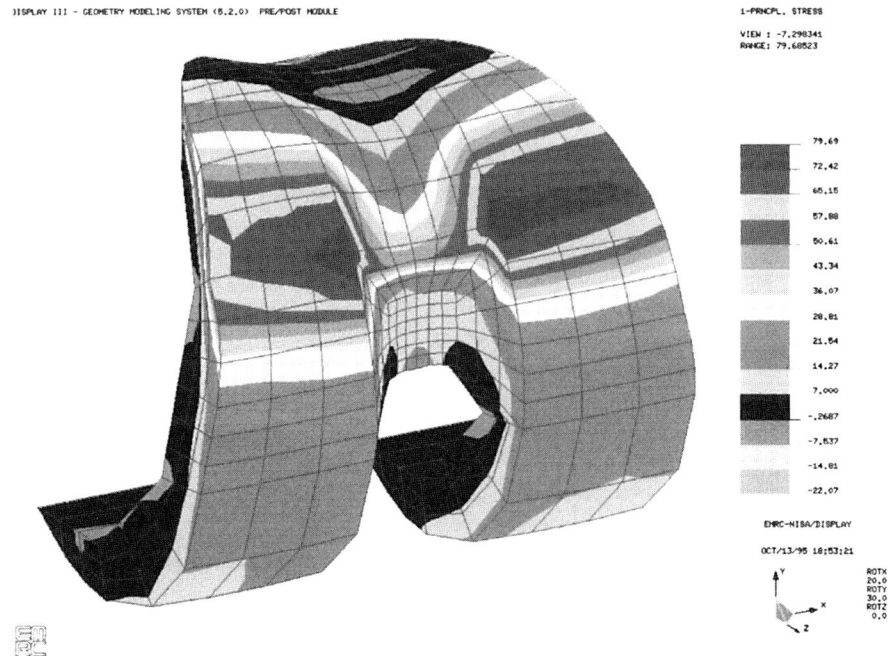

Fig. 32. 3-D smooth hybrid S1P verification model.

Table 12
Femoral Verification of all Models

Model	S1P	S3P
2 = D FEM	80	−188
2 = D BEM	81	−187
3 = D General 4	82	−132
3 = D General 9	80	−164
3 = D Smoothed 4	90	−121
3 = D Smoothed 5	64	−141
3 = D Smoothed 9	80	−101
Experimental	65	

to 90 MPa, using the standard solid hexahedron elements. The hybrid element model gave intermediate results of 80 MPa, close to the 2-D model results. Interpretation of these results leads to an interesting and unexpected conclusion. In general, the closest agreement with the experimental data came from the thick-shell element model, because the type 4 and type 9 elements are, for this geometry, overstiff, giving rise to higher-than-expected stresses. The femoral prosthesis acts like a shell, in that small bending movements are generated by the shape and loading on the condyles. The strain gage tests show that the maximum stress occurred on the lateral track, with a significant decrease toward the medial side; the lowest strains were registered on the patella track, even though this is significantly thinner than either the medial or lateral tracks. If the femoral component is visualized as a curved beam, the bending moments occurring in the patella track are lower, because of its proximity to the transverse cross-section neutral axis. Results show that the less-complicated 2-D model gave results similar to the larger and more computationally intensive 3-D models.

4.6. Fatigue and Reliability Results

Fatigue testing to 8 Mc was performed under an AP load, to simulate the patellofemoral force equivalent to normal walking. The reliability of the ceramic femoral component was determined using a multiaxial elemental strength approach incorporated into the CARES3 program (NASA-Lewis). This program for statistical analysis of strength and failure prediction of ceramic components is based on the weakest-link description of failure, which states that fracture occurs directly from pre-existing flaws. The methodology combines three major elements: linear elastic fracture mechanics, extreme-value statistics, and material microstructure. The Weibull approach and principle of independent action were used to analyze the reliability of the femoral ceramic component.

The ceramic knee was also subjected to a series of cyclic tests, starting with 1 Mc at loads of 500 N, then 1000 N, before terminating in a test of 8

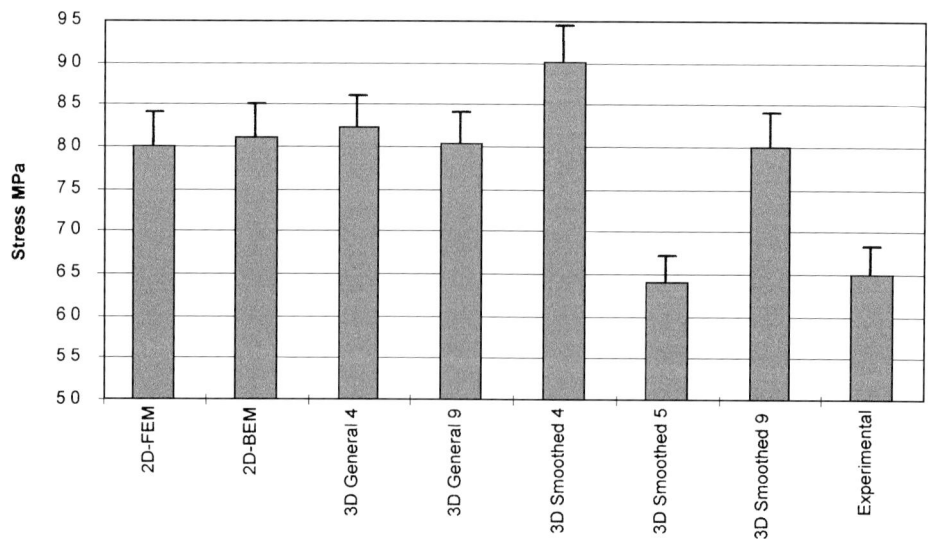

Fig. 33. S1Ps: comparison of strain gage experimental and FEA/BEM models.

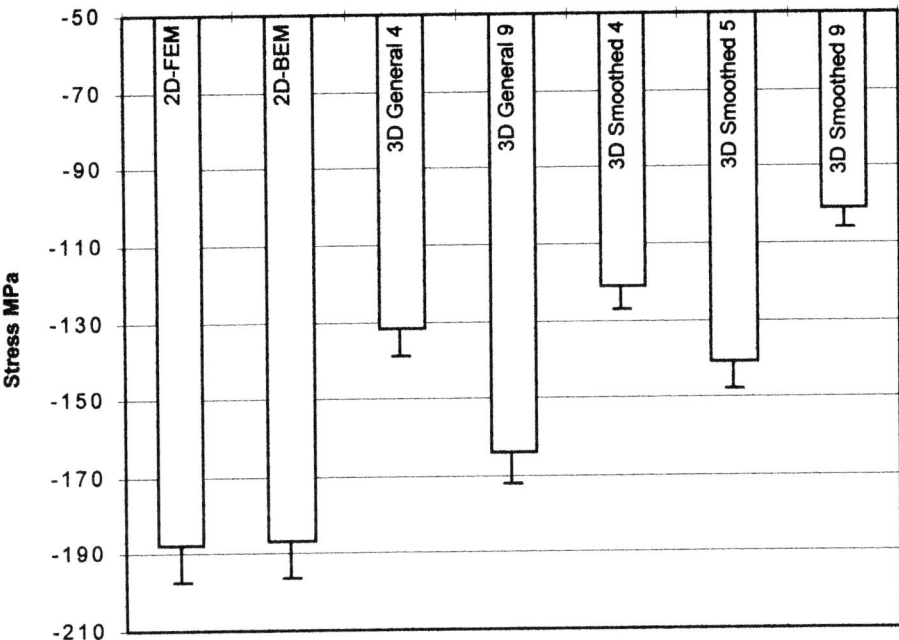

Fig. 34. S3Ps: comparison of strain gage experimental and FEA/BEM models.

Table 13
Femoral Verification 3-D Models SIPs

Position	3-D GEN 4	3-D GEN 5	3-D SMO 4	3-D SMO 9	3-D SMO 5	EXP
Medial	75	68	90	75	54	64.68
Lateral	69	63	83	71	52	60.55
Patella	58	53	68	47	56	30.8
Lat Center	27	28	37	36	38	28.98
Med Center	25	24	32	25	33	25.69

Mc at 1300 N. All tests were subjected to a cyclic ratio of 0.2. The ceramic knee was tested in the machined saddles used for the initial strain gage work. The sample was tested on an Instrom 8501 servohydraulic testing machine in a controlled environment of 23°C and 45% relative humidity. Table 14 indicates the relevant testing parameters.

The sample remained intact, and supported the combined 10 Mc, terminating after 8 Mc, at 1300 N, without evidence of crack initiation, propagation, or failure.

The static reliability data was calculated based on a sample size of 99 specimens, giving a Weibull modulus of 28.2. Batdorf coefficients for volume and surface flaws were, respectively, 10.55 and 6.71. The subcritical crack growth (SCG) part is evaluated using data obtained from Swain et al. (47). Weibull calculation used the maximum likelihood method. Both volume and surface failure were included. Reliability was calculated for the volume fracture, using a Weilbull principle of independent action, and the surface failure, using a co-planar strain energy release rate criterion, with a Griffith crack shape. The Batdorf crack density coefficient was shear-insensitive. Cyclic parameters for Mg-PSZ were provided by NASA, based on the cyclic results of Swain et al. (47). The Paris equation was used to simulated SCG.

The CARES 3 results showed that the ceramic femoral condyle, under normal loading, had a

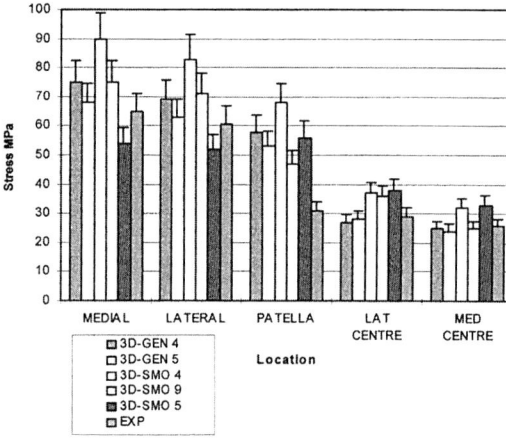

Fig. 35. 3-D stress analysis: comparison of different models at different strain locations.

Table 14
Testing Parameters

Max load	1300 N
Min load	260 N
Mean load	780 N
Cyclic ratio	0.2
Amplitude	520 N
Frequency	7.5 Hz
Waveform	Sinusoidal
Proportional gain	8.76 dB
Integral gain	0.41/S
Derivative gain	1.31 s
Cycles completed	8,000,000

probability of failure of 1×10^{-8} for 8 Mc, indicating that fatigue or ceramic reliability failure caused by the design is not a likely problem.

5. Conclusion

Based on this analysis, the major design issue is one of protecting the ceramic components from high loads that occur infrequently. In these high-load cases, the use of a shielding base plate, when temporary overload stresses may occur, will shield the ceramic from transient loads that could result in instantaneous failure.

The major stresses occurring in ceramic femoral knee prosthesis have been determined. Results indicate that the most appropriate design is a ceramic with a shielding base plate. The design has many unique features, including cross-nailing and the use of a separate, detachable base plate. The Ti base plate is integral to the design, acting as a shield to the ceramic, preventing high transient stresses, during varus–valgus loading, from reaching the ceramic. The base plate can be coated in a number of ways, so that fixation is less of a problem. In this case, if bone stocks are of good quality and the prostheses can be used as a primary replacement, then a very short stem would be recommended. However, for revision design in which bone quality is compromised, a metal stem and base plate design with cross-nailing becomes mandatory, to ensure reasonable fixation is obtained.

Acknowledgments

The authors would like to acknowledge that this kind of research could not have been initiated and successfully brought to a clinical stage without the contributions and dedicated work of the multidisciplinary team comprised of Emer. Prof. R. L. Huckstep, Dr. A. Pollack, and Dr. G. Etherington (Medical/Surgical), including Prof. M. Swain, Dr. B. Ben-Nissan, Dr. P. Lutton (Materials/Biomechanics); Dr. W. Payten, Dr. C. Bodur, Mr. D. Mercer, Dr. T-S. Liu (Engineering); S. Pratt,—ICI Advanced Ceramics (now Carpenter Inc.); R. Wright (Special Instruments). The authors would also like to acknowledge the funding given from the Australian Government DETYA-GIRD Grant, and the support given for this project, and beyond.

References

1 Mraz SJ. Human body shop. *Machine Design* 1991; 11: 90–94.
2 Lutton and B. Ben-Nissan. Biomaterials in the marketplace: focus on orthopaedic and dental applications. *Mater Technol* 1997; 12: 121–126.
3 Goodfellow J. Knee prosthesis: one step forward two steps back, *J Bone Joint Surg* 1992; 74: 1–2.
4 Insall AH. Design of the knee prosthesis, in *Surgery of the Knee* 1984; (Insall JN, ed), Churchill Livingstone, New York, pp 587–629.
5 Pope MH and Fleming BC. Knee biomechanics and materials, in *Total Knee Replacement* 1991; (Laskin RS, ed), Springer-Verlag, pp 25–38.
6 Collier JP, Mayor MB, McNamara JL, Surprenant

VA, and Jensen RE. Analysis of the failure of 122 polyethylene inserts from uncemented tibial knee components. *Clin Orthop Related Res* 1991; 273: 232–242.

7. Moran CG, Pinder IM, Lees TA, and Midwinter MJ. Survivorship analysis of uncemented porous-coated anatomic knee replacement. *J Bone Joint Surg* 1991; 6: 848–857.

8. Windsor RE, Scuberi GR, Moran MC, and Insall JN. Mechanisms of failure of the femoral and tibial components in total knee arthroplasty. *Clin Orthop Rel Res* 1989; 248: 15–20.

9. Moreland JR. Mechanisms of failure in total knee arthroplasty, *Clin Orthop Rel Res* 1988; 49–64.

10. Kilgus DJ, Moreland JR, Finerman G, and Funahushi TT. Catastrophic wear of tibial polyethylene inserts. *Clin Orthop* 1991; 273: 222–251.

11. Mintz L, Tsao AK, McCrae CR, Stulberg SD, and Wright T. The arthroscopic evaluation and characteristics of severe polyethylene wear in total knee arthroplasty, *Clin Orthop* 1991; 273: 222–251.

12. Oonishi H, Maeda A, Hamaguchi T, and Nabeshima T. Indications for cementless alumina ceramic total knee prosthesis and its limitations. *Jap J Rheum Joint Surg* 1984; 4: 311–322.

13. Oonishi H, Aono M, Murata N, and Kushitani S. Alumina versus polyethylene in total knee arthroplasty. *Clin Orthop* 1992; 282: 95–104.

14. Koshino T. Limb alignment in unicompartmental arthroplasty and clinical applications of the ceramic knee. *Curr Opin Orthop* 1994; 5: 75–80.

15. Huckstep RL. Cementless ceramic modular hip and femoral replacement. *J Bone Joint Surg* 1984; 66: 787.

16. Huckstep RL and Lutton PP. New concepts in stabilization and replacement of bone and joints. *Mater Forum* 1991; 15: 253–260.

17. Hartsock DL and Mclean AF. What the designer with ceramics needs. *Am Ceramic Soc Bull.* 1984; 63: 266–270.

18. Ben-Nissan B. Reliability and finite element analysis in ceramic engineering design. *Mater Forum* 1993; 17: 105–125.

19. Lamon J. Statistical approaches to failure for ceramic reliability assessment. *J Am Ceram Soc* 1988; 71: 106–12.

20. Huiskes R and Chao EYS. Survey of finite element analysis in orthopaedic biomechanics: the first decade. *J Biomech* 1983; 16: 385–409.

21. Beaupre GS, Vasu R, Carter DR, and Schurman DJ. Epiphyseal-based designs for tibial plateau components. II Stress analysis in the sagittal plane, *J Biomech* 1986; 19: 663–673.

22. Vasu R, Carter DR, Schurman DJ, and Beaupre GS. Epiphyseal-based designs for tibial plateau components. I. Stress analysis in the frontal plane. *J Biomech* 1986; 19: 647–662.

23. Huiskes IR, Weinans H, and Dalstra M. Adoptive bone remodelling and biomechanical design considerations for noncemented total hip arthroplasty. *Orthopaedics,* 1989; 12: 1255–1267.

24. Harrigan TP and Hamilton JJ. Optimality conditions for finite element simulation of adaptive bone remodeling. *Int J Solids Struct* 1992; 25: 23, 2897–2906.

25. Weinans H, Huskies R, van Rietbergen B, Sumner DR, Turmer TM, and Galante JO. Adaptive bone remodelling around bonded noncemented total hip arthroplasty: a comparison between animal experiments and computer simulation, *J Orthop Res* 1993; 11: 500–513.

26. Harrigan TP and Hamilton JJ. Finite element simulation of adaptive bone remodelling: A stability criterion and a time stepping method. *Int J Numerical Methods Eng* 1993; 25: 837–854.

27. Harrigan TP and Hamilton JJ. Bone remodeling and structural optimization, *J Biomech* 1994; 27: 323–328.

28. Payten WM. *Integrated computer aided design, finite element analysis and bone remodelling simulation of a modular ceramic knee prosthesis* 1996; Ph.D. Thesis, University of Technology, Sydney, Aus.

29. Huckstep RL, Pollack A, Taylor D, and Lutton PP. Design of cementless modular ceramic knee with screw fixation. *J Bone Joint Surg* 1986; 68: 336.

30. Atsui K, Tateishi H, Futani H, and Maruo S. Ceramic unicompartmental knee arthroplasty for spontaneous osteonecrosis of the knee joint. *Bull Hosp Joint Dis* 1997; 56: 233–236.

31. Lutton PP and Ben-Nissan B. Status of biomaterials for orthopaedic and dental applications. Part II: Bioceramics in orthopaedic and dental applications. *Mater Technol* 1997; 12: 107–111.

32. Lutton PP and Ben-Nissan B. Status of biomaterials for orthopaedic and dental applications. Part I: Materials, Mater. Technol 1997; 12: 59–63.

33. DeJong WF. La substance material dans lesos, *Rec Tav Chim* 1926; 45: 415–448.

34. Hench LL. Bioactive ceramics. *Ann NY Acad Sci* 1988; 523: 54–71.

35. Klawitter JJ. *Basic Investigation of Bone Growth Into a Porous Ceramic Material* 1970; Ph.D. Thesis, Clemson University, Clemson SC.

36. Kay JF and Cook SD. Biologic profile of calcium phosphate coatings, in *Hydroxylapatite Coatings in Orthopaedic Surgery* 1993; (Geesink RGT and Manley MT, eds), Raven, New York, pp 89–106.

37. DeGroot K, Klein CPA, Wolke GJC, and deBlieck-Hogervorst JMA, Calcium phosphate and hydroxyapatite ceramics, in *CRC Handbook of Bioactive Calcium Phosphates*, Vol. 2, 1990; (Yamamaro T, Hench LL, and Wilson J, eds), CRC, Boca Raton, FL, p. 3.
38. Lacefield WR. Hydroxyapatite coatings, in *An Introduction to Bioceramics* 1993; (Hench LL and Wilson J, eds) World Science, Singapore, pp. 223–238.
39. Klein LC. Sol-Gel Technology for Thin Films, Fibers, Preforms, Electronics and Specialty Shapes. 1988; Noyes, NJ.
40. Brinker CJ and Scherer GW. *Sol-Gel Science: Physics and Chemistry of Sol-Gel Processing.* Academic, London, 1990.
41. Soballe K, Hansen ES, Rasmussen HB, and Bunger C, The effects of osteoporosis, bone deficiency, bone graftings and micromation on fixation of porous-coated versus hydroxyapatite-coated implants, in *Hydroxylapatite Coatings in Orthopaedic Surgery* 1993; (Geesink RGT and Manley MT, eds), Raven, New York, pp. 107–136.
42. Lutton PP. *Computer aided development of a modular cementless hip and femoral prosthesis,* 1987; Ph.D. Thesis, University of New South Wales, Aus.
43. Bobyn JD. Optimum pore size for the fixation of porous surface metal implants by the ingrowth of bone, *Clin Orthop* 1980; 150: 263.
44. Huckstep RL. Modular cementless ceramic and titanium shoulder and humeral prosthesis. *J Bone Joint Surg* 1987; 69: 315.
45. Huckstep RL. Stabilization and prosthetic replacement in difficult fractures and bone tumors. *Clin Orthop Rel Res* 1987; 221: 12–25.
46. Standard OC. *Application of transformation toughened zirconia ceramics as bioceramics* 1994; Ph.D. Thesis, University of New South Wales, Sydney, Aus.
47. Swain MV, Huckstep RL, Tsutsumi S, and Sasaki Y. Suitability of Mg-PSZ for hip endoprosthesis articulation against high molecular weight polyethylene. *J. Adv Sci* 1991; 4: 231–240.
48. McNeice GM, Eng P, and Amstutz HC. Finite element studies in hip reconstruction, in *Biomechanics IV* (Univ. PV, ed.), 1976; University Park, Baltimore, pp. 394–405.
49. Rakotomanana RL, Leyvraz PF, Curnier a, Heegaard JH, and Rubin PJ. Finite element model for evaluation of tibial prosthesis-bone interface in total knee replacement, *J Biomech* 1992; 12: 1413–1424.
50. Rubin PJ, Rakotomanana RL, Leyvraz PF, Zysset PK, Curnier A, and Heegaard JH. Frictional interface micromotions and anisotropic stress distribution in a femoral total hip component. A finite element model for evaluation of tibial prosthesis-bone interface in total knee replacement. *J Biomech* 1993; 12: 725–739.
51. National Agency for Finite Element Models and Standards (NAFEMS). *A finite element primer* 1992; 3rd ed, NAJEMS, Bell and Bain, Ltd., Glasgow.
52. Lewis JL, Askew MJ, and Jaycox DP. Comparative evaluation of tibial component designs of total knee prostheses. *J Bone J Surg* 1982; 64: 129–135.
53. Hayes WC, Swenson LW, and Schurman DJ. Axisymmetric finite element analysis of the lateral tibial plateau, *J Biomech* 1978; 11: 21–33.
54. Ashman RB, Rho JY, and Turner CH. Anatomical variation of orthotropic elastic moduli of the proximal human tibia. *J Biomech* 1989; 22: 895–900.
55. Rohrle H, Scholten R, and Sollbach W. Analysis of stress distribution in natural and artificial knee joints on the femur side using the finite element method, in *International Conference Proceedings on Finite Elements in Biomechanics* 1980; (Simon, BR, ed), University of Arizona Press, Tucson, pp 781–794.
56. Rohrle H, Scholten R, Sigolotto C, and Sollbach W. Joint forces in the human pelvis-leg skeleton during walking, *J Biomech* 1984; 17: 409–424.
57. Harrigan TP and Harris WH. Three-dimensional non-linear finite element study of the effect of cement-prosthesis debonding in cemented femoral total hip components *J Biomech* 1991; 24: 1047–1058.

Index

Aluminum ceramics,
   dental implants, 229
   ear, nose, and throat surgery, 229, 230
   hip replacement,
      biocompatibility studies,
         bulk ceramics, 225, 226
         sarcoma induction, 228
         wear particles, 226, 228, 229
      composition and properties, 224, 225
      long-term follow-up of wear,
         artificial joint gap dimensions, 234, 235
         first-generation acetabular sockets and femoral heads, 230–232
         manufacturing aspects, 233, 234
         overview, 223, 224, 244–246
         surface treatment, 234
         surgical aspects, 233, 235
      polyethylene combination, 236–238
      safety aspects, 242–244
      socket inserts,
         interaction between socket and femoral component, 241, 242
         joining ceramic insert to metal backing, 240, 241
         metal backings, 239, 240
         overview, 238
   ocular implants, 230

Biocompatibility,
   aluminum ceramic hip prostheses,
      bulk ceramics, 225, 226
      sarcoma induction, 228
      wear particles, 226, 228, 229
   bone graft determination, 101
   calcium phosphate bone cement, 254, 255
   definition, 158
   HA-SAL2
      cell culture studies,
         bone cell colonization, 160, 161
         inflammatory cytokine release, 161
      importance for implant bonding, 158
      local tissue effects, 161

Biocompatibility *(cont.)*,
   hydroxyapatite, 52, 96
   knee, ceramic prosthesis, 313, 314
   mineralization of small implants,
      dual energy X-ray absorptiometry, 162–165
      rat tibia model, 163–165
   poly(D,L-lactide-co-glycolide) reinforced with poly(propylene glycol-co-fumaric acid) testing in rat tibia defect model,
      histologic findings, 273–277
      micro-computed tomography scanning, 273, 275, 276
      operative procedure, 271, 273
   polymethylmethacrylamate, 281, 282, 286
   poly(propylene glycol-co-fumaric acid) cement in rat tibial defect model, 299, 303
   rating of bone replacement materials, 226, 227

Bioglass,
   dental bone grafts, 147–149
   overview, 176
BioGran, dental bone grafts, 149
Bio-Oss, dental bone grafts, 143
Bone,
   cell differentiation, 96
   healing phases, 177
   interfacial remodeling reactions adjacent to bioinert implants, 230, 231
   matrix composition, 96
   mechanical properties of wet compact bone, 265, 266
   mineral content, 96, 97
   osteogenesis and healing, 97
Bone cement, *see* Calcium phosphate bone cement; Polymethylmethacrylamate; Poly(propylene glycol-co-fumaric acid); Skeletal Repair System
Bone graft, *see also* Dental bone graft,
   allograft,
      antigen destruction, 100

Biocompatibility *(cont.)*,
  allograft *(cont.)*,
    cortical allograft processing by partial demineralization and laser perforation
      biomechanical studies, 117, 118, 123, 124
      clinical application, 126, 127
      electron microscopy of demineralization, 115, 116
      histological analysis, 123
      hypotheses, 115
      immunological studies, 124–126
      kinetics of demineralization, 116, 117
      matrix factor exposure, 114
      radiographic follow-up, 122, 123
      rat transplantation studies, 118, 119
      rationale, 114, 115
      sheep transplantation studies, 119, 121–125
    donor matching, 100
    immune response, 95, 99, 100, 114
    processing,
      banking, 112, 113
      cell survival, 112
      historical perspective, 112, 113
    success rates, 111, 114
    viral infection, 100, 113, 171
  artificial materials, *see also* HA-SAL2; Hydroxyapatite,
    bioresorbable substitutes,
      bone healing, 177, 178
      indications, 171–173
      poly(propylene glycol-co-fumaric acid)-based formulations, 171, 177–180, 182–188
    ceramics, 102, 103, 106, 107, 155, 156
    composite materials, 103
    overview, 101
  autograft,
    biocompatibility, 98
    failure, 98
    limitations, 99, 171
    revascularization, 98, 99
    strength, 98
  biochemical response of materials,
    bioactive, 101, 102
    biodegradable, 101
    bioinert, 101, 102
  biocompatibility determination, 101
  historical perspective, 97, 98
  ideal properties, 95, 155, 156

Biocompatibility *(cont.)*,
  isograft, 99
  market, 171
  xenograft, cross-species, 100

Calcium acetate, filler in bioresorbable bone graft substitutes, *see* Poly(propylene glycol-co-fumaric acid), bone graft substitute with soluble calcium salts
Calcium carbonate, dental bone grafts, 143, 144
Calcium gluconate, filler in bioresorbable bone graft substitutes and cements, *see* Poly(propylene glycol-co-fumaric acid)
Calcium phosphate bone cement (CPBC),
  admixtures, 257
  applications, 258
  biocompatibility, 254, 255
  bone cell interactions, 255
  cohesion time, 256
  composition, 253, 254
  dough time, 257
  injectability, 256, 257
  mixing powder and liquid, 257
  resorption, 258
  setting times, 255, 256
  strength,
    measurement, 256
    mechanisms, 253, 254
Calcium propionate, filler in bioresorbable bone graft substitutes, *see* Poly(propylene glycol-co-fumaric acid), bone graft substitute with soluble calcium salts
Calcium sulfate,
  dental implants, 10, 12
  resorbable barrier in dental tissue regeneration, 152
Candida, colonization of dental soft lining materials,
  assays, 36, 37
  clinical importance, 36, 37
  imbibing of nutrients, 37
  inhibition studies, 37
Carbon fiber composites,
  advantages in orthopedic surgery, 203, 213
  external fixator fracture frame,
    advantages, 210, 211
    configurability, 211
    wrist fixator, 211, 213

Carbon fiber composites *(cont.)*,
  hip replacement,
    polysulfone composite for acetabular component, 209, 210
    polysulfone composite for femoral component,
      hydroxyapatite coating, 207, 209
      performance in greyhound, 204, 205
      radiography advantages, 205, 207, 213
Cervical spine fusion, *see* Spine fusion
Cervical spondylosis, treatment, 215
Cobalt-chromium-molybdenum,
  applications, 191
  hydroxyapatite coating of dental implants, 14
  nitrogen diffusion hardening,
    corrosion test, 194, 200, 202
    fatigue test, 192, 197
    hardness measurement, 192, 197
    materials, 191
    processes, 192
    surface analysis, 192, 197
    wear testing,
      knee simulator wear test, 193, 194, 197, 199, 200
      pin-on-flat wear test, 192
  surface hardening, overview, 191
Collagen, occlusive membranes in dentistry, 11, 12
Collagraft, overview, 176, 177
Coralline, dental bone grafts, 142, 143
Core-Vent implant, follow-up study, 85
CPBC, *see* Calcium phosphate bone cement
Crystalline–crystalline behavior, 25

Demineralized freeze-dried bone (DFDB), dental implants, 4, 6–8, 137
Dental bone graft,
  allograft,
    advantages, 137, 138
    demineralized freeze-dried bone, 137
    disadvantages, 138
    donors, 136
    freeze-dried bone allograft, 137
    irradiated bone, 137
  applications, 133
  autograft,
    advantages, 135, 136
    cortical bone, 135, 136
    harvesting, 136
    trabecular bone, 135

Dental bone graft *(cont.)*,
  bone morphogenetic protein therapy, 150
  composite graft systems, 150, 151
  defect degree and selection of graft material, 151
  growth factor and cytokine therapy, 149, 150
  mechanisms,
    osteoconduction, 134, 135
    osteogenesis, 133, 134
    osteoinduction, 134
  regenerative therapy,
    nonresorbable barriers, 151
    resorbable barriers, 151, 152
  synthetic bone substitutes,
    applications, 139, 140
    Bio-Oss, 143
    Bioglass, 147–149
    BioGran, 149
    calcium carbonate, 143, 144
    coralline, 142, 143
    hard tissue replacement, 144, 146, 147
    hydroxyapatite, 140–142, 150, 151
    overview, 138–140, 152
    PerioGlas, 149
    tricalcium phosphate, 140–142
Dental implant,
  bone graft materials,
    allogeneic bone processing, 4, 6–8
    alloplasts, 8–10
    alveolar ridge augmentation, 3
    autogenous bone, 4, 6
    healing phases, 3, 4
    xenografts, 8
  endosteal implant materials,
    cobalt-chromium-molybdenum, 14
    design,
      blade implants, 15
      endodontic stabilizers, 18
      root-form implants, 15–18
    hydroxyapatite coating, 14, 15
    overview, 3, 14
    titanium and alloys, 14
  follow-up studies of osseointegrated implants,
    Core-Vent implants, 85
    figures of merit for Tübingen and Göteborg implants, 78–82
    fracture forces, 87, 88
    initial failure rates, 68, 69
    International Team for Implantology implants, 82, 83

Dental implant *(cont.)*,
  follow-up studies of osseointegrated implants *(cont.)*,
    Intra-Mobile Zahn implants, 83–85
    performance criteria,
      defining, 68, 69
        esthetic and cosmetic aspects, 77, 78
        material-related criteria, 69–71
        osseointegration-related problems, 74, 75
        patient and indication-related criteria, 72
        pergingival portion, 75–77, 86, 87
        shape-related criteria, 71, 72
        surgeon-related criteria, 72–74
    plaque index, 75, 76
    Steri-Oss implant system, 85
    studies in analysis, 67, 68
    sulcus fluid flow rate, 75
    3i implant system, 85, 86
  hydroxyapatite coating,
    biocompatibility, 52
    biological composition, 49
    coating processes, 49, 50
    dissolution rate, 51
    failure, 53, 56
    interfacial strength, 52, 53, 56
    microbial colonization, 53
    rationale, 49
    resorption, 53, 56
    standards, 50, 51
    thickness, 51, 52
  light-cured resins, *see bis*-Glycidyl methacrylate
  occlusive membranes, guided tissue/bone regeneration, 10–12
  soft lining materials,
    bonding, 29
    Candida colonization,
      assays, 36, 37
      clinical importance, 36, 37
      imbibing of nutrients, 37
      inhibition studies, 37
    commercial types, 32
    composition and performance, 28, 29
    dynamic mechanical analysis,
      butadiene/styrene elastomers, 35, 36
      commercial sample analysis, 33, 34
      data analysis, 33
      elastomeric methacrylate systems, 35
      instrumentation, 32
      silicone materials, 34, 35

Dental implant *(cont.)*,
  soft lining materials *(cont.)*,
    ideal characteristics, 27, 28
    oral environment and compliance, 29
    plasticized acrylics, 28
    silicone polymers, 28
    water sorption,
      butadiene/styrene elastomers, 30, 31
      forces, 30
      polymethylmethacrylamate, 29, 30, 38–45
      silicone-based elastomers, 31, 32
      solid-state nuclear magnetic resonance, 37, 38
  subperiosteal implant materials,
    applications, 13
    hydroxyapatite coating, 14
    modeling, 13, 14
    overview, 3
    Vitallium, 12, 13
DEXA, *see* Dual energy X-ray absorptiometry
DFDB, *see* Demineralized freeze-dried bone
DMA, *see* Dynamic mechanical analysis
Dual energy X-ray absorptiometry (DEXA), mineralization of small HA-SAL2 implants, 162–165
Duofit, 239
Dynamic mechanical analysis (DMA),
  dental soft lining materials,
    butadiene/styrene elastomers, 35, 36
    commercial sample analysis, 33, 34
    data analysis, 33
    elastomeric methacrylate systems, 35
    instrumentation, 32
    silicone materials, 34, 35
  bis-glycidyl methacrylate polymerization in water,
    data acquisition, 62, 63
    glass transition temperature, 63
    instrumentation, 62
    light curing, 62
    materials, 62
    mechanical stress relaxation, 63–65

Endosteal implant, *see* Dental implant
FEA, *see* Finite element analysis
Finite element analysis (FEA), ceramic knee prosthesis,
  conclusions of analysis, 328, 329
  element type, 315
  femur, 314

Finite element analysis (FEA), ceramic knee prosthesis *(cont.)*,
    geometrical properties, 316
    interface modeling, 314, 315
    loading conditions, 316
    material properties, 315
    overview, 310, 314
    sagittal plane stresses,
        case studies, 317, 318
        gait stresses at toe-off, 317, 318, 321–324
        heel-strike to toe-off, 324, 325
    transverse plane stresses, 317, 318, 325, 327
    verification, 329, 330, 332

GBR, *see* Guided bone regeneration
GIM, *see* Granulomatous interfacial membrane
Glass–rubber transition behavior, 25
bis-Glycidyl methacrylate,
    applications, 61
    polymerization in water,
        dynamic mechanical spectroscopy,
            data acquisition, 62, 63
            glass transition temperature, 63
            instrumentation, 62
            mechanical stress relaxation, 63–65
        light curing, 62
        materials, 62
Gore-Tex,
    guided bone regeneration in dentistry, 11, 19
    nonresorbable barrier in dental tissue regeneration, 151
Göteborg implant, follow-up studies,
    figures of merit, 78–82
    initial failure rates, 68, 69
    performance criteria,
        defining, 68, 69
        esthetic and cosmetic aspects, 77, 78
        material-related criteria, 69–71
        osseointegration-related problems, 74, 75
        patient and indication-related criteria, 72
        pergingival portion, 75–77, 86, 87
        shape-related criteria, 71, 72
        surgeon-related criteria, 72–74
    plaque index, 75, 76
    studies in analysis, 67, 68
    sulcus fluid flow rate, 75
Granulomatous interfacial membrane (GIM), hip arthroplasty,
    aseptic loosening of cemented components, 281
    inflammatory cell response, 282, 283, 287

Granulomatous interfacial membrane (GIM), hip arthroplasty *(cont.)*,
    metal particle effects, 285–287
    morphology and histology in cemented hip prostheses,
        long-term surviving prostheses, 283
        short-term surviving prostheses, 282, 283
    operation failure role, 281
    polyethylene debris effects, 284, 285
    prosthetic debris sources, 281, 282
Guided bone regeneration (GBR), occlusive membranes in dentistry, 10–12

Hard tissue replacement (HTR),
    dental bone grafts, 144, 146, 147
    dental implants, 10
HA-SAL2,
    advantages in bone grafting, 167
    biocompatibility,
        cell culture studies,
            bone cell colonization, 160, 161
            inflammatory cytokine release, 161
        importance for implant bonding, 158
        local tissue effects, 161
    histology of rat tibia model, 165
    mineralization of small implants,
        dual energy X-ray absorptiometry, 162–165
        rat tibia model, 163–165
    preparation of powder and disks, 156, 167
    scanning electron microscopy, 156
Hip replacement,
    aluminum ceramics,
        biocompatibility studies,
            bulk ceramics, 225, 226
            sarcoma induction, 228
            wear particles, 226, 228, 229
        composition and properties, 224, 225
        long-term follow-up of wear,
            artificial joint gap dimensions, 234, 235
            first-generation acetabular sockets and femoral heads, 230–232
            manufacturing aspects, 233, 234
            overview, 223, 224, 244–246
            surface treatment, 234
            surgical aspects, 233, 235
        polyethylene combination, 236–238
        safety aspects, 242–244

Hip replacement *(cont.)*,
  aluminum ceramics *(cont.)*,
    socket inserts,
      interaction between socket and femoral component, 241, 242
      joining ceramic insert to metal backing, 240, 241
      metal backings, 239, 240
      overview, 238
  bioresorbable bone graft substitutes for acetabular osteolysis, 173
  carbon fiber/polysulfone composites,
    acetabular component, 209, 210
    femoral component,
      hydroxyapatite coating, 207, 209
      performance in greyhound, 204, 205
    radiography advantages, 205, 207, 213
  femoral stem design, 203, 204
  granulomatous interfacial membrane,
    aseptic loosening of cemented components, 281
    inflammatory cell response, 282, 283, 287
    metal particle effects, 285–287
    morphology and histology in cemented hip prostheses,
      long-term surviving prostheses, 283
      short-term surviving prostheses, 282, 283
    operation failure role, 281
    polyethylene debris effects, 284, 285
    prosthetic debris sources, 281, 282
  loading values in design, 244
  material combinations for articulating surfaces,
    historical perspective, 224
  metal-backed polyethylene sockets, 238
  soft tissue separations, 223
  success rates for total hip replacement, 223, 244
  zirconia ceramics, 235, 236
HTR, *see* Hard tissue replacement
Huckstep hip, 312
Hydroxyapatite,
  biocompatibility, 96
  carbonated form in bone reconstruction, 106
  dental bone grafts, 140–142, 150, 151
  dental implant coating,
    biocompatibility, 52
    biological composition, 49
    coating processes, 49, 50
    dissolution rate, 51
    endosteal implants, 14, 15
    failure, 53, 56

Hydroxyapatite *(cont.)*,
  dental implant coating *(cont.)*,
    interfacial strength, 52, 53, 56
    microbial colonization, 53
    rationale, 49
    resorption, 53, 56
    standards, 50, 51
    subperiosteal implants, 14
    thickness, 51, 52
  filler in bioresorbable bone graft substitutes, *see* Poly(propylene glycol-co-fumaric acid), bone graft substitute with soluble calcium salts
  osteogenic activity, 96
  properties for dental implants, 8–10
  tibial plateau fracture reconstruction,
    materials and methods, 103, 104
    outcomes, 104, 106
  tricalcium phosphate composite, *see* HA-SAL2

IFD, *see* Internal fixation device
IMZ implant, *see* Intra-Mobile Zahn implant
Interbody fusion device, *see* Spine fusion
Internal fixation device (IFD),
  biodegradable polymers,
    advantages, 261, 263
    complications, 263, 264
  biomechanical considerations, 265
  historical perspective, 262, 263
  metal plates, 262
  poly-L-lactide plates, 263, 264
  poly(D,L-lactide-co-glycolide) reinforced with poly(propylene glycol-co-fumaric acid),
    biocompatibility testing in rat tibia defect model,
      histologic findings, 273–277
      micro-computed tomography scanning, 273, 275, 276
      operative procedure, 271, 273
    compression-molding techniques, 268
    design considerations, 267
    extrusion techniques, 268
    hardness testing, 269
    isopropyl alcohol extraction, weight loss, 270
    materials, 268
    mechanical testing, 271, 277

Index

Internal fixation device (IFD) *(cont.)*,
poly(D,L-lactide-co-glycolide) reinforced with poly(propylene glycol-co-fumaric acid) *(cont.)*,
molecular reinforcement,
concept, 261, 262
formulations, 268, 269
molding and curing, 267, 268
objectives, 267
optimization, 269, 270
rationale, 264, 265
prospects, 277, 278
polylactic acid plates, 264
removal, 262
rigidity of fixation systems, 262
International Team for Implantology (ITI) implant, follow-up study, 82, 83
Intra-Mobile Zahn (IMZ) implant, follow-up study, 83–85
ITI implant, *see* International Team for Implantology implant

Kaiserswerther socket, 239
Knee, ceramic prosthesis,
advantages and limitations, 310, 311
biocompatibility, 313, 314
biomechanics, 309, 310
boundary element analysis and verification, 310, 329, 330, 332
design objectives, 313
fatigue testing, 332
femoral component design, 312, 313
finite element analysis,
conclusions of analysis, 328, 329
element type, 315
femur, 314
geometrical properties, 316
interface modeling, 314, 315
loading conditions, 316
material properties, 315
overview, 310, 314
sagittal plane stresses,
case studies, 317, 318
gait stresses at toe-off, 317, 318, 321–324
heel-strike to toe-off, 324, 325
transverse plane stresses, 317, 318, 325, 327
verification, 329, 330, 332
historical perspective, 310, 311
hydroxyapatite coating, 311, 312

Knee, ceramic prosthesis *(cont.)*,
indications for total knee arthroplasty, 309, 313
manufacture of partially stabilized zirconia magnesium prosthesis, 314
market for knee replacement, 309
material properties of partially stabilized zirconia magnesium prosthesis, 315, 317
porous coatings and interfaces, 311
reliability testing, 332–334
surgical options, 313, 314

Link FGK socket, 239, 241

Molloplast B, 28, 29, 32, 33

NDH, *see* Nitrogen diffusion hardening
Nitrogen diffusion hardening (NDH),
cobalt-chromium-molybdenum results, 197, 199, 200, 202
corrosion test, 194
fatigue test, 192
hardness measurement, 192
materials, 191
processes, 192
surface analysis, 192
titanium-aluminum-vanadium results, 194–196
wear testing,
knee simulator wear test, 193, 194
pin-on-flat wear test, 192

OM, *see* Osteomyelitis
OrthoFrame,
advantages, 210, 211
configurability, 211
Orthopedic implant materials, *see* Carbon fiber composites; Cobalt-chromium-molybdenum; Internal fixation device; Titanium-aluminum-vanadium
Osteomyelitis (OM), bioresorbable bone graft substitutes, 172
Osteoset, overview, 174

PE, *see* Polyethylene
PerioGlas, dental bone grafts, 149
PGA, *see* Polyglycolic acid
PLA, *see* Polylactic acid
PLGA, *see* Poly(D,L-lactide-co-glycolide)
PLLA, *see* Poly-L-lactide
PMMA, *see* Polymethylmethacrylamate

Polyethylene (PE), *see also* Ultra-high molecular-weight polyethylene,
  aluminum ceramic combinations in hip replacement, 236–238
  debris effects on granulomatous interfacial membrane, 284, 285
  metal-backed polyethylene sockets, 238
Polyglycolic acid (PGA),
  interbody fusion devices, 218, 219
  occlusive membranes in dentistry, 12
Polylactic acid (PLA),
  interbody fusion devices, 218, 219
  internal fixation devices, 264
  occlusive membranes in dentistry, 12
Poly-L-lactide (PLLA), internal fixation devices, 263, 264
Poly(D,L-lactide-co-glycolide) (PLGA),
  internal fixation device reinforced with poly(propylene glycol-co-fumaric acid),
    biocompatibility testing in rat tibia defect model,
      histologic findings, 273–277
      micro-computed tomography scanning, 273, 275, 276
      operative procedure, 271, 273
    compression-molding techniques, 268
    design considerations, 267
    extrusion techniques, 268
    hardness testing, 269
    isopropyl alcohol extraction, weight loss, 270
    materials, 268
    mechanical testing, 271, 277
    molecular reinforcement,
      concept, 261, 262
      formulations, 268, 269
      molding and curing, 267, 268
      objectives, 267
      optimization, 269, 270
      rationale, 264, 265
    prospects, 277, 278
  spinal interbody fusion devices, 218, 220, 221
Polymethylmethacrylamide (PMMA),
  disease studies in hip replacement, 281, 282, 286
  water sorption,
    kinetics, 29, 30
    measurement, 39, 40
    molecular weight effects, 38, 39
    plasticizer effects, 40–45
    solid-state nuclear magnetic resonance, 37, 38

Poly(propylene glycol-co-fumaric acid) (PPF),
  bone graft substitute with soluble calcium salts,
    cement with vinylpyrrolidone, 177, 178
    formulations and fillers, 178
    in vitro evaluation,
      compressive strength and modulus, 180, 182
      density changes, 179, 180
      scanning electron microscopy, 182
      weight loss, 179
    in vivo evaluation,
      bone healing, 183, 184
      dissolution, 183
      inflammatory response, 183
      porosity and performance, 184–186
      rat model, 182, 183
    overview, 171
    prospects, 187
  crosslinked materials,
    biocompatibility, 267
    chemistry, 265–267
  injectable bioresorbable bone cement,
    applications, 291, 292
    biocompatibility in rat tibial defect model, 299, 303
    calcium gluconate as filler, 293, 284
    comparison with other cements,
      Norian cement, 293
      polymethylmethacrylamate, 292, 293
    compressive strength, 296, 306
    degradation in vitro, 296, 303
    elemental analysis, 294–296
    formulations, 291, 293–296, 303
    fracture fixation, 292
    modulus, 296, 306
    rat fracture model of performance,
      histomorphometry, 300–302, 306
      operative procedure, 300
      radiography, 300, 301
    scanning electron microscopy, 296, 297, 303
    shelf life, 298, 299, 306
    temperature rise during cure, 298, 303
    viscisity, precure, 297, 298, 306
    working time, 298, 306
  poly(D,L-lactide-co-glycolide) reinforcement in internal fixation devices, *see* Poly(D,L-lactide-co-glycolide)
  vinylpyrrolidone cements, 177, 178, 265–267, 295, 296

Index

Polytetrafluoroethylene (PTFE), guided bone regeneration in dentistry, 11
PPF, *see* Poly(propylene glycol-co-fumaric acid)
PTFE, *see* Polytetrafluoroethylene

Rat tibia defect model,
    mineralization of small implants, 163–165
    poly(D,L-lactide-co-glycolide) reinforced with poly(propylene glycol-co-fumaric acid), biocompatibility,
        histologic findings, 273–277
        micro-computed tomography scanning, 273, 275, 276
        operative procedure, 271, 273
    poly(propylene glycol-co-fumaric acid) cement biocompatibility testing, 299, 303

Scanning electron microscopy (SEM),
    bone graft demineralization, 115, 116
    HA-SAL2, 156
    poly(propylene glycol-co-fumaric acid) bone graft substitute, 182
    poly(propylene glycol-co-fumaric acid) cement, 296, 297, 303
SEM, *see* Scanning electron microscopy
Skeletal Repair System (SRS),
    cement properties, 174
    fracture healing, 174–176
Solitary lucent bone lesion, bioresorbable bone graft substitutes, 172
Spine fusion,
    anterior fusion techniques for cervical spine, 216, 217
    clinical considerations, 217
    functions of spine, 215, 216
    interbody fusion devices,
        resorbable polymer implants,
            animal models, 219, 220
            compressive strength, 220, 221
            degradation rates, 221
            fabrication, 220
            polyglycolic acid, 218, 219
            polylactic acid, 218, 219
            poly(D,L-lactide-co-glycolide), 218, 220, 221
        types, 217, 218
SRS, *see* Skeletal Repair System
Steri-Oss implant system, 174
    follow-up study, 85

Subperiosteal implant, *see* Dental implant

TCP, *see* Tricalcium phosphate
3i implant system, follow-up study, 85, 86
Tibial plateau fracture reconstruction, *see* Hydroxyapatite,
Titanium-aluminum-vanadium
    applications, 191
    nitrogen diffusion hardening,
        corrosion test, 194, 196
        fatigue test, 192, 195
        hardness measurement, 192, 195
        materials, 191
        processes, 192
        surface analysis, 192, 194, 195
        wear testing,
            knee simulator wear test, 193, 194, 196
            pin-on-flat wear test, 192, 195, 196
    surface hardening, overview, 191
Tricalcium phosphate (TCP),
    dental bone grafts, 140–142
    dental implants, 8
    hydroxyapatite composite, *see* HA-SAL2
Tübingen implant, follow-up studies,
    figures of merit, 78–82
    initial failure rates, 68, 69
    performance criteria,
        defining, 68, 69
        esthetic and cosmetic aspects, 77, 78
        material-related criteria, 69–71
        osseointegration-related problems, 74, 75
        patient and indication-related criteria, 72
        pergingival portion, 75–77, 86, 87
        shape-related criteria, 71, 72
        surgeon-related criteria, 72–74
    plaque index, 75, 76
    studies in analysis, 67, 68
    sulcus fluid flow rate, 75

UHMWPE, *see* Ultra-high molecular-weight polyethylene
Ultra-high molecular-weight polyethylene (UHMWPE),
    knee simulator wear test, 193, 196
    metal sliding in joint implants, 191
Vario sockets, 239
Vinylpyrrolidone (VP), poly(propylene glycol-co-fumaric acid) cements, 177, 178, 265–267, 295, 296

Viscoelastic behavior,
    region A, 26
    region B, 26
    region C, 26
    region D, 26, 27
    region E, 27

VP, *see* Vinylpyrrolidone

Young's modulus, 25

Zirconia ceramics,
    hip replacement, 235, 236
    knee replacement, *see* Knee, ceramic prosthesis